EFFECTIVE MANAGEMENT IN NURSING

THIRD EDITION

Eleanor J. Sullivan, PhD, RN, FAAN
School of Nursing, University of Kansas Medical Center
Kansas City, KS

Phillip J. Decker, PhD
Barney School of Business and Public Administration
University of Hartford, West Hartford, CT

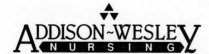

ADDISON~WESLEY
NURSING
A DIVISION OF
THE BENJAMIN/CUMMINGS PUBLISHING COMPANY, INC.

Redwood City, California • Menlo Park, California • Reading, Massachusetts • New York • Don Mills, Ontario
Wokingham, U.K. • Amsterdam • Bonn • Sydney • Singapore • Tokyo • Madrid • San Juan

Sponsoring Editor: Patricia L. Cleary
Editorial Assistant: Bradley Burch
Production Coordinator: Eleanor Renner Brown
Copy Editor: Anna Huff
Cover and Interior Designer: Irene Imfeld
Composition: Graphic Typesetting Service, Inc.
Art: Ben Turner Graphics

Library of Congress Cataloging in Publication Data

Effective management in nursing / [edited by] Eleanor J. Sullivan,
  Phillip J. Decker.—3rd ed.
      p.   cm.
    Includes bibliographical references and index.
    ISBN 0-8053-7862-6
    1. Nursing services—Administration.   I. Sullivan, Eleanor J.,
  1938–   . II. Decker, Phillip J.
    [DNLM: 1. Nurse Administrators.   2. Nursing Care—organization &
  administration.   WY 105 E275]
  RT89.S85   1992
  362.1'73'068—dc20
  DNLM/DLC
  for Library of Congress   91-26134
                                 CIP

ISBN 0-8053-7862-6

2345678910-HA-95 94 93 92

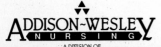

A DIVISION OF
THE BENJAMIN/CUMMINGS PUBLISHING COMPANY, INC.

390 Bridge Parkway
Redwood City, California 94065

This book is dedicated to:

Eleanor's grandmother, Alice Reed Clore,
Nursing Class of 1914, who inspired Eleanor to
enter the nursing profession; Rusti Moore-
Greenlaw, who introduced Phil to nursing;
Wendy, Colleen, Sean, Brad, and Pat, Eleanor's
children; Martha Goodrich, Phil's mother; and
Shirley Martin, who continues to inspire.

P R E F A C E

The nursing profession's first priority is competent and safe patient care. This philosophy gives direction to nurses' activities and provides a basis for intellectual, practical, and ethical decision making. By adroitly managing resources and by providing leadership to staff, the nurse manager assures the best possible environment for providing high-quality patient care.

Effective Management in Nursing is based on the above philosophical commitment. It is designed for use in a first course in nursing management, taught either in the undergraduate or graduate curriculum for both beginning and RN students, and in the nursing service setting. Additionally, any new nurse manager will find this book a practical guide to essential management concepts and skills.

This book has proved immensely popular because it is both practical and theoretical, as well as highly readable. These essential qualities have been retained and the book has been revised and updated throughout. In the third edition, substantial new content has been added in many areas.

In response to suggestions from faculty and nurse managers who use the text, new chapters have been added on: organizing care, critical thinking, managing groups and team building, enhancing employee performance, and power and politics. Also, the overall orientation has moved toward patient care management.

By using this approach, *Effective Management in Nursing* goes beyond leadership books and traditional management theory texts by providing practical assistance for developing important skills such as communication, recruiting, selecting and motivating staff, budgeting, risk management, managing conflict, and much more.

MULTIDISCIPLINARY AUTHORSHIP
The contributions of management experts often are not readily available to nurse managers. This book is unique in that the authors have drawn on the diverse expertise of management professors in schools of business and managers in private business practice, as well as that of nurse educators and nursing service administrators. This combination of theoretical knowledge and practical experience provides a rich blend of content, integrating management skills and concepts appropriate for the modern nurse manager to use in daily practice. However, each contribution has been carefully edited by the authors to conform to the goal of the book, which is to provide the best possible first course in nursing management.

NEW FOUR-PART ORGANIZATION
This new edition has been reorganized into four parts:

1. Understanding nursing management and organization—the basics of organization theory and management skills, the functions of the nurse manager, how care is organized, productivity and ethics.

v

2. Key skills in nursing management—communication, motivation, leadership, stress and time management, critical thinking, and managing groups.

3. Human resource management skills—selecting, training, and appraising staff; enhancing performance; managing absenteeism and turnover; and handling labor relations.

4. Basic survival skills for the nurse manager—budgeting, managing risk, change and conflict, and using power and politics.

This four-part framework outlines the job and its environment first, then reviews emerging issues and presents basic theoretical knowledge, and, finally, examines diverse survival skills. The overall goal is to acknowledge the primacy of patient care, accountability, quality control, and productivity enhancement. This requires the right technology, the right people, creative thinking, and above all, the successful combination of all these factors into a system that runs smoothly. In achieving this, we go beyond theoretical understanding to provide suggestions for implementing practical applications, examples, and key behavior patterns.

Introductory outlines at the start of each chapter offer a convenient reference to chapter content. In addition, each chapter concludes with a summary of key points and a current bibliography.

COMPLETE TEACHING/LEARNING PACKAGE

Unique in the field of nursing management books, *Effective Management in Nursing* is only one part of a complete teaching/learning package. Supplements have been designed to provide the maximum assistance to the instructor. The package contains an experiential skill-building workbook for students and an instructors' resource manual which includes detailed chapter outlines (for syllabi and lecture notes), explicit instructions for each exercise in the student workbook, a test bank, and master copies for overhead transparencies.

ACKNOWLEDGMENTS

The authors wish to acknowledge the contributors, as well as our research assistant, Sandra Handley; our secretaries, Marcia Pressly, Kathleen Sloan, and Patricia Walters; and at Addison-Wesley Publishing Company, Patricia Cleary, Executive Editor, Bradley Burch, Editorial Assistant, and Eleanor Renner Brown, Production Coordinator.

We owe a special debt of gratitude to the many reviewers who made comments and suggestions at various stages of the revision process. Their experience and insight have been essential to enhancing the quality and usefulness of this new edition. We would like to thank:

Judith A. Allender, RNC, MEd, MSN
Department of Nursing
School of Health and Social Work
California State University, Fresno
Fresno, CA

Jean Anderson, RN, MS
Department of Nursing
University of Rhode Island
Kingston, RI

Carolyn Brooker, MN, MS
Department of Nursing
Pittsburg State University
Pittsburg, KS

Rose Marie Chioni, RN, BSN, AM, PhD
School of Nursing
University of Virginia
Charlottesville, VA

Barbara Englehardt, RN, MN, PhD
Youngstown State University
Youngstown, OH

Mary Farley, BSN, MSN, PhD
School of Nursing
University of Colorado
Health Sciences Center
Denver, CO

Wilma Lutz, RNC, BSN, MS
Formerly of Capital University
Columbus, OH

Helen Miner, RN, BS, MSN, PhD
Department of Nursing
Southeast Missouri State University
Cape Girardeau, MO

Carolyn Schultz, RN, EdD
Department of Nursing
Pacific Lutheran University
Tacoma, WA

Eleanor J. Sullivan and Phillip J. Decker

C O N T E N T S

David P. Gustafson, PhD
Associate Professor of Management
and Organizational Behavior
School of Business Administration
University of Missouri
St. Louis, MO

Sherlyn Hailstone, RN, BSN, MSN
Vice President, Nursing
Barnes Hospital
St. Louis, MO

Judith Hibberd, RN, PhD
Associate Professor, Faculty of Nursing
University of Alberta
Edmonton, Alberta, Canada

Linda A. Knight, BS, MEd, DA
Corporate Director of Physician Services
St. Louis Children's Hospital
St. Louis, MO

June Levine-Ariff, RN, MSN, CNA
Assistant Administrator, Patient Care Services
Kenneth Norris Jr. Cancer Hospital
Los Angeles, CA

Diana J. Mason, RN, PhD
Associate Director of Nursing for
Education and Research
Beth Israel Medical Center
New York, NY

Steve Norton, PhD
Associate Professor of Management
School of Business and Economics
Indiana University at South Bend
South Bend, IN

Susan Reinhard, RN, PhD
Lobbyist, New Jersey State Nurses' Association
Trenton, NJ
and

Assistant Professor, College of Nursing
Rutgers, The State University of New Jersey
Newark, NJ

Mona Ruddy-Wallace, RN, MSN, EdD
Associate Professor, Nursing
Southern Illinois University at Edwardsville
Edwardsville, IL

Vicki Sauter, PhD
Associate Professor of Management Science
Management Information Systems
School of Business Administration
University of Missouri
St. Louis, MO

Carolyn Hope Smeltzer, RN, BSN, MSN, EdD,
FAAN
Vice President, Nursing
University of Chicago Hospitals
Chicago, IL
and
Clinical Professor
Marcella Niehoff School of Nursing
Loyola University of Chicago
Chicago, IL

Donna Lynn Smith, RN, PhD
Manager of Program Development
Long Term Care Institutions Branch
Alberta Health
Edmonton, Alberta, Canada

Marlene Strader, RN, PhD
Associate Professor of Nursing
University of Missouri
St. Louis, MO

C O N T E N T S

P A R T   1

UNDERSTANDING NURSING MANAGEMENT AND ORGANIZATION

C H A P T E R 1

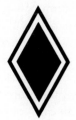

INTRODUCTION TO NURSING MANAGEMENT

KEY ISSUES FOR HEALTH CARE IN THE 1990S

KEY ISSUES FOR NURSING MANAGERS IN THE 1990S

Nurses in most health care settings today hold great responsibility to ensure that patients receive the health care that they need to lead active, productive lives. To provide high quality nursing services, it is essential to provide well-qualified nursing leadership. This is true throughout the hierarchy of nursing service and is extremely important for the position of nurse manager. It is widely accepted that the key leadership position is the first-line nursing manager since this position most directly influences the delivery of patient care. This book focuses on skills the nurse manager needs to support nursing personnel in their work. Curtin (1990) states that the organizational imperative of the 1990s will be to develop, and support, competent first-line nurse managers who are capable of helping nurses adjust to future changes. The purpose of this book is to study nursing management in the context of current health care and management theories.

◆ KEY ISSUES FOR HEALTH CARE IN THE 1990S

Several key issues will influence and create change in the delivery of health care in our society in the future. The issues center around the economics of health care, the competitive nature of the industry, the shortages of professional health care personnel, and the focus on quality outcomes and consumerism.

The nature of these changes will necessitate new and different leadership by nursing managers in the coming decade. Vaill (1989) describes our environment as a highly unstable situation that requires change to occur at a rapid and relentless pace. He draws an analogy to a state of "permanent white water" with few periods of calm water where leaders can take stock of the situation. This rapid change demands flexibility, intelligence, and new leadership expertise. Reinhard in Chapter 20 of this book reviews strategies for managing and initiating change.

The economic pressures on hospitals have been intense since the initiation of DRGs and prospective pricing for Medicare in 1983. The shift to managed care plans that control length of stay and reduce reimbursement has increased financial and competitive pressures. As the national debt continues to rise, the proportion of taxes that must go for health care continues to be a large target for Congress. Medicare reimbursement continues to be cut to all health care providers. Furthermore, health care costs for private industry create incredible burdens on companies as we move into a world economy. There are currently over 30 million Americans who work but are inadequately covered by insurance. These factors increase pressures on health care providers to provide the most efficient and economical care possible.

The reduction in reimbursement for health care puts incredible pressure on managers to focus on productivity as a way to reduce costs. The nurse manager must have a good understanding of nursing costs and have strong financial skills in budgeting and cost variance reporting. These issues are covered in depth in Chapters 10 and 19 of this book. Nurse managers must be able to reliably measure the work of nursing through nursing acuity systems to ensure that workload changes can be promptly recognized and responses can be formulated. Current staffing models require ongoing research to ensure that they are effectively utilizing the skills of professional and support personnel. The cost effectiveness of nursing care delivery systems such as primary nursing, case management, and differentiated practice will need continued study to ensure that patient outcomes are achieved as economically as possible. These issues are discussed in depth in Chapter 4.

Systems of care such as documentation, reporting, and nurse-patient communications will require review to determine if information technologies can be applied to decrease the labor-intensive nature of nursing work. In Chapter 7, Boyd reviews these systems and their current capabilities. Research in these areas is mandatory to document the systems' effectiveness in reducing cost and improving productivity. Nursing managers will be in critical positions to identify opportunities for system improvements and to help their staff adjust to future systems.

The aging of the population will create unprecedented demands for health care in the future. By the year 2050, it is expected that 33 percent of the U.S. population will be over 65 years of age, and 5 percent (16 million) will be over the age of 85 (Kutzka, 1985). Chronic diseases are now the primary condition for which our society seeks health care. The combination of the increasing numbers of elderly and the financial constraints of our government, which currently provides the insurance coverage for this group, will create increased ethical and moral dilemmas for our society and health care providers. Bartels, in Chapter 6, addresses these and other ethical concerns and provides a framework for discussion of these issues.

The increased intensity of care caused by shorter hospital stays and the aging of the population have created serious manpower issues within health care. Shortages are predicted in almost all categories of health care providers except physicians (Curtin, 1990). In 1989, 12.7 percent of all registered nurses, 8.3 percent of licensed practical nurses, and 5.7 percent of nurse aide positions were vacant (Merker and Elbein, 1990). The greatest need will be for nurses prepared at the baccalaureate and grad-

uate levels. It is projected that the current nursing shortage will continue well into the future. The nurse manager will be instrumental not only in retaining the current professional nursing staff, but also in the recruitment of new individuals. Information on the recruitment and selection of staff is covered extensively in Chapter 13 and the issue of turnover is addressed in Chapter 17.

Because of the rising cost of health care, many third-party payers, the federal government, and external review agencies such as the Joint Commission for the Accreditation of Healthcare Organizations (JCAHO) have increased their focus on quality through the continuous improvement of clinical outcomes. Statland (1989) states that quality will be the leading issue of the 1990s and the predominate issue over both technology and cost in the future. This focus on quality mirrors what is occurring in other industries in the United States. The JCAHO now requires that quality plans in nursing demonstrate a focus on continuous improvement and include measures of patient satisfaction. These changes require that nursing managers learn new ways to measure quality and new approaches in evaluating systems that result in quality care. New problem-solving techniques also will need to be learned to ensure that those involved in the production of health care services are intimately involved in and committed to continuous improvement. Chapter 21 focuses on quality and risk management; Chapter 11 covers problem solving.

The competition for patients in the health care system and the changing demand for improved service in our society have required that institutions focus on consumer satisfaction in addition to the quality of clinical outcomes. Since nurses are the largest group of health care professionals and have more contact with patients than do other employees, patients often judge the quality of care by the quality of nursing services (Bader, 1988). First-line nursing managers, by the nature of their job descriptions, are accountable to ensure that the patient's expectations of care are met. The first step in improving customer service is identifying customer expectations. This can be accomplished by surveys, focus groups, or talking to patients during rounds. After expectations have been identified, standards of performance can be established, communicated, and monitored. Extensive staff training may be necessary to ensure that the staff can meet the expectations. In an article on the application of world-class service concepts to world-class nursing, Najmaie and Modjeski (1990) identify staff training programs as critical to improving service. Staff development is covered extensively in Chapter 14.

The ability of nursing leadership in health care organizations to manage key issues will determine the future for patients and nurses and will help ensure the long range viability of our organizations. The challenges will be met through the ongoing development of nursing managers and professional staff. In Chapters 18 and 23 the importance of nursing organizations and how to form partnerships with organized nursing are reviewed.

♦ KEY ISSUES FOR NURSING MANAGERS IN THE 1990S

Covey states: "Effective management without effective leadership is, as one individual has phrased it, 'like straightening the deck chairs on the *Titanic*.' No management success can compensate for failure in leadership" (Covey, 1989: 102). He explains that leadership is the setting of the vision that is to be achieved. This senti-

ment is echoed by Vaill (1989), who feels today's business is so chaotic that only a leadership model will be successful. Waite writes: "Visionaries shape the reality of today into a vision for tomorrow and make the vision come alive. They recognize and use forces that drive change to shape a vision of the future" (Waite, 1989: 15). Nursing managers at all levels need to assess their organizational missions and the changes that are occurring in their environment to ensure that they are clearly defining and articulating a vision for their work groups. From a clear vision, the work group can establish the standards, systems, and processes that will result in quality patient care.

The manager plays an important role in facilitating the development of the standards for a work group and in role modeling behaviors that support the standards. To establish credibility, the standards established and the behavior of the manager must be congruent. Integrity is defined as a quality or state of being of sound moral principles: uprightness, honesty, and sincerity. Covey (1989) writes that integrity includes but goes beyond honesty. Honesty is telling the truth, while integrity is conforming reality to our words. Kerfoot (1990) states that the most important factor that positively influences the workplace for higher productivity and employee satisfaction is the creation of a sense of trust. Trust is developed when the manager demonstrates behaviors that support established standards. If, for example, a standard has been established for patient education, quality assurance monitoring activity should be in place to measure that goal. In addition, patient education might be a part of the orientation and performance evaluation plan for the staff. The manager might arrange for additional written educational materials to be available in the work area to be shared with patients. The manager must take a proactive approach to confront all staff who fail to meet the standard. This consistency of purpose enhances both the manager's credibility and effectiveness and the morale of the work group. Steven (1991) describes the qualities of a good leader as knowledge, integrity, ambition, judgment, communication skills, courage, stamina, organizational skills, administrative ability, and planning ability. Leadership concepts are expanded in Chapter 9 and discussed in detail throughout this book.

One of the controversies in nursing management today is the question of whether the nurse manager's greatest expertise lies in the clinical or managerial realm. McClure (1990) maintains that head nurses must be expert clinicians who are prepared to take responsibility for the care rendered on their units. Taunton, Krampitz, and Woods (1989) also hold that it is especially important that a nurse manager be an expert practitioner. This position is being challenged by other nursing management leaders who maintain that the nurse manager holds the responsibility to support the staff, who in turn are responsible for the delivery of nursing care. The change has been from a "working manager" to "manager of the staff, who manage the patient" (Manthey, 1990). This shift of responsibility is considered critical in allowing the professional nurse to be autonomous in the delivery of care. Information published by Katzin (1989) supports this position. The nurses in this study felt that one of the most important factors in job satisfaction was being allowed to exercise nursing judgment for patient care. Nurse managers must be credible clinicians in the areas they manage, but the critical factor in being an excellent nurse manager is how one manages the staff in their environment.

Health care institutions are unique, complex, social institutions that have traditionally func-

tioned as bureaucracies. Because of their hierarchical structures they often provide a work environment in which it is very difficult for the nurse to function simultaneously as both professional practitioner and employee. Kerfoot (1990) maintains that hospitals have historically been managed by industrial models of management that create tremendous job dissatisfaction and staff turnover. Rosener (1990) writes that young, educated professionals impose special requirements on the organization because they demand to participate and contribute. This position is supported by the magnet hospital work done in the mid-1980s. It was found that in hospitals where the nurses had input into decisions about their work they were more satisfied and tended to remain in their positions longer. Professional nurses must be given responsibility and authority and must hold the accountability for the patient care they deliver. Their input must be sought on matters that affect the practice of nursing in the work setting as well. The need to move to management models where the staff are empowered to make decisions seems imperative. These issues are discussed in Chapter 23.

The concept of empowerment is much easier to talk about than to implement because of the historical structure of both hospitals and nursing. Our nursing structures, because of their foundations in religion and medicine, are strongly hierarchical and controlling. Physicians continue to hold almost all of the authority for patient care. Systems have been developed based on rigid policies and procedures. Rewards and recognition have gone to managers who perform according to approved behaviors. In addition to these organizational constructs, and although not demonstrated by research, Beattie (1987) suggests that professionals such as nurses, social workers, and others in "helping" occupations demonstrate signs of co-dependency. She defines a co-dependent person as one who has let another person's behavior affect him or her and who is obsessed with controlling that other person's behavior. The co-dependent behavior pattern usually results from prolonged exposure to situations where a set of rules prevents open expression of feelings and direct discussion of problems. Cauthorne-Lindstom and Hrabe (1990) identify characteristics of co-dependents:

Powerful need to take care of others

Rigidity and perfectionism

Difficulty adjusting to change

Need to control situations and people

Denial or distortion of anger

Secret feeling of powerlessness

Dependence on others for approval

A basic sense of shame or a poor self-concept

Organizational settings, such as health care organizations, can exacerbate these tendencies in nurse managers. Such managers take accountability to fix all the problems, while maintaining all of the control. They have problems communicating difficult information to staff and frequently look for scapegoats so that they are not responsible for making employees unhappy when difficult change is required. Managers with co-dependent tendencies must recognize these behaviors and make concentrated efforts to change. Otherwise, they will be very uncomfortable with allowing the staff to make choices and decisions. Managers also must support the staff during the change process to ensure that staff with co-dependent tendencies gain insights that will allow them to change as well.

Block (1987) maintains that empowerment stems from two sources: first, from the structure, practices, and policies we support as managers who have control over others, and second, from the personal choices we make that are expressed by our own actions. Methods and approaches to problem resolution must be addressed in organizations committed to empowerment as a management philosophy. The first question that has to be asked when a problem emerges is: Who owns this problem? To correctly answer this question the organization has to have clearly identified each individual's responsibility, authority, and accountability. In a healthy nursing environment, professional nurses hold the responsibility and authority for patient care. The nurse managers are responsible for supporting the staff in their patient care activities. Nursing administration structures are responsible for supporting nurse managers in their role. Staff at all levels must have good conflict resolution skills and be able to reach consensus about decisions. Consensus exists when all members of a group can honestly state that they understand each other's points of view, that their own views are understood, and that they can support the decision of the group because it was made openly and fairly. The expectation has to be developed in the group that once consensus decisions are made they must be positively supported. It must be unacceptable for members of the group to sabotage the decision at a later time. Group decision making and meeting management are discussed in Chapter 12.

The organizational structure of nursing departments also can support or hinder the effectiveness of empowerment. Multiple layers of management make the delineation of responsibility, authority, and accountability difficult and unclear. Communication between the staff and executive levels becomes difficult, if not impossible, when excess layers of management exist. Problem solving at the appropriate level is hindered. In an ideal nursing structure, only the nurse manager would be between the top nursing executive and the staff (see Chapter 2 for more on organizational structure). In larger organizations, the maximum number of layers should be three. This concept is supported by Peters (1988) who maintains that to be successful in the future, organizations must flatten their structure to three levels, if possible, and widen the span of control to no smaller than one supervisor to 25 to 75 people.

For decentralization of decision making and empowerment to work, members of the organization must be able to take risks. The organization must develop a culture where risk taking is rewarded and failure is acceptable. The manager must convey to the staff that mistakes are to be expected in a complex environment and that human error is inevitable. Mistakes need to be analyzed when they occur to determine if the staff lacked ability or knowledge or if the error was a result of motivational issues. If the error resulted from lack of knowledge, an educational plan needs to be implemented and a follow-up plan established to ensure that the deficiency is corrected. If the mistake was inadvertent, the appropriate response is an accepting, forgiving attitude and encouraging the employee to learn from the mistake and to resume practice. Peters (1988) believes managers should go one step further and support failure actively and publicly reward mistakes in an effort to encourage faster change and innovation. We need to move from an environment where mistakes are punished to a culture where mistakes are seen as a natural byproduct of the change process.

Effective communication processes and systems are important to organizations that are striving to be successful. Nurse managers at each level must be comfortable in communicating with all members of the organization to ensure that information needed to do quality work is provided. Multiple communication mechanisms, including meetings, newsletters, open forums, and memorandums, are needed for an accurate flow of information. Managers and staff must develop effective communication strategies to support and build team commitment. These strategies include listening, being forthright about what is needed, and directing communication to the correct party. The first and most important step in effective communication is listening. Covey (1989) proposes a process called empathic listening. Empathic listening is seeking to fully understand where others are and what they need. True understanding is extremely powerful because it provides accurate information from which one can influence or problem solve. The skill of empathic listening can greatly increase managers' communication effectiveness.

Second, managers must have the courage to be forthright about what is needed from others. Clearly articulating expectations is an extremely powerful way to ensure that the needed results are achieved. Managers must be comfortable describing limits in a situation and must give their work group all of the information possible to make a decision. Another important strategy is direct communication to the individual who needs to hear the information. The practice of telling everyone about a problem except the one who is causing the problem is ineffective. The nurse manager must expect direct communication and role model this behavior to her staff for it to become a standard in the work group. Tolerating manipulative communication is counterproductive to team building.

Feedback to individuals and teams about

their work is vital to ensure achievement of a vision. Performance appraisal and coaching concepts are presented in Chapters 15 and 16. Systems of performance appraisal and feedback need to be consistent with the culture of the setting and work group. We need to strive to learn innovative approaches to performance appraisal that support professionals in their work. Staff development and training will be a critical element in successful nursing organizations of the future. Professionals need to continue to develop their clinical expertise to ensure that patient care standards can be properly established and maintained. Staff need to learn new techniques in quality improvement, interpersonal relationships, and team building.

SUMMARY

◆ A changing environment demands new management skills.

◆ Effective nursing management means quality patient care within the context of a viable health care setting.

◆ The nurse manager is accountable to clients, the staff, and the health care organization for which he or she works.

◆ The key to success in the future will be to build effective work teams.

◆ High quality clinical outcomes, cost-effective health care, and satisfied personnel and patients will be the ultimate outcome measures for nursing management.

◆ This book was written to prepare the nurse manager to meet these challenges.

BIBLIOGRAPHY

Bader, M. M. (1988). "Nursing Care Behaviors That Predict Patient Satisfaction." *Journal of Nursing Quality Assurance,* 2(3): 11–17.

Beattie, M. (1987). *Codependent No More.* New York: Harper and Row.

Block, P. (1987). *The Empowered Manager.* San Francisco: Jossey-Bass.

Cauthorne-Lindstom, C., and Hrabe, D. (1990). "Co-dependent Behaviors in Managers: A Script for Failure." *Nursing Management,* 21(2): 34–39.

Covey, S. R. (1989). *The Seven Habits of Highly Effective People.* New York: Simon & Schuster.

Cox, S. (1989). "Retention of Staff: The Head Nurse Connection." *Current Concepts in Nursing,* 2(5): 29–33.

Curtin, L. (1990). "Designing New Roles: Nursing in the '90's and Beyond." *Nursing Management,* 21(2): 7–9.

Katzin, L. (1989). "Great Head Nurses." *American Journal of Nursing,* 1(1): 42–47.

Kerfoot, K. M. (1990). "To Manage by Power or Influence—The Nurse Manager's Choice." *Nursing Economics,* 8(2): 117–119.

Kutzka, E. *Social and Health Policy on Aging.* A Report from the Policy Forum on Aging at Wingspread, March 5, 1985. Racine, WI: Johnson Foundation. P. 18.

McClure, M. L. (1990). "The Head Nurse as Clinical Leader." *Journal of Professional Nursing,* 6(2): 75.

Manthey, M. (1990). "From 'Mama Management' to Team Spirit." *Nursing Management,* 21(1): 20–21.

Merker, L. R., and Elbein, D. L. (1990). *1989 Hospital Nursing Personnel Survey Executive Summary.* Chicago: American Hospital Association.

Najmaie, H. M., and Modjeski, J. (1990). "Application of World Class Service to World Class Nursing." *Journal of Continuing Education in Nursing,* 21(2): 53–55.

Peters, T. (1988). *Thriving on Chaos.* New York: Harper and Row.

Rosener, J. B. (1990). "Ways Women Lead." *Harvard Business Review* (November–December): 119–125.

Statland, B. E. (1989). "Quality Management: Watchword for the '90's." *Medical Laboratory Observer,* 6(3): 33–40.

Steven, D. L. (1991). "Profile of a Good Manager." *Nursing Management,* 22(1): 60–61.

Taunton, R. L., Krampitz, S. D., and Woods, C. Q. (1989). "Manager Impact on Retention of Hospital Staff: Part 2." *Journal of Nursing Administration,* 19(4): 15–19.

Vaill, P. B. (1989). *Managing as a Performing Art.* San Francisco: Jossey-Bass.

Waite, Ruth M. (1989). *The Driving Forces for Change: Nursing's Vital Signs: Shaping the Profession for the 1990's.* Battle Creek, MI: W. K. Kellogg Foundation.

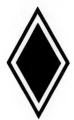

C H A P T E R 2

THE NATURE OF ORGANIZATION IN HEALTH CARE SETTINGS

We live in an organizational society, spending most of our waking hours and productive energies working toward the fulfillment of organizational goals. The justification for doing so is both rational and economic, inasmuch as we have discovered that properly organized and coordinated efforts can capture more information and knowledge, purchase more technology, and produce more goods, services, opportunity, and security than all individual efforts combined.

To achieve superior productive capability, however, an organization must depend on member behavior that is consistent with its goals. This means that individuals working in an organization must act in prescribed ways, sacrificing some of their personal freedom and autonomy. The price that people pay in loss of personal freedom must be weighed against the economic and other personal benefits they gain.

But it is a distasteful experience for most people to have little choice in the governance of their behavior, no matter how logical the reasons might be. Money alone usually provides insufficient motivation for surrendering one's autonomy. Therefore, the working relationship between organizations and their memberships must be given constant attention, and the person usually responsible for this mediating role is a manager; this activity is supervision.

This book deals with the role and functions of a particular type of manager—the nurse manager—and the contributions he or she can make to the delivery of health services in a variety of work settings. The manager's functions are vital, complex, and frequently difficult; they must be directed toward balancing the needs of the health care organization, patients, physicians, subordinates, and self. Nurse managers need a body of knowledge and skills distinctly different from those needed for nursing practice,

yet few of them have been prepared for managerial duties through education and training. Frequently they must depend on experiences with former supervisors who themselves learned supervisory techniques "in the trenches," or they must make their decisions out of some sort of instinct or common-sense reasoning and with some apprehension. Thus, there is a gap between what they know and what they need to know about managing. This book, focusing on the theory, processes, and dynamic potential of the effective nurse manager, proposes to resolve that gap in the new manager's preparation.

But the matters to be discussed must be considered within the realities of the setting in which they take place. Therefore, we first describe the role of nurse manager in terms of the most common environments in nursing, defining the organizational and environmental characteristics and constraints. To understand the nature of nursing management, we examine the structure of the institutions in which nursing is practiced and the environments in which the nurse manager and the institution function.

◆ THE NATURE OF ORGANIZATIONAL THEORY

An *organization* is a collection of people working together under a division of labor and a hierarchy of authority to achieve a common goal. Continuously working together under authority toward a goal implies management. The activities of organized people don't just happen—they are managed.

There are many types of organizations. Organizations can be grouped, for example, by product, size, ownership, or purpose. The above definition includes division of labor and a hierarchy of authority, which are subcomponents of organizational structure (Robbins, 1983). In discussing the structure of an organization, we must consider three macro components: complexity, formalization, and centralization.

Complexity concerns the division of labor in an organization, the specialization of that labor, the number of hierarchical levels, and the geographical dispersion of organizational units. *Formalization* is the degree to which an organization relies on rules and procedures to direct members' behavior; it is independent of size. *Centralization* concerns the locus of decision-making authority.

All science has as its aim the understanding, prediction, and control of an end. Organizational theory is the process of creating knowledge to understand organizational structure so that we can predict and control organizational effectiveness or productivity by designing organizations. Hence, we can design organizations so that they better achieve their goals.

The most common way modern organizational theorists analyze organizations is through a systems perspective. A *system* is a set of interrelated parts arranged in a unified whole (Robbins, 1983). Societies, automobiles, human bodies, and hospitals are systems. Systems are either closed or open. *Closed systems* are self-contained and usually can only be found in the physical sciences. This perspective has little relevance for the study of organizations. The *open system* perspective recognizes the interaction of the system with its environment. Katz and Kahn (1978) outline 10 characteristics that are common to all open systems. Understanding these characteristics helps one to conceptually understand how organizations function.

The first characteristic is *input,* or *importation of energy.* See Figure 2–1. Open systems import forms of energy from the external environment. Thus, the human cell receives oxygen and

nourishment from the bloodstream, and an organization receives capital, human resources, materials, or energy (e.g., electricity) from its environment.

The second characteristic is *throughput,* in which open systems transform the energy and materials. Just as the human cell transforms nourishment into structure, an organization can create a new product, process materials, train people, or provide a service.

The third characteristic is *output.* Open systems export some product—a manufactured substance, an inquiring mind, or a well body, for instance—into the environment.

Fourth, an organization's throughput works as a *system of cyclic events.* Organizational activities occur over and over again in a self-closing cycle, as the material that is input is transformed by throughput and results in output.

The fifth open system characteristic is *negative entropy,* which means the system reserves some of the input material so that it will be available for future use. For example, the human body stores fat that can be used for energy in lean times. Similarly, an organization can put extra money in the bank or employ extra manpower for availability in times of need.

The sixth characteristic of an open system is *information input:* the feedback and coding process. Every organization must take in information and feedback from the environment, code that information, and then store it so it can be used to predict the environment. This enables the organization to maintain a steady state, the seventh characteristic of an open system.

Sometimes called homeostasis, a *steady state* refers to the ability and desire of an organization to maintain some constancy in energy exchange. Just as the human body stays in a steady state, with no significant variation in its size and mass over time, so an organization attempts to stay in a steady state by predicting the environment and increasing or decreasing the input as information about output (market analysis) is gener-

ated. The basic principle is preservation of the character of the system.

The eighth characteristic is *differentiation*; organizational patterns tend to develop into spe-

FIGURE 2–1 THE HEALTH CARE INSTITUTION AS AN OPEN SYSTEM

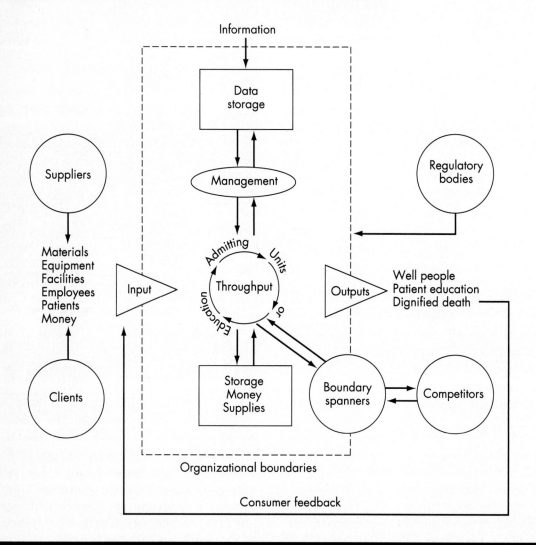

cialized subsystems for specialized tasks (e.g., the nervous system in the body). Mechanization and computerization would be considered differentiation in an organization.

Two processes combine to form the ninth characteristic: *integration/coordination*. As differentiation proceeds, it is countered by processes that bring the system together. Thus, management is an integration/coordination subsystem in an organization, just as the cerebral cortex is the integration/coordination subsystem within the human body.

The last characteristic of an open system is *equifinality*: the principle that any final goal or end can be reached by a variety of means. As open systems move and develop within their environment, they may set different goals at different times and choose different methods to attain them, but the ultimate goal of any open system is survival. The adaptability of humans for survival, for instance, represents equifinality. So does the behavior of organizations like the National Foundation for Infantile Paralysis; when its original purpose was achieved, it found another cause in order to survive.

Overall, we believe that the value of an open systems perspective is that nurse managers manage an expense center that has great control over the throughput of a product line: nursing care. They thus control, to a large extent, the viability of the organization in which they exist.

♦ THEORIES OF ORGANIZATION

The earliest recorded systematic organizational thinking was done by the ancient Sumerian civilization around 5000 B.C. The early Egyptians also dealt with this topic as did the Babylonians, Greeks, and Romans. However, organizational theory remained largely unexplored from ancient times until the Industrial Revolution (a few people did examine it—for example, Machiavelli in the 1500s). In 1776, Adam Smith (see Cannon, 1925) first established the management principles we know as specialization and division of labor.

In the late 1800s and early 1900s, other persons started to systematically think about the organization of organizations. The result today is a number of schools of thought or approaches to the organization and management of organizations. These approaches are traditionally labeled the classical, neoclassical, technological, and modern systems theories.

CLASSICAL THEORY

The *classical* approach to organizations deals almost exclusively with the anatomy of formal organization. The main thrust is efficiency through design. People are seen as operating most productively within a rational and unambiguous task/organizational design. Therefore, one designs an organization by subdividing work, specifying tasks to be done, and only then fitting people into the plan. Classical theory is built around four elements: division and specialization of labor, chain of command, structure of the organization, and span of control.

Several theorists have contributed to classical organizational thought. In 1911, Frederick Taylor wrote *The Principles of Scientific Management*. This book became an early cornerstone of management theory. In it, Taylor offers four principles of scientific management:

1. Develop a "science" for every job by studying motion, standardizing the work, and improving working conditions.

2. Carefully select workers with the correct abilities for the job.

3. Carefully train these workers to do the job and offer them incentives to produce.

4. Support the workers by planning their work and by removing obstacles (Schermerhorn, 1984).

These principles were given to maximize individual productivity.

Frank and Gillian Gilbreth added to scientific management by proposing time and motion study, the science of reducing a job to its basic physical motions. Thus, wasted movements are eliminated and incentives are based upon the newly designed job. Scientific management is the basis of job simplification, work standards, and incentive wage plans as used today.

Henri Fayol, in 1916, published *Administration Industrielle et Generale*, in which he proposed five rules of management:

1. Foresight—planning for the future, specifying goals

2. Organization—providing resources for the plan

3. Command—selecting and leading people in implementing the plan

4. Coordination—ensuring all employees' efforts fit together to achieve the goal

5. Control—verifying progress toward the goal

These rules were the basis for classical management functions: planning, organizing, controlling, and decision making. Fayol also specified 14 principles of management to be used to implement the five rules:

1. *Division of work*   The object of division of work is to produce more and better work with the same effort. It is accom-

plished by reducing the number of tasks to which attention and effort must be directed.

2. *Authority and responsibility*   Authority is the right to give orders, and responsibility is its essential counterpart. Whenever authority is exercised, responsibility arises.

3. *Discipline*   Discipline implies obedience and respect for the agreements between the firm and its employees. Establishment of these agreements binding a firm and its employees, from which disciplinary formalities emanate, should remain one of the chief preoccupations of industrial heads. Discipline also involves judiciously applied sanctions.

4. *Unity of command*   An employee should receive orders from one superior only.

5. *Unity of direction*   Each group of activities having one objective should be unified by having one plan and one head.

6. *Subordination of individual interest to general interest*   The interest of one employee or group of employees should not prevail over that of the company or broader organization.

7. *Remuneration of personnel*   To maintain the loyalty and support of workers, they must receive a fair wage for services rendered.

8. *Centralization*   Like division of work, centralization belongs to the natural order of things. However, the appropriate degree of centralization varies with a particular concern, so it becomes a question of the proper proportion. It is a problem of finding the measure that gives the best overall yield.

9. *Scalar chain* The scalar chain is the chain of superiors ranging from the ultimate authority to the lowest ranks. It is an error to depart needlessly from the line of authority, but it is an even greater one to keep it when detriment to the business ensues.

10. *Order* A place for everything and everything in its place.

11. *Equity* Equity is a combination of kindness and justice.

12. *Stability of tenure of personnel* High turnover increases inefficiency. A mediocre manager who stays is infinitely preferable to an outstanding manager who comes and goes.

13. *Initiative* Initiative involves thinking out a plan and ensuring its success. This gives zeal and energy to an organization.

14. *Esprit de corps* Union is strength, and it comes from the harmony of the personnel (Fayol, 1949: 20–41).

These rules and principles are the subject of Chapter 3.

Max Weber (1958) proposed the term *bureaucracy* (which to most of us today is a dirty word connoting long waits, inefficiency, etc.) to define the ideal, intentionally rational, most efficient form of organization. Many of Weber's suggestions for the most rational, fair, and efficient organization parallel the work of Fayol and his contemporaries.

Although the work of the scientific management theorists has been the core of industrial engineering, much of classical organizational theory has been criticized. Without considering factors such as technology, labor pool, and organizational climate and environment, there is no one best way to design an organization. Howell and Dipboye (1982) suggest that many of the classical prescriptions are not as explicit as they seem. How far, for example, should specialization be carried? At the extreme, it becomes ridiculous: thousands of very bored people doing one-minute tasks each. Thus, how far specialization should be taken is a matter of human judgment—and our "objective" principle turns out to be highly subjective. Many other criticisms have been given, most of which concern the lack of correspondence between the formal or planned organization/task and the actual organization, dehumanization of the worker, and rigidity of operation.

NEOCLASSICAL THEORY

The criticisms of classical theory led to neoclassical theory. *Neoclassical theory* takes the postulates of the classical school as given but believes these postulates are modified by people. This approach is often identified with the human relations movement of the 1930s. A major assumption of this school is that people desire social relationships, respond to group pressures, and search for personal fulfillment. Mary Parker Follet was an early advocate for the social aspects of organizations and in fact proposed the coordination of effort through mutual agreement (participative management) long before the human relations movement (see Metcalfe & Urwick, 1940).

Between 1924 and 1929, the Western Electric Company instituted a series of studies at their Hawthorne plant in Chicago that were originally designed to study scientific management principles. The first study was an examination of the effect of illumination on productivity. This study failed to find any relationship between level of illumination and production. Productivity in some groups varied at random, while in one it actually went up as illumination went down. The researchers concluded that unforeseen "psychological factors" were responsible. Further studies examined physical working conditions such as rest breaks and length of workweek. Again no relationship to productivity was found. The researchers concluded that the social setting created by the research itself accounted for the increased productivity. Workers felt special because of the attention given them as part of the research and thus worked harder. These studies led to identification of what is known as the *Hawthorne effect*—the tendency for persons to perform as expected because of special attention. Although the findings are controversial, they led to a focus by organizational theorists on the social aspects of work and organizational design.

In 1938, Barnard wrote *The Functions of the Executive,* in which he asserted that individuals cannot be coerced or bribed to do things considered unreasonable. Barnard recognized that formal authority does not work without willing participants. Later theorists, such as Maslow and McGregor, were also influenced by the Hawthorne studies and the human relations movement. These researchers proposed motivational theories to explain the link between organizational design and productivity. The work of these individuals is examined in Chapters 4 and 9.

The neoclassical theorists had a common desire to humanize classical theory without totally rejecting the structural view. All recognized the need to design a rational organizational structure, but proposed that it be done through cooperation, participation, and a view to the motivation of the individual. In a sense, these researchers bridge the gap between classical theory and systems theory. They took structure and added the individual. Systems theorists view productivity as a function of structure, people, technology, and environment.

TECHNOLOGICAL THEORY

During the 1960s a number of researchers focused their attention on the connection between technology and organizational processes. Woodward (1965), for example, surveyed 100 British manufacturing firms in an effort to find what management practices contribute to business success. She concluded that the demands of different technologies tend to shape the kind of organization that develops. Woodward categorized firms into three types of technology: unit (custom-made products), mass (large-batch manufacturing), and process production (continuous-process manufacturing). The most successful firms in her survey tended to cluster around the typical pattern in each production type.

The work of Woodward and others in this area helped make the final leap to modern systems theory, in which the organizational structure, the individual, technology, and the organization's environment all combine to determine organizational effectiveness.

MODERN SYSTEMS THEORY

An organization is a complex sociotechnical system. This concept integrates *modern systems theory.* The organization is viewed as a system that operates on certain inputs to produce certain outputs in a certain kind of environment (open systems). Modern organization theory also often relies on a conceptual analytical base, empirical research, and its integrating nature. Yet it is diverse. Examples are the open systems approach of Katz and Kahn (1978) described earlier, the decision system approach of March and Simon (1958), and the information-processing approach of Galbraith (1977).

Modern theorists ask a number of related questions. Key among them are: (1) What are the strategic parts of the system? (2) What is the nature of their mutual dependency? (3) What are the main processes in the system that link the parts together and facilitate their adjustment to each other? (4) What are the goals sought by systems? (See Scott, 1961.)

The basic part of an organizational system is the individual and the role he or she occupies. Next is the formal arrangement of functions and subparts of the organization, which is an interrelated pattern called the formal organization. Also important is the informal organization. Thus, both formal role demands from the organization and informal demands from the work group are taken into account. The physical setting is also studied.

Linking processes that are studied include role taking, communication, group processes, balance between organizational subparts, control and regulatory processes, feedback mechanisms, decision making, motivation, and leadership. Finally, goals such as organizational effectiveness, productivity, stability, and survival are studied.

Modern systems theorists view their approach as a framework for analyzing organizational behavior and effectiveness. Systems theory is an excellent method to account for general concepts of organizational functioning, but these concepts don't always lead to specific testable hypotheses. It is best to think of the systems approach as a general way of looking at organizations while we examine the specifics of organizational behavior. It is a "big picture."

Katz and Kahn (1978) view organizations as a recurrent cycle of input, transformation, and output. Organizations lack physical structure such as that of the human body. One can destroy the physical plant, but unless the articles of incorporation, charter, people (who may come and go), and job descriptions (definition of roles and authority structure) are destroyed, the organization survives. Even the goal can disappear and the organization will survive by developing new inputs, throughput, outputs, and goals. The March of Dimes is a good example. The goal of the March of Dimes was to provide care for polio victims. When polio was eliminated, the goal was irrelevant. Thus, the organization established new goals based on needs of the handicapped. The patterns of the events of organizational life are what is important. Katz and Kahn rely on role-taking and role-maintaining processes for their analysis.

March and Simon (1958) view an organization as an information-processing network with many decision points for both individual members and the organization. If we can understand those decision points and the variables or forces acting on the decision maker, we understand the most critical behavior of the system. March and Simon suggest that the classical concept of rational decision making is limited in organizations. The problem solver does not always know all the alternatives and may not have the criteria to evaluate them. These are the basic premises of rational decision making. However, decision making is rational within certain limits— "bounded rationality."

Rather than use rational decision making to optimize economic return, organizations and their members often "satisfice"—decision makers set some minimum acceptable level of return and pick the first alternative that promises to exceed this level. (See Chapter 11)

Furthermore, March and Simon suggest, instead of continually making decisions, organization members develop programs—sets of complex, organized behaviors used to respond to common environmental stimuli. These programs are why much human behavior is so predictable. Thus, March and Simon view organizational change as a process of changing the basic behavioral programs of organization members or of changing the stimuli that affect decisions.

Galbraith (1977) views an organization as a large communication system. He suggests that as uncertainty in organizations increases, the amount of communication required (or information to be processed) to keep the organization stable goes up. Thus, the organization is a system in which the goal is the reduction of uncertainty. Since all communication channels have some limit as to what they can carry, increased uncertainty (from an unpredictable environment such as that now faced by nursing with DRGs, increased health care competition, etc.) will eventually exceed the capacity of existing channels to reduce it. When this happens, it becomes necessary to (a) increase capacity or (b) reduce the quality of communication. Galbraith not only discusses strategies for increasing capacity and other methods of decreasing uncertainty, he also outlines different system types that deal with uncertainty to various degrees. One of these is the *matrix organization,* in which two distinct management systems—a departmental structure and a project or product structure—overlap. With this approach, an organization member reports to two bosses, which is a direct violation of classical rules. Yet, the matrix organization is often used in engineering and research firms because of its high information-processing capacity.

Overall, modern systems theory is a useful tool for understanding organizations. Often, it is difficult to test empirically many of the hypotheses generated by the theory, but the aim is

not to present the ideal organizational plan. The theory does recognize the vast complexity of organizations and the interactive effects of many variables. This theoretical school has made great progress in specifying what the important organizational variables are and in considering the human variables as well.

DEPARTMENTALIZATION

A bureaucratic structure, as depicted in Figure 2–2, characterizes the majority of today's health service organizations. Such a structure maintains command and reinforces authority; provides for a formal system of communication up, down, and across the facility; and buffers the caregivers from the task environment. But a bureaucratic structure is also impersonal and not always comfortable for the individuals working within it. Formal communication often takes on an autocratic, downward orientation. Even more detrimental is that the inflexibility of the structure renders individuals unable to respond to their changing environments.

Administrators structure or design health service organizations in ways intended to increase the probability of their organizations' survival and success. But they do so within differing social, political, economic, and resource climates, and they impose their own perspectives. Naturally, then, the formal structure of health care institutions tends to vary.

Characteristically, these structures take the form of a set of differentiated but interrelated functions. These broad functions are, in turn, broken down into tasks to be performed by persons in formal work groups. The decision as to how the pieces should be fitted together is usually based on the assumptions of bureaucracy.

The vertical dimension of Figure 2–2 deals with the organization's hierarchy—the lines of authority and responsibility. The organization

FIGURE 2-2 TYPICAL BUREAUCRATIC STRUCTURE, WITH SPECIAL FOCUS ON THE NURSING DEPARTMENT

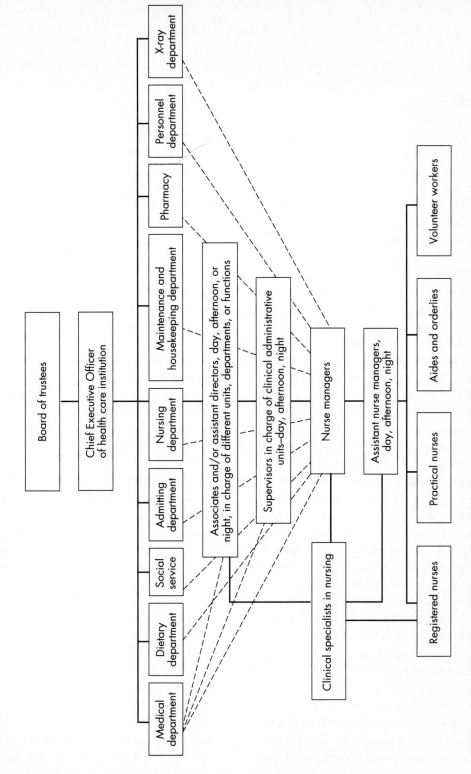

Adapted from Grace L. Deloughery, *History and Trends of Professional Nursing,* 8th ed. (St. Louis, MO: Mosby, 1977).

must be able to exercise control over the behavior of its membership, and hierarchy provides the authority for such control. On the other hand, the horizontal dimension of the chart relates to the division and specialization of labor—functions attended by specialists. The vertical dimension provides some understanding of how health care organizations use differentiation in pursuit of their goals and how differentiation results in an organizational prescription for the nurse manager.

CONTINGENCY THEORY

Health care organizations are unique with respect to the kinds of products and services they offer to their clients. However, like all other organizations, health care institutions are shaped by the same general forces. These forces stem from the environment, the kinds of technologies used in patient care, chosen strategies, organizational size, and the abilities and limitations of the personnel involved in the delivery of health care, including nurses, physicians, technicians, administrators, and, of course, patients.

Given the variety of health care "products" and patients served today, it should come as no surprise that organizations differ with respect to the environments they face, the levels of training and skills of their caregivers, and the emotional as well as physical needs of patients. It is naive to think that the form of organization best for one type of patient in one type of environment would be appropriate for another type of patient in a completely different environment. We would not expect to see the same kinds of staffing, rules and procedures, or chain of command in an inner-city substance abuse center and a suburban fertility center.

The optimal form of organization is contingent upon the circumstances faced by a particular organization. *Contingency theory* is that part

of organizational theory that seeks to establish a set of general principles for matching an organization's structure most closely to the forces of the environment, technology, people, and goals to achieve optimal organizational performance.

The *environment,* one of the most important influences on organizational structure, is defined as people, objects, and ideas outside the organization that influence the organization. These elements may be influenced in turn by the organization, but only to a slight degree. The environment of a health care institution includes patients and potential patients; third-party payers; regulators; competitors; and suppliers of physical facilities, personnel (such as schools of nursing and medicine), and equipment and medicines.

Today, virtually any health care organization must cope with an environment that is more complex, more changeable, and therefore more uncertain than the environments health care organizations faced in the past. Consequently, the health care organization of today—large or small, urban or rural, specialized clinic or major teaching hospital—must be designed to cope with more complexity and more uncertainty. Today's health care facility must be flexible, responsive, and connected with its environment to cope with this uncertainty. The structural means to achieve these abilities are discussed in more detail in this and other chapters. They include task teams, matrix designs, boundary role units, and strategic alliances such as joint ventures. James Thompson (1967) has suggested that certain identifiable persons and groups within society determine or shape an organization's purpose and influence its structure and operations. He calls these persons and groups the "task environment" and identifies four elements or clusters, shown in Figure 2–1. They include (a) clients who use the services of the organization; (b) suppliers who provide essential labor, capital, supplies, equipment, and property; (c) competitors who challenge the organization for clients or supplies; and (d) regulatory bodies such as governmental agencies, standard-setting professional organizations, collective bargaining units, and all others who might act to restructure or restrain the operation of the organization.

The relationship between the organization and its task environment is characterized by exchange, one earning resources that it may export to acquire the needed inputs from the others. The greater the need of one organization for the exports of another, the greater the control, presuming the entity has the ability to produce at the desired level.

Nested in the innermost core of the organization are the central activities or functions of the health service organization as supplied by the deliverers of health care. This core, which depends totally on a steady and predictable stream of inputs from the task environment, operates most effectively and efficiently when the traumas and uncertainties of the task environment are absent. In other words, the central activities of the health service organization must somehow be buffered from the uncertainty and instability of the environment.

In an optimal environment for the delivery of hands-on care, patients/clients arrive in a steady and predictable stream, and needed supplies are always available. Playing a role Thompson calls "boundary spanning," certain individuals (elements) serve to protect the central activities (technical core) of the organization from the uncertainties of the task environment. Boundary spanners in a hospital include personnel in purchasing or medical records, those responsible for Joint Commission on the Accreditation of Healthcare Organizations (JCAHO) liaison, and nurse managers—all of whom buffer the di-

rect caregivers from the environment, assuring to the fullest possible degree the availability of inputs.

Technology, another major influence on organizational structure, is the particular tools and methods used to provide a service or product. In health care, technology often involves the use of extremely modern advanced imaging equipment, laser scalpels, complex life support systems, bedside computing, and genetically engineered drugs. But technologies are often much less complex. A nurse who needs only common instruments such as a stethoscope and a trained eye and ear is also applying technology. Depending upon the technology used, a health care organization may require more or less coordination between staff members, strict or flexible rules for patient care, large or small departments, close supervision or autonomy. In other words, the structure of the organization depends in part on the kinds of technology used. Our health care facilities should be designed to treat each patient in an individual way; to do otherwise tends to dehumanize the patient and results in lower quality of care.

Although patients often share common complaints such as a type of disease or need for rehabilitation, they differ in terms of severity of illness, dietary needs, emotional stability, and so forth. The choice of the best technology to use to deliver health care to patients is a matter for staff nurses, physicians, and nurse managers. The issues they must consider are not just technical issues, but include economic and social issues as well.

A good definition of technology is the "tools, equipment, or materials; knowledge and skills to use them; and coordinative mechanisms and patterns of activity utilized to accomplish the organization's work" (Jelinek, Litterer & Miles, 1986: 266). Several researchers have examined the choices of technology and organizational effectiveness, including Woodward and Thompson.

According to Woodward (1965), the three main technology types are unit or small batch, mass production or large batch, and continuous process. Woodward found that the unit technology is most appropriate for firms that provide custom-designed products; mass production is usual for standardized products that are produced as individual units, such as automobiles; and continuous-process technology is most appropriate for products over which there is an extremely high degree of control and predictability, such as petroleum refining.

Which technology is most appropriate in health care? If we accept the premise that each patient has unique needs that must be assessed and individual treatment which must be prescribed and provided, then we should conclude that the appropriate technology is the unit or small batch system, or a variant of it. Such technologies are geared to address the unique needs of clients on an individual basis. Unfortunately, patients are sometimes forced through systems that tend to ignore their differences in the interests of efficiency. When this happens patient care usually suffers. We should remember, however, that most operating rooms, most surgical wings, and most convalescent centers will have similar technologies based on the usual needs of the types of patients they see. Some variations in structural elements such as span of control, hierarchy of authority, and discretion in nurses' decision making can be expected based on the extent to which the technology of the unit is small batch or continuous process.

The health care industry has room for many technologies. Something akin to mass production techniques may be appropriate in hospital laboratories wherein automated blood analyzers are employed, and continuous process may be appropriate in pharmaceutical manufacturing. Generally speaking, however, Woodward's small batch or unit production is the technology of choice in health care.

Thompson provided another useful way to think about technology in health care by focusing on the "coordinative activities and patterns of interaction" that are needed, which he termed interdependence. Three forms of interdependence were identified—pooled, sequential, and reciprocal. *Pooled interdependence* applies to situations in which two or more persons or units in an organization are linked only indirectly, through the fact that each reports to a common boss. Generally, their product is highly standardized and one unit is indistinguishable from another. Billing clerks in a hospital are an example. They need not coordinate activities with each other and need no formal mechanisms for association (although they are in the same office and will probably associate informally). A high degree of bureaucratization is appropriate.

Sequential interdependence also applies to standardized products, although there is more room for variation than with pooled interdependence. A hospital cafeteria is set up in this manner. As the customer moves down the line, food servers depend on the preceding server for the platter upon which to place the customer's selection. A high degree of information exchange and coordination are not necessary. Some specialized health clinics are also organized in this way. Patients with weight or suspected cardiac problems may be sent through a standardized regimen, one after the other, from one diagnostic center to the next. Here, too, a high degree of information exchange and coordination are not necessary. Later, of course, a physician or health care team may assemble to analyze data that were collected on a patient, identify clinical problems and develop a plan of treatment and care.

In *reciprocal interdependence,* a tremendous amount of information must be shared and processed. No one possesses it all. Furthermore, the patient may have to be sent back to a diagnostic station for more information to be obtained before a final determination can be made. Here, the course of testing cannot be completely specified at the outset, because it is determined in part by information developed in the course of treatment and care. Generally, reciprocal interdependence and unit production go hand in hand. The structure in such organizations must be designed to process high amounts of information and must be flexible, able to cope with uncertainty and change, and able to make and implement decisions almost instantaneously. Clearly the challenge of creating such a sophisticated organization that is also attuned to real world concerns such as economic constraints and shortages of skilled personnel is daunting.

Finally, the people who work to provide patient care influence the type of structure that is appropriate. People—nurses, physicians, technicians, administrators, and nonprofessionals—differ in their ability and willingness to assume responsibility for their jobs. The more highly trained and motivated these people are, the more decentralized the organization can be. Those who are less prepared to do their jobs autonomously will need guidance with closer supervision, more rules, and more regulations.

One can readily see that the choice of an organization design is an extremely complex matter. It is not surprising that tradeoffs are often necessary. While the complexity of the environment pushes the organization to have many layers and strict rules to process patients according to the needs of government regulators and third-party payors, technologies used may require

highly decentralized decision making for optimal patient care, while a tight labor market may require more bureaucracy to make sure that there is good follow through on patient needs in the face of a shortage of personnel. The nurse manager is a critical player in the choice and implementation of organizational design and should be thoroughly familiar with the issues raised in contingency theory.

◆ ORGANIZATIONAL STRUCTURE

The optimal organizational structure integrates organizational goals, size, technology, and environment. Structural reorganization often results from changes in one or more of these four factors. When organizational structure is aligned with organizational needs, it is imperceptible. When structure is not aligned with organizational needs, organizational response to environmental change is diminished; delayed, overlooked, or poor decisions are made; conflict results; and decreased organizational performance occurs. Organizational structure is an important tool through which managers can increase organizational efficiency; thoughtful reorganization should not be avoided.

Daft and Steers (1986) discuss the different structures found in modern organizations. Following is a summary of their examination of organization. Basically, all organizations fall within one of the four structures described. Most health care institutions are functionally departmentalized.

FUNCTIONAL STRUCTURE

In *functional structures,* employees are grouped in departments by task with similar tasks in the same group, similar groups in the same department, and similar departments reporting to the same manager (see Figure 2–3). In a functional structure, all nursing tasks are under nursing service, and the same is true of other functional areas. The functional structure tends to centralize decision making because the functions converge at the top of the organization.

The functional structure works best in small to medium-size organizations with few products or services. It is used where technology is routine and primary interdependence is between people within functions. Also, it works best when the environment is stable since activities are separated by functions. Coordination across functions is difficult and response time is slower. Functional structure also works best when the organizational goals concern internal efficiency, high quality service, and technical specialization, such as in health care organizations.

Functional organizations use resources efficiently, do not duplicate tasks, and simplify training because common tasks are grouped together for economy of scale. Career progression is easier and promotion can be based on func-

tional skill development. Employees identify with the department and work to excel in the functional activities.

The functional structure has several weaknesses. Coordination across functions is poor. Decisions also can pile up at the top and overload senior managers, who may be less informed regarding day-to-day operations. Responses to the external environment that require cross-function coordination are slow. General management training is limited because most employees move up the organization within functional departments. Most health care organizations meet many but not all of the criteria for a functional structure; most, however, have such a structure.

SELF-CONTAINED UNIT STRUCTURE

Self-contained unit structures are also called product line structures and, in health care, service line structures. In a self-contained unit structure all functions needed to produce a product or service are grouped together in an autonomous division (see Figure 2–4). Most

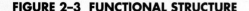

FIGURE 2–3 FUNCTIONAL STRUCTURE

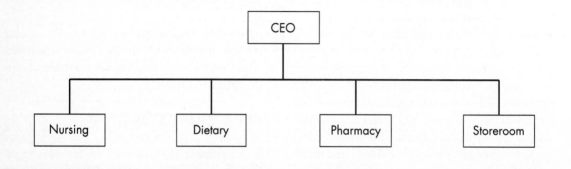

large organizations have some self-contained units. A large health care institution that acquires a smaller clinic may operate it as a self-contained unit. In a true self-contained unit structure, however, *all units are so organized.* The self-contained unit structure is decentralized and the units can be based on product, service, geographical location, or type of customer.

Self-contained unit structure is preferred in situations where the organization is large and complex, because the same activity can be assigned to several self-contained units. The self-contained unit structure is extremely appropriate when environmental uncertainty is high and the organization requires frequent adaptation and innovation.

One of the strengths of the self-contained unit structure is its potential for rapid change in unstable environments. Since each division is specialized and outputs can be tailored, high client satisfaction can be achieved. High coordination across functions occurs; employees identify with the unit and compromise or collaborate with other unit functions to meet unit goals and reduce conflict. Service goals receive priority under this organizational structure because the employees see the product line as the primary purpose of their organization.

The major weaknesses of the self-contained unit structures include duplication of resources and lack of in-depth technical training and specialization. Coordination across product lines is difficult in a self-contained unit structure; divisions operate independently and often compete. Each service line (which is independent and autonomous) has its own nursing staff and competes with other service lines for their nursing staffs.

FIGURE 2–4 SELF-CONTAINED UNIT STRUCTURE

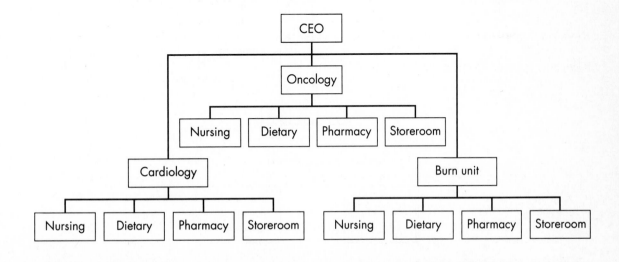

HYBRID STRUCTURE

When an organization grows, it typically organizes some self-contained units and some functional units; the result is a *hybrid organization* (see Figure 2–5). The strengths of the hybrid structure are that it provides simultaneous coordination within product divisions while maintaining the quality of each function, that there is greater alignment between corporate and division goals, and that the organization can adapt to the environment and still maintain efficiency. The organization can obtain economy of scale by centralization and adaptability and innovation within functions by making them self-contained.

Hybrid structures have two basic weaknesses. One is conflict between top administration and divisions. Second, managers often resent administrators' intrusions. The build-up of large corporate staffs to oversee divisions and provide functional coordination across divisions puts increasing pressure on the product units.

MATRIX STRUCTURE

The *matrix* organization is a unique structure and is rare because of its complexity. When organizations find that neither functional, nor product-line, nor hybrid structures work, they often organize into a matrix. The unique aspect of a matrix is that both product and functional

FIGURE 2–5 HYBRID ORGANIZATIONAL STRUCTURE

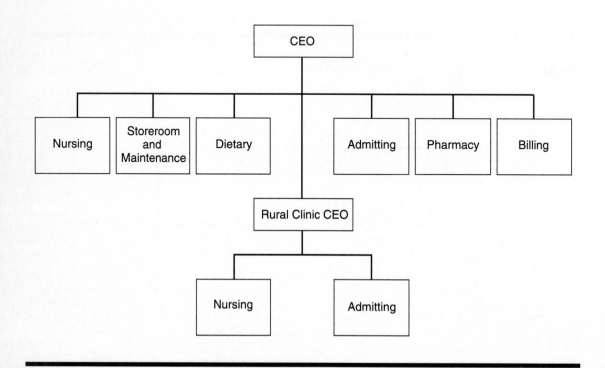

structures are implemented simultaneously (see Figure 2–6). Rather than separate functional and product structures, this structure overlaps both.

In a matrix structure, separate executives are responsible for each side of the matrix. Within the matrix, department heads report to both the functional and the product manager. They may receive conflicting demands from the matrix managers and often must resolve the conflict themselves. Matrices tend to exist where strong outside pressures exist for a dual organizational focus on product and function.

The matrix is appropriate in an environment that is highly uncertain and changes frequently but also requires organizational expertise. A major weakness of the matrix structure is the dual authority, which can be frustrating and confusing for departmental managers and employees. Excellent interpersonal skills are required from the managers involved. A matrix is time-consuming because frequent meetings are required to resolve problems and conflicts; the structure will not work unless participants can see the big organizational picture over their own functional area. Finally, if a matrix is imple-

FIGURE 2–6 MATRIX ORGANIZATIONAL STRUCTURE

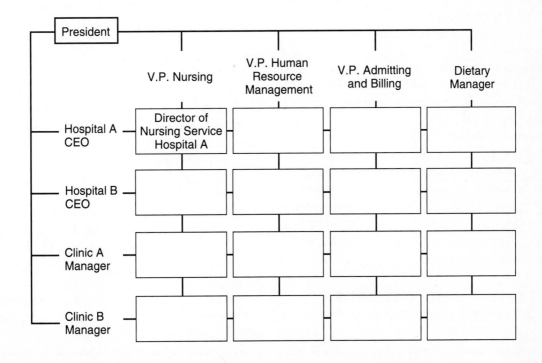

mented and the dual pressures do not continue, the side of the matrix more closely aligned with organizational objectives becomes dominant.

When complex structures such as hybrid or matrix structures are implemented, integrating mechanisms must be included in the organizational structure. Integrating structures enhance coordination across departmental boundaries. These may not be apparent on the organizational chart, but they include information systems, planned meetings, schedules, liaison roles, and task forces.

STRUCTURES UNIQUE TO HEALTH CARE

The typical health care organizational structure is the result of historical isolation and the complex relationships that exist between the formal authority of the health care organization and the authority of its medical staff. Consequently, a health care organization frequently has parallel structures rather than one organizational structure. The medical staff usually is separate and autonomous from the organization.

This results in an organizational dilemma: two lines of authority. One line extends from the governing body to the CEO and then to the managerial structure; the other line extends from the governing body to the medical staff. These two intersect in departments such as nursing in which decision making involves both managerial and clinical elements. Health care institutions with a functional structure and separate medical governance are termed *parallel structures*.

♦ TYPES OF HEALTH CARE ORGANIZATIONS

Health care organizations can be categorized as: (a) acute care institutions; (b) long-term care institutions; (c) ambulatory care organizations; (d) home health care agencies; and (e) temporary health care services. In addition, they may be private or public and proprietary or nonprofit. Most health care institutions and agencies are not for profit, but this picture may be changing with the recent development of proprietary, or for profit, hospitals or chains of hospitals. Some of these institutions specialize in one area of health care, such as alcohol treatment, but most function as general hospitals.

The largest number of health care organizations in this country today are acute care hospitals. Some hospitals are private, most of which have been founded by religious organizations, while others are public and are owned and operated by local, state, or federal governmental agencies—for instance, Veterans' Administration hospitals or state mental hospitals.

Many hospitals, regardless of other characteristics, also serve as teaching institutions for physicians, nurses, and other health care professionals, but the term *teaching hospitals* commonly designates those hospitals with a house staff of residents on call 24 hours a day. This is in comparison to a community hospital, with only physicians in private practice on the staff. These private physicians tend to be less accessible than a house staff, so the medical supervision of patient care differs. For the staff and supervisory nurses, patient care also will differ in the two types of institutions.

The growth of long-term care institutions has paralleled the increase in the elderly population. Today more people are living longer and living with poorer health, thus increasing the demand for long-term care.

Health care is also provided in ambulatory care settings, the home, and by agencies that provide personnel for temporary service. Ambulatory care providers are similar to hospitals in that they may be private (emergency aid facility) or public (county health department clinic) and proprietary (physician's office) or not for profit (church-operated screening clinics).

The trend toward home health care has also grown in recent years. Inflation and cost containment, for one thing, have forced hospitals and third-party payers to examine critically the length of patient stay. The result has been earlier discharge of patients and a more acutely ill patient population returning home. Further, more people are surviving life-threatening illness or trauma and thereby needing care. Visiting nurse associations (nonprofit, private), local health departments (nonprofit, public), temporary service agencies (proprietary, private), as well as departments of acute care hospitals all provide home health care. The largest growth, however, has occurred in private (for profit and not for profit) home care agencies. Services provided by home care agencies are primarily nursing, but some larger agencies also offer other professional services such as physical therapy or social work.

The temporary service agencies have grown in response to nursing shortages. These agencies provide nurses and other health care workers to hospitals that are temporarily short-staffed as well as providing private duty nurses to individual patients. Some hospitals rely a great deal on these agencies to provide staffing when staff shortages and variations in the patient census make scheduling difficult and inefficient.

Multihospital systems are becoming increasingly common. Nursing homes, psychiatric facilities, HMOs, and home care agencies are also often part of the multiunit systems.

Multi-institutional arrangements take many forms (Freund & Mitchell, 1985): (a) *formal agreement,* where two or more institutions engage in a joint program while maintaining responsibility for separate actions or services; (b) *shared services,* where clinical or administrative functions common to two or more institutions

are carried out cooperatively; (c) *consortia on planning or education,* where groups of institutions meet together and with health systems agencies to determine which institutions will provide specific services to the community; (d) *contract management,* in which an outside management firm contracts to take over day-to-day responsibility for managing an organization (no change of ownership occurs); (e) *leasing,* similar to contract management, but the management firm regulates not only day-to-day operations but policy as well; (f) *corporate ownership with separate management,* where a corporation owns several institutions and contracts for their administration with independent firms; and (g) *complete corporate ownership,* where a corporation owns and manages several institutions.

Multiunit systems can integrate horizontally or vertically. In a horizontally integrated system the units provide the same or similar services. In a vertically integrated system the units provide different services. An example of the latter would be a system with a health maintenance organization (HMO), psychiatric hospital, acute care hospital, and nursing home.

Freund and Mitchell (1985) suggest that although these arrangements have been highly touted, the final verdict on performance/efficiency will have to await the test of time and empirical studies. The authors have delineated the possible benefits and constraints of such organizations; these are displayed in Figure 2–7.

The nurse manager may be responsible for supervising patient care in all of the various types of health care organizations described. The knowledge of organizations and management principles presented here is applicable in all health care settings. Because most nurses are employed in hospitals, however, the examples focus primarily on nursing management in hospitals. When appropriate, other health care settings are also discussed.

FIGURE 2–7 MULTI-INSTITUTIONAL BENEFITS/CONSTRAINTS FOR NURSING

I. BENEFITS

Economic:
- Access to capital to finance new programs, services, and continuing education.
- Support for otherwise failing institutions.
- Program start-up costs spread over larger base.

Improved Technology:
- Corporate production of patient education and training aids.
- Corporate-wide computerized cost accounting, patient care information, and patient classification systems.
- Availability of new, sophisticated patient care equipment.

Diversification:
- Market analysis for special projects.
- New programs/services involving nursing (surgical centers, home health programs, wellness centers, child day care, hospice programs), bringing enhanced career mobility within the same corporate structure.
- Nonhealth lines of business, such as uniform companies for staff purchase at lower than market prices.

Fringe Benefits:
- Stock option purchases at reduced rates.
- End-of-year stock bonuses.
- Vested retirement system through corporation that is transferable with relocation.
- Continuing education for nursing staff and management.
- Educational leave program.
- Financial rewards for writing and publication.
- Awards (with monetary value) for community services and excellence.
- Attractive insurance and tax deferral benefits.
- Benefits transferable if relocate within the system.

Professional:
- Improved registered nurse ratio.
- Increased number of clinical specialists and nurse researchers.
- Decentralized nursing organizations.
- Specialists attracted to rural areas.
- Upward mobility for nursing staff.
- Systemwide mobility.

II. CONSTRAINTS

Reduced Autonomy:
- Nurse executive autonomy reduced, especially in regard to institutional governance and diversification.
- Nurse executives have not recognized their corporate responsibility; tend to be myopic toward their own institution.

Quality:
- Rapid expansion without the necessary resources and personnel results in current staff overload and reduction in quality initially.
- Reduced registered nurse mix due to regional determination of standard registered nurse mix.
- Consultants have no ongoing influence in given institution.

Reprinted with permission of Anthony J. Janetti, Inc., publisher, *Nursing Economics*, 3 (Jan./Feb. 1985): 30.

◆ THE DEPARTMENT OF NURSING

Nursing is the largest department in any hospital. At its head is the nursing service administrator, who is called the nursing administrator, director of nursing, vice-president for nursing, or one of many other titles designating the chief nurse executive. The nursing director has at least one assistant for every period of the day, since the nursing department is staffed around the clock. Each nursing department has clinical specialists in such areas as maternity, pediatrics, and the operating room, and every clinical service usually has more than one division with a nurse manager in charge. There may also be staff positions in such areas as inservice education and recruiting. Special nursing units include medical, surgical, pediatric, obstetric, psychiatric, operating room, recovery room, emergency room, and intensive care. Figure 2–8 illustrates an organizational chart for the typical decentralized nursing service.

A recent phenomenon in the structuring of nursing departments has come from the desire to democratize decision making in hospitals, especially among the nursing staff. These innovations may simply take the form of participative decision making (which is discussed in Chapter 11), but more elaborate systems known as shared governance also have begun to be developed.

Shared governance is a system that allows staff nurses significant input into major decisions about nursing practice. These systems are usually built on a foundation of primary nursing, peer review, and some provision for clinical advancement. Most shared governance systems are designed along the lines of academic or medical governance models: Nurses elect a "congress" that represents all nurses. Operating

under the congress may be a council (human resources) in charge of staffing levels, recruitment, and retention and a council (nursing care) in charge of care standards, audit criteria, research, and staff education.

Some shared governance systems incorporate elected advisory boards for each service and/or clinical department. From these boards is elected a senate or congress that meets several times a year to decide larger issues.

The ultimate outcome of shared governance is that nurses participate in a democratic forum to control their own practice within the health care system. The assumption is that nursing staffs, like medical staffs, will predetermine the clinical skills of staff nurses and monitor the work of each through peer review, while deciding other practice issues through elected forums.

Such systems should increase job satisfaction and lower turnover among those nurses who wish to participate in deciding the direction of their practice. However, it may also lower satisfaction for the inevitable minority who do not wish to participate in democratic forums or spend the time in the meetings and the other group work required of a democratic shared governance system. Nevertheless, efficiency may be improved by such systems as nurses take charge of their units/divisions/practice and move away from reliance on float pool or agency nurses to fill the gaps. Patient care should improve when nurses control their own practice. Many hospitals are examining such systems and weighing the costs and benefits. Only time will give us the answers to the economic questions. We feel, however, that regardless of the economic outcomes, such systems are good for nursing and allow nurses to gain an equal voice not only in nursing practice but also in health care.

FIGURE 2-8 DECENTRALIZED NURSING SERVICE

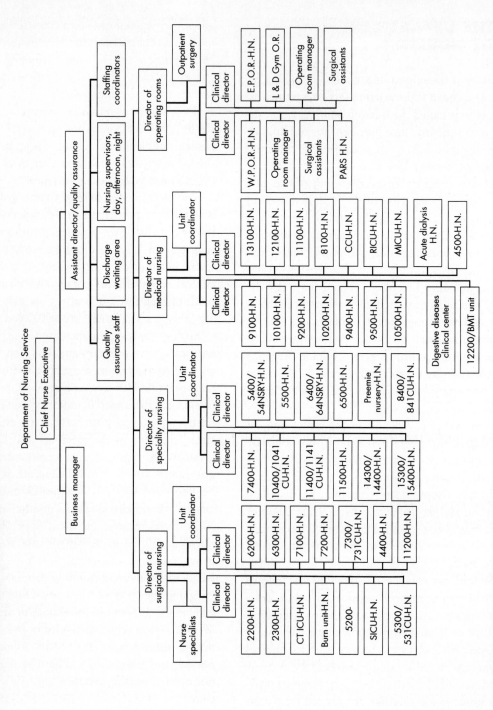

BOX 2-1
FACTORS REDUCING EFFECTIVENESS IN HEALTH CARE ORGANIZATIONS

From an open systems viewpoint, organizational effectiveness means sensing a change in the environment, inputting and digesting relevant information, using that information rather than organizational past history to make creative decisions, changing the throughput according to those decisions while managing undesired side effects, outputting new products or services in line with perceived environmental demands, and obtaining feedback on the change.

The following are points at which these processes could fail, thus reducing effectiveness:

1. Failure to sense environmental changes in a timely manner
2. Misperception of environmental changes
3. Failure to attempt to gain a market share in innovations until all or almost all the competition has done so
4. Failure to transmit relevant information to organization decision makers
5. Failure to foster creative decision making
6. Failure to recognize assumptions inherent in decisions made internally or by external change agents/consultants
7. Failure to convert the production system completely to the change
8. Failure to realize that simply announcing change doesn't make it happen
9. Failure to allow participation in change by organization members responsible for implementation
10. Failure to recognize and deal with the inevitable resistance to change
11. Failure to ensure that all subsystems change as needed
12. Failure to communicate to the environment that change is taking place so that the product or service can be exported in a timely manner
13. Failure to obtain feedback
14. Failure to use the feedback to modify the change

◆ ORGANIZATIONAL EFFECTIVENESS IN HEALTH CARE TODAY

It is difficult to define organizational effectiveness, especially in a service industry such as health care. Do we look at the number of patients processed or the outcomes? In teaching hospitals, do we look at curing patients or providing learning for interns and nurses? We must recognize that open systems have multiple functions and exist within environments that provide uncertainty and that their effectiveness may be measured by their ability to survive, adapt, maintain themselves, and grow. Viewed through a systems perspective, effectiveness comes to be defined by how well an organization copes with its environment. Nothing could be more meaningful for health care today.

Many factors today make it difficult for bureaucratically structured organizations to be effective. A bureaucracy's strength is its capacity to manage routine and predictable activities in a stable and predictable environment with its well-defined chain of command and rules. But many organizations, especially in health care, are not well equipped to deal with today's rapid and continuous environmental change. In addition, growth introduces complexity in a bureaucratic pyramid. Increased administrative overhead, tighter controls, rigid rules, and greater impersonality all result from increased organization size. Increased diversity also results from growth. Today's environment demands diverse, highly specialized competence that is often incompatible with a bureaucracy's hierarchy and rigidity. Also needed today is a change in managerial philosophy. New concepts of people and their values, needs, and reactions to uses of power are needed. Finally, innovative, nonstatus quo thinking must be integrated into organizational decision making. Any organization designed to deal with a stable environment where organizational processes are rigid or based on past history will not react effectively to environmental pressures. In fact, many have not survived.

It is difficult, though, to view health care today in a stable, predictable environment. Organizational effectiveness for health care institutions in today's environment entails, therefore:

1. *Adaptability*—the ability to solve unique problems quickly in reaction to a changing environment

2. *A sense of organizational purpose*—knowledge and insight as to where an organization is headed and why. This is shared by all members of the organization.

3. *Ability to test reality*—the ability to search out, accurately perceive, and correctly interpret the environment and its implications for the organization.

4. *Integration*—the ability to ensure that all organizational subparts are integrated and not working at cross purposes (see Schein, 1980).

SUMMARY

♦ We live in an organized society where individuals balance lack of personal freedom in furthering organizational goals with the economic and personal benefits of increased productivity. Managers mediate the process in which individuals surrender autonomy for other benefits.

♦ Organizations are open systems that operate much like the human body. Their ultimate goal is to survive, and they change various resources (people, capital, supplies) into services.

♦ Organizations produce goods and services that are exchanged for the resources required to survive. Many factors influence the organization's performance (e.g., patients, suppliers, competitors, governmental regulatory bodies, physicians, third-party payers, and the labor market).

♦ Organizations can be viewed as social systems consisting of people working in a predetermined pattern of relationships toward a goal. The goal of health care organizations is to provide a particular mix of health services.

♦ The four schools of organizational theory are classical, neoclassical, technological, and modern systems.

♦ Within the organization, an authority structure is created that determines the formal communication system and guides the organizational activities. This structure can be examined on two dimensions: horizontal and vertical.

◆ The optimal organizational design is suggested by contingency theory.

◆ The four types of departmentalization in organizations are functional, self-contained unit, hybrid, and matrix.

◆ The five types of health care institutions are acute care, long-term care, ambulatory care, home health care, and temporary health care. They may be private or public, proprietary or nonprofit.

◆ Nursing is the largest department of a hospital, includes many units, and can be centralized or decentralized.

◆ The nurse manager interacts with patients and staff to manage a nursing unit. Accountability in nursing means responsibility for providing high quality patient care and acceptance of the consequent praise or blame. Difficulty arises when one's decision about what is best for the patient conflicts with others' (physicians' and administration's) beliefs.

◆ Organizational effectiveness is a difficult concept in health care today. Innovation and creative problem solving are needed and must be fostered.

Daft, R. L., and Steers, R. M. (1986). *Organizations*. Glenview, IL: Scott, Foresman.

Fayol, H. (1949, English version). *General and Industrial Administration*. London: Pitman.

Freund, C. M., and Mitchell, J. (1985). "Multi-Institutional Systems: The New Arrangement." *Nurs Econ*, 3 (Jan.–Feb.): 24–31.

Galbraith, J. R. (1977). *Organizational Design*. Reading, MA: Addison-Wesley.

Galbraith, J. R. (1982). "Designing the Innovating Institution." *Organizational Dynamics* (Winter): 5–15.

Howell, W. C., and Dipboye, R. L. (1982). *Essentials of Industrial and Organizational Psychology*. Homewood, IL: Dorsey.

Jelinek, M., Litterer, J., and Miles, R. (eds.). (1986). *Organizations by Design: Theory and Practice*. Plano, TX: Business Publications. P. 266.

Katz, D., and Kahn, R. (1978). *The Social Psychology of Organizations*. New York: Wiley.

March, J. G., and Simon, H. (1958). *Organizations*. New York: Wiley.

Metcalfe, H. C., and Urwick, L. (editors). (1940). *The Collected Papers of Mary Parker Follet*. New York: Harper.

Robbins, S. P. (1983). *Organizational Theory*. Englewood Cliffs, NJ: Prentice-Hall.

Schein, E. H. (1980). *Organizational Psychology*. Englewood Cliffs, NJ: Prentice-Hall. Chapter 13.

Schermerhorn, J. R., Jr. (1984). *Management for Productivity*. New York: Wiley.

Scott, W. G. (1961). "Organization Theory." *J Acad Mngmt*, 4(1): 7–26.

Taylor, F. W. (1911). *The Principles of Scientific Management*. New York: Harper & Brothers.

Thompson, J. D. (1967). *Organizations in Action*. New York: McGraw-Hill.

Weber, M. (1958). In: *From Max Weber: Essays in Sociology*. Gerth, H., and Mills, C. W. (editors). New York: Oxford University Press.

Woodward, J. (1965). *Industrial Organization: Theory and Practice*. London: Oxford University Press.

BIBLIOGRAPHY

Barnard, C. I. (1938). *The Functions of the Executive*. Cambridge: Harvard University Press.

Cannon, E. (editor). (1925). *Adam Smith, an Inquiry into the Nature and Causes of the Wealth of Nations*. 4th ed. London: Methuen. Originally published in 1776.

THE FUNCTIONS OF A NURSE MANAGER IN A HEALTH CARE SETTING

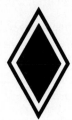

MANAGEMENT FUNCTIONS
Planning
Organizing
Controlling
Decision Making

LEVELS OF MANAGEMENT

MANAGEMENT FUNCTIONS FOR THE FIRST-LEVEL MANAGER
Planning
Organizing
Controlling

This chapter discusses the functions of a supervisor (nurse manager) in a health care setting with particular attention to the traditional functions of management. In addition, it provides an introduction to some of the more current functions of human resource management and reviews some of the functions that are especially characteristic of health care settings, such as multiple bosses, role conflict, and patient care management. Figure 3–1 illustrates many of the environmental, institutional, and human factors that converge on the nurse manager.

♦ MANAGEMENT FUNCTIONS

Supervision can be defined as the process of getting work done through others—done properly, on time, and within budget. Throughout this book the terms *supervision* and *management* are used interchangeably although, conceptually, management can be viewed as a broader role that goes beyond direct supervision of people to include the deployment of resources to accomplish organizational ends. Management functions can be defined as follows:

1. *Planning:* Determining the long- and short-term objectives (ends) of the institution or unit and the actions (means) that must be taken to achieve these objectives.

2. *Staffing:* Selecting the personnel to carry out these actions and placing them in positions appropriate to their knowledge and skills.

3. *Organizing:* Mobilizing human and material resources so institutional objectives can be achieved.

4. *Directing:* Motivating and leading personnel to carry out the actions needed to achieve the institution's objectives.

5. *Controlling:* Comparing results with predetermined standards of performance and taking corrective action when performance deviates from these standards.

6. *Decision making:* Identifying a problem, searching for solutions, and selecting the alternative that best achieves the decision maker's objectives.

This chapter gives special attention to planning, organizing, and controlling for the nurse manager, with less attention to staffing, directing, and decision making, as these are covered elsewhere.

PLANNING

Planning is always important since the future is uncertain, especially in such areas as the health care field, where environmental factors are rapidly changing. Planning is a four-stage process: (a) establish objectives (ends); (b) evaluate the present situation and predict future trends and events; (c) formulate a planning statement (means); and (d) convert this into an action statement.

One can usually differentiate between strategic planning and contingency planning, although in both cases a similar process is used. *Strategic planning* refers to determining the long-term objectives of the institution and the policies that will be used to achieve these objectives; such planning is carried out primarily by the chief administrative head and/or the board of directors in a health care institution. Although lower level managers are not directly involved in strategic planning, they are affected by the strategic plan since it will determine both the objectives they must achieve and the means by which they can do so. A manager's effectiveness is directly related to her or his knowledge of the institution's strategy and its application to the unit for which the manager is responsible.

FIGURE 3–1 FACTORS AFFECTING THE NURSE MANAGER

**Institutional
Structure**

Authority structure
Means of departmentalization
Span of control
Centralization vs. decentralization
Integrative systems
Control and measurement system
Recruitment and selection system
Reward system

**Environmental
Factors**

Economic
Legal/governmental
Market/competetive
Technological
Social/personnel

Work Social Structure

Institutional culture
Norms/sentiments/beliefs
Rituals
Language
Socialization processes
Roles/role conflict
Status system
Organizational climate

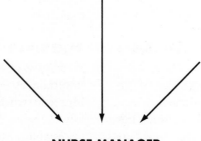

NURSE MANAGER

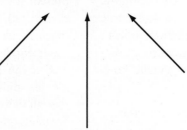

**Institutional
Objectives**

Product/service
Productivity/efficiency
Social
Human resource
Goal displacement
Participation in goal setting

People

Values/assumptions
Background
Status
Motivation
Learning style
Group processes/cohesiveness

**Task/Technology
Factors**

Nature of tasks
Physical layout of workplace
Work design
Medical/nursing science
Process technology
Computer system

Contingency planning refers to identifying and dealing with the many problems that interfere with getting the work done. This requires advance identification of the department's or unit's objectives, the contingencies that may prevent the achievement of these objectives, and how the work can be organized or assigned to prevent these contingencies from getting out of hand.

SETTING OBJECTIVES. Contingency planning essentially flows from strategic planning. Since the latter involves establishing objectives as well as policies to achieve them, a discussion of institutional objectives is in order. These objectives can be categorized into four general areas: product/service, efficiency, social, and human resource.

PRODUCT/SERVICE. For health care facilities this is the most important area because of its relationship to patient care. What patient care needs will be directly satisfied by the institution? What types of patients are to be served? What types of services will be offered? Some health care facilities also set goals (objectives) in the areas of teaching and/or research. The relative importance of each of the above depends on such factors as whether the institution is a private or public facility, whether it is affiliated with a university or some other type of institution, and its size and geographical location.

EFFICIENCY. This refers, of course, to efficiency in the performance of the institution's work. How many resources are required per unit of care—for instance, the number of nurses per patient day? How much time is expended per procedure? How many square feet are allocated per service? How will the efficiency of the unit be measured (e.g., average hospital stay, oc-

cupancy rates, within budget, hours of nursing care required for a given mix of patients)? Outside agencies such as third-party payers and governmental agencies are particularly concerned with these matters, in view of the rapid growth in health care costs over the last 10 years.

SOCIAL. Objectives in this area relate to meeting the obligations that have been established by the community or society in which the institution resides. Will the institution actively seek to be a good citizen or will it merely meet its minimal obligations by obeying the letter of the laws governing its behavior? It should be noted that hospitals themselves possess considerable political power through such lobbying organizations as the American Hospital Association and the American Medical Association and may therefore influence the laws under which they are regulated.

HUMAN RESOURCES. This has to do with the efforts that will be made to satisfy employee needs to maintain their commitment to the objectives of the institution. Will specific objectives be set in the areas of nurse manager/supervisor development and employee attitude and satisfaction?

Figure 3–2 shows the mission statement of one university-affiliated private hospital, which presents the nature of the institution and the direction in which it plans to go in the future. It is followed by the philosophy statement and an annual corporate goals and nursing service objectives statement (see Figures 3–3 and 3–4). It also includes some specific objectives needed to achieve these overall goals. Obviously, goal statements for non–university-affiliated hospitals or community hospitals that focus on secondary care might be very different. Goal statements need to be reviewed periodically to keep them realistic and consistent with environmental trends.

Statements of goals, as in Figure 3–3, focus thinking on the future, on what might happen in the future, and on how present activities help to move the institution toward these goals. Institutions with such specific goals are called proactive institutions; their administrators spend much of their time on future events and on preparing the institution to deal with those events. Institutions without clear goals are reactive institutions—ones that tend to operate on a day-to-day basis and spend much of their time and attention on "firefighting" instead of "fire prevention."

These same principles can be utilized by first-level managers. For example, Barnes Hospital in St. Louis recently developed a nursing service strategic planning model that fits with the current hospital process. The process incorporates the corporate strategy, assessment of the nursing service department, planning sessions with the clinical service division chiefs, and any assessments of new business lines that may have been completed during the previous year. The key groups assessed in the environment assessment include patients, families, physicians, staff, internal hospital departments, and the local and national nursing issues. In assessing the external environment, the nursing service focused mainly on corporate directions and evaluation of corporate issues to determine department applicability. Examples of issues assessed would be the aging population, clinical service strengths, phy-

---

FIGURE 3-2 MISSION STATEMENT OF BARNES HOSPITAL, ST. LOUIS, MISSOURI

◆ To be dedicated to excellence and international health care leadership in affiliation with an outstanding medical school.

◆ To serve as one of the world's pre-eminent providers of health care, engaging in a full range of services, including primary, secondary, and tertiary acute patient care.

◆ To provide resources necessary to serve as a national and international institution for medical education at all levels and for applied research in the biosciences.

◆ To strive towards ensuring the availability of compassionate, cost effective, quality health care services throughout the metropolitan region.

◆ To provide an environment that is conducive for the medical staff members to practice to the extent of their qualifications in accordance with bylaws, rules, and regulations approved by the Hospital Board of Directors.

◆ To provide employees with a high quality of working life, including equitable compensation and benefits, and opportunities to achieve their full potential as individuals and as members of the health care team.

◆ To meet the financial requirements of the institution necessary to remain fiscally viable.

Used by permission of Barnes Hospital, St. Louis, Missouri.

sician relations, etc. The second component of the environment assessment is the market assessment. Future directions for consumer relations were examined, patient satisfaction surveys were summarized, and public expectations of nursing care were reviewed. Manpower availability for nursing was included in the market assessment. Both national trends and Barnes Hospital nursing service recruitment data for the past four years were examined. The entry-into-practice issue was also addressed, as were the quality directions for the hospital as a whole.

A physician evaluation of the nursing services provided would also be important to include in a market assessment.

In assessing the nursing department as a whole, the nursing service reviewed several issues. The current employee attitude survey and actions taken to correct deficiencies were reviewed. Area salary and benefit surveys were examined to determine the nursing service position. The latest Joint Commission recommendations and their progress in meeting the deficiencies were reviewed. Other active nursing

---

FIGURE 3-3 HOSPITAL NURSING SERVICE PHILOSOPHY

Nursing is the individualized process of caring for and supporting patients as they progress through the changing levels of health.

♦ We are committed to the development of patient-centered nursing care and the accountability of individual professional nurses for specific patient care through the nursing process. This process includes assessment of patients' health care problems, establishing nursing diagnosis, planning for and instituting goal-directed nursing activities, and critically evaluating the effectiveness of that care on a continual basis.

♦ We support the dignity of the individual and believe that patients have the right to respectful care. We believe that nurses are patients' advocates, who participate in communications relative to the various aspects of patient care and the coordination of that care. Collaboration with other health care professionals and support of therapeutic medical treatment is recognized as essential throughout the process of care. We believe that patients and/or their important others should be included in the development and evaluation of their care.

♦ We are committed to health teaching that promotes an optimum level of functioning. We believe that discharge planning, which provides for the transition from hospital to community, is an integral part of the patient's plan of care.

♦ We believe that professional growth of nurses is related to the development of competency in nursing practice and the acceptance of responsibility for one's own actions and judgments. We provide experiential and educational opportunities that support professional growth and recognize that research activities are necessary to the continued development of nursing practice.

♦ In response to expressed health needs of the community, we accept the responsibility to share relevant knowledge and information. We recognize the community has the right to expect that care be provided in a manner that demonstrates concern for cost effectiveness.

Used by permission of Barnes Hospital, St. Louis, Missouri.

FIGURE 3-4 CORPORATE GOALS AND NURSING SERVICE OBJECTIVES

I. PATIENT CARE DELIVERY

Goal A: To develop a coordinated continuum of care.

♦ Objective 1: To expand the heart transplant program by implementation of Mechanical Assist Program.

♦ Objective 2: To explore the feasibility of developing a Comprehensive Critical Cardiology Service (CCCS).

♦ Objective 3: To develop a geriatric psychiatric program.

♦ Objective 4: To develop systematic process for organ retrieval in support of the organ transplant program.

♦ Objective 5: To further develop the Epilepsy program on Neurosurgery.

♦ Objective 6: To explore the development of a Cooperative Care Unit.

♦ Objective 7: To assist in the development of a plan to create a center of excellence in pulmonary medicine.

♦ Objective 8: To develop an outpatient Psychiatric Day Hospital.

♦ Objective 9: To develop an outpatient center for cardiac assessment and screening.

♦ Objective 10: To develop an outpatient diabetic center.

♦ Objective 11: To develop a plan for centralized outpatient facility for medical therapies or diagnostic procedures.

♦ Objective 12: To investigate the feasibility of developing a comprehensive outpatient treatment facility for dermatology patients.

♦ Objective 13: To assist in the development of a sports medicine rehabilitation program.

♦ Objective 14: To develop a business plan for Obstetrics following the movement of patients to Regional.

Goal B: To Improve the efficiency and effectiveness of operations.

♦ Objective 1: To develop, where appropriate, intermediate care units for patients who do not need intensive care but need more than general ward care and to evaluate effectiveness.

♦ Objective 2: To design cost-effective nursing care delivery practices and systems.

♦ Objective 3: To determine nursing care cost information per DRG.

♦ Objective 4: To implement nursing portion of computerized pharmacy information system.

♦ Objective 5: To ensure quality patient care through the establishment of standards and revision of documentation and quality monitoring systems.

Goal C: To identify new markets and improve the awareness, utilization, and value exchange of services.

♦ Objective 1: To promote Cardiology services.

service committees such as Career Ladder and Nurse Practice Committee efforts were incorporated. During the organizational assessment component, the nursing department's relationships with other hospital departments and with the local and national nursing community in the areas of education, research, and publishing were explored. The expectation was to develop a three-year departmental plan. An objective for nurse managers was set up on their divisions to identify issues to be addressed for the next three years. The nurse managers would have to be knowledgeable of the corporate strategy, the nursing department goals and objectives, and any clinical service activities that affect their area.

For a division assessment, the following items were thought to be important: patient care delivery systems, quality scores, staff development, patient/physician satisfaction, staff satisfaction, support department evaluation, physical plant assessment, equipment needs identification, and clinical practice changes that would be affecting the area. Division planning is expected to be a participative process where unit goals and objectives would be set and prioritized, and action plans developed. It is clear that division planning fits in with both the departmental and hospital planning. And nurse managers will be expected to do such planning in the future (Hailstone, 1987).

One common problem for many institutions, especially those without clear-cut operational goals, is goal displacement. Goal displacement means that a hospital unit pursues its own narrowly defined goals rather than the overall goals of the institution. Sometimes goal displacement manifests itself as excessive enforcement of rules (or excessive concern over the means of the unit) rather than the ends of the institution; this is especially likely to occur in bureaucratically organized institutions or when the official goals of the institution are general and ambiguous. Such ambiguity often results when there is difficulty in achieving agreement among units as to the institution's overall goals, so that each unit pursues its own goals.

It is not only important for an institution to establish objectives, but also each individual in the institution should be involved in the process. One popular technique for doing this is what is known as *management by objectives* (MBO) (Ordiorne, 1965). MBO involves several stages. Ideally, the first stage is the determination of the overall objectives of the institution. These objectives are shared with subordinates, who then formulate objectives for their particular units. These latter objectives are discussed by the subordinates and their managers to be sure that overall and unit objectives are congruent.

Once the objectives are formulated, the subordinate works on developing a plan (means) to achieve them. Measures of achievement are predetermined, and feedback as to whether or to what degree the objectives are achieved is given to the subordinate at specified intervals. Periodic subordinate/supervisor review of the MBO plan is useful so that corrective action may be taken. In some cases adjustment of the objectives (up or down) may be necessary; in other cases changes will be made in the means used to achieve them.

Both academicians and management practitioners have raised questions as to the effectiveness of this technique. The literature shows that MBO is usually more effective in improving employee satisfaction and morale than in improving employee productivity, but MBO can nevertheless serve as both a planning and a control technique. It tends to work best in situations where there are clear-cut institutional objectives; top administrators are committed to lower level participation in goal setting; individual and measurable tasks are involved; performance feedback can be given; considerable trust exists between the supervisor and the subordinate; true participation in objective setting is afforded; and the subordinate is highly motivated toward achievement. Some would argue that the above situation represents a very favorable work environment and that MBO is likely to work best where it is needed the least. Nevertheless, objective setting (see Chapter 11) is an important supervisory function.

EVALUATING AND PREDICTING. The second stage in the planning process is evaluation of the present situation and prediction of future events. From a strategic planning point of view, this stage requires an evaluation of the internal and external environment of the institution. The former calls for evaluating the present strengths and weaknesses of the institution. What activities does the institution perform well or poorly? Present activities and the policies relating to them might be grouped into the following categories: patient care/teaching/research; physical facilities; human resources; budgets (financial development); organizational system; technological capabilities; auxiliary services; finance/accounting; and management/administrator reputation.

The factors in the external environment that must be evaluated, along with some examples of their effects on health care institutions, are shown in the list below.

External Environment Factors	Some Effects on Health Care Institutions
Economic	
Inflation	Increased costs of equipment
State of the economy/business cycle	Decreased elective surgery/fewer beds filled during recessions
Fiscal/monetary policies	Availability of government funds to support health care, cost of funds for expansion, tax rates on for-profit hospitals
Legal/Governmental	
Health care regulation	Professional standards review Organization law State review of rates State certificate of need for opening new facilities Reimbursement mechanisms
Health care support	Related to fiscal policies—support for research, teaching in health care
Legal liabilities	Increased malpractice suits
Accreditation agencies	Must meet JCAHO and state division of health criteria or lose governmental support
Market/Competitive	
Non-health care competitors	Emergence of new services or elimination of unneeded services
Changes in patient needs	Home health care services
Changes in population—e.g., aging	Increased demand for long-term health care facilities
Substitute products	Emergency aid facilities
Technological	
Changes in technology	Need for retraining
Cost of new technology	Increased cost of hospitalization

continued

External Environment Factors	Some Effects on Health Care Institutions
Social/Personnel	
Availability and cost of personnel	Nursing shortage/surplus
New opportunities for women	Nurses demand more participation in decision making
Changing attitudes toward health care, death, physical fitness	Increased number of sports injuries Holistic health care "Right-to-life" movement Living wills

After both the internal and external environments of the institution have been evaluated, specific policies can be formulated. These are expressed in the list below, with questions on the left and possible answers, choices, or observations on the right.

Policy Questions	Health Care Examples
What services will be offered by the organization?	Types of patient care Teaching Research
What kinds of patients will be served?	Children, the aged, special conditions
How will these services be delivered?	Free-standing treatment facilities such as emergency aid clinics, surgical centers, and outreach programs
How will these potential patients be informed about the services offered?	Note the recent advertising by organizations providing alcoholism treatment, billboards advertising emergency aid facilities
How will these services be priced?	Percentage of indigent patients served, relationship with Blue Cross, Medicare, Medicaid, HMOs.

How will the institution be financed?	Sources of funds for new building/wing/special care facilities
On what basis will the institution choose to compete? What will be emphasized? What kind of care? What patient mix of acuity levels?	General, specialties, trauma, referral, pediatrics

From these general policies come specific allocations of resources to achieve institutional goals. Procedures, rules and regulations, schedules, and budgets are established as part of the overall institutional plan.

ORGANIZING

Once a strategic plan is established, the organizational structure to carry out that plan must be established. Figure 3–1 shows the many factors (e.g., organizational structure, environment, background of employees) that influence the institution's functioning. The plan determines what tasks need to be performed to achieve the goals.

These tasks are then subdivided into subtasks. It is such division of labor/specialization—e.g., one person to give the medications, another to transport patients off the unit—that brings efficiency to an institution.

These tasks, however, need to be coordinated. One way to do this is by grouping them into departments, such as nursing and housekeeping. Departmentalization can be based on product or service (maternity, psychiatric); type of client (elderly, children); functions (accounting, finance, housekeeping); process (operating room, radiology); time (evening/night nurse); or geography (emergency).

AUTHORITY AND POWER. The most important means of coordination is the authority structure of institutions. According to Scott and others (Scott et al., 1967), authority involves certain kinds of rights that are possessed by members of the institution. There are two general types of authority rights: the right to allocate institutional tasks and the right to evaluate the performance of these tasks. These evaluations affect the rewards and sanctions received by employees from the institution.

A variety of individuals may possess these rights. Whether a person has these rights can be determined by the answers to two questions: Would the person A allocating institutional tasks or evaluating the performance of these tasks be negatively evaluated by her supervisors for doing so? Would the person B to whom the tasks have been assigned be negatively evaluated for noncompliance with these orders? If the answer to the first question is no and the answer to the second question is yes, then we can say that A has authority rights over B.

Allocation rights can be exercised either by direction or by delegation. The first would include specifying how a task is to be performed, and the second would leave to the subordinate how the task is to be performed. The latter type of allocation is most commonly found in institutions employing professionals.

Evaluation rights are broken down into three stages: criteria setting, sampling, and evaluating. In institutions employing professionals, such as health care facilities, the profession itself frequently establishes the criteria by which an individual should be evaluated, but it is usually the manager's right to sample work behavior and then compare this behavior with the established standard.

A second theory of authority is the "zone of indifference" theory developed by Barnard and elaborated by Simon (Simon, 1976). This theory places less emphasis on the institution as a source of authority and focuses more on the relationship between the supervisor and subordinate and on the sources of power that the former has over the latter.

French and Raven have classified sources of power into five main categories: reward, coercive, legitimate, expert, and referent (French & Raven, 1959). *Reward* and *coercive* power have to do with the ability of the supervisor to mediate positive or negative rewards for the subordinate, including such items as pay, recognition, work schedule, duties, and continued employment. *Legitimate* power relates to the belief that the supervisor has the right to give commands; it is frequently based on acceptance of the social system. *Expert* power refers to the belief by the subordinate that the supervisor has superior knowledge in this particular area. *Referent* power refers to the degree to which the subordinate identifies with the superior and therefore patterns his or her behavior accordingly.

Nurse managers have reward and coercive power over their subordinates. Many newer staff nurses tend to believe that the nurse manager also has legitimate power over them. Expert and referent power would more likely come after nurse manager and staff nurse have worked together for some time. More experienced nurses might also share expert and referent power with the nurse manager over the newer staff nurses. The more types of power a supervisor has over a subordinate, the greater the control that supervisor has. This makes it extremely important for nurse managers to be selected on the basis of their technical expertise and personal leadership qualities, including their ability to serve as a role model.

BUREAUCRACIES. Although authority is the most common means used to link the tasks, people, and technology of the organization, other integration techniques are also used. Rules and regulations, for instance, are especially important within the bureaucratic type of organization. The bureaucratic organization consists of a set of positions arranged in a hierarchical manner, wherein each position holder has formal duties with a high degree of specialization and a formally established system of rules and regulations that governs his or her decisions and actions. Individuals are employed on the basis of professional or other qualifications rather than political, family, or other connections, and the person seeks this particular position as a career. In this "ideal" type of organization, bureaucratic officers hold their positions because of their expertise; they apply the rules and regulations in an impersonal manner, without favoritism, to make rational decisions and achieve administrative efficiency.

Bureaucracy is often used pejoratively to connote an institution where excessive enforcement of rules leads to inefficiency. The major problem that most bureaucratic institutions face is a form of goal displacement, where the energies of the participant in the unit are focused more on enforcing the rules than on providing service to the clients; this is not an unusual situation within public health care institutions. Nevertheless, the bureaucratic model is still followed in parts of most health care institutions, especially in support and administrative departments.

Other commonly used means of integration, especially among different units within the institution, according to Jay Galbraith, include direct contact, liaison roles, task forces (temporary committees), teams (permanent committees), integrating personnel, integrating departments, and, finally, matrix organizations (Galbraith, 1977). For example, nursing committees can be viewed as an integrating force. Galbraith, as well as Jelinek and colleagues, discuss these means of organizing in some depth (Galbraith, 1977; Jelinek, Litterer & Miles, 1981).

CONTROLLING

Control involves establishing standards of performance, determining the means to be used in measuring performance, evaluating performance, and providing feedback of performance data to the individual so behavior can be changed.

MBO, presented earlier as a planning device, can also be considered as a control mechanism. First, it entails determining objectives (standards) against which performance can be measured. Second, specific measures have to be established to determine whether these objectives are met. Third, the actual accomplishment of the objectives would be measured in relation to the standard and this information would be fed back to the individual. Then corrective action could be taken as indicated.

The MBO process is a rather mechanistic system that is applicable to only a limited range of tasks and situations. It involves a lot of self-control, and many health care organizations rely heavily on internalized "self-control." This type of control depends heavily on proper selection and training of individuals to ensure that they have the capability and desire to behave in the manner required by the organization to accomplish its tasks. Especially important to self-control are the socialization processes that cause persons to internalize the values of their profession and accept a code of behavior. Socialization as a means of control is useful in health care organizations because continuous monitoring of behavior is difficult.

SOCIALIZATION. There are five important stages in the socialization process (Klein & Ritti,

1984: 128–131). The first stage is *anticipatory socialization,* during which individuals acquire what they believe to be the attitudes, values, and beliefs of the group to which they hope to belong. Some of this learning, unfortunately, comes from the myths that are presented in the media and from contacts with individuals in these occupations. Consider, for instance, how the numerous television series on hospitals have often encouraged would-be nurses to develop erroneous conceptions (e.g., subservience) about nursing as a profession.

The second stage involves *learning* in a pre-socializing institution such as a school of nursing. During this period, which culminates for most nursing professionals in graduation and passing the licensure examination, an individual becomes more aware of the real norms of the profession. The third stage comes with *recruitment,* when the institution seeks individuals who already possess the skills and values desired by the institution. Proper selection makes the job of the nurse manager in the health care facility easier.

The next stage, *institutional socialization,* introduces individuals to the norms and values of the particular institution in which they are employed. "Reality shock" occurs when individuals find that the norms and values of the "aspired-to" group are different from those learned in the first two stages and anticipated for the third stage. This results in feelings of helplessness, powerlessness, frustration, and dissatisfaction (Schmalenberg & Kramer, 1979).

The final stage of socialization is sometimes referred to as *"the rite of passage."* It occurs when a person is accepted into full membership status and is committed to the actual norms and values of the institution.

Schmalenberg and Kramer perceive four phases in the role transformation from student to staff nurse: honeymoon phase, followed by shock, recovery, and resolution stages. They argue that the subcultures of school and work have different values and norms. In nursing schools, "the dominant values transmitted are comprehensive, total patient care with individualization and family involvement. Use of judgment, autonomy, cognitive skills, and decision making are strongly promulgated in this system. In the work subculture, the emphasis is on the value of providing safe care for all the patients. Organization, efficiency, cooperation, and responsibility are highly valued" (Schmalenberg & Kramer, 1979: 1).

During the honeymoon phase the new graduate is pleased with the first job as a "real nurse" and focuses on learning the routines of the hospital, perfecting her skills, and becoming accepted by other staff. The second stage begins when the graduate finds that some of the values taught in school are not as highly valued in the work setting. In the recovery stage the nurse begins to tolerate some of the aspects of the situation that before seemed intolerable. The final phase involves constructive resolution of the conflict between work and school values.

An effective and understanding nurse manager can help new nurses deal with this socialization process and facilitate the sharing of experiences in resolving the conflict. Newly graduated nurses need to understand the universal nature of the process they experience and be allowed to express and explore their feelings with others.

MANAGERIAL SURVEILLANCE. A second type of control system is managerial surveillance, which involves both direct observation of subordinate behavior and indirect observation through records. The amount of control from this source is related to the authority structure of the organization. For some types of managerial situations in a health care facility, control through direct observation may be very important: in emergency rooms, units with a large number of beginning nurses, highly technical areas that lack experienced personnel, or units with a number of nonprofessional staff such as nursing assistants. In units staffed by highly qualified and experienced professionals, managerial surveillance through direct observation may be less important.

Related to managerial surveillance is the "span of control" of the supervisor, or the number of individuals for whom the supervisor is directly responsible. Narrow spans of control, with only three to five subordinates, allow for a great degree of control, while spans of control for over ten employees make it difficult to control each subordinate by direct observation. Some of the factors that allow for wider spans of control include very routine work, well-trained subordinates, a highly capable manager, personal assistants, stable operations, similar functions among subordinates, highly formalized tasks, and spatially dispersed subordinates (Van Fleet & Bedeian, 1977). When the individuals being monitored are physically isolated or dispersed, direct observation is obviously difficult.

A number of sources of information are frequently used for indirect observation—among them budgets, schedules, time sheets, activity reports, statistical reports, patient surveys, narcotic reports, and patient charts. The types of information available are specific to each institution as are the standards used to evaluate that information.

The more sources of power that a supervisor has over a subordinate, such as reward, coercive, legitimate, referent, and expert, the more likely it is that the supervisor will be able to control the subordinate's behavior and direct it toward the accomplishment of institutional objectives. Rules and regulations also serve as a source of control, especially in situations where these rules and regulations have been internalized. Reliance on this means of control is most common in those parts of the institution that have a bureaucratic structure.

PRINCIPLES OF CONTROL. Whatever method is used to control the performance of others, the manager should be aware of several principles of control. The first one has been referred to by Klein and Ritti as "setting the fox to watch the henhouse" (Klein & Ritti, 1984: 482). In this situation, individuals themselves provide their supervisors with the information that will be used to evaluate their performance. It is relatively easy for them to modify or in some other way manipulate the information, because it is subjective or judgmental and therefore not easily detectable. When such self-reported data are used for evaluation, caution is advised.

Another important principle is the notion that "measured behavior" drives out "unmeasured behavior." If a supervisor focuses on specific, measurable aspects of the job in giving feedback to an individual, it may drive out unmeasured (and unrewarded) behavior.

Finally, there is what has been referred to as the "paradox of control" (Dalton, 1971). In attempting to control others, an individual may impose new requirements on them. This leads to countermeasures by the controllee, either to avoid this control, to modify the information, or even to seek substitutes for the desired action. This leads to countermeasures by the controller, and the whole process can become a vicious cycle. Frequently greater control over the behavior of others can be gained by giving up control—giving people greater freedom and trusting that they will do what is desired.

DECISION MAKING

Decision making permeates all aspects of the manager's job (Chapter 12). It includes: (a) identifying a problem; (b) establishing the criteria used to evaluate potential solutions to the problem; (c) searching for alternative solutions/actions (recognizing that no action is always an alternative; (d) evaluating the alternatives; and (e) selecting a particular alternative. This process can take place in a second (e.g., deciding to whom you will give a certain task) or may take place over months or even years (e.g., choosing a career, a spouse, or a new job).

March and Simon have pointed out that in using this approach to decision making, decision makers tend to use a simplified model of the real situation and to seek satisfactory rather than "optimal" solutions (March & Simon, 1964). Most decision makers establish some minimum criteria as to the acceptability of a decision and then search for a solution that meets this minimum acceptability.

◆ LEVELS OF MANAGEMENT

The lowest, or first, level of management is supervisors, such as nurse managers or head nurses, who are directly responsible for supervising the work of the nonmanagerial personnel reporting to them. Managers at other levels, such as middle nurse managers (MNMs) and chief nurse executives (CNEs), have managers or supervisors reporting to them. Figure 2.3 gives examples of these levels.

Katz argues that a manager needs three types of skills: technical, human relations, and conceptual (Katz, 1974). *Technical* skills involve method, procedures, and techniques and a knowledge of work being performed in the organization. *Human relations* skills relate to the ability to motivate and lead others and to manage conflict. *Conceptual* skills require analytical thinking and being able to perceive trends and to conceive of the organization as whole. Conceptual skills are required in strategic planning. Generally, human relations skills are very important on all levels of management, while technical skills are most important at the lower levels of management and conceptual skills are most important at the top levels of management.

Technical skills are very important to the nurse manager. McClure states: "Head nurses must be expert clinicians who are prepared to take responsibility for the care rendered on their units. This requires understanding and assessment of patient needs and staff abilities on a day-to-day basis" (McClure, 1990: 75). Figure 3–5 shows tasks performed by first-line managers in acute care hospitals of Los Angeles County, California, and shows the complexity of the first-line manager's job. According to Patz, Biordi, and Holm, human relations skills are the most critical skills for MNMs (Patz, Biordi & Holm, 1991). Higher level managers such as CNEs must focus on long-term issues and therefore need conceptual skills. They are most likely to interact with people both within and outside the organization, while the nurse manager is responsible for day-to-day direction and control of a small group of nursing personnel.

All managers, from the chief executive officer of a hospital to the head nurse, perform the managerial functions of planning, organizing, controlling, and communicating. All managers are responsible for the performance of other people and must create and maintain environments in which the tasks of the organization can be achieved. The following section focuses on some of the managerial functions important to the nurse manager.

◆ MANAGEMENT FUNCTIONS FOR THE FIRST-LEVEL MANAGER

Particularly relevant to the first-level manager's position are the functions of planning, organizing, and controlling; most of the time, for the person in this position, these involve dealing with contingencies. Since the nurse manager's job is to maintain the highest possible level of patient care while at the same time meeting other conflicting goals such as staying within budget, keeping staff satisfied, and so on, it is important to consider those factors referred to as contingencies, which prevent these goals from being achieved. Gellerman (1975) defines contingencies as those unplanned interruptions, unanticipated events, and inconvenient or awkward circumstances that prevent the work from being accomplished. Much of the content here on planning, organizing, and controlling for the nurse manager stems from Gellerman's ideas. He states:

FIGURE 3–5 TASKS OF FIRST-LINE NURSE MANAGERS

The following nineteen tasks were selected by more than 50 percent of the respondents to a survey conducted by Anita L. Beaman (1986). These represent the common tasks of the first-line managers in acute care hospitals of Los Angeles County, California, as perceived by the Director of Nursing Service.

◆ Assist inservice to prepare orientation schedule.
◆ Discuss progress of orientee with inservice.
◆ Decide when orientation is complete.
◆ Write counseling reports and discuss with employee.
◆ Discuss the need for termination.
◆ Terminate employees after obtaining approval.
◆ Submit time schedules for three shifts.
◆ Assign specific patients and teams for 7 to 3 shifts.
◆ Make recommendations regarding the budget to nursing administration.
◆ Calculate nursing hours and justify or explain.
◆ Call in extra help (when manager is on duty).
◆ Prepare reports regarding budget variances.
◆ Make daily patient rounds.
◆ Attend and participate in first-line nursing management meetings.
◆ Conduct meetings with own staff for the purposes of problem-solving and educating.
◆ Set goals for individual area.
◆ Participate in setting goals for the nursing department.
◆ Discuss unit problems with physicians regularly.
◆ Participate in all levels of quality assurance activities including designing studies, collecting data, and preparing reports.

A. L. Beaman, "What Do First-line Nursing Managers Do?" *J Nurs Adm,* 16(5) (1986): 8.

Planning, for a supervisor, means identifying the most probable sources of contingencies in advance. . . . Organizing, for a supervisor, means making sure that when contingencies occur . . . his/her subordinates are ready for them. This means that they are properly equipped and in the right places at the right times; and above all that they are properly trained. Controlling means making sure that contingencies are properly dealt with, and—when necessary—intervening in the subordinate's work to prevent a contingency from getting out of hand (Gellerman, 1975: 1).

The fundamental principles of the nursing process—assessing, planning, implementing, and evaluating—are very similar to the management concepts of planning, organizing, and controlling, as shown in Figure 3–6.

PLANNING

Contingency planning is very difficult because of the crisis nature of hospital work and the unknowns involved in patient care. Nevertheless, the nurse manager must try to be aware of the contingencies that may prevent the work from being accomplished. For instance: new, inexperienced, part-time or temporary staff, who do not know the policies and procedures of the institution well and may not be very committed to it; tardiness or unexpected absenteeism, which leaves the unit short of personnel (holidays, weekends, or vacations); staff tardiness from lunch or breaks; excessive demand for space when the division is at full capacity; new residents who need to be oriented; unexpected number of critical care patients; physician requests for special services; patients scheduled to be in two or more places at the same time; unavailability of staff, especially for evenings and nights; unavailability of medications, supplies, or equipment at the right time; staff quitting without giving notice.

Once aware of possible contingencies, the nurse manager must be alert to detect their occurrence before they are out of control. This involves nursing rounds at the beginning of each shift and thereafter as needed. A good nurse manager attempts to make frequent but brief contacts with subordinates to determine whether the work of the unit is progressing satisfactorily. It is important to remember the word *brief*. Personal interchanges are best left to breaks, lunch hours, or other social occasions. Also one can be seduced into spending extra time with subordinates if they are working on an interesting task. If the subordinate is adequately handling a particular situation, then the nurse manager should be elsewhere, making sure that a problem is not starting up at another location.

Making rounds also enables the nurse manager to assess patient care and staff performance on the unit. She can assess the quality of care being provided, a staff member's organizing abilities and interpersonal skills, team cohesion, and individual patient status. "Paper patrolling," such as reviewing records, budgets, and performance data, can also ensure that work is being performed satisfactorily. A nurse manager should develop a system of "red flags" that show that work is not being done correctly, on time, or within budget. Such things as patterns of absenteeism or lateness, direct nursing care hours versus overhead, patient days volume, use of medical-surgical supplies or pharmacy items, or failure to fill out reports (including patient charts) adequately can indicate a potential problem. This review should be done periodically to enable early correction of problem situations.

Finally, what activities are necessary to prevent problems from happening and what are the plans for dealing with problems once they have occurred? For example, does the unit have plans on dealing with certain kinds of disasters—ex-

FIGURE 3–6 COMPARISON OF TASKS OF CLINICAL NURSE AND NURSE MANAGER

I. ASSESSMENT

Clinical nurse
- Observe the patient/client and his/her environment.
- Communication skills. Art of listening and interviewing.
- Collect facts, identify priorities.

Nurse manager
- Observe staff reactions to policies and objectives.
- Observe needs of community–priorities in health-care–manpower trends and availability of resources.
- Communication skills. Art of listening and interviewing.
- Collect facts, identify priorities.

II. PLANNING

Clinical nurse
- Interpret in the light of clinical knowledge and the facts.
- Set short-and long-term goals for the patient and his/her family.
- Decide how to solve problems, keeping in mind quality of care, safe care, and the nursing policies laid down.
- Involve the patient and his/her family in the plan of care, and other disciplines as required, in order that there is coordination and progress toward similar goals.

Nurse manager
- Interpret mission/goals in the light of "managerial" knowledge and the facts.
- Set short-and long-term goals for service.
- Decide how to solve problems, keeping in mind quality of care and safe care, and revise policies if necessary.
- Involve the staff and other disciplines in order that there is coordination of planning and progress toward similar goals.
- Innovate/be creative.

III. IMPLEMENTATION (ORGANIZATION)

Clinical nurse
- Set the plan into action, taking into account:
  The patient's ability to help himself/herself.
  Professional resources.
  Equipment available.
- Meet teaching needs–of patient, family, nursing and other students.
- Organize for continuity of care.
- Provide team leadership and an environment in which good work can be done.

Nurse manager
- Set the plan into action, taking into account:
  The amount of delegation that can be safely undertaken.
  Professional resources.
  Time available.
- Meet teaching needs–development of staff–orientation of new staff to fulfill their respective roles.
- Organize for continuity in providing a service.
- Provide leadership in the area of responsibility and an environment in which good work can be done.
- Organize the budget.
- Consumer relations.

IV. EVALUATION (CONTROL)

Clinical nurse
- Analyze results of implementation of plan for patient and family.
- Consider changes that have taken place that necessitate reassessment.
- Consider quality of care provided, alongside the standards and policies that have been agreed upon.
- Identify areas of nursing practice that require revision of research. Communicate the need together with a suggestion for action to appropriate level of institution.
- Communicate changes in planning that may be required to keep patient/client, colleagues, and other professionals informed.

Nurse manager
- Analyze results of implementation of plan in consultation with those delivering nursing care.
- Consider changes that are necessary and the case for re-planning or adjustment of the plan.
- Consider quality of care provided alongside the standards and policies that have been agreed upon. Take action where needed.
- Facilitate clinical nurses and managers to undertake research projects and critique practice.
- Communicate changes in planning that may be required to keep staff and other professionals informed.

Based on M. Schurr, "Getting it Together", *Nursing Times*, 75 (August 30, 1979): 1472–1473. Used with permission.

ternal disasters, for instance, that increase demand for unit space, or snow or floods that prevent employees from getting to work, or internal disasters such as fire or loss of power?

ORGANIZING

Organizing means having qualified people and the right materials, information, and equipment needed to deal with contingencies. The last three items are specific to an organization and the type of services it provides. It is important for the nurse manager to identify these needs and make sure that subordinates have the resources available. Backup materials and equipment are especially important. It is also critical for the nurse manager to be aware of the state of the unit's equipment.

Having qualified personnel at the right time and place to take care of the division's work is one of the most important responsibilities of the nurse manager. The manager needs to be sure not only that the unit personnel have the knowledge and ability to do the job, but also that they are familiar with the policies and procedures of the specific unit. This is frequently achieved through training, which must be an ongoing process to ensure adequate patient care. Refresher (or developmental) training may also be indicated so that seldom used but important skills such as cardiopulmonary resuscitation are retained. Just as ball players have spring training and firefighters hold fire drills, so must nurses and nursing support staff periodically rehearse appropriate behavior in specialized situations; they should also understand the reasons behind the policies, procedures, rules, and regulations in the organization. Sometimes these do not make sense to new or inexperienced personnel. Helping staff nurses to understand the "why"

behind policies frequently leads to greater compliance with institutional requirements.

Another important aspect of organizing is scheduling—making sure that persons with the appropriate skills are available on each shift. Obviously, scheduling is very much affected by the institution's policies. In some institutions scheduling is centralized, while in others the nurse manager is responsible. In the former the nurse manager would have to work closely with the centralized scheduler to make sure that adequate personnel were available. In the latter situation, the nurse manager would need to develop scheduling skills.

Proper scheduling includes knowing in advance the capabilities, availability, needs, and desires of the unit personnel. A nurse manager must anticipate needs, estimate when additional personnel will be needed, and have backup personnel plans. Knowing about each person's knowledge, skill, home situation, and even his or her "biological clock" can help ensure the availability of adequate personnel to meet contingencies. Working out potential substitutions in advance can help to reduce conflicts in crises. Scheduling is discussed in Chapter 4.

In addition to the above, the nurse manager must help each staff nurse to organize time and activities. Time management (see Chapter 11) is an important aspect of this. Techniques for improving time management are as important to the staff nurse as they are to the nurse manager. Nurse managers can demonstrate effective time management by example.

Patient care is organized according to the type of delivery system used in the unit. Generally, there are different means of organizing the tasks of nursing and these methods lead to different problems for the nurse manager. See

Chapter 4 for a complete discussion of nursing care delivery methods.

CONTROLLING

Controlling means that the nurse manager must monitor the performance of her subordinates and take corrective action when performance deviates from the established standards. Thus nurse managers take corrective action when contingencies are about to or have gotten out of control.

One specific concern is when to take corrective action, or intervene, and how to intervene. An effective nurse manager intervenes when a specific policy, procedure, rule, or regulation has been or is likely to be violated; when there is danger to the patient or personnel; when the subordinate is overloaded or does not possess the necessary skill, information, or authority to act properly; or when there is threat to the property of the institution. For example, the nurse manager would intervene upon observing a staff nurse using incorrect procedures that might affect the patient's health and safety. The nurse manager would also help in emergency situations where the staff nurse was overloaded. On the other hand, the nurse manager may delegate handling of certain contingencies by assigning specific duties to other individuals.

The act of controlling, intervening, or correcting the behavior of a subordinate can be a frustrating experience for both controller and controllee. Too frequent intervention may lead subordinates to lose confidence in themselves or lead to less risk-taking behavior. But failure to intervene can lead to serious problems.

Both nurse managers and subordinates should know in advance the situations or "trigger points" that call for nurse manager intervention. Subordinates should also know under which conditions the nurse manager is willing to provide assistance to ensure that a situation remains under control. It is necessary to stress the importance of frequent patrolling whether it be nursing rounds or "paperwork patrolling." The nurse manager should spend as much time as possible on prevention of problems rather than on later corrective action.

This chapter has focused on the traditional functions of management, namely, planning, organizing, and controlling. Frequent references have been made to other chapters in the book that focus on some of the other functions of management, especially the modern functions of motivation, leadership, and human resource management. The rest of the book presents emerging issues in nursing management (productivity, change, ethics, and chemical dependency); the modern functions of management (communication theory, decision making, leadership, and motivation); human resource management (recruitment, selection, training, and performance appraisal); and other aspects of management appropriate for nursing (budgeting, risk management, conflict management, and labor unions).

SUMMARY

♦ Management is the process of getting work done through others, done properly, on time, and within budget. Traditionally, management functions have included planning, staffing, organizing, directing, controlling, and decision making.

♦ Planning is a four-stage process: establish objectives, evaluate the present situation and predict future trends, formulate a plan, and convert this into action.

♦ Objectives can be categorized into four general areas: product/service, efficiency, social, and human resource objectives. Predicting trends must be done inside and outside the organization. These objectives can be used in MBO systems to guide action.

♦ Once a plan is formulated, an organizational structure must be established to carry out the plan. Organizations are organized by task, department, client, time, and/or geography.

♦ The most important means of coordination is the authority structure. Authority involves two general types of rights: allocation of tasks and evaluation of performance. Furthermore, direction can be exerted from other sources besides legitimate power: reward, coercion, expert, and referent power.

♦ Roles and role definitions help define the authority structure of an organization.

♦ Socialization is the process of fitting people into the roles and informing them of the rules inherent in any authority structure. Socialization includes five stages: anticipatory socialization (beliefs), learning in a presocialization institution (school), recruitment, institutional socialization, and the final "rite of passage." Nurse managers should facilitate the socialization process.

♦ Managerial surveillance (through observation of behavior or records) is a key to control. The manager's span of control may determine the amount of time available for surveillance.

♦ Measured behavior tends to drive out unmeasured behavior. Staff will do what is focused on by the manager and/or what is rewarded.

♦ Nurse managers plan, organize, direct, and control, as do all managers.

BIBLIOGRAPHY

Christen, J. W. (1987). "The Changing Nature of First-line Supervision." *Health Care Supervisor,* 5(2): 65–70.

Dalton, G. W. (1971). "Motivation and Control in Organizations." In: *Motivation and Control in Organizations.* Dalton, G. W., and Lawrence, P. R. (editors). Homewood, IL: Irwin-Dorsey. P. 4.

Douglass, I. M. (1984). *The Effective Nurse: Leader and Manager.* 2nd ed. St. Louis: Mosby.

French, J. R. P., and Raven, B. (1959). "The Bases of Social Power." In: *Studies in Social Power.* Cartwright, D. (editor). Ann Arbor: University of Michigan Institute for Social Research. Pp. 150–167.

Galbraith, J. R. (1977). *Organization Design.* Reading, MA: Addison-Wesley.

Gellerman, S. (1975). *Leader's Guide to Accompany . . . "Effective Supervision: Planning, Organizing and Controlling."* Rockville, MD: BNA Communications. P. 1.

Gillies, D. A. (1982). *Nursing Management: A Systems Approach.* Philadelphia: Saunders.

Hailstone, S. (1987). Interview with Sherlyn Hailstone, Associate Vice President, Nursing Service, Barnes Hospital, St. Louis, MO (May).

Jelinek, M., Litterer, J. A., and Miles, R. E. (editors). (1981). *Organizations by Design: Theory and Practice.* Plano, TX: Business Publications.

Katz, R. (1974). "Skills of an Effective Administrator." *Harvard Business Review,* 52: 90–101.

Klein, S. M., and Ritti, R. R. (1984). *Understanding Organizational Behavior.* Boston: Kent. Pp. 128–131.

McClure, M. L. (1984). "Managing the Professional Nurse. Part II. Applying Management Theory to the Challenges." *Journal of Nursing Administration* 14(3): 11–17.

McClure, M. L. (1990). "The Nurse Executive: The Lead as Clinical Leader." *Journal of Professional Nursing,* 6(2): 75.

Manthey, M. (1980). *The Practice of Primary Nursing.* Boston: Blackwell.

March, J. G., and Simon, H. A. (1964). *Organizations.* New York: Wiley.

Marriner, A. (1984). *Guide to Nursing Management.* 2nd ed. St. Louis: Mosby.

Ordiorne, G. (1965). *Management by Objectives*. New York: Pitman Publishing.

Patz, J. M., Biordi, D. L., and Holm, K. (1991). "Middle Nurse Manager Effectiveness." *Journal of Nursing Administration,* 21(1): 15–24.

Rowland, H. S., and Rowland, B. L. (1985). *Nursing Administration Handbook*. 2nd ed. Germantown, MD: Aspen Systems Corporation.

Schmalenberg, C., and Kramer, M. (1979). *Coping with Reality Shock*. Wakefield, MA: Nursing Resources. P. 1.

Scott, W. R., et al. (1967). "Organizational Evaluation and Authority." *Administrative Science Quarterly,* 12: 93.

Simon, H. A. (1976). *Administrative Behavior*. 3rd ed. New York: The Free Press. P. 126.

Van Fleet, D. D., and Bedeian, A. G. (1977). "A History of the Span of Management." *Academy of Management Review,* 2: 364.

van Servellen, G. M., and Mowry, M. M. (1985). "DRGs and Primary Nursing: Are They Compatible?" *Journal of Nursing Administration,* 15(4): 32–36.

C H A P T E R 4

ORGANIZING CARE

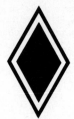

DELIVERY SYSTEMS
        Differentiated Practice
        Case Management
        Primary Nursing
        Team Nursing
        Functional Nursing
        Total Patient Care
        Product-Line Management

STAFFING AND SCHEDULING
        Philosophy
        Productivity
        Accreditation Requirements
        Staffing Approaches
        Flexible Scheduling
        Supplemental Staffing
        Patient Classification
        Computerized Scheduling

ORGANIZATIONAL CULTURE

Few aspects of clinical practice are more significant to nurses than the way in which they deliver care. The essence of nursing rests in how nurses care for patients, and the way in which nurses provide service revolves around issues such as care delivery, staffing, scheduling, patient classification, and organizational culture. Organization of nursing care is impacted by pressures from multiple sources. The ever-present scarcity of nursing resources combined with the drive to continuously reduce health care costs dictate that nursing care must be provided with optimal efficiency. Consumers of nursing service expect a high level of quality, as defined by the consumer. Nursing research gives evidence that patients must become partners and active participants in the care they receive for effective disease prevention and health promotion (Dienemann, 1989).

A critical objective for nurses is organizing work in a manner that is effective and personally gratifying (Porter-O'Grady, 1986). No single way exists to achieve effective, satisfying care delivery. However, key factors contributing to success are decision-making authority for direct caregiving nurses and effective methods of communicating with colleagues, other health care providers, and administrators.

◆ DELIVERY SYSTEMS

For decades, nursing administrators have examined nursing care delivery systems and have debated pros and cons of various methods of providing care (e.g., primary nursing, team nursing, functional nursing, and, more recently, differentiated practice models). The impetus created by demands of health care consumers, third-party payers, and nurses themselves has resulted in a need to carefully and cautiously examine problems in health care systems. The cornerstone of any nursing care delivery system must be a careful but efficient analysis of that system and the needs of its consumers, practitioners, and payers.

The following case study involving a 125-bed specialty hospital illustrates this point. The staff mix was 30 percent RN, 30 percent LPN, and 40 percent nursing assistants. Registered nurses were responsible for documentation and team leading. Nursing assistants and LPNs carried patient loads and delivered direct care. Patients, physicians, and allied health staff complained about continuity of care, communication problems, and failure to meet direct care needs. Following the retirement of the vice-president of nursing, an internal candidate was promoted to the position. After one week in the position, she decided that the system needed an updated, current method of nursing care delivery. She reached this conclusion through a careful review of the literature, which indicated that many facilities were adopting a case management approach. The new system was designed to provide coordination of health care from preadmission to postdischarge, goals that were attained according to case presentations in the literature. Although the system was carefully implemented, it failed. A nursing consultant reviewed the system and found that several problems consistently had been identified by the nurses, physicians, and allied health staff of the hospital, none of which were corrected by the identified method of case management. The new vice-president of nursing had designed and implemented a new system, based on a valid method of nursing care delivery, that failed to remedy critical underlying problems specific to the hospital.

Several methods of nursing care delivery are discussed, and benefits and pitfalls of each are articulated. No method is perfect, and the latest and newest, of course, is not necessarily the best. Nurse executives are urged to carefully consider the characteristics, needs, and demands of their own systems prior to adopting any delivery method.

DIFFERENTIATED PRACTICE

Rather than a specific method of nursing care delivery, *differentiated practice* is a basis underlying models of nursing practice. In differentiated practice, nursing roles vary according to the outcomes or competencies. Three models of differentiated practice exist: education based, assessment based, and all professional. The *education-based* model uses educational preparation (baccalaureate or associate degree) as the foundation for role descriptions. The *assessment-based* model combines educational preparation, abilities, experiences, and past performance as a foundation for roles. Finally, in the *all-professional* model, only baccalaureate-prepared nurses are involved in patient care roles (Murphy & DeBack, 1990).

CASE MANAGEMENT

Developed in response to a need to more effectively coordinate patient care throughout the health care system, *case management* is a method of nursing care delivery in which a professional nurse maintains responsibility for patient care from admission through and following discharge. In case management, nurses coordinate care for a small group of patients, monitor implementation of the interdisciplinary plan of care, and maintain communication with third-party payers and referral sources. A key factor distinguishing case management from other nursing care delivery systems is that the nursing case manager's accountability for care coordination transcends unit and service boundaries (Zander, 1988a).

The New England model of case management (Zander, 1988b) involves critical paths based on diagnosis-related groups (DRGs) and expected patient outcomes. The case manager follows patient progress through the system and accounts for variances from the critical path. The case manager may not provide direct nursing care but supervises the direct care provided by licensed and unlicensed nursing personnel. Registered nurses become eligible for case manager positions after completing a course in leadership and finance.

Related to the need to create efficient yet effective hospitalizations, case management has been adopted by numerous facilities. The model has been applied to various settings, including acute care, rehabilitation, and home health care (Whitman, 1991).

PRIMARY NURSING

Conceptualized and implemented during the late 1960s at the University of Minnesota Hospitals, *primary nursing* was designed to place the registered nurse back at the patient's bedside (Manthey, 1980). Merker and Elbein (1989) found that 32.1 percent of hospitals surveyed used primary nursing (see Figure 4–1). Primary nursing continues to be the means of nursing care delivery at many health care facilities. Although primary nursing systems vary, the underlying principle is that the registered nurse maintains a caseload of "primary" patients for whom the nurse designs, implements, and is accountable for the nursing care plan. In the system at Rush–Presbyterian–St. Luke's Medical Center (Chicago), the primary nurse selects a primary caseload and an associate caseload. All patients have a primary and one or more associate nurses identified. For example, when patient Doris Smith is admitted to a unit, Nurse Jones selects her as a primary patient. Nurse Jones assesses Ms. Smith and identifies a nursing care plan with her. Nurse Jones reports off to Nurse Monahan, who continues implementation of the care plan designed by Nurse Jones. Nurse Osco, on the 11:00 P.M.–7:30 A.M. shift, disagrees with the plan of care, but implements it, recommending that it be altered. Nurse Jones maintains accountability for Ms. Smith's care plan, educational program, and discharge planning throughout Ms. Smith's hospitalization.

Primary nursing enables nurses to provide directly the patient care for which they were educated, without the need to delegate care or supervise nonprofessional staff (Christman, 1980). Threats to continuity of care are minimized, as the registered nurse is accountable on a 24-hour-a-day basis for the patients' nursing care plan. However, since primary nursing

places the registered nurse in the role of direct care provider, more professional staff and fewer nonprofessional staff are required for successful implementation. This has led to the criticism that primary nursing is costly and is an inefficient use of scarce professional nurse resources (Horvath, 1990). This concern seems to be without solid foundation, as reports of implementation indicate that costs do not increase and may even decrease with primary nursing (McCausland et al., 1988). Another concern with primary nursing is that it complicates physician rounds because no single nurse on the unit knows all the patients. The response to this criticism by proponents of primary nursing is that, although the physician has to look for the primary nurse and may have to complete rounds

FIGURE 4–1 NURSING CARE DELIVERY SYSTEMS UTILIZATION, APRIL 1989

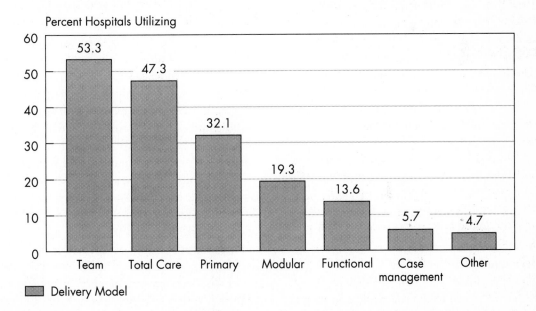

Merker and Elbein. AHA, Hospital Nursing Personnel, 1989.

with more than one nurse, the information the physician receives will be more accurate, comprehensive, and timely than if the nurse who accompanied the physician was less informed about specific patients. Given the ever-rising acuity level of hospitalized patients, it is not likely with any nursing care delivery system that one nurse could keep informed on all patients.

TEAM NURSING

Used by a majority of U.S. hospitals (Merker & Elbein, 1989), *team nursing* is the delivery of nursing care by nursing staff of various educational preparations. The team is led by a registered nurse and may include other registered nurses, licensed practical nurses, and nursing assistants. Team members provide direct patient care under the direction of the team leader, who is responsible for communicating with physicians and allied health personnel and for resolving problems encountered by team members. In team nursing, the nurse manager supervises the patient care teams and frequently rounds with the physicians. The nurse manager oversees implementation of nursing care plans for all patients on the unit (Kron & Gray, 1987).

Effective team nursing requires strong communication skills on the part of all team members; a key aspect of team nursing is the nursing care conference, in which the team leader reviews each patient's plan of care and progress with all team members (Marriner-Tomey, 1988). A disadvantage is that the time the team leader spends with patients is limited and, therefore, much of the team leader's information on patient status, problems experienced, and progress comes from team members. An advantage of team nursing is that patient care needs requiring more than one staff member, such as patient transfers from bed to chair, are more easily met than in primary nursing, where the primary

nurse must go find another to assist with the transfer.

Potential problems with team nursing are role confusion and resentment. The nursing assistants and professional staff may view the role of the team leader as more focused toward "paperwork" and less directed at the physical needs of the patient. Strong, effective delegation skills are required for the team leader. Problems in communication and delegation are common reasons that team nursing becomes less effective than desired. For example, work sampling studies reflected that while 24 percent of the work time of nursing assistants was classed as nonproductive, only 11 percent of the registered nurses' time was spent on nonproductive or personal activities (Hinshaw, 1989).

FUNCTIONAL NURSING

Commonly practiced during the 1950s in response to a national nursing shortage, *functional nursing* continues to be used in a few hospitals (Merker & Elbein, 1989). In functional nursing, tasks are divided, with one nurse assuming responsibility for specific tasks (e.g., medication administration, catheterizations, and baths and linen changes) (Marriner-Tomey, 1988). Functional nursing delivery systems were adapted to health care from Taylor's time and motion studies, which stressed control, quality, and efficiency. The advantage of functional nursing is clearly identifiable in the example of an intravenous therapy team. The IV team nurse is responsible only for IV starts and monitoring. As a consequence, clinical expertise is developed, and the accuracy, efficiency, and quality of intravenous therapy become higher than if all nurses are responsible for their own IVs. The major disadvantages of functional nursing are problems with continuity, absence of a holistic view of the patient, and the possibility that care may become rigid and mechanical. Additionally, communication is difficult when there are so many with whom to communicate, and it is easy to "pass the buck" and fail to assume responsibility for errors in care delivery.

TOTAL PATIENT CARE

The original form of nursing care delivery was *total patient care,* in which a nurse was responsible for all aspects of one or more patients' care. In Florence Nightingale's time, this required the provision of all care for a ward of patients. Twenty-four-hour accountability was not routinely necessary, as patients were sometimes left without care at night (Dolan, 1958). During the 1920s, total patient care, or case nursing, was common (Marriner-Tomey, 1988). Compliance with physician's orders was routine and was the basis for the method of nursing care delivery. In total patient care, nurses worked directly with the patient, family, physician, and allied health staff in implementing a plan of care.

PRODUCT-LINE MANAGEMENT

Originally conceived at Proctor and Gamble for Lava soap in 1928 (Lyonski, 1985), *product-line management* has been adapted to the health care setting. In product-line, or service-line, management, a product manager is accountable for production efficiency, marketing, and product outcome and is empowered to make the decisions necessary to effect product success (McDaniel & Gray, 1980). As applied to health care, product-line management requires the definition of "products," such as rehabilitation, women's health, or arthritis care. Specific areas of service need are identified for targeted marketing. The product manager remains accountable for cost-effective "production" of the service (Yano-Fong, 1988).

Product-line management attempts to resolve issues such as ineffective interdisciplinary problem resolution that have become long-standing within traditionally organized health care facilities (Bird, 1988). In one 350-bed hospital, rehabilitation and acute care services were organized along traditional departmental lines (see Figure 4–2). One problem involved relationships between nursing and occupational therapy. Patient therapy sessions for occupational therapy started at 8:15 A.M. For the patients to arrive in occupational therapy on time, the nurses began waking them at 5:00 A.M. Patients were hurriedly dressed, prepared for breakfast, and transported to therapy. Patients complained of fatigue, and progress in the rehabilitation program was not as expected. The program was reorganized to a product-line system (see Figure 4–3). Following the reorganization, the product-line manager implemented a practice of having occupational therapists arrive on the nursing units prior to breakfast, for dressing and feeding programs. Activity of daily living programs became more effective, patients conserved energy, and staff, both nurses and occupational therapists, expressed a high degree of satisfaction with the revised policy.

Although adopting a product-line management approach does not alter the direct delivery of nursing care, it may impact the flow of communication within the hospital. A perceived risk with product-line management is that nursing may be removed from the direct formal communication path found within the division of nursing (Hesterly & Robinson, 1988). This risk seems to be minimal in relation to the benefits of effective interdisciplinary problem resolution and cost control that occur in organizations changing to product-line management (Summers, Naderman, Turnis, Lynn, Rechlin, Hentges & Roche, 1988; Watkins, 1989).

♦ STAFFING AND SCHEDULING

PHILOSOPHY

With the multiplicity of pressures on nurse managers to admit, care for, and discharge sicker patients in shorter periods of time, the need for an effective staffing mix and pattern is essential. Staffing is probably the most pressing issue facing nursing managers. Ensuring sufficient numbers of nurses, effective quality of nursing care, and keeping costs down are the essence of the role of the nursing middle manager. Staffing goals are:

1. Project patient care needs

2. Evaluate the level of quality provided

3. Provide the numbers and mix of nursing staff needed

4. Anticipate availability of nursing staff

5. Provide low-cost, high quality nursing care

Balancing the quantity of staff available with the numbers needed and the desired cost and quality of care requires a well-defined philosophy of staffing.

PRODUCTIVITY

More is not always better. In one small community hospital, the nursing care hours average 9.6 to 10.0. There are frequent patient and family complaints about the organization of care and the level of care provided, with specific comments about the length of time required to answer patient requests. In contrast, in a large for-profit nursing home in southern Illinois, the residents speak highly of the care provided, although nursing care hours are consistently

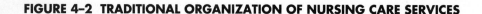

FIGURE 4–2 TRADITIONAL ORGANIZATION OF NURSING CARE SERVICES

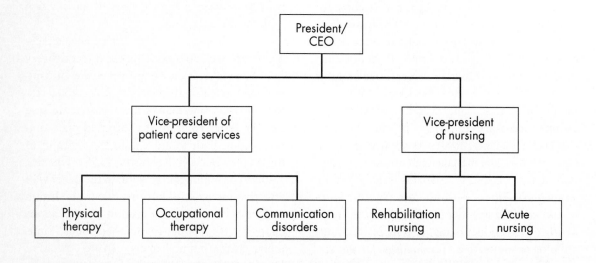

under 2.0. The difference between the two facilities lies in leadership and expectations of productivity, rather than in a simple provision of more nursing staff.

The nurse executive must identify the productivity level expected of staff, which will require a correlation between the acuity level and nursing care hours. See Chapter 10 for more on productivity. The formula for nursing-care hours calculation is illustrated below.

$$\text{Nursing-care hours (NCH)} =$$

$$\frac{\text{Number of staff} \times 8 \text{ hours}}{\text{Patient census}}$$

ACCREDITATION REQUIREMENTS

The Joint Commission on Accreditation of Healthcare Organizations (JCAHO) requires that staffing levels be based on a determination of patient acuity. Additionally, the nursing JCAHO surveyor will review staffing levels and identify if such levels are sufficient for patient care requirements, staff expertise, unit geography, support services, and method of patient care delivery. JCAHO does not identify a specific level of nursing-care hours; however, some accreditation groups do specify a minimal level of staffing. For example, the Commission on Accreditation of Rehabilitation Facilities (CARF) requires that a minimum of 5.5 hours of nursing care be provided by rehabilitation nurses for inpatient rehabilitation programs.

STAFFING APPROACHES

To determine staffing requirements, the nursing manager must examine patterns in patient care needs. The care demands on a surgical unit, for example, will be heaviest early in the morning,

FIGURE 4-3 PRODUCT-LINE SYSTEM OF NURSING CARE SERVICES

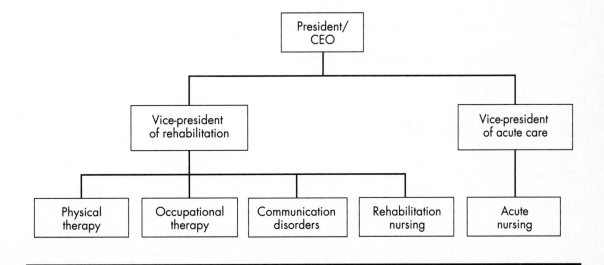

prior to the start of the surgical schedule, and late in the afternoon, after patients return from the operating room. On a medical unit, care needs are heaviest in the morning, during physician rounds and morning care. In rehabilitation programs, care needs are greatest before early morning, when therapy schedules start; at noon, when patients return to the unit for lunch; and after therapy schedules end in the afternoon. In contrast to schedules with definite patterns, the labor, delivery, and emergency room areas cannot predict when patient care needs will be most intense. By examining patient care needs, the nurse manager can determine a basic staffing plan. A sample basic staffing plan is illustrated in Table 4-1. Determination of full-time equivalents based on a factor of 1.4 is included in Table 4-2. This staffing plan, based on an average census of 26, results in estimated nursing care hours of 6.15:

Average daily census: 26
Direct care total: 20 × 8 hours/shift
Nursing care hours = 20 × 8/26 = 6.15

FLEXIBLE SCHEDULING

The nursing shortage has made flexible staffing patterns increasingly necessary. Combinations of 8-, 10-, 12-, and 16-hour shifts and creative staffing strategies such as weekender programs are common. Displayed in Table 4-3 is an example of a unit's flexible schedule patterns. Flexible patterns can present a major challenge in creativity, and in some cases a mathematic challenge to nursing managers. The use of 8-, 12-, and 16-hour shifts is fairly straightforward. Problems with combined staffing patterns include nurse fatigue and the perception that nurses are always coming and going, with no standard intershift report times. Advantages are that the flexible times may better meet patient care needs and maximize the availability of nurses. Ten-hour shifts provide greater overlap between shifts but can increase salary expenses by as much as 25 percent.

Difficulties in covering weekends with minimal levels of qualified nurses have existed for decades. However, the nurse shortage and the rising acuity of patients served have intensified

TABLE 4–1 BASIC STAFFING PLAN FOR A 30-BED MEDICAL UNIT

| | Leadership | | | | | Totals | |
Shift	H.N./Asst. H.N.	R.N.s	L.P.N.s	N.A.s	Unit clerk	Direct care	Staff
Day	1	5	2	2	1	9	12
Evening	1	4	2	2	1	8	10
Night	0	2	0	1	0	3	3
Total	2	11	4	5	2	20	25

the need to provide quality care over weekends. This has been addressed through weekender programs, in which nurses agree to work every weekend for full-time benefits and/or full-time salary.

SUPPLEMENTAL STAFFING

Some answers to staffing problems are nursing staff agencies, float pools, and nurse extender roles. Staffing agencies are available in most urban areas, but charges may be excessive. If used, agency nurses require orientation to the facility and should work under the supervision of an experienced in-house nurse. Additionally, the nurse manager must verify valid licensure and current malpractice insurance for agency nurses and should recognize that the use of agency nurses may compromise continuity of care. Internal float pools of nurses can provide supplemental staffing resources at a substantially lower cost than agencies, but will not correct the continuity of care concern.

Nurse managers also are supplementing nursing care through the employment of nurse extenders. These roles are nonprofessional and usually do not provide direct nursing care. Rather, nurse extenders complete non-nursing tasks and allow nurses time to assume direct care. Emptying trash cans, running for supplies, distributing linens, and passing trays are all indirect activities that take nurses away from the patient's professional care. Nurse extenders assume these activities, in addition to transporting patients to and from radiology and other departments. At Rush–Presbyterian–St. Luke's Medical Center in Chicago, for example, the unit technician is a nurse extender position. The role was implemented in 1988 and has provided nurses with additional time for direct patient care.

PATIENT CLASSIFICATION

Providing sufficient staffing for quality care is an issue fraught with subjectivity. Few nurses ever feel that their unit is well staffed or would volunteer to float to another unit to prevent overstaffing. More often, nurses perceive that there is never enough time in a shift to fully meet

TABLE 4–2 CALCULATION OF FULL-TIME EQUIVALENTS

Shift	Leadership H.N./Asst. H.N.	R.N.s	L.P.N.s	N.A.s	Unit clerk	Totals Direct care	Staff
Day	1.0	7.0	2.8	2.8	1.4	12.6	15.0
Evening	1.0	5.6	2.8	2.8	1.4	11.2	13.6
Night	0	2.8	0	1.4	0	4.2	4.2
Total	2.0	15.4	5.6	7.0	2.8	28.0	32.8

their patients' needs. Consequently, nursing managers must be able to determine accurate staffing needs and justify the use of scarce nursing resources. Patient acuity and classification systems were developed to meet these needs. Systems of patient classification are designed to provide an objective format for determining workload requirements; the JCAHO requires that nursing staffing decisions be based on an acuity or patient classification system. Patient classification systems also provide information tracking for budgeting and productivity analyses, and some systems are formatted to additionally serve as care plans and as a basis for costing out nursing care. Various patient classification systems and their applications, advantages, and disadvantages are discussed in this section.

Adopting a patient classification system is often a difficult and costly proposition, requiring time studies and workload sampling of the units on which the system will be used. Institutional systems differ substantially, with policies, procedures, and practices impacting nurses' workload and, therefore, direct and indirect care time. For example, a patient classification system may take into account that nurses pick up trays after completion of a meal as part of indirect care. In a health care institution where nurses pick up trays and place them on dietary carts, there is no difficulty with this assumption. However, in one hospital, nurses pick up trays and also are responsible for scraping uneaten food off of each plate, rinsing the dishes, stacking them, and placing them in an area near die-

TABLE 4–3 FLEXIBLE SCHEDULING WITH A MIX OF 12-HOUR AND 8-HOUR SHIFTS

Name	S	S	M	T	W	T	F	S	S	M	T	W	T	F	S	S	M	T	W	T	F	S	S	M	T	W	T	F	S	S	M	T	W	T	F	S	S	M
Grover, B.	D	D		D	D	D	D			D	D	D		D	D		D	D	D	D				D	D	D		D	D		D	D	D	D				
Minami, K.	E	E		E	E	E	E			E	E	E		E	E		E	E	E	E				E	E	E		E	E		E	E	E	E				
Lewis, C.	N	N		N	N	N	N			N	N	N		N	N		N	N	N	N				N	N	N		N	N		N	N	N	N				
Burch, B.			D				D	D	D			D	D			D				D	D	D			D	D			D						D	D	D	
Friedman, A.			E				E	E	E			E				E				E	E	E			E				E						E	E	E	
Kenney, L.			N				N	N	N			N				N				N	N	N			N				N						N	N	N	
Ohlson, M.	7	7			7	7	D		D				7	7		7	7	D		D			7	7	D		7	7			D							
Hom, L.			7	7			7	7	D	D				7	7			7	7	D	D				7	7			7	7								

tary service. This illustrates why it is necessary to individualize the program and tailor it to the hospital in which it will be used prior to implementation. Table 4-4 contains an analysis of various patient classification systems.

COMPUTERIZED SCHEDULING

Packages such as GRASP© may be of use to the nurse manager. A disadvantage with computerized programs is the difficulty in individualizing the schedule.

GRASP©. In 1968, three nurses and a physician set out to find a tool to measure nursing workload. The system, published in 1970, was originally called PETO. The effort to validate PETO resulted in the 1976 system known as the Grace Reynolds Application and Study of PETO (GRASP). GRASP is one of the forerunners of patient classification systems and is used in over 500 health care facilities. GRASP is based on the concept that 85 percent of nursing activities can be identified through the areas in the example shown in Table 4-5 (Meyer, 1978). Ordinal data on patient care needs are obtained with GRASP, which provides greater information and a truer estimate of nursing staff needs than can be accommodated in systems centered on nominal data, such as the classifications between categories 1, 2, 3, and 4. The reliability and validity of the GRASP system have been carefully studied (Meyer, 1978; Santopoalo, 1986), and the system incorporates interrater reliability testing to verify continued accuracy of the data.

The GRASP system operates as a multidimensional, nursing management, information system package and includes management reporting, staffing/scheduling, budgeting, cost identification, and quality evaluation. The patient classification portion of the system may be implemented in either a manual, pen-and-paper fashion or computerized. The data sheets con-

TABLE 4–4 PATIENT CLASSIFICATION SYSTEMS

System	Year developed	Number of facilities using	Ordinal/ nominal data	Computerized or manual	Time to implement	Approximate cost
Medicus©	1970	600	nominal	either	6 months	$10,000
ARIC©	1970	200	ordinal	either	1 year	$12,000
GRASP©	1978	500	ordinal	either	1 year	$20,000
Self-deficit	1980	1	ordinal	computerized	6 months	$ 5,000
Riverside	1983	100	nominal	either	1 year	$20,000

TABLE 4–5 COMPONENTS OF GRASP

Rehab example

Assessment: (Circle each shift) Patient	1	2	3	4	5	6	7	8	9	10	11	12
Assessment/Update assessment	3	3	3	3	3	3	3	3	3	3	3	3
Planning: (Circle each shift)												
1. Update/Revise care plan/Problem list	2	2	2	2	2	2	2	2	2	2	2	2
Knowledge deficit: (Circle as applicable)												
1. Planned teaching	2	2	2	2	2	2	2	2	2	2	2	2
2. Reinforce teaching	6	6	6	6	6	6	6	6	6	6	6	6
Self care deficit - nutrition: (Circle highest applicable)												
1. Feeds self independently	2	2	2	2	2	2	2	2	2	2	2	2
2. Feeds self with assistance by personnel/family	4	4	4	4	4	4	4	4	4	4	4	4
3. Total feed or self feed with dysphagia training	24	24	24	24	24	24	24	24	24	24	24	24
4. Total feed by staff/feeds self with constant supervision	9	9	9	9	9	9	9	9	9	9	9	9
5. Tube feeding continuous/bolus	6	6	6	6	6	6	6	6	6	6	6	6
Self care deficit - toileting: (Circle highest applicable)												
1. Incontinent care - toilet/BSC with constant supervision	12	12	12	12	12	12	12	12	12	12	12	12
2. Toilet with assist/BSC/bedpan/urinal	8	8	8	8	8	8	8	8	8	8	8	8
Self care deficit - bathing/hygeine/grooming: (Circle highest applicable)												
1. Total care by staff	6	6	6	6	6	6	6	6	6	6	6	6
2. Moderate care by staff	3	3	3	3	3	3	3	3	3	3	3	3
3. Minimal care by staff	2	2	2	2	2	2	2	2	2	2	2	2
Operation in safety												
1. Restraint	4	4	4	4	4	4	4	4	4	4	4	4
2. Monitor the wandering patient	10	10	10	10	10	10	10	10	10	10	10	10
Other direct: (Circle as applicable)												
1. Assistive devices	4	4	4	4	4	4	4	4	4	4	4	4
2. Accucheck	3	3	3	3	3	3	3	3	3	3	3	3
3. Empty foley/leg bags/drainage collection containers	1	1	1	1	1	1	1	1	1	1	1	1
4. Simple dressing change/remove staples/sutures/steri strips	2	2	2	2	2	2	2	2	2	2	2	2
5. Complex dressing/decubitus care	7	7	7	7	7	7	7	7	7	7	7	7
6. I & O calculation/calorie count	1	1	1	1	1	1	1	1	1	1	1	1
7. Nourishment/supplement feedings/diabetic snacks	1	1	1	1	1	1	1	1	1	1	1	1
Direct care:	10	10	10	10	10	10	10	10	10	10	10	10
Evaluation: (Circle each shift)	2	2	2	2	2	2	2	2	2	2	2	2

Unit PCH Note: Time values on chart have been increased to reflect time for all unlisted activities.

Total PCH												

tain patient care requirements, which the nurse completes; the data instruments may be tailored for the patient population requirements of the unit. The classification data sheets are completed each shift for each patient on the unit. They are taken to a centralized location and tallied, and the information is transposed to staffing requirements.

The cost of implementing the GRASP system varies depending on the size of health care facility and whether or not the system is computerized. If it is computerized, cost can be substantial and will easily fall within the capital expenditure range of any budget.

As with cost, the time required for implementation of the GRASP system varies according to the size of the facility. Often, cost is seen as the major limitation to adopting a system such as GRASP. However, when one considers the years of experience associated with the tool's development, the cost is realistic and worthwhile. Using GRASP has several advantages. The system was developed by nurses and can be individualized to fit the facility. It has been tested for validity and reliability, and a mechanism for interrater reliability checks is included. Finally, GRASP enables nurses to track and account for patient education, conferences, and non-direct care activities.

MEDICUS©. One of the first patient classification programs developed, Medicus, originated in 1969. It continues to be used in over 300 health care facilities. The concept underlying Medicus is the classification of patients into categories: 1, 2, 3, and 4. Patients classified as a 4 require the greatest intensity of nursing care. Using this nominal level data results in a clustering of patients into categories; the nursing care requirements are defined in terms of average

hours of care per category. For example, on a 22-bed acute medical unit with an average patient rating of 3.5, the hours of nursing care required might be 6.8. Nurses responsible for direct care delivery rate patients by 37 variables on the Medicus system daily (Lee et al., 1990).

As with GRASP, the cost of Medicus varies with the decision to computerize the classification system. The system is available in either a manual or a computerized mode. It has been applied to a wide variety of nursing specialty areas, including intensive care, mental health units, and rehabilitation. Other disciplines, such as pharmacy, also have attempted to adopt and modify the tool (Day, Mason, and Reeme, 1986).

ARIC©. Developed by the Sisters of Mercy Health Corporation in 1970, the Allocation, Resource Identification and Costing (ARIC) system is a computerized patient classification tool. ARIC incorporates admission, discharge, and transfer information from each patient along with the classification information. Several features of ARIC make it a unique patient classification tool. Staffing reports are generated based on the patient classification information entered. The reports identify actual versus needed staffing, the level of productivity, and staff exceeding workload (Edwardson, Bahr, and Serote, 1990).

THEORY-BASED PROGRAMS. Dorthea Orem's self-deficit theory has been developed into a patient classification system used at Mississippi Methodist Rehabilitation Center (Jackson, Mississippi). The system classifies patients into four categories of care requirements. The system is computerized, and patients are reclassified every shift. Although based on work sampling, reliability of the system has been affected by the failure to incorporate a mechanism for interrater reliability checks. Samples from the system are included in Table 4-6.

INTEGRATION OF CARE PLAN AND CLASSIFICATION SYSTEM. A difficulty with many patient classification systems is that completion of the daily assessments, data entries, and staffing calculations requires scarce nursing time. At Riverside Medical Center (Kankakee, Illinois), nursing administrators computerized a manual classification system based on the factor of one point per minute of patient care requirement and integrated it with the interdisciplinary plan of care (Adams and Duchene, 1985). The system works through a light pen–selectable series of computer screens in which the primary nurse or team leader identifies patient care needs. Each selection corresponds with staffing requirements based on work sampling studies. The system calculates an estimate of indirect nursing care time and factors in patient admissions and discharges. For each shift, the system identifies requirements for nurses and unlicensed caregivers. A principal advantage of Riverside's system is that the nurse enters care requirements only on admission and as changes in care routines occur.

◆ ORGANIZATIONAL CULTURE

The environment in which nurses practice is affected by the leadership style and expectations of the health care facility's chief executive officer and governing board (Hershey and Blanchard, 1988). Even an ideal nursing care delivery system with computerized patient classification tools and advanced scheduling strategies will be ineffective in retaining and recruiting qualified professional nurses if the organizational culture is not similarly progressive and humanistic.

In assessing organizational culture, nursing administrators consider the history and tradition of the organization. Is the organization receptive to new concepts, suggestions, and innovations, or is it experiencing "paradigm paralysis" (Peters, 1989)? As an example, during the 1960s, rehabilitation theory focused on re-socialization of individuals with disabling conditions. Proponents of re-socialization recommended that beds be placed on opposite head walls in the rooms. Also during the 1960s, patients admitted to rehabilitation were required to be in stable medical condition. Since the advent of DRGs, however, patients in more acute conditions are being admitted to rehabilitation. Many require the use and availability of oxygen and vacuum suction. Renovation of the patient rooms requires that every wall be piped, at double the cost that would be experienced if the bed configuration was altered. Failure of the organization to change the paradigm is indicative of a lack of openness to other innovations. At the rate health care is changing, receptivity to creativity and participatory decision making is essential for a healthy work environment for professional nurses.

In assessing the organizational climate, the nursing manager examines the value system of the organization as indicated by the hiring preferences of the chief executive officer and the nursing administrator. An organization in which nursing leaders are innovative, creative, and energetic will tend to operate in a fast-moving, goal-oriented fashion. In contrast, if humanistic, interpersonal skills are sought in candidates for leadership positions, the characteristics of the organization will be focused on human resources and employee and patient advocacy (Hershey and Blanchard, 1988). Addi-

TABLE 4–6 SAMPLE DESCRIPTORS FROM THE SELF-DEFICIT THEORY CLASSIFICATION SYSTEM

Category	Descriptor	Capabilities	Nursing care required
Level 0	Independent	Patient has required knowledge skills, judgment, willingness. Patient performs appropriately and consistently.	No nursing assistance needed
Level 1	Minimally dependent	Has basic knowledge, adapts to personal situation. Usually willing to do most activities, requests assistance as needed. *Limitations/deficits* May have difficulty remembering some aspects or making decisions about care.	Obtaining and setting up materials and equipment. Standby supervision, guidance, and support in making judgments and regarding priorities. Provision of complex or infrequent prescribed medical/nursing measures or treatments.
Level 2	Moderately dependent	Some basic knowledge, is learning and developing skills in rehabilitation program. Performs 50 percent or more care independently or with equipment. *Limitations/deficits* May not always make safe decisions, may not remember or be willing to engage in self-care on a consistent basis.	Assistance with activities of daily living, transportation, and to complete care. Requires teaching, guarding, supervision, and emotional support.
Level 3	Heavily dependent	Usually aware and willing to cooperate in care activities. *Limitations/deficits* General lack of knowledge of what and how to do. May have cognitive intelligence, communication, emotional deficits. Medical condition/treatment pose limitations and require special observation and care. Physical inability to move or perform.	Requires assistance for most of care. Requires close supervision.
Level 4	Totally dependent	*Limitations/deficits* Unable to engage in self-care due to medically unstable health.	Almost constant nursing monitoring and care required. Patient has to be monitored for an extended (24-hour) period.

tionally, the culture within the organization includes common practices, procedures, and policies. Organizations that require decision-making ability and empower nurses to participate in determining their practice environment will retain nurses who desire a substantial degree of autonomy. Systems involving participatory management and shared governance create organizational climates that reward decision making, creativity, independence, and autonomy.

Organizational culture also is evident in the values expressed in high-level positions and leadership meeting agendas. It is common for organizations to have a vice-president of finance, but rare for those same agencies to have a vice-president of quality. This indicates a clear but unspoken commitment to the bottom line with less attention to quality. Likewise, few board of directors meetings occur without a lengthy and substantial presentation on the financial condition of the institution. However, board meetings rarely have difficult discussions on the quality of care, morale of employees, and satisfaction of patients. Harry (1990) has suggested that organizations address quality issues and spend less time on finances to implement continuous quality improvement. The information that the board of trustees, the chief executive officer, and the vice-presidents consider crucial becomes the values of the organization.

As the health care environment continues to evolve, it is essential that organizations adopt consumer-sensitive cultures and enable accountability and decision making by nurses. If consumers are required to go to the nursing administrator for decisions and responses to concerns, the organization will frustrate consumers and fail to meet their expectations.

An organizational culture that values creativity, innovation, and participatory decision mak-ing will retain and recruit independent, accountable professionals. Additionally, in response to consumer demands for fast attention to concerns and questions, organizations that empower nurses to make decisions will better meet consumer requests.

SUMMARY

♦ Patient care delivery systems are critical in nursing; no best method exists.

♦ Several methods of delivery exist. Differentiated practice means that nursing roles vary according to education, experience, or skill. Case management helps coordinate care throughout the health care system. Primary nursing allows the nurse to maintain a caseload of patients. Team nursing is the delivery of care by a staff of various educational preparations. In functional nursing, tasks are divided and nurses specialize by task.

♦ Staffing is probably the most pressing issue facing nursing managers. Expected productivity level, acuity level, and nursing hours must be determined. Numerous approaches are available.

♦ Flexible staffing patterns have become increasingly necessary due to the nursing shortage.

♦ Adopting a patient classification system is often difficult and costly. Methods such as GRASP, Medicus, and theory-based programs are available.

♦ Organizational culture is affected by and affects nursing care delivery.

BIBLIOGRAPHY

Adams, R., and Duchene, P. (1985). "Computerization of Patient Acuity and Nursing Care Planning: New Approach to Improved Patient Care and Cost-Effective Staffing." *Journal of Nursing Administration,* 15(4): 11–17.

American Hospital Association (1984). "AHA's New Data Shed Light on Hospital Staffing." *American Journal of Nursing,* 84: 809.

American Hospital Association (1988). *Hospital Research Educational Trust Health Care Statistics.* Chicago: American Hospital Association.

Bird, G. (1988). "Product-Line Management and Nursing." *Nursing Management,* 19(5): 46–48.

Christman, L. (1980). "Accountability with an All-RN Nursing Staff." In: *All RN Nursing Staff.* Alfano, G. (editor). Wakefield, MA: Nursing Resources.

Day, D., Mason, M., and Reeme, P. (1986). "Using a Nursing-Workload Index to Validate Hospital Pharmacy Productivity." *American Journal of Hospital Pharmacy,* 43: 909–912.

Dienemann, J. (1989). "Theoretical Perspective in Organization Science for Nursing Administration." In: *Dimensions of Nursing Administration.* Henry, B., Arndt, C., DiVincenti, M., and Marriner-Tomey, A. (editors). Boston: Blackwell Scientific Publications. Pp. 159–174.

Dolan, J. (1958). *Goodnow's History of Nursing.* Philadelphia: W. B. Saunders.

Edwardson, S., Bahr, J., and Serote, M. (1990). "Patient Classification and Management Information Systems as Adjuncts to Patient Care Delivery." In: *Patient Care Delivery Models.* Mayer, G., Madden, M., and Lawrenz, E. (editors). Rockville, MD: Aspen Publishers. Pp. 293–313.

Harry, M. (1990). *The Nature of Six Sigma Quality.* Detroit, MI: Motorola.

Hershey, P., and Blanchard, P. (1988). *Management of Organizational Behavior: Utilizing Human Resources.* 5th ed. Englewood Cliffs, NJ: Prentice-Hall.

Hesterly, S., and Robinson, M. (1988). "Nursing in a Service Line Organization." *Nursing Management,* 18(11): 32–86.

Hinshaw, A. (1989). "Programs of Nursing Research for Nursing Administration." In: *Dimensions of Nursing Administration.* Henry, B., Arndt, C., DiVincenti, M., and Marriner-Tomey, A. (editors). Boston: Blackwell Scientific Publications. Pp. 251–296.

Horvath, K. (1990). "Professional Nursing Practice Model." In: *Patient Care Delivery Models.* Mayer, G., Madden, M., and Lawrenz, E. (editors). Rockville, MD: Aspen Publishers. Pp. 213–235.

Kron, T., and Gray, A. (1987). *The Management of Patient Care.* Philadelphia: W. B. Saunders.

Lee, T., Cook, E., Fendrick, A., Shammash, J., Wolfe, E., Weisberg, M., and Goldman, L. (1990). "Impact of Initial Triage Decisions on Nursing Intensity for Patients with Acute Chest Pain." *Medical Care,* 28(8): 737–745.

Lyonski, S. (1985). "A Boundary Theory Investigation of the Product Manager's Role." *Journal of Marketing,* 49: 26–39.

McCausland, M., et al. (1988). "Primary Nursing in a Psychiatric Setting." *Nursing Economics,* 6(6): 297–301.

McDaniel, C., and Gray, D. (1980). "Product Manager." *California Management Review,* 23: 87–94.

Manthey, M. (1980). *The Practice of Primary Nursing.* St. Louis, MO: C. V. Mosby.

Marriner-Tomey, A. (1988). *Guide to Nursing Management.* 3rd ed. St. Louis, MO: C. V. Mosby.

Merker, L. R., and Elbein, D. (1989). *Hospital Nursing Personnel Survey Executive Summary.* Chicago: American Hospital Association.

Meyer, D. (1978). *GRASP©: A Patient Information and Workload Management System.* Morgantown, NC: MCS.

Murphy, M., and DeBack, V. (1990). "Myths and Realities." In: *Current Issues and Perspectives on Differentiated Practice.* American Organization of Nurse Executives. Chicago: American Hospital Association. Pp. 5–16.

Peters, T. (1988). *Thriving on Chaos.* New York: Harper and Row.

Porter-O'Grady, T. (1986). *Creative Nursing Administration: Participative Management into the 21st Century.* Rockville, MD: Aspen Systems Corporation.

Porter-O'Grady, T. (1990). *Reorganization of Nursing Practice: Creating the Corporate Venture.* Rockville, MD: Aspen Systems Corporation.

Santopoalo, R. (1986). "Developing a Patient Classification System (PCS) in a Rehabilitation Setting Using the GRASP© System." *Rehabilitation Nursing,* 11(2): 20–24.

Summers, P., Nadermann, N., Turnis, R., Lynn, P., Rechlin, R., Hentges, J., and Roche, A. (1988). "Quality Management: Program Design." *Nursing Clinics of North America,* 23(3): 665–670.

Watkins, B. (1989). "Evaluation of Process and Product Life Cycles in a Hospital Setting." *Nursing Management,* 20(5): 81–90.

Whitman, M. (1991). "Case Management in Head Injury Rehabilitation." *Rehabilitation Nursing,* 16(1): 19.

Yano-Fong, D. (1988). "Advantages and Disadvantages of Product-Line Management." *Nursing Management,* 19(5): 27–31.

Zander, K. (1988a). "Nursing Case Management: Resolving the DRG Paradox." *Nursing Clinics of North America,* 23(3): 503–520.

Zander, K. (1988b). "Nursing Case Management: Strategic Management of Cost and Quality Outcomes." *Journal of Nursing Administration,* 18(5): 23–30.

PRODUCTIVITY

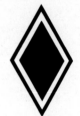

Americans invest billions of dollars in health care each year; in return they expect health care providers to give an accounting of how the money is spent and with what result. As health care cost inflation continues to increase at a rate greater than the overall rate of inflation, consumers and policy makers demand decreased health care costs and waste, more careful allocation of scarce resources, and evidence that the care given is of adequate quality.

These externally imposed financial constraints have made health care facilities much more attentive to their productivity in recent years. Nursing is one health care service that is subjected to productivity evaluation. Nursing not only comprises the largest single group of health care providers, but also can account for 50 percent or more of the operating budgets of institutions such as hospitals and nursing homes. Because of their size, nursing services are likely to be reduced in an attempt to cut budgets because percentage reductions in nurses can appear small in relation to reductions in other smaller departments. Consequently, the definition and measurement of nursing productivity have become a high priority for most nursing managers.

Unfortunately, nursing productivity is an ill defined concept. In this chapter the concept of productivity is reviewed, and ways of defining and measuring nursing productivity are discussed. The chapter concludes with specific strategies a nursing manager might use to improve productivity.

♦ WHAT IS PRODUCTIVITY?

ECONOMIC/INDUSTRIAL DEFINITIONS

As an economic concept, productivity describes the relationship between the output of an industry and the resources required to produce that output (output per input). It is measured by a number of different methods, the most common being the labor productivity statistic. Labor productivity measures the dollar value of output per person-hour used to produce the output; this gives a simple estimate of whether industries are becoming more or less efficient in their production methods. But this single factor output/input ratio fails to take into account possible reasons for increases or declines in efficiency other than the cost of labor or how hard employees work. A total factor productivity measure can be used to account for the contribution of inputs other than labor. Other relevant inputs include, for example, the introduction of new technology, increases in the cost of raw materials, and substitution of equipment or supplies.

DEFINING PRODUCTIVITY IN HEALTH CARE

Finding a definition of productivity for health care is more complex than determining whether only labor or all relevant factors should be used to measure input. Fundamental questions remain about what should be considered an input. Moreover, there is considerable debate about how output should be measured.

HEALTH CARE INPUTS.   Inputs present fewer measurement problems than outputs. Inputs include the labor, materials, and equipment used in the production of services; they usually can be measured in physical units such as hours of labor; dollars spent on equipment, remodeling, or building expense; and supplies used. But the measurement of some inputs is not as simple as it seems. Nursing personnel, for example, is not a homogeneous group since nurses vary in level of education, experience, and skill. Some of the differences in educational level and experience may be reflected in different pay rates. Yet any two nurses with equivalent education and years of experience are likely to differ considerably in their efficiency and ability to perform a quantity of work. Methods for quantifying differences in skill level are rudimentary.

THE HOSPITAL'S PRODUCT. As difficult as it may be to adequately define input, defining the output of health care is even more problematic. Until recently, hospital output was most frequently defined as patient days, i.e., the total number of days all patients were hospitalized in a facility over a period of time (Feldstein, 1971). Then it was realized that some patient days require the use of many more resources than others. A day of care for a transplant patient is much more costly than a day of postpartum care, for example. It became necessary to consider some new definitions of output.

Most of the new conceptions of hospital output assume that the hospital has more than one product (patient days)—that it is instead a multiproduct firm. Currently, most attention is focused on refining the meaning of *patient days* by using the concept of case mix, a set of methods for clustering patients into groupings that are homogeneous with respect to the use of resources. Factors used to cluster patients have included diagnosis, prognosis, utilization, organ system, hospital department, and patient demographic characteristics (Hornbrook, 1982). The best known of these case-mix measures is the Diagnosis Related Groups (DRGs) system that groups patients into 468 resource-use groups using information about diagnosis, age, and the use of certain procedures. Using the DRG case-mix measure, the hospital could potentially produce 468 distinct products that vary from one another in the cost of production. Each DRG is weighted to represent the average cost of providing care to patients in that category. While

there are many arguments about the validity of the resource clusters produced by the DRG system, it or a case-mix method similar to it is likely to remain in use since it provides greater precision in measuring hospital output.

OUTPUT OR OUTCOME? Case-mix measures have refined how output quantity is measured, but they do not address output quality. Estimating the quality of health care services is a particularly vexing problem. In purchasing goods such as household appliances and automobiles, the consumer is usually able to judge the quality of a product by inspection or by referring to a consumers' guide to that product. If a manufacturer consistently puts out inferior goods, consumers can express their quality preferences by not purchasing the product.

The purchase of health care services is fundamentally different. Because health care is a service, production and consumption of the service are simultaneous events. The consumer cannot return a defective product and often cannot reverse the effects of poor service. Furthermore, no consumers' guide to health care services exists, and most consumers cannot or do not have time to learn how to evaluate health care services. Instead, the health care consumer must rely on the ethical obligation of the professional to exercise sound judgment in making decisions about the type and quantity of health care required.

To protect further the interests of the consumer, therefore, health care output is increasingly being defined in terms of quality as well as the quantity of services. The goal is to describe output as a quality-adjusted output, or an outcome.

Quality adjustments of outputs can be made in one of two ways: in terms of the soundness of the process of care used to produce the output or the quality of the output itself. The soundness of the process of care is generally the most convenient to measure, but it is based on the assumption that a demonstrable link exists between the care activities performed and the outcome achieved by the patient. Is there, for example, a verifiable cause and effect relationship between pre-operative teaching and improved recovery following surgery? If the link between process and outcome is demonstrated, evidence that the best process was used constitutes evidence of the quality of the service. While researchers have made much progress in demonstrating these links in nursing care, the work proceeds at a relatively slow pace.

The alternative to measuring the care process is to assess the quality of the output (i.e., the outcome of care) directly. Measuring outcome is both difficult and expensive. It is difficult because the ultimate outcome of many episodes of illness or care and treatment encounters is not known for some time after the care ceases. It is expensive since it may entail locating the patient after the care and treatment ends to perform special evaluations. Finding a meaningful indicator of quality that is also easy to measure is likely to be a key task for the next decade.

♦ WHAT IS NURSING PRODUCTIVITY?

As the prior discussion indicates, there are two basic approaches to measuring productivity. The economic/industrial concept views productivity as the ratio of work output to work input: units of output/units of input. This approach comes out of the scientific management tradition of the 1920s, which asked the question: How can we design processes and procedures to produce the product most efficiently? The use of scientific management principles in nursing is found in the development of patient classification systems for measuring nursing workload.

Although the principles of scientific management have been applied to nursing productivity, a second, more comprehensive model for evaluating productivity is currently being advocated in the health care and nursing literature. This model attempts to place productivity within a systems framework and incorporates the concept of effectiveness as well as efficiency. Jelinek and Dennis (1976) were among the first to articulate the concept in nursing when they used an open systems model (see Figure 5–1) showing the relationships between inputs, processes, and outputs and suggested that it is also necessary to consider the influence of the environment in which the first three elements exist.

Inputs include the number and type of nursing personnel, equipment, and supplies used and the capital costs incurred in providing care. Processes include all of the activities and resources required to convert inputs into output. Output represents the "product" resulting from the application of processes and inputs. The environment is everything external to the organization over which the nursing manager has little control, including labor laws, health care financing policies, and personnel licensing laws.

In addition to developing a framework for understanding nursing productivity, Jelinek and Dennis (1976) proposed that in defining nursing productivity, we must be as concerned about the quality as the quantity of output.

The concept of productivity encompasses both the effectiveness of nursing care, which relates to its quality and appropriateness, and the efficiency of care, which is production of nursing output with minimal resource waste (p. 3).

This definition is consistent with standard economic definitions of productivity and also takes into account some special characteristics of nursing services (Edwardson, 1986). There is an increasing tendency to incorporate both efficiency and effectiveness into the operational definition of the output of health care organizations (AMSI, 1980).

Effectiveness of the hospital's output refers to the safety, appropriateness, and excellence of care and encompasses the issues of health status changes, patient outcomes, and patient satisfaction (AMSI, 1980). Efficiency refers to a state in which the inputs and methods used to produce a product or service result in the maximum feasible output (Pauly, 1970).

These two approaches to defining productivity offer practicing nurses a difficult choice. On the one hand, nurses are drawn to the simplicity and easy measurement of industrial definitions of the concept but are repulsed by the way industrial models reduce the complicated process of care to crude output/input ratios. On the other hand, nurses' professional instincts draw them to the comprehensive definitions of productivity that incorporate estimates of effectiveness. But they are fully aware that in the real world there is limited time and money to devote to evaluation.

◆ MEASURING NURSING PRODUCTIVITY

A number of performance measures are currently being used to evaluate the productivity of nursing services. Although some do not meet the strict definition of productivity as a ratio of output per input, they do provide the nursing manager with important information about the efficiency of nursing care delivery.

FIGURE 5-1 NURSING PRODUCTIVITY FRAMEWORK

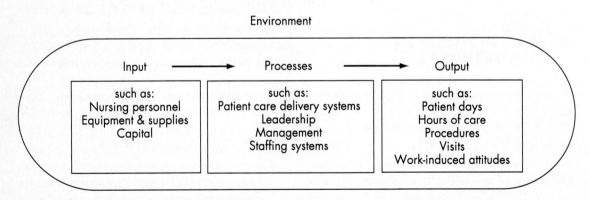

Adapted from R.C. Jelinek and L.C. Dennis, *A Review and Evaluation of Nursing Productivity* (Bethesda, MD: Health Resources Administration, 1976), DHEW Publication No. HRA 77-15.

RESOURCES PER PATIENT DAY

Nursing hours per patient day is a commonly used indicator of labor productivity that is simple and easily understood. As shown in Figure 5–2, it is calculated by totaling the paid hours for nursing personnel for a period of time and dividing that total by the total number of patient days for the same time period. To accurately reflect the true cost of nursing care, the total paid hours should include the fringe benefit hours (e.g., vacation, holiday, and sick hours used)

FIGURE 5–2 CALCULATING RESOURCES USED PER PATIENT DAY

I. NURSING HOURS PER PATIENT DAY

$$\frac{\text{Total paid hours for nursing personnel for time } X}{\text{Total number of patient days in time } X}$$

Direct nursing hours per patient day

$$\frac{\text{Total paid hours for nursing personnel providing direct care in time } X}{\text{Total number of patient days in time } X}$$

II. NURSING SALARY COSTS PER PATIENT DAY

$$\frac{\text{Total payroll expenses for nursing personnel in time } X}{\text{Total number of patient days in time } X}$$

Direct nursing care salary costs per patient day

$$\frac{\text{Total payroll expenses for providing direct nursing care in time } X}{\text{Total number of patient days in time } X}$$

---

and the paid hours for nursing administrators as well as the hours required for direct patient care.

While nursing hours per patient day is one of the oldest and most frequently used performance measures, it attributes productivity and all changes in productivity from one time period to another to a single input: the number of hours of nursing care. It fails to consider any changes that may have been made in the process of care or in the supplies and equipment used—changes that may have increased or decreased the efficiency or effectiveness of care. It also fails to consider changes that may have been made in the skill level of the staff providing the care, the type and intensity of patient days being considered, or the quality of the patient days being produced.

Another very similar performance measure is nursing salary costs per patient day. It is a slightly more refined measure, however, in that the use of salary costs provides some information about the skill mix of the staff. Nursing salary costs per patient are calculated by totaling the actual salary costs for nursing personnel and dividing by the total patient days for the same time period.

STANDARDIZING PATIENT DAYS. Both nursing hours per patient day and salary costs per patient day are useful measures of labor productivity (i.e., personnel costs per unit of output), but only if the nature of the patient day is held constant. If the nature of the patients cared for on a unit changes, it is difficult to know whether productivity changed unless an adjustment is made. Consider a nursing unit that provided the same number of hours of care in two time periods. If the level of patient acuity or dependence remained the same during the two time periods, labor productivity would remain unchanged. But if the overall level of patient dependency on nursing care increased in the second time period, labor productivity would have increased.

One way to factor in patient dependency levels is to standardize patient days using information from the patient classification system designed to measure nursing workload. Patient days can be standardized by substituting the required hours of care as calculated by the patient classification system for patient days. Productivity ratios can then be calculated as shown in Figure 5–3. If desired, the required hours of care can be divided by 24 hours to produce required days of care. Such standardization of the nature of the patient days produced improves the validity of comparisons of nursing hours and nursing salary costs per patient day in two or more monitoring periods.

DEGREE OF OCCUPATION

Another common productivity indicator is the degree to which the nursing staff is occupied.

FIGURE 5–3 RESOURCE USE PER STANDARDIZED PATIENT DAY

I. NURSING HOURS PER STANDARDIZED PATIENT DAY

$$\frac{\text{Total paid hours for nursing personnel for time } X}{\text{Total Required hours (or days) of care in time } X}$$

II. NURSING SALARY COSTS PER STANDARDIZED PATIENT DAY

$$\frac{\text{Total payroll expenses for nursing personnel in time } X}{\text{Total required hours (or days) of care in time } X}$$

Nursing managers regularly measure degree of occupation on a very informal basis using a "busyness scale." The nursing manager observes the unit staff and makes a judgment about whether the number of staff available is sufficient to handle the workload.

While this procedure may appear to be too informal to be valid, many believe that a skilled and experienced charge nurse or head nurse can, in fact, be a very finely tuned measurement instrument of staffing adequacy. This assumption has led to at least one method for assessing degree of occupation—i.e., staffing adequacy—more systematically. Williams and Murphy (1979) have developed a tool for assessing staffing adequacy that requires the charge nurse to answer a series of questions about the activity level on the unit that day (e.g., number of admissions and surgeries) and to judge the adequacy of the number of staff assigned and of the care given.

Some researchers question, however, whether degree of occupation is a valid productivity measure. It could be argued that a fully occupied staff is not necessarily a productive staff if the work is poorly organized and sequenced or if the support services and equipment available are inadequate for allowing the staff to perform efficiently. The staff may be exceedingly busy and understaffed using current practice models, but that does not preclude the possibility that there is considerable room for improving the quantity and quality of care given without increasing costs (Edwardson, 1986).

UTILIZATION RATES

One of the best known performance measures used in nursing is the ratio of required to actual staffing levels. This performance measure is produced by most nurse staffing systems based on patient classification.

To obtain information for calculating utilization rates, the patient classification system used for nurse staffing is used to predict the amount of care each patient will require in the near future (usually one or two shifts hence). The time required by all patients on a unit is summed and then labeled "required hours of care." Additional time is factored in for indirect care activities (e.g., charting, making referrals), unit maintenance activities, and the nurses' break time. At the end of the shift for which the prediction was made, the actual hours of nursing time paid are calculated. The utilization rate is then calculated as:

$$\frac{\text{Required hours of care}}{\text{Nursing hours paid}}$$

Table 5–1 shows an example of how utilization rates ("productivity") are frequently reported in nursing management information systems. The actual hours of care provided are subtracted from the required (or predicted) hours of care to give a variance. The percentage of productivity is then calculated by dividing the required hours of care by the actual hours provided and then multiplying the quotient by 100.

A productivity rate of 100 percent indicates that the actual hours of care matched the required hours. A rate greater than 100 percent indicates that actual hours were less than required, while a rate less than 100 percent shows that more hours of care were provided than were required. Most institutions set acceptable productivity ranges of 85 percent to 115 percent.

While these rates are perhaps the single best day-to-day control monitor available to nursing managers, they are more appropriately called a utilization rather than a productivity indicator unless certain assumptions are made about required hours of care. Compared to standard economic definitions of productivity, the required to actual hours of care ratio has an input measurement (actual hours) but does not have a commonly used output measurement.

REQUIRED HOURS OF CARE AS AN OUTPUT. The required/actual ratio is useful as a productivity measure only if the nursing service assumes or has demonstrated that the required number of nursing hours can provide the quantity and quality of care that the health care institution wishes to provide. In other words,

TABLE 5–1 EXAMPLE OF A PRODUCTIVITY MONITORING SYSTEM

Cost center	Hours (or FTEs)			Percentage product
	Required	**Actual**	**Variance**	
432	45	45	0	100%
433	45	42	3	107%
343	45	48	–3	94%

the use of staff utilization ratios to judge productivity is based on one very important, but frequently unacknowledged, assumption: The standard hours of care used by the patient classification system to calculate required nurse hours are assumed to provide the desired level of service.

To be used as an output indicator, the required hours of care should be thought of as targeted hours of care—i.e., the hours of care required to produce the desired level of quality of care. To affirm the validity of targeted hours as a proxy (substitute) measure of the desired output, the nursing department either needs to use the research findings of others to show that a certain amount of care produces the desired results or must do its own evaluation studies to demonstrate that care of a given level of quantity and quality can be produced by a given number of nursing care hours. In other words, the targeted hours of care are used as a substitute for direct measures of the quantity and quality of nursing care output.

An example from a maternity service illustrates the point. Assume that a maternity service has determined that five hours of professional and two hours of nonprofessional nursing care during the postpartum period meets the outcome standards set by the service (see Figure 5–4). By a careful evaluation of outcomes, the providers of this maternity service have determined that patients are discharged in a reasonable number of days and that the mothers are satisfied with their care and are able to care for themselves and their infants. The complication rate also is judged to be adequate. If a nursing service provides this type of evidence that it is able to meet the institution's own standards of care, then targeted hours of care could quite legitimately be substituted as an indicator of output—the appropriate quantity and quality of care (Edwardson, 1986).

The process for calculating the productivity of the unit is shown in part II of Figure 5–4. When the actual hours of care provided match the target, productivity is 100 percent, but when

---

FIGURE 5–4 EXAMPLE OF THE USE OF TARGETED HOURS OF CARE AS AN OUTPUT INDICATOR

I. OUTCOME STANDARD
Average length of stay = 2.9 days
Knowledge and skill
    90% score above 90% on a post-teaching test of knowledge
    98% give satisfactory return baby bath demonstration

Satisfaction
    90% satisfied or very satisfied on satisfaction questionnaire

Complications
    2% postpartal and newborn infection rate
    50% of mothers continue breast feeding at least one month

II. CALCULATING PRODUCTIVITY
These standards can be met at 7 hours of care per patient day. Therefore, productivity can be calculated as follows, using hypothetical actual hours of care provided.

a. $\dfrac{Target}{Actual} = \dfrac{7}{7} = 100\%$

b. $\dfrac{Target}{Actual} = \dfrac{7}{7.9} = 89\%$

c. $\dfrac{Target}{Actual} = \dfrac{7}{6.5} = ?$

actual hours exceed the target, productivity falls below 100 percent. A problem arises in calculating productivity when the actual hours provided are fewer than the target. Although most institutions would calculate productivity as 108 percent in this case, there is a question about whether this is a legitimate calculation. When the actual use of staff is less than the targeted level, it suggests that the standards used to establish the target are too high or that the organization is willing to compromise its standards with unknown consequences. For these reasons, some have suggested that productivity levels should never exceed 100 percent unless the clinical service can show that the care process has been made more efficient by using new methods or new equipment and that the quality of the outcome has not suffered.

♦ IMPROVING NURSING PRODUCTIVITY

Having reviewed and critiqued some common indicators of nursing performance and suggested ways to improve them, we now consider how the manager can improve nursing productivity. As the productivity model in Figure 5–1 suggests, productivity gains may be made at two points: through changes in the use of inputs and through changes in the care process. Changes to elements of the environment are largely beyond the control of the nursing manager, at least in the short run.

CHANGES IN USE OF INPUTS

Inputs include the raw materials, manpower, supplies, and equipment used to provide a service or produce a product. Little attention has been given to the "raw material" of nursing ser-

vices since it is a little disconcerting to think of patients and clients as raw material. Nurses have traditionally had little control over the type of patients presented to them. Recent activities among health care institutions to identify areas of excellence and market those selected services to potential consumers may change all that. Increasingly, nursing departments and individual nursing practitioners are marketing their services as well, thereby exerting some influence over the type of patients for whom they care.

MATCHING SUPPLY WITH DEMAND. The most costly input in the provision of nursing care is the labor. Therefore, greatest productivity gains can be achieved by careful selection and use of personnel. The most readily available method for controlling the use of labor inputs is to use patient classification data to measure requirements for care and then schedule nursing personnel to meet the expected demand.

Before patient classification systems (PCSs) were developed, the number of nursing staff scheduled was determined by global staff-patient ratios (often one nurse to three or four patients). These global standards were insensitive to differences in care requirements among patients; some patients required more care than available with fixed staff-to-patient ratios and some required less (Giovannetti, 1978).

PCSs are designed to recognize this variation by grouping patients into categories with similar nursing care requirements. Using concepts that derive from the scientific management theoretical framework, it is assumed that work can be subdivided into specific functions that vary as to length of time and skill required to perform them.

After specific functions have been identified, it is necessary to measure the time required to care for patients needing different combinations of tasks. Three basic approaches are taken toward work measurement. PCSs of the tasking type use a long and comprehensive list of tasks, each with an associated time requirement. Patients can then be categorized into groups (usually four or five groups are identified) depending on the time required to complete all of the tasks identified for them.

Factor PCSs use only a few tasks (e.g., bathing, feeding, and ambulation) that have been shown to be critical indicators or predictors of the amount of care required. Patients are categorized into four or five groups on the basis of whether they demonstrate one or more of the critical indicators. The average amount of time required to care for patients in each category is then measured. Finally, prototype PCSs use broad descriptive statements to describe patients in groups requiring similar amounts of care (Giovannetti, 1979).

Regardless of the type of PCS, the most important characteristic is that it is valid and reliable. Invalid or unreliable patient classification systems not only will lead to inappropriate use of nursing personnel, but also can lead to dissatisfaction among the staff. Staff members may attempt to undermine systems that are perceived to be inaccurate. The validity and reliability of a PCS can only be maintained through regular monitoring and adjustments to changing conditions.

Once the nursing manager is convinced that the PCS produces valid and reliable data, the system can be used to classify patients from one to three times per day. Classification tools consist of descriptions or checklists of the variables used in classifying patients. The decision about how often patients are classified is made by the nursing division based on a number of considerations, including the degree of change in pa-

tients' conditions from shift to shift and the ability of the staffing system to make changes in staff allocation.

After the nursing care requirements of each patient have been measured, the total time required by all patients on the unit is calculated according to the methods specified by the PCS. This total time becomes a prediction about the amount of time that will be required to care for that set of patients one or two shifts hence.

To determine the number of staff members needed to care for these patients in the subsequent shift, divide the total time required by eight (the number of hours worked by each nurse per shift). The number of staff members required is then compared to the number who have been scheduled to work that shift minus any known absences.

The key to efficient resource use is to match the required and available staff. If more nurses are needed than are scheduled, the nursing manager needs to identify other nurses who can work that shift by calling upon a float pool, unscheduled employees, or a substitute nurse service. If more nurses are scheduled than are needed, the nursing manager may need to ask some of the staff to float to other units with greater need or not come to work that day.

MAKING STAFF SUBSTITUTIONS. As noted earlier, because of differences in education, skill, and experience among individual nurses, the nursing labor input usually does not exist in homogeneous units. Some differences are reflected in salary differences. Many would argue that it is logical to take advantage of these differences in payment rates. To the casual observer, it would seem that employing more nonprofessional staff who receive lower salaries should reduce personnel costs. Increasing the number of LPNs and nursing assistants in relation to the number of RNs, for example, would result in more available hours of personnel time per patient day with no increase in cost.

There are, however, theoretical arguments for and against staff substitution as a method for improving nursing productivity. Adherents of the scientific management tradition predict that productivity will be greatest when the work of providing care to individual patients is divided into its component parts and the tasks assigned to staff members according to their ability. Tasks are assigned to the least costly personnel category capable of doing the task; the most qualified individuals are assigned only those tasks requiring their special expertise. Supporters of the human relations theoretical framework, on the other hand, argue that knowledge workers such as nurses will be most satisfied, and therefore most productive, when they are allowed to perform "whole tasks," i.e., to provide total patient care for a caseload of patients. They argue against dividing the work into component parts and assigning isolated tasks to individuals.

In addition to conflicting theoretical predictions of what division of labor will be most productive, the empirical evidence is also inconclusive. Unfortunately, some experiments with increasing the proportion of professional to nonprofessional staff were done in conjunction with the introduction of primary nursing (Dahlen, 1978; Marram, Barret & Bevis, 1979; Nenner, Curtis & Eckhoff, 1977; Osinski & Powals, 1980). The use of two experimental treatments simultaneously makes it impossible to sort out which of the reported changes are attributable to alterations in skill mix, which to the change in the mode of care, and which to a combination of the two. Other studies of all-RN or predominantly RN staffing have been uncontrolled case studies rather than experiments (e.g., Burt,

1980; Hinshaw, Scofield & Atwood, 1981; Miller, 1980).

Although acknowledged methodological problems exist in the study of skill mix in the provision of nursing care, a situation with a high proportion of professional staff has several reputed advantages. First, it has been reported that such a situation leads to greater patient satisfaction (Abdellah & Levine, 1958) and better coordination and quality of care (Georgopoulous & Mann, 1962; Miller & Bryant, 1965). Two other studies suggest that it may be relatively costly to use nursing assistants because nursing assistants require greater supervision and more instructions. They have been found to be occupied only 65 percent to 73 percent of their scheduled work time as opposed to RNs, who were occupied 92 percent to 100 percent of the time (Christman, 1978; Clark, 1977).

These findings suggest that providing nursing services in a health care institution may be too variable and unpredictable to take full advantage of the theoretical economies to be achieved by assigning tasks to the least qualified individual capable of performing them. Although there is tentative evidence that high professional to nonprofessional ratios may be no more costly, and frequently less costly, in terms of salary costs and turnover rates (Burt, 1980; Corpuz & Anderson, 1977; Dahlen, 1978; Forseth, 1980; Hinshaw, Scofield & Atwood, 1981; Marram, Barret & Bevis, 1979; Marram, Flynn, Abaravich & Carey, 1976; Miller, 1980; Nenner, Curtis & Eckhoff, 1977; Osinski & Powals, 1980), methodological problems in some of the available literature make it essential that investigation continue.

The current shortage of nurses and continuing financial pressures on health care facilities have led nursing managers to search for new methods for extending the professional nurse.

The reader is referred to the growing body of literature about differentiated practice (Johnson, 1988; Koerner, Bunkers, Nelson & Santema, 1989).

CONTROLLING THE USE OF SUPPLIES AND EQUIPMENT. The nurse manager also can control input costs by wisely using supplies and equipment. One method is to compare the cost and features of roughly equivalent supplies and equipment, selecting products that have the desired qualities at the lowest cost. At times, the individual manager or the institution's purchasing department may be able to use competitive bidding procedures in which vendors submit bids as a method for obtaining the lowest cost.

Once supplies and equipment have been purchased, cost can be controlled by using them wisely. For example, the nursing manager can implement systems that carefully monitor the use of supplies to reduce waste and prevent theft. Increasing cost sensitivity among nursing personnel is another method. One nurse manager was able to produce large savings simply by placing price tags on chargeable supplies. Nurses in the study hospital discovered that they could substitute less costly items and avoid using some items altogether with no untoward effects (McVay, 1983).

CHANGES IN THE CARE PROCESS

Finding ways to improve productivity by making changes in the care process allows the nursing manager to use his or her creativity to the fullest. Jelinek and Dennis (1976), in their comprehensive review of the literature on nursing productivity, called the care process the "technology of nursing." According to their definition, technology "comprises all methodologies employed in converting inputs into outputs" (p. 12). In this concept of productivity, technology includes the physical and managerial organization of nursing services, leadership and supervision, patient care delivery systems, staffing and scheduling practices, care planning and documentation procedures, and the performance of nursing activities themselves. Clearly, there are many opportunities to experiment with methods for improving the quantity and quality of nursing care given.

SELECTED EXAMPLES. It would be impossible to give examples of all of the possible methods for changing the process of care. The following few, however, are representative.

A frequently used method for improving the process of care is to alter the work schedules of nurses. Using restructured workweeks—such as four 10-hour shifts, three 12-hour shifts, or special weekend schedules—has been reported to improve staffing efficiency while also meeting some nurses' needs for leisure time (Huey, 1981; Hutchins and Cleveland, 1978; Kent, 1972; Mills, Arnold & Wood, 1983). Job sharing or job pairing, in which two individuals divide one full-time position, is another possible scheduling modification.

Some have suggested that nursing could become more productive if nurses were to give up some rituals of nursing care. "Rituals" include those routine activities such as linen changes and vital signs monitoring that are sometimes completed out of habit and without regard for the individual patient's need for them. Of course, some activities may appear to be unnecessary, but habitual behavior may be required to protect the institution from possible liability. A careful needs evaluation may enable a nursing unit to free time for more important work.

Other changes in the direct care process may lead to improvements in the quantity and quality of care delivered. Experiments with new approaches to common clinical problems such as incontinence and situational confusion may be fruitful. Investigating alternative modes of nursing care delivery such as primary nursing, case management (McIntosh, 1987), or other restructuring methods (Bennett & Hylton, 1990; Brett & Tonges, 1990; Malloch, Milton & Jobes, 1990; Olivas, Del Togno-Armanasco, Erickson & Harter, 1989) and using new or improved products or equipment can have positive results in some cases.

DOCUMENTING CHANGES. Regardless of the nature of the changes made in the process of care, it is essential that the changes and their consequences are measured and evaluated. Without careful documentation, it may be impossible to convince others that the innovations introduced are safe, effective, and efficient.

Consider the example of one nurse midwifery clinic. Several years ago the staff of the clinic decided that they could be more efficient if they replaced an individual approach to early prenatal teaching and orientation to the clinic with a group approach. After some time it became apparent that the clientele, who represented several ethnic groups and some with limited command of English and little formal education, was too diverse to make group teaching practical. Class members frequently were forced to wait while the instructor attended to language or other unique needs of individuals. Original estimates of a one-hour class turned into several actual hours, attendance dropped, and concerns grew about the women's ability to care for themselves in early pregnancy.

The staff of the clinic decided an evaluation of the patient teaching program was in order. By totaling the cost of staff time (including the time of staff who were largely unoccupied during the class) and the cost of the unused clinic rooms and comparing them with the attendance rate and knowledge outcomes, it became clear that the group approach for this set of patients was inappropriate and at least as costly. The clinic reverted to the one-on-one teaching strategy.

To evaluate the effects of changes in process, therefore, the nursing manager should include cost and outcome data collection as a part of all clinical studies. This is a less formidable task than it may appear. Cost accounting methods are well understood and relatively easy to apply. Most financial officers are eager to assist managers in performing cost analyses. While outcome evaluation can be difficult, studies of outcome, when they are used for managerial purposes, need not meet all of the rigorous criteria applied to research studies.

CALCULATING COSTS. Costs can be calculated using one of two approaches. In some cases it will be necessary to estimate only the direct costs of the change, such as costs associated with changes in the brand of a product used or introduction of a new record-keeping system.

In other cases the relevant unit of analysis is an episode of care or a patient stay. The manager must estimate the total cost of nursing care for patients affected by the change in practices. Fortunately, data available from the PCS can also be used to compute the nursing care costs for individual patients and groups of patients.

Table 5–2 presents an example of how this is accomplished. First, patients are classified in the usual manner. It is important that the classification for each patient is recorded in a retrievable fashion such as on the patient record or on a computer file. After discharge the total hours of care are totaled and multiplied by the hourly nursing care salary cost (total salary costs/total number of paid hours). Then all indirect nursing costs are added in. Indirect nursing costs include the unit's share of the expenses of nursing administration, staff development, the cost of operating the physical plant, and similar non–patient-specific expenses. These costs are generally prorated on a per-patient-day cost basis (total indirect costs/number of patient days). To ob-

tain an average cost for all patients being studied, the total cost of each patient's care is totaled and divided by the number of patients in the sample. The average costs before introduction of the innovation can then be compared to costs after its introduction to identify cost savings.

TABLE 5–2 COST ESTIMATION EXAMPLE

	Day of stay	Hours for each patient served					
		A	B	C	D	E	F
1. Apply workload measurement system	1	3	5	4	5	3	2.8
	2	2.8	5	4	4.9	3	2.8
	3	2.5	4.8	4	4.9	2	2
	4	2.5	4.6	3	4.6	2.3	
2. Add hours of care for length of stay	5	2.3	4.6	3			
		13.1	24.0	18	19.4	10.3	7.6
3. Assign hourly cost of nursing care to individual patients (e.g., $16/hour)		× $16	× $16	× $16	× $16	× $16	× $16
		$209.6	384	288	310.4	164.8	121.6
4. Add indirect costs (e.g., $20/patient day)		$309.6	484	388	390.4	244.8	181.6

5. Calculate average cost per case

   A. Add total cost for all relevant patients

$ 309.60
     484.00
     388.00
     390.40
     244.80
     181.60

$1,998.40

   B. Divide sum by number of patients $1,998.40/6 = $333.07

MEASURING OUTCOME. Measuring the effects of a change in practice can be more difficult. In a few cases, a change in the process of care may have been evaluated in a research study reported in the literature. If that is true, the nursing unit may be able to replicate the outcome measurement made in the original study.

In most instances, however, the nursing staff must design its own outcome evaluation method. The first question to ask in developing an evaluation strategy is: What is the outcome that should be measured? The answer lies in what the innovation is intended to do, what the possible untoward consequences could be, and what the institution can afford to measure. In evaluating a new method for caring for incontinent patients, for example, intended outcome could be to reduce the number of times the patients are incontinent and reduce skin breakdown. Outcome criteria then would include the number of incontinent episodes per day and the degree of skin excoriation. Untoward consequences might include unsightly garments or decreased patient autonomy. Procedures for evaluating patients' emotional responses could be used to evaluate such potential untoward results. In the incontinence example, each proposed outcome could be measured during the hospitalization at a relatively modest cost.

But the nursing staff may also want to know the long-term outcome of their new care strategy. This implies that patients will need to be located after hospital discharge and outcome measurements made at that time—a potentially costly procedure. There are several ways to complete this type of evaluation with little cost to the unit. One approach is to enlist a nurse researcher interested in the problem. Another is for the unit staff to apply for external grant funding to perform their own evaluation. Finally, it may be possible to get information about patient outcome from colleagues working in other settings. Sending evaluation forms or conducting telephone interviews with nurses working in home care or in long-term care settings can provide the needed outcome data.

USING COST AND OUTCOME DATA. Once cost and outcome data are gathered, the nursing manager must relate one to the other to come to a conclusion about whether the innovation was beneficial. One method for doing this is by using a decision model proposed by Fishman (1975) for applying cost-effectiveness analysis to evaluation studies in a service setting.

As shown in Figure 5–5, the decision-making strategy relies on comparisons of the cost and results of two methods for accomplishing a goal. Any option that produces equal or superior results and costs less or any option that produces superior results for equal cost should be chosen. Similarly, any option that produces inferior results for equal or greater costs should be rejected. Ambiguity arises when a superior result costs more or when the costs and results are equal for the two options. In these cases, the decision would depend on a value judgment about the importance of the goals to be achieved by the options in question relative to other organizational objectives. An ambiguous choice situation may also inspire the staff to identify third and fourth options for achieving the same objective at a somewhat lower cost.

The evaluation strategy for assessing the effects of changes in the process of care described here is but one of several that could be used. Whichever evaluation method is selected, it is important that it be selected before an innovation or change in the process of care begins. Unless planned in advance, the manager will lack the data to determine whether the change did or did not enhance productivity of the nursing unit.

Overall, these are just a sampling of the kinds of things nurse managers can do in concert with administrative staff and physicians to find ways to deliver quality care while meeting an institution's financial objectives.

The American public demands and is entitled to information about the efficiency and effectiveness of the health care services provided to them. The nursing profession can do one of two things: (a) develop methods for demonstrating its own value as a health care discipline, or (b) wait for others to do that evaluation. The choice seems clear. The profession must move to define the product of nursing services, provide scientific evidence of the links between nursing intervention and patient outcome, and then use professional and scientific knowledge about productivity to affect health care policy.

SUMMARY

♦ Productivity is a concept that describes the relationship between inputs and outputs.

♦ Productivity refers to the resources used to produce a product or provide a service and

FIGURE 5–5 COST-EFFECTIVENESS MATRIX

		Cost of Program A relative to Program B		
		A is less costly	A is as costly	A is more costly
Effectiveness of Program A relative to Program B	A is less effective	?	choose B	choose B
	A is as effective	choose A	no	choose B
	A is more effective	choose A	choose A	?

Adapted form D. Fishman, *Development and Testing of a Cost-Effectivenes Methodology for CMHC's* (Springfield, VA: National Technical Information Service,1975), NTIS Nos. PB 246-676 and PB 246-677.

BOX 5-1

Sovie (1985) has developed a list of strategies that can be used to manage nursing resources in hospitals more productively.

1. Do more with no more. Reduce specialized staff and return some activities assigned to other departments to nurses. For example, many institutions support IV teams at considerable cost yet there is no evidence to indicate patient welfare is thus enhanced. This may require an all-RN staff, however, if done by staff.

2. Use generic care plans. If one to two hours of nursing hours are required for each patient care plan, and an institution uses generic care plans judiciously, several nurse full-time equivalents (FTEs) could be saved.

3. Develop new flow sheets to streamline documentation. Since nurses may spend up to 40 percent of their time documenting patient care, bedside flow sheets with appropriately labeled sections may contribute to efficient use of nursing time.

4. Use group counseling and teaching methods to meet patient and family needs. In selected circumstances, group methods may be much more effective than the traditional one-on-one approach. For example, group methods could be used for discharge instructions for patients in the same DRG or to provide baby care instruction for new mothers.

5. Package nursing programs and infomation. Any common presentation, such as orientation to the unit or preparing a family to take a patient home, could be put on video or print media. Medication fact sheets can be prepared.

6. Separate nursing charges from room charges. Patient classification systems allow average hours of nursing care per category to be developed. This will allow nursing to become a unit cost center where costs can be compared across health care institution or unit per DRG. Furthermore, nursing costs per DRG could be used in incentive programs.

7. Increase use of ambulatory surgery facilities and day of surgery admissions programs. This has happened already. For these programs to funciton effectively, nursing must work closely with medical staff.

8. Effectively manage materials and shared services. Every entrepreneur knows the importance of inventory control and lower price/same quality subsititution. Nursing has not yet learned this.

9. Think "competitive marketing" and "consumer choice." Nurses have never viewed their services as a consumer choice, but it is. Nurses represent the institution and form its image to the patients and family, who go back to the community and share their experiences.

10. Develop new products. By taking on the philosophy of wellness rather than acute care, one can think of all kinds of new marketable programs/services in the health promotion business.

11. Create a learning culture with staff. Economics, accountability, marketing, change management, productivity, cost containment, networking, and, especially, human resource management are only a few of the many topics on a potential learning agenda.

12. Maximize the contributions of professional nursing through participative management, effective staff organization, professional recognition, and shared governance programs.

13. Consider matrix staffing. Unit-based nurses have traditionally accepted that floating within their own service may be required to meet nursing care requirements. However, in matrix staffing, nurses develop or are hired for competencies in at least two services and can float between services.

14. Develop and use nursing productivity standards and implement control systems. Productivity standards per DRG are essential to efficient use of staff and control of overtime.

to the quantity and quality of that product or service.

♦ It has been difficult to measure productivity in health care in general and nursing in particular because of the unique nature of the service provided and a lack of consensus about how best to measure output.

♦ Standardizing the nature of patient days (output) and estimating the validity of measurements made by patient classification systems are just two of the simple modifications that can improve the validity of current methods for evaluating productivity.

♦ Nursing productivity can be enhanced by making changes in the use of inputs and in the processes used to deliver care.

♦ Nurse managers can improve the use of inputs by matching the supply of staff with the demand for care, by carefully evaluating the consequences of staff substitutions, and by controlling the use of supplies and equipment.

♦ Demonstrating the relative productivity of nursing services is the responsibility of every nurse manager.

BIBLIOGRAPHY

Abdellah, F., and Levine, E. (1958). "Developing a Measure of Patient and Personnel Satisfaction with Nursing Care." *Nursing Research, 5*: 100–108.

American Management Sciences, Inc. (AMSI). (1980). *Productivity and Health.* Bethesda, MD: Office of the Assistant Secretary of Health. DHHS No. (HRA) 80-14028.

Bennett, M. K., and Hylton, J. P. (1990). "Modular Nursing: Partners in Professional Practice." *Nursing Management, 21*(3): 20–24.

Brett, J. L. L., and Tonges, M. C. (1990). "Restructured Patient Care Delivery: Evaluation of the ProACT Model." *Nursing Economics, 8:* 36–40.

Burt, M. L. (1980). "The Cost of All-RN Staffing." In: *All-RN Nursing Staff.* Alfano, G. (editor). Wakefield, MA: Nursing Resources. Pp. 87–90.

Christman, L. (1978). "A Micro-Analysis of the Nursing Division of One Medical Center." *Nursing Digest, 6*(2): 83–87.

Clark, E. L. (1977). "A Model of Nursing Staffing for Effective Patient Care." *Journal of Nursing Administration, 7*(2): 22–27.

Corpuz, T., and Anderson, R. (1977). "The Evanston Story: Primary Nursing Comes Alive." *Nursing Administration Quarterly, 1*(2): 9–50.

Dahlen, A. (1978). "With Primary Nursing, We Have It All Together." *American Journal of Nursing, 78:* 426–428.

Edwardson, S. R. (1986). "The Cost-Quality Tradeoff in Productivity Management." In: *Patients and Purse Strings—Patient Classification and Cost Management.* Shaffer, F. A. (editor). New York: National League for Nursing. Pp. 259–271.

Feldstein, M. S. (1971). *The Rising Cost of Hospital Care.* Washington, DC: Information Resources Press.

Fishman, D. (1975). *Development and Testing of a Cost-Effectiveness Methodology for CMHC's.* Springfield, VA: National Technical Information Service. NTIS Nos. PB 246-676 and PB 246-677.

Forseth, J. (1980). "Does RN Staffing Escalate Medical Care Costs?" In: *All-RN Nursing Staff.* Alfano, G. (editor). Wakefield, MA: Nursing Resources. Pp. 103–110.

Georgopoulous, B. S., and Mann, F. C. (1962). *The Community Hospital.* New York: Macmillan.

Giovannetti, P. (1978). *Patient Classification Systems in Nursing: A Description and Analysis.* Washington, DC: U.S. Government Printing Office. DHEW Publication No. HRA 78-22.

Giovannetti, P. (1979). "Understanding Patient Classification Systems." *Journal of Nursing Administration, 8*(2): 4–9.

Hinshaw, A. S., Scofield, R., and Atwood, J. R. (1981). "Staff, Patient, and Cost Outcomes of All-Registered Nurse Staffing." *Journal of Nursing Administration, 11*(11 & 12): 30–36.

Hornbrook, M. C. (1982). "Hospital Case Mix: Its Definition, Measurement and Use: Part I. The Conceptual Framework." *Medical Care Review, 39*(1): 1–43.

Huey, F. (1981). "The Demise of the Traditional 5–40 Workweek?" *American Journal of Nursing, 81:* 1138–1141.

Hutchins, C., and Cleveland, R. (1978). "For Staff Nurses and Patients—The 7–70 Plan." *American Journal of Nursing, 78:* 230–231.

Jelinek, R. C., and Dennis, L. C. (1976). *A Review and Evaluation of Nursing Productivity.* Bethesda, MD: Health Resources Administration. DHEW Publication No. HRA 77-15.

Johnson, J. H. (1988). "Differences in the Performances of Baccalaureate, Associate Degree, and Diploma Nurses: A Meta-Analysis." *Research in Nursing and Health,* 11: 183–197.

Kent, L. A. (1972). "The 4–40 Workweek on Trial." *American Journal of Nursing,* 72: 683–686.

Koerner, J. G., Bunkers, L. B., Nelson, B., and Santema, K. (1989). "Implementing Differentiated Practice: The Sioux Valley Hospital Experience." *Journal of Nursing Administration,* 19: 13–20.

McIntosh, L. (1987). "Hospital-Based Case Management." *Nursing Economics,* 5: 232–236.

McVay, E. (1983). *Lost Supply Charges: Would Visible Price Tags Reduce Their Number?* Unpublished master's thesis. University of Minnesota, Minneapolis, Minnesota.

Malloch, K. M., Milton, D. A., and Jobes, M. O. (1990). "A Model for Differentiated Nursing Practice." *Journal of Nursing Administration,* 20: 20–26.

Marram, G., Barret, M. W., and Bevis, E. M. (1979). *Primary Nursing: A Model for Individualized Care.* St. Louis, MO: C. V. Mosby.

Marram, G., Flynn, K., Abaravich, W., and Carey, S. (1976). *Cost-Effectiveness of Primary and Team Nursing.* Wakefield, MA: Contemporary Publishing.

Miller, P. W. (1980). "Staffing with RNs." In: *All-RN Nursing Staff.* Alfano, G. (editor). Wakefield, MA: Nursing Resources. Pp. 91–95.

Miller, S. J., and Bryant, W. D. (1965). *A Division of Nursing Labor: Experiment in Staffing a Municipal Hospital.* Kansas City, MO: Community Studies.

Mills, M. E., Arnold, B., and Wood, C. M. (1983). "Core-12: A Controlled Study of the Impact of 12-hour Scheduling." *Nursing Research,* 32: 356–361.

Nenner, V. C., Curtis, E. M., Eckhoff, C. M. (1977). "Primary Nursing." *Supervisor Nurse,* 8(5): 14–16.

Olivas, G. S., Del Togno-Armanasco, V., Erickson, J. R., and Harter, S. (1989). "Case Management: A Bottom-Line Care Delivery Model. Part 1: The Concept." *Journal of Nursing Administration,* 19(11): 16–20.

Osinski, E. G., and Powals, J. G. (1980). "The Cost of All RN Staffed Primary Nursing." *Supervisor Nurse,* 11(1): 16–21.

Pauly, M. V. (1970). "Efficiency, Incentives and Reimbursement for Health Care." *Inquiry,* 7: 114–131.

Sovie, M. D. (1985). "Managing Nursing Resources in a Constrained Environment." *Nursing Economics,* 3(3): 85–94.

Williams, M. A., and Murphy, L. N. (1979). "Subjective and Objective Measures of Staffing Adequacy." *Journal of Nursing Administration,* 9(11): 21–29.

ETHICS IN HEALTH CARE

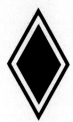

◆ PREVALENCE OF ETHICAL ISSUES

The practice of nursing is a moral enterprise based on a commitment to provide care. Throughout history, nurses have confronted ethical dilemmas. Traditionally, issues such as confidentiality and informed consent have required the nurse's attention to safeguard patient rights. These issues are with us still and require even more focus, as the complexity of care and treatment makes interpretation more important.

Innovations in health care technology give today's professionals the tools to keep bodies alive almost indefinitely. As we question even the definition of life and the definition of death, we face many decisions fraught with ethical dilemmas. Treatment provides cure or comfort and at the same time often costs a great deal physically, financially, and emotionally. Our clients require assistance to make difficult decisions and to balance the costs and benefits in terms of their own beliefs and values. Nurses address intrapersonal and interpersonal conflicts in their daily practice. Nurse managers face these same dilemmas and in addition must address the ethical implications of their management decisions. The ability to address ethical issues is at the heart of the practice of nursing today.

◆ ETHICS IS INTEGRAL TO NURSING MANAGEMENT

How we operate in a management role is influenced by our beliefs and values and the experiences that form us as individuals and as leaders. Our personal values as well as the values of the profession in which we have been socialized define responsibilities to our clients and to society. The American Nurses Association *Code for Nurses* (Figure 6–1) and its interpretive statements and the ANA social policy statement (available from ANA) provide a framework for making ethical decisions from the point of view of the profession. The AHA Patient's Bill of Rights clarifies rights for patients in institutional settings and implies an obligation on the part of the nurse to assist the patients in securing them.

In these documents, it is clear that the nurse manager has an obligation to:

1. Provide safe and respectful care

2. Not discriminate

3. Assure privacy and confidentiality

4. Ensure that the patient has enough information for informed consent

5. Support continuity of care

6. Safeguard the public from unethical or illegal practice

7. Support the welfare of the nursing profession

8. Follow physician's orders

9. Support the policies of the hospital

10. Maintain conditions of employment conducive to high quality care

11. Collaborate with other health professionals

12. Act in accord with one's own values

13. Promote efforts to meet the health needs of the public

What is obvious as one scans the list is that in the process of meeting one obligation the nurse may become unable to meet another. Consider the case of an AIDS patient who requests that the nurse not inform his spouse of the diagnosis. This creates a conflict between the duty of safeguarding the client's right to privacy and the duty to protect the public health.

Another dilemma occurs as nurses are faced with an agonizing decision regarding whether to go on strike. The ANA *Code for Nurses*, statement 9, states: The nurse participates in the profession's efforts to establish and maintain conditions of employment conducive to high

---

FIGURE 6-1 AMERICAN NURSES ASSOCIATION CODE FOR NURSES

I. PREAMBLE

The *Code for Nurses* is based on beliefs about the nature of individuals, nursing, health, and society. Recipients and providers of nursing services are viewed as individuals and groups who possess basic rights and responsibilities, and whose values and circumstances command respect at all times. Nursing encompasses the promotion and restoration of health, the prevention of illness, and the alleviation of suffering. The statements of the *Code* and their interpretation provide guidance for conduct and relationships in carrying out nursing responsibilities consistent with the ethical obligations of the profession and quality in nursing care.

II. CODE FOR NURSES

1. The nurse provides services with respect for human dignity and the uniqueness of the client unrestricted by considerations of social or economic status, personal attributes, or the nature of health problems.

2. The nurse safeguards the client's right to privacy by judiciously protecting information of a confidential nature.

3. The nurse acts to safeguard the client and the public when health care and safety are affected by the incompetent, unethical, or illegal practice of any person.

4. The nurse assumes responsibility and accountability for individual nursing judgments and actions.

5. The nurse maintains competence in nursing.

6. The nurse exercises informed judgment and uses individual competence and qualifications as criteria in seeking consultation, accepting responsibilities, and delegating nursing activities to others.

7. The nurse participates in activities that contribute to the ongoing development of the profession's body of knowledge.

8. The nurse participates in the profession's efforts to implement and improve standards of nursing.

9. The nurse participates in the profession's efforts to establish and maintain conditions of employment conductive to high quality nursing care.

10. The nurse participates in the profession's effort to protect the public from misinformation and misrepresentation and to maintain the integrity of nursing.

11. The nurse collaborates with members of the health professions and other citizens in promoting community and national efforts to meet the health needs of the public.

American Nurses Association, Inc. (For a complete statement of standards write the Publications Fulfillment Center, 2420 Pershing Road, Kansas City, Missouri 64108.)

quality nursing care, while the obligation to provide safe care requires that we not abandon the patient.

Conflicting obligations are a major source of stress for nurses, and without help in addressing them, they are also a source of nurse burnout (Cameron, 1986). Ethical dilemmas, by definition, seldom have right or wrong answers. The nurse manager can deal with them by preparing herself and his or her staff to participate in decision making. A knowledge of the theories and principles of biomedical ethics and a model for decision making will assist in analyzing issues and in the ability to articulate ethical positions.

◆ ETHICAL APPROACHES

The field of biomedical ethics is a fairly new one that has become more important as health care decisions have emerged into the public arena. The abortion debate, questions related to stopping feeding for Nancy Cruzan, and brain death legislation are examples of issues from the health care arena that have spurred public interest in ethical decision making. Philosophers, theologians, and social scientists are now contributing to the analysis of ethical issues.

Theories and principles used to address biomedical problems are drawn from the discipline of moral philosophy. Biomedical ethics applies these philosophical concepts to problems encountered in the delivery of health care. Deontology and teleology are two theoretical approaches frequently used to address issues in biomedical ethics.

Deontology (derived from the Greek word *deon*, meaning duty) focuses on duties or obligations and holds that the features of actions themselves determine whether they are right or wrong. It assumes that certain universal principles or rules are inherently good or right, inde-

pendent of their consequences. Examples of such duties are "tell the truth," "do not kill," and "keep promises."

Teleology (derived from the Greek term *telos*, meaning end), also called utilitarianism, gauges the rightness or wrongness of actions by their ends or consequences. The basic principle is that of utility. It asserts that the goal of morality is to produce the maximum benefits and minimum harm for the greatest numbers. Right conduct and duty are defined in terms of what is good or that which produces goods (Beauchamp & Childress, 1989). Whether we consider the good or harm in terms of the individual, family, or society will influence the decisions we make.

Codes of ethics and philosophical frameworks for professions have been developed by applying these theoretical bases to the practice of the professions. Thus, the philosophical premise chosen defines the obligations or duties of the professions. Leah Curtin has proposed the concept of human advocacy as a philosophical foundation for nursing practice. Since the purpose of nursing is the welfare of other human beings, she posits that the end or goal of the profession is a moral, not a scientific one. The "good" that it seeks involves our relationships with other human beings. "The wise and human application of our knowledge and skill is the moral art of nursing" (Curtin, 1979: 130). This ideal of advocacy is based on our common humanity, our common needs, and our common rights. To operate as an advocate, we need to understand both the clinical and moral dimensions of the issues our patients and we, as professionals, are facing. Diseases have a physiological impact and they damage our humanity as well. Our abilities to be independent, to act freely, and to exercise our right to make choices are influenced by both medical problems and by the bureaucratic institutions with which the client must interact when he or she is ill.

The nurse in this advocacy role has a responsibility to provide appropriate information, to assist patients to make decisions within their value system, and to help them find meaning and purpose in the issues they must confront.

These philosophical positions provide divergent frameworks for addressing ethical dilemmas, i.e., defining which right or obligations apply or identifying the harm or good produced by the action. The principles addressed in the next section help conceptualize issues to make them understandable.

♦ PRINCIPLES OF BIOMEDICAL ETHICS

Principles of biomedical ethics provide concepts and language that can be used to identify issues, to reflect on them, and to articulate the ethical positions we take. A concept is "an abstraction or generalization that helps attach meaning to a phenomenon which is observed in the clinical setting" (Rossman-Jillings, 1985: 52). It helps us to recognize what is occurring. If we say a patient is in shock, a fairly representative picture will appear in our minds. In the same way, if we identify an issue as one of patient autonomy, an entire range of questions will arise. Respect for persons as a basis for practice underlies the principles of autonomy, nonmaleficence, beneficence, and justice.

THE PRINCIPLE OF AUTONOMY

Autonomy is derived from the Greek terms *autos* (self) and *nomos* (rule) and is defined as self-rule or self-governance. Personal autonomy is "being one's own person, without constraints either by another's action or by psychological or physical limitations" (Beauchamp & Childress, 1989: 59). This principle requires that we respect individuals in our care as autonomous agents who have a right to control their own lives. To make one's own decision requires accurate information; thus, informed consent is based on the principle of autonomy. Nurses often encounter situations where a person has not received information or has not heard or remembered it. We are frequently in the position of providing information to patients, seeking information for them, or letting them know that they have a right both to receive information and/or to refuse treatment. Differences of opinion between patients and families or among caregivers arise as we ask questions such as: "Should we tell him he has cancer?" "Does she know that the treatment will be painful and expensive and may be futile?"

In the spirit of respect for autonomy, we must help people to be involved to the extent they are able in decisions that affect them. To be self-governing, one must be competent to act. Competency assessment is a critical feature in determining who makes decisions. In cases of incompetency or emergency, health care professionals act in the "best interest" of the person.

When possible, we reflect the patient's values in these decisions. The competent patient has the right to decide, even if the outcome of refusing treatment may be death. For example, Jehovah's Witnesses refuse blood transfusions because in their belief system risking their eternal souls is a greater threat than death.

It is difficult to allow someone to make a decision that is "noncompliant" or likely to be harmful from our point of view. However, because of the risk of paternalism, to override their decision we need to have *strong* evidence that the person is indeed incapable. *Paternalism,* or parentalism, is a term that refers to doing what is in the "best interest" of those for whom we are providing care. It presumes that we know what is in their best interest. Health care professionals have acted in accordance with this concept out of good will. The human rights movement in this country brought with it a major focus on individual rights. Since that time the value of patient autonomy has become increasingly important.

The right to privacy and confidentiality also arise from the principle of autonomy. The issue of AIDS has created some new questions regarding confidentiality: "How can I protect the health of other hospital staff without disclosing the person's diagnosis?" "Who has the right to information in the medical record?" In these instances, the right to autonomy and confidentiality needs to be weighed against the health and well-being of others. Autonomy is a basic right, but it is not overriding in all cases.

THE PRINCIPLE OF NONMALEFICENCE

Nonmaleficence is the principle that requires that we "do no harm." This is often considered a most stringent duty for the health professional. Our contract with society requires that we provide safe care. To act in accordance with this principle, we must act thoughtfully and competently. "Due care" requires that we have adequate knowledge and skill to perform the tasks we undertake. The American Nurses Association *Code for Nurses* states that "the nurse maintains competency in nursing."

The concept of harm can extend to infliction of emotional and financial costs as well as of pain, death, or disability. Dilemmas occur when differing perceptions of harm arise. Death may be perceived by the staff as the worst option but the patient may disagree, or vice versa. In the case of chemotherapy administration or trans-

plantation, it is obvious that pain and illness are harms that one may choose to sustain to prevent the even greater injury of profound illness or death.

THE PRINCIPLE OF BENEFICENCE

Beneficence—the doing of good–is on the same continuum as the principle of nonmaleficence. It is more active, however, and requires action that contributes to the welfare of others. It also includes prevention and removal of harm. Mercy, kindness, and charity are concepts related to the principle of beneficence.

The first tenet of the ANA *Code for Nurses* states, "The nurse provides services with respect for human dignity and the uniqueness of the client. . . ." This means that to not provide available services would be a breach of this professional obligation and the principle of beneficence.

There have been years of discussion regarding whether a nurse has an obligation to provide care to patients having abortions when the nurse believes it is wrong. The outcome of these discussions most often is that a nurse may transfer to another unit where abortion is not routinely encountered. However, in the short term, if one is assigned to the patient, the nurse may not abandon the patient. This discussion exemplifies the higher obligation to do no harm, or nonmaleficence.

Beneficence and nonmaleficence are extreme ends of the same scale. The distinction between the two comes in the degree of activity required to act. The nursing profession has a special contract to provide care for the sick. Our active involvement in providing or arranging for appropriate care is an act of beneficence.

NONMALEFICENCE ⟷ BENEFICENCE
To do no harm   To do good

THE PRINCIPLE OF JUSTICE

Justice, in concept, is often equated with fairness or, more precisely, "desert"—giving each his or her right or due. To receive a license to practice nursing is fair because you earned it by study and effort.

Distributive justice—the just distribution of burdens and benefits in society—is a recurring theme in health care today, as advanced technology and increased cost control create challenges for many policy decisions. Resource allocation discussions have increased in recent years with the recognition that available resources are not limitless. On an individual level, establishing the criteria for receiving an organ for transplant is an example of a discussion of justice. On a macroeconomic level, issues are addressed with questions such as: Is there a right to health care? What does that right mean? The uninsured and underinsured have been added to the ranks of the disenfranchised who cannot obtain health care. Policymakers discuss a "safety net" and/or providing catastrophic insurance to assist those whose resources are expended.

Nurse managers participate in decision making regarding institutional programs that will be developed or discontinued. They participate in budget development and strategic planning. Because they wear the "two hats" of institutional administrator and nursing manager, they must consider the obligation to provide quality care as well as the necessity to operate in a cost-effective manner so the institution can continue its mission.

Nurse managers address justice questions as they consider staff mix and the percentage of staff assigned to each shift and as daily assignments are made. Judgments reflect the needs of the clients, the skills of the nursing staff, and the determination as to how the best care can be provided. The ANA *Code for Nurses* says that these decisions will be made "unrestricted by considerations of social or economic status, personal attributes, or the nature of health problems." For most nurses, *their* best interest would come into play if, with two equally ill people—one of them a "bag lady" and the other, the hospital's director—they had to decide who was assigned the best qualified staff. Beliefs and values and self-interest do play a role in many decisions.

Therefore, nurse managers need to be aware of their own values and biases. We are human as well as professional, and we make value decisions all the time. We can make our decisions more consciously, but probably not perfectly. Since there are seldom clear "right" answers, but rather options to be weighed, a model for decision making can help us analyze the ethical issues we confront.

◆ A MODEL FOR ADDRESSING ETHICAL ISSUES

Most models for ethical decision making utilize the nursing process and incorporate the principles of biomedical ethics discussed in the last section. Crisham (1985) developed and refined a model for decision making based on her work with hundreds of staff nurses in acute care settings. The model is a tool that can be used to clarify the issues when nurses face conflicting obligations. It outlines a process for identifying and articulating a position so nurses can clarify their concerns in the process of decision making.

The model involves five steps represented by the mnemonic MORAL:

M = massage the dilemma

O = outline options

R = review criteria and resolve

A = affirm position and act

L = look back

To illustrate the steps of the model, we review the case of Mrs. Y.

CASE STUDY

The nurse manager of an intensive care unit identified an ethical dilemma when the staff nurses caring for Mrs. Y said that she was communicating verbally and nonverbally (by resisting treatments) a wish that she be allowed to die. As her condition worsened, they anticipated that a cardiac arrest might occur and they believed it would be abusive to the patient to perform resuscitation efforts. But there was no "do not resuscitate" order in the medical record; until an order could be obtained, they were obligated by policy to initiate resuscitation efforts.

When Mrs. Y's sons were approached with this information, they indicated that a discussion of death would take away Mrs. Y's hope and thus might actually hasten her death. They wanted all possible efforts to sustain her life continued. As discussions were occurring between the nursing and the medical staff, Mrs. Y's condition worsened. She slipped into a coma and was unable to communicate.

How does the nurse manager address this dilemma?

MASSAGE THE DILEMMA

The first step, as in any process, is to be aware that an ethical dilemma exists. Nurses feel less discomfort when they are able to identify the specific conflict. *Massaging the dilemma* (or collecting data) helps one to identify the dilemma and who is, or who should be, involved in the process of decision making. Collecting all the relevant data possible is the most crucial component in ethical decision making.

It is important to remember that conflicting wishes and values may occur among several parties—patient, family, nurse, doctor—or a conflict may exist *within* the nurse's own values. A dilemma means that one believes there are reasons to do two opposing actions. Phrased another way, reasons exist to do and to not do the same thing, e.g., to respect the patient's wishes and to not violate institutional policy. In this case, the nurse manager's conflicting obligations are to:

1. Do no harm (not abuse)

2. Provide treatment (good)

3. Support the patient's autonomy and act according to his or her wishes

4. Support the family in a crisis time

5. Follow orders and hospital policy (e.g., to resuscitate since there was no order to the contrary)

6. Assist staff to act professionally and to make an ethical decision

In collecting data for decision making, some issues for consideration are:

1. What is the prognosis?

2. Who has the information regarding the prognosis?

3. Who can make the decision?

4. Was Mrs. Y competent when she indicated her wish to die?

5. What are the relationships among family members?

6. Can the sons represent Mrs. Y's best interest?

7. How capable are the sons of making the decision? Are they "in denial" regarding their mother's prognosis?

8. Can hospital policy be of assistance in this instance?

9. What is my primary obligation as a nurse manager?

As the nurse manager attempts to unravel the confusion, it is helpful to consider the nursing options and the manager's tools. Ultimately, nurses cannot write a "do not resuscitate" order, but they participate with others (e.g., family, physicians, chaplains) in the decision making. Nurses have concerns about the family system and the survivors as well as the dying patient and her autonomy. In this dilemma, the nurse manager's goal becomes to assist the decision makers and the family to share their information and their values in the hope of arriving at a consensus.

OUTLINE OPTIONS

Outlining the options can be done with staff involvement to help them (the staff) clarify the options available and the consequences of their potential actions. Options may include:

1. Do nothing

2. Discuss the medical diagnosis, prognosis, and medical plan with the primary physician

3. Discuss with the family their perceptions of diagnosis and prognosis, their values and beliefs, and what their mother would have wanted; this may include questions such as

what is quality of life for her—is it awareness, productivity, spending time with grandchildren, etc.?

4. Discuss the nurses' values and clarify their rationale for not wanting to resuscitate; clarify whose "best interest" they are representing

5. Schedule a care conference with the family, nurses, physicians, and whoever else may be helpful, e.g., minister, chaplain, social worker

REVIEW CRITERIA AND RESOLVE

To determine appropriate actions, one needs to weigh the options generated against the principles or primary values of those involved. Crisham (1985) provides a decision matrix (Figure 6–2) that includes the principles as well as practical considerations. The alternatives (options) listed in the preceding section can be put on this graph and weighed against the criteria the nurse manager believes are important. Value considerations for the nurse manager may include: respects staff, acts fairly, etc. Practical considerations such as legal impact, effectiveness, and likelihood of success can also be included in the grid.

A plus (+) or minus (−) grid or applying numerical weighting can give the nurse a visual indication of the positive and negative outcomes of various choices. Many ethical decisions are approached by weighing options, because there is seldom one right or wrong answer when dealing with an ethical dilemma. Listening and attempting to understand the values of the parties involved is essential to collaborative decision making.

Different individuals assess positives and negatives differently and weigh choices differently. Thus, the tool, when used with staff, can help in understanding the frame of reference of those involved.

AFFIRM POSITION AND ACT

Once one has decided the next appropriate action, a strategy needs to be developed. Literature in biomedical ethics indicates that knowing the correct action does not have a great deal of influence on whether health care workers act in accordance with what they believe to be correct. To enhance appropriate action, one may look at the organizational forces that assist or impede an action plan.

Questions to be considered in planning for action in Mrs. Y's dilemma include:

1. Are the nurses able to risk stating their opinion and rationale?

2. What are the consequences of following and not following institutional policy?

3. Will the physician be willing to attend a conference?

4. Can we "live with" all potential outcomes of the conference?

5. Do we need additional resources to assist with the process?

Planning the specifics of the conference is part of the nurse manager's facilitating role in

FIGURE 6–2 DECISION MATRIX

Options	Values							Practical considerations		
	Patient autonomy	Beneficence	Nonmaleficence	Staff autonomy	Interdisciplinary relationships	Family comfort	Compliance with policy	Reduce legal risk	Time	Clarity of issues
Do nothing	−	−	−	−	NA	+	+	+	+	−
Discuss with M.D.	+	+	+	−	−	?	+	+	−	±
Discuss with family	+	+	+	±	NA	+	NA	+	−	±
Discuss with nurse	+	+	+	+	−	±	NA	+	−	±
Schedule a care conference	+	+	+	+	+	±?	+	+	+	+

P. Crisham, MORAL: "How Can I Do What's Right?" *Nursing Management* (March 1985):16,3.

ethical decision making. The manager can help the staff determine the appropriate time, place, and participants that will allow them to participate in decision making and to feel supported. Participating in the conference also will help the staff develop new skills they can use in dealing with future dilemmas.

LOOK BACK

In Mrs. Y's case, the staff had a care conference. During the conference, it became clear that the family was acting on information obtained weeks earlier and was assuming that if treatment were successful, Mrs. Y would have two years or more of "normal" life. The nurses and doctors had seen her failing and becoming infected and septic. They now believed that the best they could do would be to prolong a painful and brutal process of dying. When family members were able to hear the new prognostic information, they agreed that extraordinary efforts would cause more harm than any possible good and agreed that if Mrs. Y arrested, she should not be resuscitated. Mrs. Y died a few days later.

In this instance, the resolution was successful in that it prevented harm to Mrs. Y and promoted the good of respect and participation for all involved. If disagreements persist, however, one may need to recycle through the process to define the problem, generate options, and identify consequences with all the decision makers. The nurse manager also may involve resource people to assist with the problem-solving process.

APPLYING THE MODEL TO MANAGEMENT DECISION MAKING

As a nurse manager addresses dilemmas in her management practice, the same grid format that lists options, values, and practical considera-

tions can be used as a basis for reflection. Additional values such as fairness, honesty, supporting staff autonomy and growth, or improving interdisciplinary relationships can be included. These can be listed along with the ethical principles that we applied to cases or they can replace them on the decision matrix, depending on what values are applicable to the situation.

The field of business ethics addresses issues such as corporate responsibility, conflict of interest, and honesty in dealing with consumers. The nurse manager addresses relationships with staff and colleagues, responsibility to the patients and to the organization, cost effectiveness, and sometimes community relations in management decisions and supervisory relationships. Articulating the issues clearly, defining the issue one wishes to achieve, and analyzing its impact are a way of increasing the consciousness with which we make decisions. It also enhances our ability to articulate the rationale for directions we intend to pursue.

◆ SPECIAL ISSUES FOR THE NURSE MANAGER

PROVISION OF SAFE CARE

The primary ethical obligation of the nurse manager is to provide safe care. With the increasing complexity of care and the increasing complexity of technology, the nursing staff requires sophisticated assessment skills and up-to-date knowledge about new treatments and procedures. The skills discussed in Chapter 14 on training and education are important for nurse managers to use in addressing patient care from the perspective of "at least, do no harm" (nonmaleficence). The development of patient education skills allows the nurse to support patients in caring for themselves and also provides information essential for autonomous decision making.

CONFRONTING UNSAFE PRACTICE

The "due care" standard requires the nurse manager to deal with the unsafe or impaired practitioner. The nurse manager needs to know the institution's procedures for addressing issues of safety and professional conduct—whether the impaired practitioner is a nurse or other health care professional. It is also crucial to remember that "respect for persons" underlies all the principles of biomedical ethics. To deal humanely and gently while providing accurate data requires the nurse manager to employ the best communication and leadership skills while confronting this most painful issue.

SUPPORTING PATIENT AND STAFF AUTONOMY

To address ethical issues, we must know our own values and goals. This knowledge assists us in articulating our own positions when we take an ethical stand. It also increases objectivity and the possibility of helping the client or staff member make decisions related to *their own* value system, not ours. We need to avoid parentalism. Language that identifies the "noncompliant" patient sometimes provides a clue that we are facing a value system that differs from our own. A patient's definition of "quality of life" and ours may be greatly disparate. To act as an advocate, the nurse must understand patient values and support patient decisions. "So often by trying to do what we think is right by our value system, we trespass upon the authenticity of the person" (Curtin, 1979: 132). The nurse manager must hear and understand the values and goals of the staff to avoid "trespassing" on the individuality of staff and colleagues, as well.

ETHICS EDUCATION AND RESOURCE MANAGEMENT

Since ethical issues are commonly discussed in our institutions, many facilities have created resources to deal with them. These resources can provide education, consultation, and support.

Individuals who can be of assistance are line supervisors and staff resources such as clinical specialists or ethics consultants. Also, many institutions now have ethics committees whose purposes are to develop policies that protect patient rights and to provide education and consultation for difficult cases. Most committees are interdisciplinary and thus can supply objectivity as well as an overview of the process to ensure "due care" in decision making.

Ongoing staff education and discussion of ethical issues when a crisis is not looming are effective tools in preparing the staff to address ethical dilemmas when they do arise. Formal classes as part of inservice education will provide a framework for discussion. Open discussion of ethical dilemmas at staff meetings will help identify issues and patterns of issues that occur frequently.

An effective method for approaching ethical issues is to use "ethics rounds." These interdisciplinary rounds include nursing staff and members of other disciplines who interact with patients and personnel in a unit. Principles can be presented and discussed or cases can be retrospectively reviewed and discussed. Through this process, participants develop a common language as well as an awareness of one another's values, which are then known and understood when a difficult issue arises. As staff members gain skills and awareness, ethical issues are often identified at an earlier stage and crises are more often averted. The goal of ethics education is to develop in the staff skills they can use to handle issues that arise in professional practice.

By initiating educational opportunities, the nurse manager indicates that such issues are open to discussion and are an important part of nursing practice. By listening and participating in problem solving and/or soliciting additional resources, the manager makes it possible for the staff to risk raising an issue.

The nurse manager who knows his or her own values, who respects staff members, and who expects high quality care is the nurse manager who creates an environment in which ethical issues can be addressed and resolved. The time and skill required to resolve conflict and encourage creative problem solving are scarce resources in the nursing department. The capable nurse manager, therefore, is the institution's best asset in developing professional, ethical nursing practice.

SUMMARY

♦ Beliefs, values, and experiences influence one's ethical decision making.

♦ The nursing profession has delineated its code of ethics in the American Nurses Association *Code for Nurses*. Along with the interpretive statements (available from ANA), the *Code* guides nurses' ethical decision making.

♦ Ethical principles include autonomy, non-maleficence, beneficence, and justice.

♦ Use of a model for addressing ethical issues assists the nurse in the process of decision making.

♦ The nurse manager has additional ethical dilemmas including obligations to provide safe

care, confront unsafe practice, support patient and staff autonomy, manage resources, and provide ethics education to staff.

♦ The staff's ability to deal with ethical issues is directly related to the nurse manager's skills in conflict management, willingness to allow risk taking, and support of staff acting in a professional manner.

♦ Nurse managers communicate interest in ethical issues by assisting staff in generating alternatives and developing strategies for action.

BIBLIOGRAPHY

American Nurses Association (ANA). (1976). *Code for Nurses with Interpretive Statements*. Kansas City, MO: ANA.

Aroskar, M. (1980a). "Anatomy of an Ethical Dilemma: The Theory and Practice." *American Journal of Nursing*, 80 (April): 628–634.

Aroskar, M. (1980b). "Establishing Limits to Professional Autonomy: Whose Responsibility?" *Nursing Law and Ethics*, 1 (May): 5.

Aroskar, M., and Davis, A. J. (1983). *Ethical Dilemmas and Nursing Practice*. Norwalk, CT: Appleton-Century-Crofts.

Beauchamp, T., and Childress, J. F. 1989. 3d ed. *Principles of Biomedical Ethics*. New York, Oxford: Oxford University Press.

Beauchamp, T., and Walters, L. (1982). *Contemporary Issues in Bioethics*. 2d ed. Belmont, CA: Wadsworth.

Cameron, M. (1986). "The Moral and Ethical Component in Nurse-Burnout." *Nursing Management*, 17 (April): 4.

Cranford, R. E., and Daudera, A. E. (1984). *Institutional Ethics Committees and Health Care Decision-Making*. Ann Arbor, MI: Health Administration Press.

Crisham, P. (1985). "MORAL: How Can I Do What's Right?" *Nursing Management*, 16 (March): 3.

Curtin, L. L. (1979). "The Nurse as Advocate: A Philosophical Foundation for Nursing." *Advances in Nursing Science*, 1 (April): 1–10.

Curtin, L. L. (1982). "Ethics in Nursing Administration." In: *Contemporary Nursing Management*. Marriner, A. (editor). St. Louis, MO: C. V. Mosby. Pp. 41–46.

Deciding to Forego Life-Sustaining Treatment: A Report on the Ethical, Medical and Legal Issues in Treatment De-

cisions. (1983). President's Commission for the Study of Ethical Problems in Medicine and Biomedical and Behavioral Research.

Fry, S. T. (1986). "Moral Values and Ethical Decisions in a Constrained Economic Environment." *Nursing Economics,* (July–August). Vol. 4(4), pp. 160–164.

Gortner, S. R. (1985). "Ethical Inquiry." In: *Annual Review of Nursing Research.* Vol. 3. Werley, H., and Fitzpatrick, J. (editors). New York: Springer.

Hunt, R., and Arras, J. (1977). *Ethical Issues in Modern Medicine.* Palo Alto, CA: Mayfield.

Ketefian, S. (1985). "Professional and Bureaucratic Role Conceptions and Moral Behavior among Nurses." *Nursing Research,* 34(4): 248–253.

Mappes, T. A., and Zembaty, J. S. (1986). *Biomedical Ethics.* 2d ed. New York: McGraw-Hill.

Mayberry, M. A. (1986). "Ethical Decision Making: A Response of Hospital Nurses." *Nursing Administration Quarterly,* 10(3): 75–81.

Nelson, J. B. (1976). *Human Medicine.* Minneapolis, MN: Augsburg Publishing.

Rossman-Jillings, C. (1985). "Concepts Relevant for Critical Care Nursing: The Knowledge-Practice Connection." *Critical Care Nurse,* 5: 2.

Yarling, R. R., and McElmurry, B. J. (1986). "The Moral Foundation of Nursing." *Advances in Nursing Science,* 8(2): 63–73.

P A R T   2

KEY SKILLS IN NURSING MANAGEMENT

C H A P T E R 7

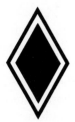

COMMUNICATION AND INFORMATION SYSTEMS

Communicating clearly, effectively, and successfully is critical for the nurse manager. Therapeutic communication skills, typically used in patient situations, are not sufficient in a complex management environment. To be an effective leader, the nurse manager must be able to successfully use the techniques of communication to express ideas and plans both verbally and in writing and to be able to listen attentively and accurately to others. This is no small task. The success of management strategies depends upon effective communication because managers work through others, and their ability to do so makes effective management possible.

Developing management communication skills may be compared to learning other complex skills. For example, patient teaching is a complex skill that requires knowledge about human behavior, disease processes, and patient learning. The same is true with developing communication skills. Communication involves knowledge of management and communication theories, people, and the context of organizations.

♦ COMMUNICATION MODELS

Early communication models focused on the transmission of messages from senders to receivers. For example, the *Shannon-Weaver model* (see Figure 7–1) was considered to be the standard explanation of business communication (Shannon & Weaver, 1949). The sender encodes and transmits a message; the receiver receives and decodes the message. A message also may be returned. This model is important historically because it depicted the complexity of communication and defined communication as a process involving give and take between the participants.

This model is limited because it focuses on the sender's ability to prepare messages and ignores inferences that the receiver makes. Furthermore, the Shannon-Weaver model indicates that the receiver's message follows the sender's, when, in fact, communication may be occurring concurrently (Timm, 1986). There also are no provisions for nonverbal communication, which makes up a large portion of most exchanges (Asante, 1980).

FIGURE 7–1 THE SHANNON-WEAVER COMMUNICATION MODEL

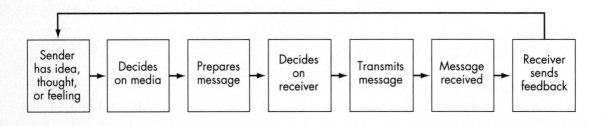

Sender has idea, thought, or feeling → Decides on media → Prepares message → Decides on receiver → Transmits message → Message received → Receiver sends feedback

Communication is a management strategy that involves choosing the most appropriate messages and sending them through the best channels (Shelby, 1988). The nurse manager rarely has unlimited control over the messages that are sent. However, it is usually possible for the manager to choose the content, organization, style, and presentation of a message. Practicing management communication involves understanding the impact of communication on employee behavior. If managers identify the possible types of messages, choose the best among them, and send the messages through the most appropriate channel, they should increase the probability of successful communication. Shelby (1988) has developed a model to enhance these elements.

The *strategic choice model* (Shelby, 1988) is helpful to managers. Shelby advocates using four steps in making choices about communication (see Figure 7–2). The first is to analyze and determine communication goals, which serves two purposes, task and social. The task goal involves the purpose in communicating: providing information, influencing others, or enlisting collaboration. The social purpose has to do with managing credibility. The sender can reduce threat or uncertainty, as well as generate good will.

The next step is to identify the options available regarding content, organization, style, presentation, and channels. The manager chooses whether the message should be a written (e.g., in house newsletter) or oral presentation (e.g., an announcement at a meeting). If the purpose is to tell or get information to and from staff members, internal memoranda, reports, procedure manuals, agency newsletters, and brochures are some of the usual channels. If the purpose of the communication is to sell, meetings may be appropriate.

The third step is to consider the receiver's probable response. The nurse manager assesses receiver variables such as staff knowledge level, personality factors, needs, attitudes, beliefs, values, and how new messages are perceived and situational variables such as interpersonal climate, organizational culture, technology, and environmental issues.

The last step in the strategic choice model is to evaluate the force or success of the communication options. Will the message be effective and meet the original communication task and social goals? Is the choice an efficient one? The

---

FIGURE 7–2 APPLIED STRATEGIC CHOICE MODEL

I. IDENTIFY COMMUNICATION GOAL

- ◆ Task
  - ◆ Tell/understand
  - ◆ Sell/buy
  - ◆ Collaborate
- ◆ Social
  - ◆ Credibility

II. IDENTIFY OPTIONS
- ◆ Content
- ◆ Organization/strategy
- ◆ Style
- ◆ Presentation
- ◆ Channel

III. ASSESS PROBABLE RESPONSE (+/–)
- ◆ Relevant receiver variables
- ◆ Relevant situational factors

IV. ASSESS RELATIVE FORCE
- ◆ Effectiveness
- ◆ Efficiency
- ◆ Quality

amount of time and resources involved in preparing and sending the communication should be evaluated when considering efficiency. Is the quality of the communication consistent with the significance of the message?

Another influential communication **model** is the Targowski-Bowman model, a **comprehen-**sive, useful framework for understanding communication within a management setting (Targowski & Bowman, 1988). Figure 7–3 shows

FIGURE 7–3 THE TARGOWSKI-BOWMAN COMMUNICATION MODEL: COGNITIVE MANAGEMENT APPARATUS

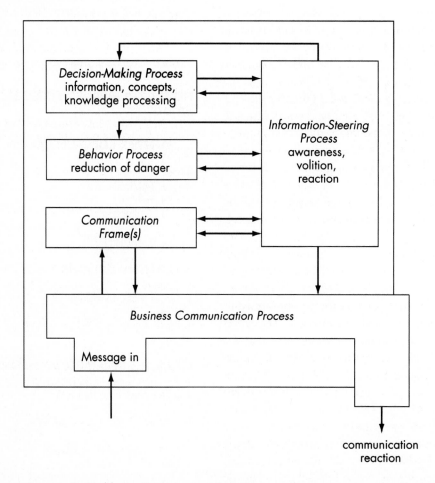

The Targowski-Bowman Communication Model: Cognitive Management Apparatus

that communication does not occur in a vacuum and information is received from a variety of sources. The aspect of the human brain responsible for processing communication is called the *cognitive management apparatus.* Within it are four linking processes: (1) the *information-steering process,* the system that manages the transmission of data, (2) the *decision-making process,* the system that categorizes information and determines the importance of knowledge, (3) the *behavior process,* the system that determines what actions need to be done to process the information, and (4) the *business communication process,* the system that generates the messages from the sender and interprets messages from the receiver. Environmental conditions, the individual's knowledge of the situation, and the quality of the communication are important. Communication consists of interactions between the senders and various influences, not just the sending and receiving of messages.

According to Targowski and Bowman, messages are composed of communication frames. These frames consist of the actual message and additional information (called reflecting information) such as nonverbal behavior that comes from the information-steering process. For example, nurse manager Stevens has decided to inform staff nurse Martin that her days off have been changed from Thursday and Friday to Saturday and Sunday. The message is worded in an apologetic manner (communication frame) because Ms. Stevens knows that Ms. Martin has already made plans for her time off (additional information).

The actual message sent has meaning to both the sender and receiver. Hopefully, it is the same for both. However, words and messages may have many meanings that are determined by cultural understandings and defined within the im-

mediate environment. Meanings differ because of culture, the immediate environment, and word definition with some messages being more important than others. According to Targowski and Bowman, messages having many meanings result in a layering of meanings. For example, choosing to communicate over the telephone may indicate that the message is less important than communicating in person. On the other hand, a telephone message communicates an urgency that is not communicated by a later appointment or memo.

Figure 7–4 shows the 10 different layers through which communication is sent. The *physical link,* the actual physical connection be-

FIGURE 7–4 THE TARGOWSKI-BOWMAN COMMUNICATION MODEL: LAYER-BASED LINKS

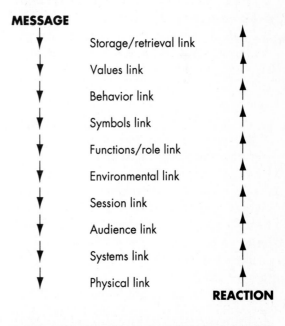

MESSAGE

Storage/retrieval link

Values link

Behavior link

Symbols link

Functions/role link

Environmental link

Session link

Audience link

Systems link

Physical link

REACTION

tween sender and receiver, is the most basic level, through which the actual message is communicated. This link may be either "immediate" or "recorded" sight and/or sound: voice, printed word, or other electronic link. When a nursing supervisor contacts a staff nurse on the telephone, a spoken physical link has been established.

The *systems link* represents the actual system used in establishing the physical link, as well as existing attitudes of both the sender and receiver toward the system involved. These systems include radio, TV, print media, face-to-face (verbal and nonverbal), electronic mail, and other electronic media. For example, many people find electronic answering machines useful and efficient mechanisms while others dislike telephoning people who use that physical device for communication.

The *audience link* involves audience selection and appropriateness for a particular message. A manager sharing personal feelings about a proposed organizational change with a friend who is a staff nurse within the organization prior to the formal announcement is an example of an inappropriate choice of audience. The size of the audience and the perceived knowledge and attitude of the audience are important as well.

The *session link* deals with the space and time of the communication. Messages can be delivered on a "real-time" exchange or a "store-and-forward" exchange. Face-to-face meetings, telephone conversations, computer conferences, and video conferences are real-time exchanges. Letters, reports, electronic mail, and voice mail, on the other hand, are store-and-forward exchanges. Some people prefer real-time messages to store-and-forward messages.

The *environmental link* accounts for the effect of the immediate environment. For example, a supervisor communicates differently when

in the more public nurses station than when in his or her own office.

The *functions/role link* is the first link that does not deal with physical factors; it deals with the effect of sender and receiver roles on the message. Formal roles (supervisor) and informal roles (charismatic leader) are included, as are economic and status differences.

The *symbols link* deals with the meaning of the language. Ideally, sender and receiver share the same symbol system. Since language includes both verbal and nonverbal behaviors, misinterpretation of the meaning of either the verbal or nonverbal message can have a profoundly negative effect on communication. The obvious example is two people who do not speak the same language. A more subtle example is communication between people from different cultures.

The *behavior link* includes evaluating observed behavior. In this link interpreting the consistency of verbal and nonverbal behavior becomes important. Targowski and Bowman point out that when the verbal and nonverbal messages contradict each other, the receiver is more likely to believe the nonverbal message.

The *values link* accounts for the impact of a person's cultural and personal values. Both nurses and nurse managers value quality health care. However, their conceptions of what is quality health care may vary. For a staff nurse, quality health care may mean hiring additional staff, but for the nurse manager, it may mean reorganizing the delivery of care.

The last link is the *storage/retrieval link*. It is a different type of link from the others. It concerns previous experiences of the sender and receiver: Sender and receiver may base their current communication on previous communications or previous experiences with similar situations. For example, a new nurse who came from a unit with a very authoritarian head nurse may interpret constructive criticism by a manager as "not being liked" by the manager or "being told what to do." The best planned communication may be misinterpreted because of the receiver's experiences in the storage/retrieval link.

Conceptualizing communication using the Targowski-Bowman model allows the nurse manager to analyze multiple aspects of communication. This model is still being tested but has support (Bowman, 1990; Targowski, 1990; van Hoorde, 1990). According to the authors, any message must pass through all 10 links as illustrated in Figure 7–4 as it is transmitted and received. Using this approach to examine communication, the nurse manager can determine both obvious and subtle effects on communication.

♦ FACTORS INFLUENCING MANAGEMENT COMMUNICATION

Several factors should be considered when applying Shelby's strategic choice model and the Targowski-Bowman communication management model. These factors are important in understanding the influence of the functions/role, symbols, behavior, and values links; they are gender, culture, and organizational climate.

GENDER

Studies indicate that gender impacts many aspects of communication. In patriarchal societies, women are assigned attention-giving roles and males are assigned attention-getting roles (Chodorow, 1978). These findings suggest that during communication activities, females are more concerned about subordinates and good will and males are quick to challenge others (Bradley, 1981). Nurses' orientation to service and institutions' expectation that nurses are there to serve others reinforces dysfunctional communication. As nurse managers climb the corporate ladder, more and more of their colleagues are men. This presents a particular dilemma. In one study when male and female subjects read the same speech, the male speakers were perceived "as more honest, as doing a better job in giving the facts, and as better justifying the conclusions by the facts than women" (Aries, 1987: 166). In other studies that examined gender and communication expertise, even when performance was held constant, men were seen as more knowledgeable than women (Deaux, 1985; Wallston & O'Leary, 1981). These researchers believe that expectations are higher for women than for men when performing the same communication behavior; therefore, men will be perceived to have higher "expertise."

In another study (Leet-Pellegrini, 1980), men talked longer and, as a result of dominating the conversation, were perceived to be more influential. Some speculate that women avoid "power behaviors," which lowers their prestige but increases their credibility, goodwill, and fairness (Kenton, 1989).

Kramer (1978) suggests a male is likely to be more dynamic than an equally knowledgeable female speaker. However, females who assume a male speech pattern may be criticized as being overbearing by both males and females. There are no easy solutions for either male or female nurse managers. Ideally, all levels of management should have an equal gender mix so that any negative effects would be neutralized. However, in reality nursing is 97 percent female. The best approach is to identify the effects of gender on all management communication and use that information when communicating.

SOCIETAL CULTURE

The workforce will contain many more minorities by the year 2000 (Hanamura, 1989; Foster, Jackson, Cross, Jackson & Hardiman, 1988). Fifty-three percent of the workforce is now made up of women and minorities and 15 percent is made up of immigrants. Management within the health care industry must address this cultural diversity. Since effective communication is the basis of effective management, attention to the influence of culture on communication is vital.

The cultural effects of communication are complex because different cultures represent language differently. Some cultures may use different sounds for the same words. Cultural attitudes, beliefs, and behaviors all affect communication. Since individuals are products of their culture, their behavior is also culture-bound in their work environment. Such elements as body movement, gestures, tone, and spatial orientation are culturally defined and a great deal of misunderstanding results from the participants' lack of understanding of each other's cultural expectations. For example, Asians are more concerned about role expectations than is the typical American. Asians take great care in exchanges with superiors so that there is no conflict or "loss of face" for either person.

Managers should consider specific problems related to cultural interpretation of messages. This requires the nurse manager to understand the cultural heritage of her employees. Once communication problems are identified, strategies can be developed to promote intercultural understanding and communication (Masterson & Murphy, 1986).

ORGANIZATIONAL CULTURE

In organizations, cultures evolve over time that affect individual and group behavior in predictable, though often subtle, ways (Buono, Bowditch & Lewis, 1985) (see also Chapter 8). Organizational culture is similar to societal culture in that both are pervasive and powerful forces that shape behavior (Wilkins, 1984). Analysis of organizational culture is particularly important for a manager who is new to the organization.

Three components of organizational culture impact communication and should be examined: *customs, objective and subjective culture,* and *climate.* Each organization has its own *customs,* which are the "glue" that holds the organization together. These customs are the traditional ways of carrying out organizational responsibilities. Often called "the way we do things," they include specific patterns of beliefs and expectations that emerge over time. As a result of these beliefs and expectations, a shared understanding of the "work world" emerges (Buono, Bowditch & Lewis, 1985). For example, at one institution, an employee Christmas program had become a custom. Even though the program required hours of preparation, many of them during employees' work time, administration supported it intensely. A new administrator recommended that the program be canceled because the institution was unusually short of nursing staff. On the surface, this seems like a reasonable action; however, most of the staff were quite upset. Had the administrator analyzed the organization's customs and their meanings prior to her recommendation, she could have anticipated the staff response.

Objective organizational culture includes the trappings created by the organization such as physical settings, office locations and decor, and even computer access. *Subjective organizational culture* refers to common beliefs, assumptions, or expectations held by organizational members. It also includes the group's perception of the organization's environment, norms, and values. Managers need to be aware that there are shared beliefs within organizations and that they often center around organizational "heroes."

Organizational climate is different from either customs or objective/subjective culture. Organizational climate is a "measure of whether people's expectations about what it should be like to work in an organization are being met" (Schwartz & Davis, 1981: 33). Climate concerns whether employee beliefs and expectations are being met. For example, in one institution, the nursing administrator is very traditional and autocratic. In the institution across the street, the nursing administrator is more democratic and involves the staff in more decision making. When employees from both institutions were asked whether they were involved in decisions as appropriate, they both responded favorably. Thus, employees in the first institution expected an autocratic leader and those in the second expected a more democratic leader. Climate was rated high in each institution regardless of amount of staff involvement or other cultural issues.

Within any organization, there are also likely to be *subcultures,* groups who have a common belief system that distinguishes them from the majority, and *countercultures,* groups who reject the beliefs of the dominant culture. A manager communicating with members of these groups should consider the influence of their beliefs. If a health care institution is hiring agency nurses, it would be expected that their beliefs, expectations, and behaviors would be different from those of nurses employed full-time by the

organization, and they may develop a subculture. Nurse's aides who are being phased out of a health care institution would be a likely group to form a counterculture.

♦ EFFECTIVE COMMUNICATION THROUGH HUMAN INTERACTION

PRINCIPLES OF EFFECTIVE COMMUNICATION

Once a manager understands the components and the processes of management communication and then considers the factors that influence communication, techniques of communication can be chosen. There are many useful techniques that can produce effective communication. When any of these techniques are used, the following principles should be kept in mind.

Principle one: Information giving is not communication. Communication requires that the participant share a mutual interaction, with the receiver providing feedback to the sender.

Principle two: The sender is responsible for clarity. Frustration with others' actions is built into the manager's job, and nursing management is no exception. However, this frustration can be reduced if the nurse manager makes messages to staff clear. Remember, the responsibility for communicating ideas clearly is the manager's, not the staff person's.

Principle three: Use simple and exact language. In both written and spoken communication, words used precisely and in the simplest terms possible are more likely to be understood. This means selecting explicit words in terms of the listener's (not the sender's) experience.

Principle four: Feedback should be encouraged. The best way to be sure a message has been accurately interpreted is to obtain feedback; lack of it is a common reason for misunderstanding. Feedback received may not be complimentary, or the ideas of the receiver may be in conflict with those of the sender. Nurse managers also must learn how to evaluate feedback, putting it into the total picture so that any disturbing aspect can be dealt with constructively.

Principle five: The sender must have credibility. The personal and professional credibility of the information giver is important in effecting the desired outcome. Being trustworthy, reliable, and competent are characteristics of a credible professional. Remember the rule, "Say what you mean and mean what you say."

Principle six: Acknowledgment of others is essential. The nurse manager may sometimes be reluctant to acknowledge the contributions of others because of fears of their responses; this is especially likely to be true if work is viewed as competitive. However, if the employment atmosphere is one of cooperation and individual contributions are viewed as complementary, acknowledgment is encouraged.

Principle seven: Direct channels of communication are best. The more people through whom the message must be filtered, the more opportunity for distortion. Additionally, face-to-face communication is preferable to written and phone communication. Immediate feedback is obtained, thereby reducing the chances for misunderstanding. You can also read the body language and facial expressions of the other person in a face-to-face discussion.

Adherence to all of the above principles can save time for the manager. In contrast, distorted communication and misunderstandings usually result in unproductive use of time, poor patient care, and frustration for both staff and managers. Settling problems after they have occurred

takes more time than preventing them through clear and appropriate communication.

ORAL COMMUNICATION

Oral communication is both verbal and nonverbal. All nonspeech communication that transmits information about the message and the relationship of the communicants is nonverbal communication. It consists of four areas: (a) kinetics, or the body movements and gestures that accompany speech; (b) spatial relationships between communicants; (c) paralanguage, or nonlanguage verbalizations that affect speech, including pitch, tone, timing, pace, and voice; and (d) cultural attributes and appearance, including clothing, grooming, and hairstyle.

The nonverbal message comes through more powerfully and effectively when there is incongruence between what is actually said and the nonverbal message. Generally, the listener will believe the nonverbal message. *This incongruence is the most significant difficulty in communicating effectively.*

The nurse manager often acts as a conduit and a filter for communication between others and staff. The ability to assist both parties to understand and work with each other is probably the greatest asset the manager can possess. For this, the manager needs skill in both written and oral communication.

The nurse manager also must consider nonverbal aspects of communication in presenting oneself and in observing others. Posture, dress (including such items as a stethoscope in one's pocket), mannerisms, and gestures all contribute to the way others "hear" the manager's words in the context of nonverbal cues. Although people generally think they pay close attention to someone's words, the context and the nonverbal elements set the stage, and words have impact only as they relate to the setting. When the verbal and nonverbal messages are incongruent, the listener will attend to the nonverbal. Therefore, the nurse manager must attend to the nonverbal behaviors of subordinates, peers, and superiors and consider the total picture of words and their meaning within that context.

The importance of the interaction between verbal and nonverbal communication cannot be overemphasized. You must know not only what to say, but also how to say it. Studies have shown that managerial effectiveness is greater when the manager is sensitive to how messages are communicated and relates positively to employees (Sorenson & Savage, 1989).

LISTENING

Central to communicating is listening effectively. Although much has been written in recent years about active listening skills as they pertain to therapeutic skills with patients, little attention has been focused on the need for effective listening skills for nurse managers. The difficulty in receiving messages as the sender intended them lies in the fact that one must decode the message within one's own frame of reference. This includes both verbal and nonverbal elements as well as the listener's past experiences, attitudes, biases, and preconceptions regarding the sender.

Along with the problems that most people have in listening effectively, the nurse manager has additional barriers to overcome. One of these is the complexity of her responsibility and the diversity of the nurse manager's relationships with staff and colleagues in daily interactions. Another barrier is the nursing setting with all the accompanying stimuli that often overload the nurse manager, whose attention is demanded by a number of people and in several places and situations simultaneously. This may create a lack of confidence on the part of others

that the manager is really listening and responding to them.

Actually, to learn active listening skills *requires paying more attention to another's message than to forming a response.* The listener must pay attention to the words, expressions, gestures, and context of the message and check out with the speaker impressions of the message. Here are several active listening principles:

1. Find a place to talk with a minimum of distractions or interruptions.

2. Sit or stand so that you can look directly at the other person.

3. Listen to words but pay closest attention to nonverbal cues.

4. Ask questions to develop points further.

5. Be empathic—try to put yourself in the other's place.

6. Obtain feedback for your impressions of the other's thoughts or feelings.

7. Acknowledge positive contributions of the other.

8. Respond to the other's message and meaning.

9. Be patient.

Muller (1980) reported positive results when nursing service administrators used active listening techniques in meetings with hospital employees. The administrators stated that increased feelings of being understood were reported by the staff when the former practiced active listening.

WRITTEN COMMUNICATION

A combination of written and spoken communication is often used by the nurse manager in day-to-day management tasks. The nurse manager's skills must include the ability to receive oral or written information, decode that information, select information to give to appropriate people, and present that information in an effective way, written or oral, to the required person(s). Generally, the nurse manager is responsible for the written work of staff members and must be able to assist them in expressing information clearly and accurately. One example is incident reports.

Most written communication in management is formal and includes (a) preparation of employee records and materials, job descriptions, performance appraisals, or anecdotal notes; (b) documentation of activity reports or justification reports; (c) a record of committee activities, including agenda and minutes; or (d) development of written policies and procedures for the unit or institution.

The nursing clinician who becomes a manager is familiar with the need for documentation since a large part of the job in patient care is to document observations, patients' subjective reports, nursing actions, and patient responses to procedures, treatments, or medications. Similarly, the nurse manager uses anecdotal notes—"critical incidents," as they are frequently referred to—in assessing staff performance. The critical incident technique is an effective way to document events as they occur without a formal structure. It reduces both the occurrence of "selective remembrance" and the influence of personal bias in appraisal. Skill in using accurate, precise language to report specific behavior is essential.

The nurse manager also frequently needs to explain current unit conditions and future unit needs. This requires written justification reports requesting specific resources and supporting data to justify the request. Included in the report

is the background of the situation, rationale to explain the need, and specific details of how resources will be utilized. Last, but not least, the benefit the needed resource will have for the institution is explained.

Memos are one way the nurse manager communicates with others. Although the manager sometimes does this carelessly, one must remember that a memo is a written representation of the author to others, and the organization, clarity, style, tone, and content will be judged accordingly. Following are key behaviors to remember in writing memos:

1. Analyze the situation by determining the subject, the purpose, the form, the audience, and the voice.

2. Closely analyze the needs of the audience and the impact of possible types of voice.

3. Use this analysis to decide on the particular writing skills to be used, such as what words to use, what thoughts or sentences to write, what kinds of material to include or exclude, and how it should be organized.

4. Select words that are appropriate to the audience and are objective. Don't use "nursing jargon" when writing to non-nurses.

5. Use sentence tone to convey meaning: e.g., for a command, say directly what you expect without being overbearing or, conversely, don't ask if people want to do what you are asking such as, "No one will go to lunch before 11 A.M." (too harsh) or "Does anyone object to going to lunch after 11 A.M.?" (too lenient). "Lunch hours should be scheduled after 11 A.M." is just right.

6. Refer to yourself by title ("Sue Brown, RN") and include your position if writing outside

your unit; refer to the audience by their titles, "nursing staff."

7. Arrange material logically by presenting the topic, purpose, what needs to be done, rationale, and time frame.

8. Include enough detail to inform but not too much to confuse or overwhelm.

DISTORTED COMMUNICATION

In any communication, distortions can arise. The sources of the communication may be the origin of the distorted message. The sender may write or speak without adequate reasoning or use inadequate or very strong, judgmental words. The speaker may be too fast or too slow or the receiver may be busy or distracted. The sender may use words unfamiliar to the receiver or spend so much time on detail that the receiver misses the main point. Consider the following example, in which the sender uses inadequate words at an inappropriate time.

> Supervisor (speaking to nurse manager): "Ms. Green, your unit's absenteeism is too high."

Ms. Green can interpret this message several ways: her staff is missing work more often than those on other units; the supervisor thinks the absentees are not really ill; or Ms. Green is doing something she should not or is not doing something she should, thereby causing her staff to call in sick.

Ms. Green responds by becoming defensive and thinking to herself, "I'd like to see her manage these people and take care of all our sick patients," or, "It isn't my fault people get sick."

If the supervisor offers her comment as she is passing through the unit on a busy day and if she does not sit down with Ms. Green to discuss possible underlying problems and how they can work together to solve them, the problems will remain and Ms. Green will now see her supervisor as an adversary. This will set the tone for their next interaction. Given the previous interaction, Ms. Green may be reluctant to report future staff problems, especially if they might reflect negatively on her.

As discussed previously, the context of the interaction significantly determines its meaning and result. *Where, why,* and *how* an interaction occurs is as influential in the outcome as *what* was said. Since the sender is the initiator of the interaction, he or she is often responsible for selecting the time and place—two usually controllable aspects of the context.

The sender can reduce the amount of distortion in the message by choosing words that clearly express the intended meaning, by speaking in a manner that can be easily understood, and by selecting an appropriate time and place for the interaction. The sender cannot control many aspects of the situation but can try to minimize distortion.

The receiver has less control over the situation because he or she receives an already developed message and responds to it; consequently, the receiver has more opportunity for distorting the message. In fact, the receiver's attitude toward the sender and perception of the meaning of the message bias the message even before it is sent. The receiver is also influenced by past experiences with the sender and others. One hears it said, for instance, that a particular employee who cannot get along with a supervisor seems to "have a problem with authority figures," the connotation being that the person has displaced residual feelings toward someone in authority in the past, to the supervisor in the present situation. The receiver then selectively listens, with one's biases and preconceptions acting as filters to allow in only the words that fit with predetermined expectations.

Douglass suggests that commonality of experiences influences the effectiveness of communication and that the greater the number of common experiences, the more likelihood that the sender and receiver will effectively communicate with each other (Douglass, 1984). For instance, if the nurse manager has a lifestyle similar to those of staff, they will be more likely to understand her words and actions accurately. In turn, the nurse manager will be more likely to present ideas in a way that staff will understand.

Several obstacles prevent people from making themselves understood in written communication. The nurse manager should try to avoid the following:

Clutter—excessive use of language and statements that simply get in the way, complicate, and confuse

Poor word choices—difficulty in choosing words that are varied (to create interest) and precise (to say what we mean)

Unnatural language—the tendency to resort to pompous, pretentious language

Lack of organization—the lack of both perception (seeing the "whole") and discipline in putting information together in a plan with order and sequence

Poor style and structure—difficulty in linking words in a cohesive pattern and in rhythmically linking thoughts that are grammatically well structured (Max, 1985: 51)

These obstacles can be identified and removed quite easily. Clutter can be identified by looking for extraneous language and unnecessary information. Poor word choices can be avoided by selecting language to say precisely what you

mean. Varying expressions adds interest. Unnatural language can be eliminated by the use of language that is current and simple, not archaic and contrived. Organizing your thinking before planning what you are going to write helps develop your message in a logical sequence. Poor style and structure can be avoided by checking grammar and varying the form (Max, 1985).

ASSERTIVENESS

Once a message is formulated properly, one aspect of communication that may be critical in sending it is assertiveness. *Assertiveness* is a term that describes behaviors that a person can use to stand up for oneself and one's rights without violating the rights of others. One can be assertive without being aggressive. It is especially appropriate for nurses and nurse managers to learn to assert themselves within a system that has encouraged nurses' subservience. In health care, women must not only learn to be assertive in general, but especially so in relation to hospital administrators and physicians, who are often very powerful men.

Melodie Chenevert (1988) identifies "Ten Basic Rights for Women in the Health Professions." They are:

1. You have the right to be treated with respect.

2. You have the right to a reasonable workload.

3. You have the right to an equitable wage.

4. You have the right to determine your own priorities.

5. You have the right to ask for what you want.

6. You have the right to refuse without making excuses or feeling guilty.

BOX 7-1
DISTORTION IN WRITTEN COMMUNICATION

There is ample opportunity for distortion in the complicated process of sending, receiving, and responding to messages, as demonstrated by the following correspondence between a plumber and an official of the National Bureau of Standards (Donaldson & Scannell, 1979).

Bureau of Standards
Washington, D. C.
Gentlemen:
    I have been in the plumbing business for over 11 years and have found that hydrochloric acid works real fine for cleaning drains. Could you tell me if it's harmless?

                Sincerely,
                Tom Brown, Plumber

Mr. Tom Brown, Plumber
Yourtown, U.S.A
Dear Mr. Brown:
    The efficacy of hydrocholoric acid is indisputable, but the chlorine residue is incompatible with metallic permanence!

                Sincerely,
                Bureau of Standards

Bureau of Standards
Washington, D.C.
Gentlemen:
    I have your letter of last week and am mightily glad you agree with me on the use of hydrochloric acid.

                Sincerely,
                Tom Brown, Plumber

Mr. Tom Brown, Plumber
Yourtown, U.S.A
Dear Mr. Brown:
    We wish to inform you we have your letter of last week and advise that we cannot assume responsibility for the production of toxic and noxious residues with hydrochloric acid and further suggest you use an alternate procedure.

                Sincerely,
                Bureau of Standards

Bureau of Standards
Washington, D.C.
Gentlemen:
    I have your most recent letter and am happy to find you still agree with me.

                Sincerely,
                Tom Brown, Plumber

Mr. Tom Brown, Plumber
Yourtown, U.S.A
Dear Mr. Brown:
    Don't use hydrochloric acid, it eats the hell out of pipes!

                Sincerely,
                Bureau of Standards

For communication among more than two people, the chance of distortion increases proportionally.

BOX 7-2
INTERNAL FRAMES OF REFERENCE

It is useful for people who work together to understand others' perspectives and what each person considers important and why. Culbert and McDonough (1980) propose that people align their self-interest with the needs of their job and that if each employee understands and respects the others' alignments, the likelihood of inaccurate projection of meanings onto others is minimized. An alignment is a "lens" through which an individual views and interprets all organizational events. This alignment determines how a person will perform and relate to organizational events.

A technique developed by Mitchell (1986) helps employees develop an appreciation of each others' alignments. This exercise is best conducted by a person who has knowledge and skills in group dynamics and small group behavior. The leader presents a brief description of alignment theory and then asks each participant to respond to 12 open-ended questions (see "Internal Frames of Reference," below). Once finished, each person shares their responses. This exercise brings an increased understanding of co-workers that helps decrease the amount of inaccurate conceptualizations of messages.

DIRECTIONS: PLEASE ANSWER THE FOLLOWING QUESTIONS.

Personal or Life Symbols

1. What are you trying to prove or demonstrate to yourself and what are you trying to demonstrate to others? Why (is this important)?
2. How do you want to be remembered by the people who are close to you (e.g., what motto would you like to have carved on your tombstone)?

3. What about you is most often misunderstood or misinterpreted by others?
4. Who were some persons who have been important role models for you, both positive and negative, and in what ways are you like them and unlike them?

Career Category

5. What specialty do you wish to pursue? Please tell why. If you are not in this field now, explain how you plan to get into it.
6. What do you want to accomplish in that specialty?
7. What honor or monument would you like to have symbolize your success in that specialty? Why would this consititute a personal hallmark?
8. If you could custom design your work/professional role, what would it be?

Current Work or Organizational Category

9. What word or short phrase would you use to best describe (in the context of your present association with this work group): (a) you, (b) you as other see you, and (c) you as you would like to be seen?
10. Describe the work experiences with this team that were most (a) satisfying or personally rewarding or (b) frustrating or unpleasant.
11. If you could spend more time doing "exactly what you want to do" in this work setting, what changes would you make in your present activities?
12. What is the next lesson you need to learn (with respect to this work group or work project) and how do you plan to do so?

7. You have the right to make mistakes and be responsible for them.

8. You have the right to give and receive information as a professional.

9. You have the right to act in the best interest of the patient.

10. You have the right to be human.

She states that nurses have these basic inalienable rights but that each individual is responsible for acquiring these rights for herself; no one is responsible for "giving" them to anyone else (Chenevert, 1988).

Assertive behavior is situation specific and can be differentiated from nonassertive and aggressive behavior in which participants respond in a certain manner regardless of the situation. As the manager develops skill in clear, accurate, and honest expression of ideas and feelings, others are encouraged to respond in kind. Consider the following example.

Ms. Jones, nurse manager, enters Mr. Wilson's room to find him scowling. He promptly states, "That stupid nurse forgot my medicine *again*!" Ms. Jones could respond in one of the following ways:

1. "There, now, don't worry, I'm sure it will be all right."

2. "Oh, really! Well, I'll take care of her!"

3. "Tell me what you missed and I'll check on it."

If she uses the first response, Ms. Jones negates the patient's rights with a verbal pat on the head. She is responding nonassertively and accepting responsibility for her staff nurse's actions even without finding out the facts. With the second response, she assumes the staff nurse is to blame and plans to chastise the nurse. This is aggressive behavior. The third response indicates she has heard the patient and is going to take action in his behalf, but she has done this without taking the blame herself and without blaming others. She has accepted his emotional response without reacting to it.

Often people who learn assertive communication report a decrease in stress. Another benefit is the increased likelihood to respond at the appropriate time. With nonassertive behavior, the person often attempts to avoid problems by remaining silent, although still angry; the aggressive person responds to the emotional aspect of the situation, thereby alienating others. But the assertive person responds appropriately to the specific situation and at the appropriate time. Participants may not agree with each other's responses, but they clarify what the other's position is and accept the other's right to differ.

Open, direct, and timely interactions between employees encourage problem identification and facilitate problem solving and decision making. Assertive communication techniques are valuable tools for the nurse manager in carrying out these tasks.

Assertiveness in any situation employs several rules that guide behavior (Smith, 1975). They are:

1. Avoid overapologizing.

2. Avoid defensive, adverse reactions such as aggression, temper tantrums, backbiting, revenge, slander, sarcasm, and threats.

3. Use body language that is appropriate to and matches the verbal message (e.g., eye contact, body posture, gestures, facial expression).

4. Accept manipulative criticism while maintaining responsibility for your decision.

5. Calmly repeat a (negative) reply without justifying it.

6. Be honest about feelings, needs, ideas. Use "I" statements.

7. Accept and/or acknowledge your faults calmly and without apology.

♦ SPECIAL TYPES OF HUMAN INTERACTION COMMUNICATION

Communication channels utilized by the nurse manager may be downward, upward, or diagonal as demonstrated in Figure 7–5. Downward communication (between a manager and a subordinate) is often directive and includes specific instructions for the subordinate. Upward communication is often reporting, while lateral communication is most often discussion and negotiation.

COMMUNICATION WITH SUBORDINATES

Depending on the institution's policies, the nurse manager's responsibilities may include selecting, interviewing, counseling, and disciplining employees; handling their complaints; and settling conflicts. The principles of effective communication are especially pertinent in this relationship because good communication is the adhesive that builds and maintains an effective work group.

To give directions and achieve the desired results, however, the nurse manager needs to de-

FIGURE 7–5 COMMUNICATION CHANNELS

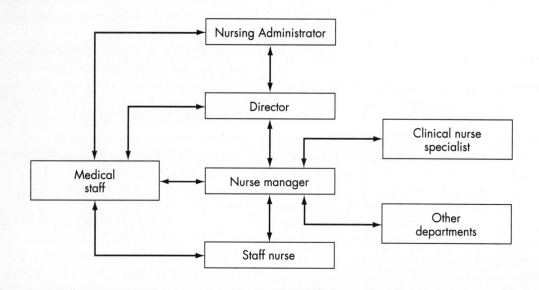

velop a "message strategy." The strategies suggested below should help to increase the chance of effective responses from others.

Know the context of the instruction. Be certain you know exactly what you want done, by whom, within what time frame, and what steps should be followed to do it. Be clear in your own mind what information a person needs to carry out your instruction, what the outcome will be if the instruction is carried out, and how that outcome can or will be evaluated. When you have thought through these questions, you are ready to give the proper instruction.

Get positive attention. Avoid the factors that can interfere with effective listening. Informing the receiver(s) that the instructions will be given is one simple way to try to get positive attention. Highlighting the background, justification, or the importance of the instructions may also be appropriate.

Give clear, concise instructions. Use a nonoffensive/nondefensive style and tone of voice. Be precise, and give all the information needed to carry out your expectations. Follow a step-by-step procedure if several actions need to be completed.

Secure verification through feedback. Make sure the receiver has understood your specific request for action. Ask for a repeat of the instruction.

Give follow-up communication. Understanding does not guarantee performance. Follow up to determine the outcome of your instruction, and give feedback to the receiver.

As stated earlier, direction giving is *not* communication. However, if the manager receives an appropriate response from the subordinate, communication has occurred.

The nurse manager is responsible both for the quality of work life of individual employees and for quality of patient care of the entire unit. To carry out this part of the job, the nurse manager can utilize communication principles by acknowledging the needs of individual employees, especially if the needs conflict with needs of the unit; by speaking directly with those involved; and by stating clearly and accurately the rationale for the decisions made.

COMMUNICATION WITH SUPERIORS

The manager's interaction with higher administration is comparable to the interaction of the manager and subordinate except that the manager is now the subordinate. Upward communication also is shown in Figure 7–5. The nurse manager must recognize that higher administration is responsible for the consequences of decisions made for a larger area, such as all of nursing service or for the entire institution. However, the principles used in communicating with subordinates are equally appropriate. Managers must state their needs clearly, explain the rationale for requests, suggest benefits to the larger unit, and utilize the appropriate channels. They must also be prepared to listen objectively to the response of their supervisors and be willing to consider reasons for possible conflict with needs of other areas. This is, of course, a description of an ideal communication between nurse manager and supervisor, with both participants practicing good communication skills. The manager can serve as role model to both subordinates and supervisors by consistent and daily use of appropriate communication skills.

COMMUNICATION WITH MEDICAL STAFF

Communication with the medical staff is often difficult for the nurse manager because of the nature of the physician/nurse relationship: (a) the medical staff, although not employees, have enormous power in the health care setting; (b) the historical relationship of physicians and nurses is that of superior and subordinate; and (c) a gender disparity exists within both professions, with a great preponderance of male physicians and female nurses.

In addition, the medical staff is in itself diverse. The medical staff may consist of physician employees, interns, residents, physicians in private practice, and consulting physicians. Some physicians, such as pathologists, radiologists, and anesthesiologists, work on a contractual basis. Obviously, the principles of effective communication are very important in interactions with the medical staff. For more on the nurse manager's role in working with physicians, see Chapter 24.

COMMUNICATION WITH OTHER HEALTH CARE PERSONNEL

The nurse manager has the overwhelming task of coordinating the activities of a number of personnel with varied levels and types of preparation and different kinds of tasks. The patient may receive regular care from a respiratory therapist, a physical therapist, a dietitian, etc. The nurse manager must utilize considerable interactional skill in communicating with personnel and managers in other departments; in this situation the communication moves in a horizontal or diagonal direction (see Figure 7–5), depending upon whether the nurse manager is communicating with managers of other departments (at the same level on the hierarchy as the nurse manager) or directly with staff in other departments. As previously discussed, horizontal communication usually follows formal channels, while diagonal communication is more often informal.

In interacting with persons from other departments, the nurse manager must recognize and respond to the differences between the goals of their departments and her nursing unit. This recognition can help the nurse manager to search for commonality of purpose.

COMMUNICATION IN PUBLIC RELATIONS

The nurse manager is a visible sign of the institution's image. Appearance, manner of speaking with groups as well as with individuals, and nonverbal communication (body movements, tone, timing, pace, voice, and pitch) convey powerful messages about the ability of the institution to provide competent and professional care. In today's competitive health care environment, it is critical that every message about the institution be professional. Obviously, it also must depict an accurate image of the institution.

♦ INFORMATION SYSTEMS

The acceptance of computers in nursing has paralleled that in the business community. In the 1960s, most health care institutions were introduced to computers to support general accounting systems, such as patient billing and payroll. Larger institutions purchased both the hardware and software to perform these functions with the anticipation that they would be easy to install and maintain. Because these systems were very expensive, smaller institutions shared services with similar organizations. By the 1970s, computer technology supported activities of individual departments. It was during this decade that the concept of hospital information systems (HIS) was born. Bedside computing may be our future. Computers are now used in two ways: patient monitoring/care and data communication within the institution.

PATIENT MONITORING

One of the first applications of computers in patient care was patient monitoring. By the early 1980s, almost all coronary and intensive care units did some type of computer monitoring of patients' vital signs, cardiac output, and blood gas changes (Curtin, 1982). In the early 1990s, computer monitoring of patients was expanded to general hospital areas, long-term care facilities, and outpatient settings (Pulliam & Boettcher, 1989).

The primary functions of such systems are to record the patient's progress and alert the nurse to any significant changes. While some computer-monitor systems record the patient's progress on paper, many also transmit the information to monitors at the nursing station, clinic, or physician's office. Where there are such monitors, the computer may print a notice on the monitor to alert the nurse when a change occurs and also may sound an alarm to indicate a significant change.

While almost all current systems simply provide information to a health professional for action, some equipment has been developed that not only detects undesirable trends, but also analyzes them and automatically administers medication appropriate to the problem (Edwards, 1982; Squire, 1982).

Such developments facilitate the nurse's efforts to handle unexpected or poorly defined problems. However, these developments also present challenges. It is crucial that the nurse manager, by developing training programs, help the staff become skilled in the use of computer equipment. If the nurses are not trained in its usage, the highly technical monitoring equipment will not provide the intended efficiencies. However, the nurse manager must provide more than training in the technical aspects of the equipment. She must, in addition, provide support so the staff nurses feel comfortable with the equipment; if the nurses are not comfortable with the equipment, their anxiety may frighten or demoralize the patient, and the intended increase in quality of care will not be achieved.

In addition, the nurse manager needs to be sure that the use of computers does not dehumanize care. She needs to monitor computer use by staff nurses to ensure that they rely on the equipment as an aid to the nursing function, not as a replacement for the interpersonal aspects of patient care. These aspects are the essence of nursing care and are essential, because not everything that is relevant to know about a patient appears on a monitor, and equipment can break (Dumont, 1985; Hales, 1985).

PROVISION OF CARE

Computers are also being used to help nurses provide patient care. For example, computers are being used to monitor and, in some cases, control the intake and output systems to which patients might be connected. Brimm (1987) describes the use of computers in critical care that not only monitor heart rate, blood pressure, and temperature, but also perform calculation and non-invasive measuring of cardiac output, transcutaneous oxygen, partial pressure oxygen saturation, and hemodynamic parameters such as vascular resistance. In addition, computers are being used to regulate the pressure, volume, and flow rate of ventilators to ensure that they deliver adequate volumes of gas. Further applications include the control of fluid resuscitation, anesthesia, serum glucose levels, arterial pressure, and energy expenditure (Andreoli & Musser, 1985; Roncoli, Brooten & Deliveria-Papadopoulos, 1986). Computer programs are available to help the nurse evaluate symptoms and to develop nursing diagnoses (Mehmert, 1987; Ryan, 1985).

Computers also are being used to help educate the patient regarding his or her health needs (Sinclair, 1985). Some systems help the nurse to explain post-hospitalization procedures to patients; others are interactive programs designed to help patients increase their awareness of good health habits.

Computers also are increasingly being used to assist in surgery. For example, computers assist in arteriography and angiography and help regulate autotransfusions during open heart and vascular surgery. Computers are used as well to facilitate diagnostic procedures and reconstructive surgery (Paquet, 1982).

PATIENT RECORDS: CHARTS, CARE PLANS, AND KARDEXES

The patient chart is a tool intended not only to identify and record important attributes of a patient's condition, but also to provide an account of the care given. With the increased complexity of health care delivery, including more tests, protocols, and procedures, the quantity of information in that medical chart has exploded. In most noncomputerized systems, each time new data are recorded, they are entered as independent events. This results in a sequential listing of events, not the integrated description of the patient's responses necessary for the delivery of professional health care. The patient's problems and symptoms are likely to be randomly scattered throughout the protocol descriptions, test results, and nursing notes. Because it is often difficult to locate and integrate these data, their cumulative implications are often underevaluated or missed. Furthermore, the pressures of legal liabilities, quality assurance investigations, audits, and research have mandated more attention to patient records.

Computerization makes the increased information easier to use. In most systems, the computer is able to rearrange data from the chart in any form useful to health care professionals. For example, using a computer, a nurse could isolate and examine the history of symptoms that a patient experienced during a stay (or previous stays). Or the nurse could investigate the effects of specified regimens on a particular symptom by relying on those same sorting and summarizing capabilities of the computer.

Some institutions are experimenting with bedside terminals for online charting (Hendrickson & Kovner, 1990). Nurses enter patient data and charting at the bedside terminal. Early findings suggest that nurses spend as much time charting when using bedside terminals as with the paper and pen method but they are more accurate. Physicians, however, do not like the system as well because they want to have all available information on a written chart to review before they enter the patient's room.

Care plans can be developed more easily with a computer for several reasons. First, nurses can be more efficient in recording their observations and developing appropriate plans because the system provides standard screens with standard choices. Having all possible options in front of them during planning not only simplifies the process, but it also reduces the likelihood that some factor might inadvertently be left unrecorded. An example of a nursing assessment menu is shown in Figure 7–6. Second, the nurse is made aware of changes that require her intervention as soon as possible because information from ancillary departments and some monitoring equipment is sent to the nursing station automatically. This allows a change in the care plan without delay. Third, computerization allows for some analyses (sorting of information in the patient record) to be done by the computer which provides the nurse with the necessary information to help in developing the care plan. Because the nurse can isolate the necessary information, trends or peculiarities can be identified. An example of a computer generated care plan is shown in Figure 7–7.

Computerized kardexes are also being tried in some institutions. This computer system prints a kardex-type work plan for communicating information at report. As a result of this type of system, less time is used in report at the change of shifts and the accuracy of information is increased. This system has been particularly helpful during the nursing shortage while temporary agency nurses are working on unfamiliar units (Hendrickson & Kovner, 1990).

FIGURE 7–6 NURSING ASSESSMENT MENU

PAGE NUMBERS FOR NURSING ORDERS

Basic Care
1. General Hygiene–excluding facial hygiene.
2. Facial hygiene.
3. Pressure area and sore care.
4. Aids for relief of pressure.
5. Position.
6. Mobility.
7. Intake–diet.
8. Intake–fluids.
9. Observation charts.
10. Observations.
13. Recordings.

Tests
20. Urine tests (ward).
21. Urine tests (laboratory).
22. Tests–excretary (except urine) and blood.
26. Swabs and aspirates.
28. Biopsies.
30. X-ray investigations.
35. Investigations–excluding x-rays.
39. Bovey day cases.

Treatments
40. Alimentary canal–upper.
41. Cardiac therapy.
42. Dialysis.
43. Genito-urinary tract–catheters.
44. Urology.
45. Genito-urinary tract–excluding catheters.

47. Infusion therapy.
48. Intestinal tract.
50. Orthopaedic–traction.
51. Orthopaedic–plaster.
52. Orthopaedic–exercise and appliances.
53. Ear, nose and throat.
56. Respiratory tract–inhalations.
57. Respiratory tract–excluding inhalations.
58. Skin–topical applications.
59. Skin–non topical.
60. Bandages.
61. Clips, sutures, clamp and rod.
63. Drains.
64. Dressings.
66. Packs.
67. Operation or investigation.
69. Treatments and applications–hot and cold.

Miscellaneous
70. Patient/relative tuition.
71. Patient/relative appointments, etc.
72. Therapy, clinics, visits and domiciliary services.
73. Transfer and transport.
74. Handicaps, etc.
75. Special precautions.
76. Reminders to nurse in charge.
77. ⎫
78. ⎭ Nursing problems (printed on care plans).
79. Sensitive problems (not printed on care plans).

C. Astbury, "Nursing Care Plans: Aspects of Computer Use in Nurse-to-Nurse Communication." In: *Medinfo–83 Seminars*, O. Fokkens et al., editors. © IFIP-IMIA; North-Holland, 1983. By permission of Elsevier Science Publishers BV, Amsterdam.

FIGURE 7–7 NURSING CARE PLAN

CARE PLAN			

```
                          CARE PLAN
                                                  08-03–PAGE 1 END
4436-02 MYERS MARTHA R          24Y BROWN JC            PT CLASS: 02
CUR DIAG:  ABDOMINAL PAIN                          MED INFO:
```

SURGERY:
SURGERY DATE/TIME: DAYS-STAY 06   POST-OP   POST-PARTUM
ALLERGIES FOOD: CITRUS FRUITS AND MILK PRODUCTS
ALLERGIES MED/OTHER:
PATIENT PROBLEM: HEARING IMPAIRMENT–USES HEARING AID   ISOLATION:

PROCEDURES-TESTS		08	09	10	11	12	13	14	15
0011	GB SERIES–RULE OUT GALLSTONES	ONCE	X							
A	NO SMOKING DURING PREP	CONT								
B	DELAY DIET AND FLUIDS EXCEPT SMALL AMTS OF H2O WITH NECESSARY PO MEDS	SFT 3 & 1								

ACTIVITY/MISCELLANEOUS										
0002	BLOOD PRESSURE BID	BID		X						
	PT CARE SUPPORTIVE ASSISTANCE	CONT								
A	SELF PERSONAL HYGIENE & FEEDING	CONT								
A003	LOW FAT DIET	CMEALS	X				X			

NURSING PROBLEMS/NURSING ACTION										
A002	PROBLEM 1–UPPER RT ABD PAIN	CONT								
A	OBSERVE AND REPORT TYPE OF PAIN, ONSET, DURATION, CONSTANCY AND SEVERITY	CONT								
B	OFFER PAIN MEDICATION PRN AS ORDERED	PRN								
C	RECORD RESULT OF MEDICATION	CONT								

LONG AND SHORT-TERM GOALS										
A004	SHORT-TERM GOAL–REASONABLE RELIEF FROM PAIN AND NAUSEA	CONT								

SOCIO-PSYCHOLOGICAL NEEDS										
A007	ANXIETY DUE TO IMPENDING TESTS ENCOURAGE VERBALIZATION OF FEELINGS	CONT								

TEACHING PLANS										
A006	EXPLAIN ALL TESTS AND TEST PREPARATIONS	ONCE	X							

NURSING OBSERVATIONS

```
                              VISIT CONDITION              SHIFT
4436-02 MYERS MARTHA R      K36752    RV    G    WED 08-03 –   1
```

TRAINING AND EVALUATION

Computerized instruction is an invaluable tool for nurse managers who need either to transmit new information to their staff or review acquired information. With the proliferation of microcomputers came increasing opportunities for interactive systems to facilitate teaching and practice of nursing functions. Such technology allows the nurse to practice a wide range of skills, such as calculation of fractional medication dosage, without jeopardy to the patient. Furthermore, the technology provides a variety of modes, from programmed learning to graphic, interactive simulations of nursing situations. One system, for example, provides a self-learning program on the physical assessment and clinical interpretation of arterial pulses. Another system helps nurses become proficient in calculating drug dosages by presenting clinical problems (with explanations) and providing pharmacological information and simple mathematical formulas as references, on which students can practice.

These computerized instructional systems can be an asset to the nurse manager. The advantages lie primarily in their flexibility in allowing learners to proceed at their own pace, their infinite patience in repeating material for individual users, and their non-judgmental approach to instruction. Furthermore, as the amount of nursing information continues to explode, computerized instructional packages help everyone keep pace, and computerized databases of nursing information will provide a ready source of instructional material. Finally, computers will allow more effective dissemination of information to nurses in remote areas who might not have continuing education or inservice programs available.

SCHEDULING AND STAFFING

Scheduling is one of the nurse manager's most frustrating and least fulfilling activities (see Chapter 4). No matter how much effort the manager puts into juggling the resources and policies to determine working hours, he or she is not likely to arrive at a stable schedule or, according to nurses, one that is both flexible and fair. The problem in developing a schedule is that there is generally too much information for one person to handle. However, the computer's specialty is just that: handling a lot of information systematically. This makes it a natural to help in the scheduling function.

The first step in developing a schedule, of course, is to analyze the need for nursing care in a particular unit. This step is, in part, dictated by institutional standards. It is also influenced by the current and expected demands for various types of nursing personnel occasioned by the patient mix of the unit. The computer can help with this latter requirement. The computer can determine each patient's current nursing needs by screening his or her record for assessment indicators and determining the illness acuity. This needs analysis can be helpful not only for the specific time period for which the schedule is being created, but also for long-term staffing. By analyzing the historical needs per type of patient as well as needs determined by patient mix, the nurse manager can better estimate how many of what types of nurses are needed to handle the expected load of the unit. (See Chapter 4 for more on classification systems to determine nursing care requirements.)

If the computer does not include historical data, then such information must be entered as input by the nurse manager (see Figure 7–8). Once the accumulated workload needs have

FIGURE 7–8 WEEKLY STAFF REQUIREMENTS

Unit Number _____

Staffing Categories

(Administrators include head nurse and assistant head nurses)

	S	M	T	W	T	F	S
Min. # administrators (SUP) shift 1 (beg. 7 AM)							
Desired # administrators (SUP) shift 1							
Min. # administrators (SUP) shift 2 (beg. 3 PM)							
Desired # administrators (SUP) shift 2							
Min. # administrators (SUP) shift 3 (beg. 11 PM)							
Desired # administrators (SUP) shift 3							

(Exclude head nurse and assistant head nurse in RN counts)

	S	M	T	W	T	F	S
Min. # RN staff shift 1 (beg. 7 AM)							
Desired # RN staff shift 1							
Min. # RN staff shift 2 (beg. 3 PM)							
Desired # RN staff shift 2							
Min. # RN staff shift 3 (beg. 11 PM)							
Desired # RN staff shift 3							

	S	M	T	W	T	F	S
Min. # LPN staff shift 1 (beg. 7 AM)							
Desired # LPN staff shift 1							
Min. # LPN staff shift 2 (beg. 3 PM)							
Desired # LPN staff shift 2							
Min. # LPN staff shift 3 (beg. 11 PM)							
Desired # LPN staff shift 3							

Staffing Categories (cont.)

	S	M	T	W	T	F	S
Min. # aide staff shift 1 (beg. 7 AM)							
Desired # aide staff shift 1							
Min. # aide staff shift 2 (beg. 3 PM)							
Desired # aide staff shift 2							
Min. # aide staff shift 3 (beg. 11 PM)							
Desired # aide staff shift 3							

	S	M	T	W	T	F	S
Min. # secretaries shift 1 (beg. 7 AM)							
Desired # secretaries shift 1							
Min. # secretaries shift 2 (beg. 3 PM)							
Desired # secretaries shift 2							
Min. # secretaries shift 3 (beg. 11 PM)							
Desired # secretaries shift 3							

Minimum Requirements for Skill Categories in Combination

	S	M	T	W	T	F	S
Min. # SUP + RNs shift 1 (beg. 7 AM)							
Min. # SUP + RNs shift 2 (beg. 3 PM)							
Min. # SUP + RNs shift 3 (beg. 11 PM)							
Min. # SUP + RN + LPNs shift 1 (beg. 7 AM)							
Min. # SUP + RN + LPNs shift 2 (beg. 3 PM)							
Min. # SUP + RN + LPNs shift 3 (beg. 11 PM)							
Min. # SUP + RN + LPN + aides shift 1 (beg. 7 AM)							
Min. # SUP + RN + LPN + aides shift 2 (beg. 3 PM)							
Min. # SUP + RN + LPN + aides shift 3 (beg. 11 PM)							

From L. Douglas Smith and A. Wiggins, "A Computer-Based Nurse Scheduling System," *Computer and Operations Research*, pp. 195-212, New York: Pergamon Press, 1977.

been established, the computer can consider the actual scheduling question. A nurse manager would use the nursing needs, the institutional policies in regard to nurse scheduling, and the numbers and qualifications of available staff as input to the system. Many systems have additional flexibility and can accept information about the preferences of nurses and their past schedules or performance to help obtain a schedule that meets not only the requirements, but also the preferences of the nursing staff (see Figure 7–9).

Once given these data, the computer, much like a nurse manager, juggles the demands of the unit against the supply of nursing personnel for that unit. One difference between the approaches that the computer and the nurse manager use is that the computer can consider all possible options and their value before choosing a given schedule. Further, the computer is impartial and can weigh many more factors at any given time than can the nurse manager.

An example of a schedule that might result from computer evaluation of the staffing needs is shown in Figure 7–10. It obviously looks very much like one prepared by hand. The nurse manager does not need to rely on the capabilities of the institution's computer to perform these tasks. Some relatively low-cost microcomputer packages can provide help in setting staffing levels.

In summary, it is advantageous to use computers for scheduling functions. Nurses are often more satisfied with their schedule, primarily because they perceive that they are being treated more fairly. Also, unlike most nurse managers, the computer can easily balance all the necessary information for even the largest of units. Further, because the computer can consider the needs for personnel beyond any one unit, it can evaluate opportunities for sharing personnel with other units to improve the overall efficiency of nursing coverage. Finally, the computer can handle the complexities associated with flextime and split shifts that are almost impossible to consider by hand; this capability can make the unit a more desirable working place (Fitzpatrick, Farrell & Richter-Zeunick, 1987).

SUPPLIES AND MATERIALS MANAGEMENT

Nurse managers and materials managers frequently clash because the former contend that supplies are not available when needed while the latter contend that too many supplies are not being used but kept in inventory. The resulting conflict stems from the perspectives of the two positions. The computer, with its almost limitless capability for weighing many factors simultaneously, organizing data, and preparing reports, can be an effective tool for resolving conflict between the two perspectives.

A computerized inventory system has two purposes: (a) to generate efficient inventory policies that could be considered for implementation and (b) to maintain control over how supplies are being used. To meet these goals, the system must be able to keep accurate records of the supplies being used in each unit as well as to determine when to place an order for more supplies. The system must be able to forecast usage of supplies, determine the time at which reordering should occur, and determine the total amount of an item that should be ordered at any given time. Furthermore, the system must be able to analyze each item or group of items separately to determine if different ordering policies are warranted for different supplies.

The differences among systems center on how the forecasting of future demand is computed and on how the removal of products from

FIGURE 7-9 PROTOTYPE

Employee Data Form for Shift Scheduling

1. Name __Blank, L__   2. Employee Number _____10886_____
3. Classification _____1_____   (1-head nurse, 2-assistant head, 3-RN, 4-LPN, 5-NA/ORD, 6-Sec.)
4. Unit Number _____215_____
Number of Shifts to be Assigned Weekly:
5 Minimum __3__   6. Desired __5__   7. Maximum __6__
8. Number of weekends can work between weekends off _____1_____
Length of work stretch (consec. days):
9. Min. (usually 2) __2__   10. Max. (usually 6) __6__
11. Shift Rankings (1: beg. – 7 AM; 2: beg.– 3 PM; 3: beg.– 11PM)
(If hired for straight shifts, specify first choice only)
First Choice _1__   Second Choice __3__   Third Choice _2__
12. Allocate 10 aversion points among choices of shift (aversion points must *increase* in value from 1st to 2nd to 3rd choice – let first choice aversion be 9999 if on straight shifts).

First Choice   Second Choice   Third Choice
Aversion__0__   Aversion __5__   Aversion __5__
13. Indicate preference for the first day off in a week prior to a weekend off. (2=Mon.; 3=Tues.; 4=Wed.; 5=Thurs.; 6=Fri.)

First	Second	Third	Fourth	Fifth
Choice_2__	Choice_3__	Choice__4__	Choice__6__	Choice__5__

14. Indicate preference for the second day off in a week following a weekend off.

First	Second	Third	Fourth	Fifth
Choice__6__	Choice__2__	Choice__4__	Choice__3__	Choice__5__

15. Indicate preference for day-off pairs midweek. [Usual alternatives are (2,3), (3,4), (4,5), (5,6), (2,5) (2,6), (3,6).]

First Choice Pair_3_,_4_; Second Choice_2_,_3_; Third Choice_4_,_5_; Fourth Choice_5_,_6_; Fifth Choice_2_,_6_; Sixth Choice_3_,_6_; Seventh Choice_2_,_5_.
16. Cumulative number of holidays due __0__
17. Cumulative number of vacation days due __0__
18. Current value of shift aversion index __5__
19. Current value of day-off aversion index __2__
20. Number of times shifts worked to date:
Shift 1__0__   Shift 2__0__   Shift 3__0__
21. Shift worked on last day of previous month __1__
22. Number of weekends worked since last weekend off__1__
23. Last day off previous week __6__
24. Remarks:

Adapted from L. Douglas Smith and A. Wiggins "A Computer-Based Nurse Scheduling System,"*Computer and Operations Research*, pp. 195-212. New York: Pergamon Press, 1977.

inventory is controlled and audited. Some systems require that demand be input by the nurse manager; she must make an educated guess on what the patient mix will be over time and what

supplies are warranted for that mix. In other systems, demand is computed on the assumption that the same usage of supplies that was observed in the most recent similar period will con-

FIGURE 7-10 SCHEDULE RESULTS

Schedule for period beginning June 10, 1973

	10 Su	11 Mo	12 Tu	13 We	14 Th	15 Fr	16 Sa	17 Su	18 Mo	19 Tu	20 We	21 Th	22 Fr	23 Sa	24 Su	25 Mo	26 Tu	27 We	28 Th	29 Fr	30 Sa	1 Su	2 Mo	3 Tu	4 We	5 Th	6 Fr	7 Sa	Ro/%m	WE	RG	RM*	RF
1. Hale	D	D	D		D	D	D		D	D	D		D	D	D		D	D	D		D	D	D		D	D				50	0	0	26
2. Collins	D		D	D	D	D		D	D	D		D	D	D		D	D	D	D		D	D	D	D	D		D	D		50	0	0	12
3. Smith	N	–	–	–		N	N	N	N	N	N		N	N	N		N	N	N	N	N		N	N	N	N			51	0	0	28
4. Palmer	N	N		N	N	N	N	B		–	–	–	–	–		N	N	N	N		N	N	N	N					0	0	0	28
5. Jones	N	N	N						N	N		N	N	N	N	•	•	•	•	N	N								51	40	40	28
6. Peabody	DE	D		E	E	E	E		E	E		D	D	D	D		N	D	D	D	D		D	D	•			26	48	5	5	28
7. Penna	DN	N	N		D	D	D	•	–	–	C		N	N	N		N	D	D	D	D		D	D	D			27	48	5	5	28
8. Clark	DN	•	–	–	–	–	•	D	D	D		N	N	N		N	D	D	D	D		D	D	D	D		D	D	23	50	12	12	28
9. Cunkle	DR		N	N	D	D		D	D	D	D		D	D		D	C	C	C		E	E	E	E		D	D	D	27/10	50	0	0	28
10. Myers	DR	D	D	D		N	N	D		D	D		D	D	E	E		E	E	E	E		D	D					28/9	50	0	0	28
11. Hill	DR	D	D	D		D	E	E	D	D	D		D	C	C	C		N	D	D	D		N	D	D				25/20	51	0	0	28
12. Andrews	E	E	E		E	E	E	•	•	–	E	E		E	E	E	E		E	E	E		E	E	E		E	E		50	10	10	28
13. Sutherland	E	E	E	E		E	E	•	•	–	E	E	E		E	E	E	E		E	E	•	•	H	–	–	–	–	–	51	35	35	28
14. Levine	E	E	E	E	E		E	E	E		E	E	E			E	E	E		E	E	E	E		E	E	E	E	50	0	0	28
15. Anderson	D	D	D	D		D	D	D		D	D	D	D		D	D	D	D		D	D	D		D	D		53	0	0	8
16. Green	DE	D	D	D	D	D		D	D		E	E	E	E		D	D	D	D		D	D		E	E	E		27	51	0	5	28
17. Majors	N		N	N	N	N	N		N	–	–	–	–	•	•	–	N	N	N	N		N	N	N	N				6	6	28
18. Greenberg	DE	D	E	E		D	D	•	•	B	–		D	D	D	D		D	C	C	C		E	E		E	E	D	D	25	50	13	13	28
19. Waxman	DR		D	D	D		D	D	D		N	N	N	N		D	E	E		D	D	D		D	D	D		26/10	50	0	0	28
20. Hagen	DE	D	D	D		E	E		D	D	D	D	•		D	D	D	D		D	D	D		D	E	E		D	D	24	51	11	11	28
21. Pearlman	DE	E		D	D	D	D		•	D	D	D		D	D	E	E		D	D	D		D	D	D		D	D	23	50	5	6	28
22. Wilson	DE		D	D	D	D		E	E	E	E		D	D	D		D	D		•	D	D	D	D	E		25	51	5	5	28
23. Grycz	E		E	E	E	E	•	E	E	E	•	E	E	E		E	E	E	E	•	E	E	E	•	E	E	D		50	5	5	28
24. Rapley	E	E	E	E		E	E	E	E		E	E	E	E		E	E	E		E	E	E	E		E	D	E		50	0	0	28
25. James	E			E			E	E	E					E	E	E	E										50	0	0	28
26. McCarry	N	N	N			N	N	N	N			N	N	N	N			N	N	N	N			N	N				0	0	28
27. Barkan	N	N	N			N	N	N	N		N	N	N			N	N	N	N			N	N	N	N				0	0	28
28. Downing	N		N	N	N	N	N		N	N	N	N	N		N	N	N	N	N			N	N	N	N			0	0	28
29. Gammer	D		D	D	D	D		D	D	D	D	D		D	D	D	D		D	D	D	D			0	0	28
30. Mitchell	D	D	D	D	D		D	D	D	D		D	D	D	D		D	D	D	D					0	0	28
31. Liary	E	E	E		E		E		E		E	E		E		E		E		E	E	E			0	0	28
32. Santos	E	E		E	E	E	E		E	E	E	E		E	E	E	E		E	E	E	E		0	0	28

RNS

	Su	Mo	Tu	We	Th	Fr	Sa	Su	Mo	Tu	We	Th	Fr	Sa	Su	Mo	Tu	We	Th	Fr	Sa	Su	Mo	Tu	We	Th	Fr	Sa
Nite	2	2	2	2	2	2	2	2	2	2	2	2	2	2	3	2	2	2	2	2	2	2	2	2	2	2	2	2
Day	3	6	5	6	6	6	4	3	6	5	5	6	6	3	3	6	7+6	5	5	4	4	7+6	6	6	6	6	3
Even	2	3	3	4	3	2	2	3	3	3	3	3	3	3	3	3	3	3	3	2	2	3	4	3	3	3	2

RN + LPN

	Su	Mo	Tu	We	Th	Fr	Sa	Su	Mo	Tu	We	Th	Fr	Sa	Su	Mo	Tu	We	Th	Fr	Sa	Su	Mo	Tu	We	Th	Fr	Sa
Nite	2	3	3	3	3	3	2	2	3	3	3	3	3	2	2	3	3	3	3	3	2	2	3	3	3	3	2
Day	5	9	9	9	9	10+5	5	5	8	7	7	8	6	5	9	9	8	8	9	5	5	9	9	9	9	10+6
Even	4	6	6	5	6	5	4	4	6	5	5	6	5	4	5	6	5	5	5	5	4	4	6	6	5	6	5	4

Total

	Su	Mo	Tu	We	Th	Fr	Sa	Su	Mo	Tu	We	Th	Fr	Sa	Su	Mo	Tu	We	Th	Fr	Sa	Su	Mo	Tu	We	Th	Fr	Sa
Nite	4	5	5	5	5	5	4	4	5	5	5	5	5	4	4	5	5	5	5	5	4	4	5	5	5	5	5	4
Day	6	10	11	11	11	11	6	6	9	9	9	9	9	6	10	11	10	10	10	6	6	10	11	11	11	11	7
Even	4	7	7	7	7	5	4	7	6	7	7	7	5	5	7	6	7	6	7	5	4	7	7	7	7	7	5

*Request: Vacation, C Hospital business, B Birthday, H Holiday off tinue over some future period. The remainder of the systems have a forecasting component that analyzes trends in past usage of supplies for a particular mix of patients at a particular time of year and bases the forecast on the assumption that these conditions will continue. Similarly, packages differ on how the request for items is entered into the system and on how much control there is over reporting of items on that system.

COMMUNICATION WITH PHARMACY, LABORATORY, AND RADIOLOGY

While the major benefits to nursing of a computerized system are the reduced time spent doing paperwork and the associated increase in time available for professional nursing functions, computers are also helpful when nursing is interfacing with support units such as pharmacy, laboratory, and radiology. Computers can increase the effectiveness of the interface between nursing and these units by making the communications clearer and more uniform and can increase the efficiency of the interface by reducing the amount of time spent in this function.

In many health care institutions, nurses are responsible for record keeping related to medication orders and administration; in smaller institutions they might also be responsible for dosage preparation and medication inventory. A computerized system can help in the record keeping and can be used to request medication from the pharmacy (see Figure 7–11).

FIGURE 7–11a OBTAINING MEDICATION INFORMATION FROM A PHARMACY PROFILE

■   PHARMACY ACTIVE ORDER PROFILE 07-30–1200

PATIENT NAME	AGE	SEX	NSTA	ROOM-BED	PATIENT-ID	WEIGHT	SURG DT/TM

▶MYERS MARTHA R ◀24Y   F   4C   4436-02   803254   110 LB

  ALLERGIES-FOOD: CITRUS FRUITS AND MILK PRODUCTS

▶ALLERGIES-MED/OTHER: PENICILLIN

  PATIENT PROBLEMS: HEARING IMPAIRMENT-USES HEARING AID

CURRENT DIAG: POSSIBLE CHOLECYSTOLITHIASIS   MED INFO:

ORDER	PROC	RT	FREQUENCY	START DT/TM	LAST DT/TM	DOSAGE	ORDERING DOCTOR
0015	14652	▶IM	Q4HPRN	07-29 1400		50MG	BROWN JC

    ▶DRAMAMINE   50.000MG/1ML INJECTION

DIMENHYDRINATE   SEARLE

| 0016 | 17854 | ▶IM | Q4HPRN | 07-29 1400 | 08-01 1400 | 50MG | BROWN JC |

    ▶DEMEROL   50.000MG/1ML INJECTION

    MEPERIDINE HYDROCHLORIDE   XXXXX

Page 1

The nurse's interface with such systems varies. In one system, pharmacy personnel collect and use carbon copies of physicians' medication orders; they input the information into the system. Then, at regular intervals, the pharmacy makes the requested medication available to the nurses for administration. The only paperwork necessary for the nurse is to complete a form that is returned to the pharmacy indicating that the medication has been administered or, if not, why not. All other record keeping is done on the computer at the pharmacy.

If the charts are computerized, the orders to the pharmacy are placed automatically when the physician enters instructions. Alternatively, the nurse might simply enter the information on a terminal at the nursing station. Whatever the form of input to the system, computerized pharmacy systems allow for better auditing of medication (Long, 1982).

The computer also creates an easily accessible record of medication patterns and reasons for failure to maintain those patterns. For example, in some systems, the nurse receives medication

---

FIGURE 7–11b ENTERING MEDICATION ORDERS

```
■      PHARMACY IV ORDER ENTRY    07-29–1030
PATIENT NAME          PTID/RMBD        ORDERING DOCTOR
MYERS MARTHA R        4436-02          BROWN JC               SURG:
CURR DIAG:  POSSIBLE CHOLECYSTOLITHIASIS                      MED INFO:


►024       SOLUTION–SELECT ONE FROM BASE SOLUTIONS BELOW OR ENTER OTHER SOLUTION
►14        VOLUME 1 = 1000CC  2 = 500CC  3 = 250CC  4 = 100CC  OTHER  ►           ◄
                   ENTER X BESIDE ADDITIVES TO INCLUDE IN ORDER
                         ►******A D D I T I V E S******◄
►◄ KCL 40 MEQ                          ►◄AMINOPHYLLINE 500 MG
►◄ BERROCA-C 500 4 CC                  ►◄KEFLIN 10M
►◄ BERROCA-C 2 CC                      ►◄SODIUM PENICILLIN C 5 MG
►◄ MVI CONCEN 5 CC                     ►◄ADDITIONAL ADDITIVES
                         ►******B A S E  S O L U T I O N******◄
01 = 5% DEX & 2% SOD CHL               11 = 50% DEX INJ
02 = 5% DEX INJ                        12 = 5% DEX EL-LYTE #75
03 = 5% DEX % .45% SOD CHL             13 = 5% DEX/ASCOR-B-SOL
04 = 5% DEX IN LACT RING INJ           14 = 2.5% DEX I& .45% SOD CHL
05 = LACTATED RINGERS INJ              15 = AMMON CHL IN W 2.14%
06 = SOD CHL INJ .9                    16 = 10% DEX & .9% SOD CHL
07 = 10% INV SUGAR IN ELECT 2          17 = SODIUM LACTATE INJ
08 = DEX & .9% SOD CHL                 18 = 5% SOD BICARBONATE
09 = 5% DEX EL-LYTE #48                19 = 6% SOD BICARBONATE
10 = 10% DEX INJ                       OTHER=►
```

Page 1

BHIS (Unisys)

prepackaged for each patient and must return the package after the medication has been administered. If the medication was not given, the nurse must state those reasons on the package. These packages, when returned to the pharmacy, provide data to be used as input into the pharmacy system. These data can be accessed easily for evaluating a particular patient, all patients in a particular unit, all patients in a particular diagnostic category, or all patients receiving that medication. More important, these summaries can be provided in a matter of minutes.

Computerized systems can be designed to include as part of the pharmacy system a "library" of drug information that can be reviewed to determine the expected side effects of medication, drug interactions (especially synergistic ones), and associated nursing requirements. Or, the nursing unit may have a stand-alone system, such as "Nursing Pharmacology," on which they can check the compatibility of drug interactions, drug dosages, time infusion rates, etc. Such systems can also prepare instructions for patients when they leave the hospital, including the purpose for each drug, its possible side effects, appropriate dietary or activity instructions, and effects that should be reported to the physician.

Laboratory and radiology systems have similar advantages from the nursing perspective. Entering an order into the patient's chart automatically alerts the appropriate unit to schedule a test. Once the test has been scheduled, some systems will send a pretest regimen for the patient or reminders of schedules to the nursing station. In many cases, these studies are analyzed by a computer and the results are routed immediately to the nursing station, entered into the patient's chart, and summarized for review by the nurse and physician.

Such computerized systems tend to decrease errors because they have better and more sys-

tematic checks than manual operations, they reduce the amount of nursing time spent away from patient care, and they reduce the amount of waste due to errors. However, they can also have some disadvantages, which need the attention of the nurse manager. The most significant problem is how the nurses react when the computer is not available for use. Many nurses, even those who were at the hospital before computerization, forget the necessary procedures for ordering medication, X-rays, and tests without the computer. Since computer failures are a reality in all organizations, the nurse manager must prepare the staff for this situation. Furthermore, the manager must ensure that appropriate regimens are being followed even if, because of computer failure, nurses are not able to receive "reminders."

The second problem associated with these systems is more subtle: the absence of human interaction between the unit and other units on a regular basis. Sometimes, smoothly operating systems exist because people can relate to people in the other unit on a one-to-one basis. If all the communications are electronic, then those relationships and the value they add to the system are lost. Thus, if such relationships are necessary for operations, the nurse manager must foster them in other ways.

◆ NURSING INFORMATION SYSTEMS

Each application previously identified, as well as some others, can be used independently. However, computerization is more effective when an integrated system is in place through which the various units communicate. An integrated system such as this is referred to as a nursing information system (NIS), a hospital information system (HIS), or a medical information system (MIS).

A nursing information system is one that assists the nurse in determining a nursing diagnosis and developing a nursing care plan, recommends interventions, and determines evaluation strategies. An NIS also provides the nurse manager with a way to determine the number of patient care hours needed based on patient acuity. Since the patient's chart is in the system, documentation can be done on the computer. The cost of patient care can usually be determined by the NIS, also. A nursing information system was developed for use at Mercy Hospital in Davenport, Iowa (see Figure 7–12). A computerized system was selected that was user friendly, that had the capability for full order entry, that had the potential for a patient acuity system, and that could be used for nursing diagnosis-based care planning (Mehmert, 1987). Additionally, the system was able to determine staffing needs.

◆ HOSPITAL INFORMATION SYSTEMS

The highest level of hospital information systems allows all of the previous possibilities plus uses the computer to analyze trends in overall patient responses and to develop care plans. This level is referred to as a total hospital information system. The benefits of such a system are illustrated in Figure 7–13, which shows how a typical patient's information flows through the system.

The HIS has several important advantages for the nurse. First, HIS facilitates reading and understanding of both the physician's instructions and the nursing care plans. Since all entries use standard forms, the chart documents have a uniform format that makes them readable and clear. This reduces the ambiguity that often re-

sults from handwritten observations and instructions. Second, the system allows results from tests and radiology to be available to the nursing staff as soon as possible, thus reducing the delay that is often characteristic of manual systems and allowing the nurse to make changes in care plans as early as possible. Third, it facilitates the discussion of patient care between shifts because care plans and test results are available in an easily followed format for consideration. Fourth, it provides reminders of care needs such as medication administration or special preparation for tests. Fifth, it facilitates the preparation of care reports. Finally, it improves the utility of the patient chart not only because of the previously stated advantages, but also because the computer itself can perform some analyses on the information to highlight abnormalities that need attention or peculiarities that arise in response to patient care.

Figure 7–14 illustrates the changes that would be experienced by the staff as a result of conversion to an automated system. In the manual system, the nurse spends substantial time completing paperwork, waiting on the telephone, and running errands. With a computerized system the nurse has only to enter the information on the terminal and all of the paperwork is completed and all orders are sent automatically. Further, the total system eliminates problems in reading reports and delays in sending or receiving orders and decreases the errors made in calculations because the human interaction in these areas is minimized.

◆ NONHOSPITAL SYSTEMS

Computers also can be used in nursing outside of the hospital environment, such as in home health care. Historically, the use of computers in the nonhospital environment has followed the

FIGURE 7–12 NURSING INFORMATION SYSTEM MODEL

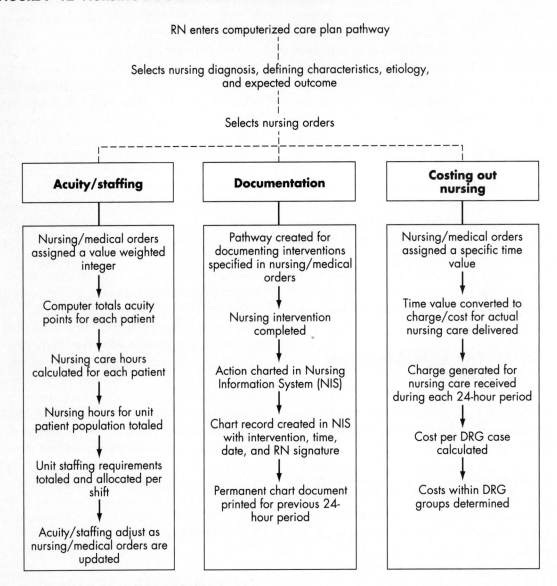

RN enters computerized care plan pathway

Selects nursing diagnosis, defining characteristics, etiology, and expected outcome

Selects nursing orders

Acuity/staffing	Documentation	Costing out nursing
Nursing/medical orders assigned a value weighted integer	Pathway created for documenting interventions specified in nursing/medical orders	Nursing/medical orders assigned a specific time value
Computer totals acuity points for each patient	Nursing intervention completed	Time value converted to charge/cost for actual nursing care delivered
Nursing care hours calculated for each patient	Action charted in Nursing Information System (NIS)	Charge generated for nursing care received during each 24-hour period
Nursing hours for unit patient population totaled	Chart record created in NIS with intervention, time, date, and RN signature	Cost per DRG case calculated
Unit staffing requirements totaled and allocated per shift	Permanent chart document printed for previous 24-hour period	Costs within DRG groups determined
Acuity/staffing adjust as nursing/medical orders are updated		

© Department of Nursing, Mercy Hospital, Davenport, Iowa. April 1986, Rev. 1/87.

FIGURE 7-13 INFORMATION TRANSFER IN A HOSPITAL INFORMATION SYSTEM

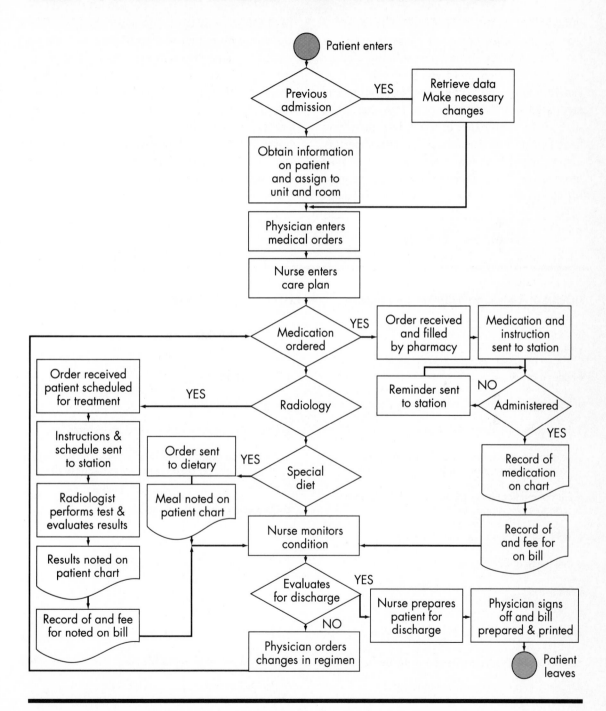

same pattern as that in hospitals. The early use was in the development of financial and accounting records through which the agency could track patients and employees as well as generate bills. Over time, computerization has facilitated the management of staff as well. Also, with greater confidence in computers, managers have begun to use them to track nurses' performance, thereby allowing them to evaluate staff more fairly. This, in turn, has reduced the need for close monitoring; nurses often do not need to check in with their supervisors daily and so can spend more time with their patients.

More recently, computers have also been used by nurses in patient care. Nurses can keep uniform notes on patient changes, thus providing more reliable observation records and care plans. Based on these developments, nurses in home health care will probably soon be deriving the same benefits from computerized systems that nurses in hospitals do now. Nurses will have available a base of information for refer-

---

FIGURE 7-14 COMPARISON OF MANUAL AND AUTOMATED SYSTEMS

I. MANUAL

- Physician order.

- Check chart.

- Stamp pharmacy request with patient plate.

- Transcribe order to requisition.

- Telephone pharmacy regarding STAT. Have STAT request taken to pharmacy.

- Fill out medication card or sheet. (Calculate schedule and stop time.)

- Add medication to patient kardex.

- Tell nurse of STAT order.

II. AUTOMATED

- Physician order.

- Check chart.

- Sign on to terminal.

- Enter medication order via pharmacy pathway.

- Requisition prints in pharmacy. New order prints on unit (bells on both printers ring because of STAT).

- Give copy of new order to nurse.

Problems

1. Legibility

2. Number of forms handled on nursing unit.

3. Error potential on schedule calculated.

4. Delay in pharmacy receiving request.

Solutions

1. All reports legible.

2. None used to enter order.

3. Calculated automatically.

4. Immediate notification.

ence, the capability to communicate with other professionals, and access to extensive training packages.

♦ SURVIVING WITH COMPUTERS

One purpose of a computerized system is to reduce the amount of paperwork done by nurses and thus facilitate patient care. Wolfe (1990) suggests two simple steps to remember when instituting computerization. The first is defining the computing needs of the unit (based on goals) and the second is choosing the appropriate hardware and software configuration. The key to surviving with computers is to remember those facts.

The nurse's and nurse manager's jobs will change as a result of computerization. For example, the nurse manager will not need to dedicate as much attention to scheduling and hence will have more time and energy for improving the interworking relationships and the efficiency and effectiveness of the unit and for developing better educational programs for the unit staff. The nurse and nurse manager will spend less time being clerks and more time being professionals.

SUMMARY

♦ Effective communication skills are essential tools for the nurse manager in managing personnel. These skills, like many others, can be learned.

♦ Effective communication is based on a theoretical understanding and application of management communication.

♦ Communication channels operate as both direct (formal) and indirect (informal) lines in an organization.

♦ Effective communication through human interaction involves understanding principles of effective communication, using verbal and nonverbal techniques, listening, and developing assertive behavior.

♦ Communication can be easily distorted. It is important to use exact language to present congruent verbal and nonverbal messages, and to consider the context in all communication.

♦ Communication between the nurse manager and subordinates, superiors, and physicians revolves around their mutual tasks.

♦ The nurse manager conveys the institution's image of competency and professionalism to the public.

♦ Computers are used in health care institutions for patient monitoring and care as well as for scheduling, training, and evaluation. Computers also are used to order and record pharmacy supplies, laboratory tests, radiology orders, and supplies and materials management.

♦ Nursing information systems (NISs) are used in some institutions, and hospital information systems may include an NIS. These systems integrate all computer use in one system.

BIBLIOGRAPHY

Aries, E. (1987). "Gender and Communication." In: *Sex and Gender*. Shaver, P., and Hendrick, C. (editors). Newbury Park, CA: Sage Publications. Pp. 149–176.

Andreoli, K., and Musser, L. (1985). "Computers in Nursing Care: The State of the Art." *Nursing Outlook,* 33(1): 16–21.

Asante, M. (editor). (1980). "Intercultural Communication: An Inquiry into Research Direction." In: *Communication Yearbook 4.* New Brunswick, NJ: Transaction Books. Pp. 401–410.

Bowman, J. (1990). "Response to Johan van Hoorde." *Journal of Business Communication,* 27(1): 71–74.

Bradley, P. (1981). "The Folk-Linguistics of Women's Speech: An Empirical Investigation." *Communication Monographs,* 48: 73–90.

Brimm, J. (1987). "Computers in Critical Care." *Critical Care Nursing Quarterly,* 9(4): 53–56.

Buono, A., Bowditch, J., and Lewis, J. (1985). "When Cultures Collide: The Anatomy of a Merger." *Human Relations,* 38(5): 477–500.

Chenevert, M. (1988). *STAT, Special Techniques in Assertiveness Training for Women in Health Professions.* 2d ed. St. Louis, MO: C. V. Mosby.

Chodorow, N. (1978). *The Reproduction of Mothering.* Berkeley, CA: University of California Press.

Cook, M., and McDowell, W. (1975). "Changing to an Automated Information System." *American Journal of Nursing,* 75: 46.

Culbert, S., and McDonough, J. (1980). *The Invisible War: Pursuing Self-Interests at Work.* New York: Wiley.

Curtin, L. (1982). "Nursing: Patient Care and Computers. How They Work Together." *Nursing Management,* 13: 25.

Deaux, K. (1985). "Sex and Gender." *Annual Review of Psychology,* 36: 49–81.

Donaldson, L., and Scannell, E. (1979). *Human Response Development: The New Trainer's Guide.* Reading, MA: Addison-Wesley. Pp. 47–48.

Douglass, L. (1984). *The Effective Nurse.* 2d ed. St. Louis, MO: C. V. Mosby.

Dumont, E. (1985). "The Computer Doesn't Have a Heart!" *Journal of Gerontological Nursing,* 11(4): 48.

Edwards, L. (1982). "Computer-Assisted Nursing Care." *American Journal of Nursing,* 82(7): 1076.

Fitzpatrick, T., Farrell, L., and Richter-Zeunick, M. (1987). "An Automated Staff Scheduling System That Minimizes Payroll Costs and Maximizes Staff Satisfaction." *Computers in Nursing,* 5(1): 10.

Foster, B., Jackson, G., Cross, W., Jackson, B., and Hardiman, R. (1988). "Workforce Diversity and Business." *Training and Development Journal,* 42(4): 38–42.

Hales, G. (1985). "A Different Perspective." *Computers in Nursing,* 3(5): 194.

Hanamura, S. (1989). "Working with People Who Are Different." *Training and Development Journal,* 43(6): 110–114.

Hendrickson, G., and Kovner, T. (1990). "Effects of Computers on Nursing Resource Use." *Computers in Nursing,* 8(1): 16–22.

Kenton, S. (1989). "Speaker Credibility in Persuasive Business Communication: A Model which Explains Gender Differences." *Journal of Business Communication,* 26(2): 143–157.

Kramer, C. (1978). "Male and Female Perceptions of Male and Female Speech." *Language and Speech,* 20(2): 151–161.

Leet-Pellegrini, H. (1980). "Conversational Dominance as a Function of Gender and Expertise." In: *Language: Social Psychological Perspective.* Giles, H., Robinson, W., and Smith, P. (editors). New York: Pergamon. Pp. 97–104.

Long, G. (1982). "The Effect of Medication Distribution Systems on Medication Errors." *Nursing Research,* 31: 182.

Masterson, B., and Murphy, B. (1986). "Internal Cross-Cultural Management." *Training and Development Journal,* 40(4): 56–60.

Max, R. (1985). "Wording It Correctly." *Training and Development Journal,* 39(3): 50–51.

Mehmert, P. (1987). "A Nursing Information System." *Nursing Clinics of North America,* 22(4): 943–953.

Mitchell, R. (1986). "Team Building by Disclosure of Internal Frames of Reference." *Journal of Applied Behavioral Science,* 22(1): 15–28.

Muller, P. (1980). "Using an Active Listening Model." *Supervisor Nurse* 11(April): 44–46.

Paquet, J. (1982). "OR Computers: The Future Is Today." *Today's OR Nurse,* 4(1): 10.

Pulliam, L., and Boettcher, E. (1989). "A Process for Introducing Computerized Information Systems into Long-Term Care Facilities." *Computers in Nursing,* 7(6): 251–257.

Roncoli, M., Brooten, D., and Delivoria-Papadopoulos, M. (1986). "A Computerized System for Measuring the Effect of Nursing Care Activities on Clinical Indices of Energy Expenditure." *Computer Methods and Programs in Biomedicine,* 22(1): 53–60.

Ryan, S. (1985). "An Expert System for Nursing Practice: Clinical Decision Support." *Computers in Nursing,* 3(2): 77.

Schifiliti, C., Bonasoro, C., and Thompson, M. (1986). "LOTUS 1-2-3: A Quality Assurance Application for Nursing Practice, Administration and Staff Development." *Computers in Nursing,* 4(5): 205.

Schwartz, H., and Davis, S. (1981). "Matching Corporate Culture and Business Strategy." *Organizational Dynamics* (Summer): 30–48.

Shannon, C., and Weaver, W. (1949). *The Mathematical Theory of Communication.* Urbana, IL: University of Illinois Press.

Shelby, A. (1988). "A Macro Theory of Management Communication." *Journal of Business Communication,* 25(2): 13–27.

Sinclair, V. (1985). "The Computer as a Partner in Healthcare Instruction." *Computers in Nursing,* 3(5): 212.

Smith, M. (1975). *When I Say No, I Feel Guilty.* New York: Bantam.

Sorenson, R., and Savage, G. (1989). "Signaling Participation through Relational Communication." *Group and Organizational Studies,* 14(3): 325–354.

Squire, P. (1982). "Monitoring a Sick Pattern." *Nursing Mirror,* 20: 154.

Targowski, A. (1990). "Beyond a Concept of a Communication Process." *Journal of Business Communication,* 27(1): 75–86.

Targowski, A., and Bowman, J. (1988). "The Layer-Based, Pragmatic Model of the Communication Process." *Journal of Business Communication,* 25(1): 5–24.

Timm, P. (1986). *Managerial Communication.* Englewood Cliffs, NJ: Prentice-Hall.

van Hoorde, J. (1990). "The Targowski and Bowman Model of Communication: Problems and Proposals for Adaptation." *Journal of Business Communication,* 27(1): 51–70.

Wallston, B., and O'Leary, V. (1981). "Sex and Gender Make a Difference: The Differential Perceptions of Women and Men." *Review of Personality and Social Psychology,* 2: 9–41.

Wolfe, K. (1990). "Computerized Information Management." *AAOHN Journal,* 38(4): 186–188.

Wilkins, A. (1984). "The Creation of Company Culture: The Role of Stories and Human Resource Systems." *Human Resource Management,* 23(1): 41–60.

MOTIVATING STAFF

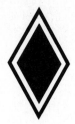

The term *motivation* comes from the Latin word *movere*, which means "to move." All human behavior is motivated by something; very little human behavior is completely random or instinctive. Most human behavior is goal directed: People do things for some reason, to get a certain result. The reasons may not always seem logical or rational, but they do tend to be systematic and, hence, behavior is relatively predictable. This is quite fortunate because it makes the study of motivation possible, particularly from an organizational point of view. While the concepts discussed in this chapter are relevant to human behavior in general, the chapter focuses on motivational problems frequently encountered by nurse managers in motivating staff members.

◆ WHY MOTIVATE PEOPLE?

Motivation is unquestionably important in health care institutions because, like in any other organization, people are required to function effectively if they are to provide adequate patient care. This implies that a health care institution must motivate qualified personnel to seek employment in the institution and then motivate them to remain on the job. Continual turnover means continual recruiting and training costs, inconvenience, and disruption of staff functions. (Recruitment, selection, and retention of staff are discussed in Chapters 13 and 17.) Once nursing staff are on the job, it is the nurse manager's responsibility to motivate them to produce both high quantity and high quality of work.

In addition, an understanding of motivational processes is essential for a more complete understanding of such other factors as leadership, job design, and incentive systems (e.g., salary, bonus) as they relate to employee performance and satisfaction. Indeed, most other techniques and programs are designed primarily to influence motivation, including both individual and group performance. The question for the nurse manager is how to utilize these tools most effectively to motivate effective nursing performance.

◆ WHAT MOTIVATES PEOPLE?

All motivational theories are concerned with three things: (a) what mobilizes or energizes human behavior; (b) what directs behavior toward the accomplishment of some objective; and (c) how such behavior is sustained over time. The relative utility of all motivational theories depends upon their ability to explain motivation adequately, to predict with some degree of accuracy what people will actually do, and, finally, to suggest practical ways of influencing employees to accomplish organizational objectives.

There are some distinct differences among motivational theories, however, that allow them to be classified into at least two different groups: content theories and process theories. In general, *content theories* emphasize individual needs or the rewards that may satisfy those needs, whereas *process theories* emphasize *how* the motivation process works to direct an individual's effort into performance.

◆ CONTENT THEORIES OF MOTIVATION

INSTINCT THEORIES
Content theories generally take two different forms: instinct theories and need theories. *Instinct theories* are much older, dating from the

1890s. While some early theorists saw instincts as purposive and goal directed, other instinct theorists defined the concept more in terms of blind, mechanical action. However, all of them characterized instincts as inherited or innate tendencies that predispose individuals to behave in certain ways. One version of the instinct theories dates from Sigmund Freud, who noted that individuals are not always consciously aware of their desires and needs. Thus, Freud's theory focused on the notion of unconscious motivation (1949).

In the early 1920s, however, instinct theories came under increasing attack on several grounds. First, the list of instincts had grown to well over 6,000, making it very difficult to pinpoint the specific motivation for a given behavior in terms of one or even some combination of instincts. Second, while every individual was assumed to have a complete set of instincts, researchers became increasingly aware that these instincts varied in strength across individuals. However, the relative strength of various instincts did not seem to be strongly related to subsequent behavior. Finally, some psychologists began to question whether Freud's unconscious motives were really instinctive or were, in fact, learned behaviors.

This last criticism led, in part, to the development of a second class of content theories focusing on the concept of learned needs. While there are many *need theories,* the most notable are those of Abraham Maslow, Clayton Alderfer, and Frederick Herzberg.

NEED HIERARCHY THEORY

Maslow (1943; 1954) attempted to bring a greater degree of order to the concept of needs by restricting the list to only five needs and organizing them into a hierarchy of prepotency, meaning that the needs were assumed to operate in a particular order. A lower level need is prepotent or controls behavior until it is satisfied, and then the next higher need energizes and directs behavior. The hierarchy, from the lowest to the highest level, is as follows: (a) physiological needs (e.g., hunger, thirst), (b) safety needs (i.e., bodily safety), (c) belongingness or social needs (e.g., friendship, affection, love), (d) esteem needs (e.g., recognition, appreciation, self-respect), and (e) self-actualization (e.g., developing one's whole potential).

Maslow's need theory is frequently used in nursing to provide an explanation of human behavior. A patient's needs are viewed in this hierarchical order, with nursing care directed toward meeting the lower level needs before addressing higher needs. Although Maslow's theory provides an explanation of human needs, it is not very useful in management, where predicting behavior and directing appropriate change is the focus.

EXISTENCE-RELATEDNESS-GROWTH THEORY

Alderfer (1969; 1972) has suggested three, rather than five, need levels: (a) existence needs (including both physiological and safety needs), (b) relatedness needs (Maslow's belongingness or social needs), and (c) growth needs (including the needs for self-esteem and self-actualization). His ERG (existence–relatedness–growth) theory is similar to Maslow's in assuming that the satisfaction of needs on one level activates the next higher level need. Alderfer suggests, however, that frustrated higher level needs cause a regression to and re-emphasis upon the next lower level need in the hierarchy.

In addition, Alderfer's model suggests that more than one need may be operative at any point in time. While it is somewhat less rigid than Maslow's hierarchy, it presents little that is new or substantially different. The criticisms of Maslow's theory in management are applicable to Alderfer's modified need hierarchy theory as well.

TWO-FACTOR THEORY

Herzberg's two-factor theory explains motivation as identical to job satisfaction (Herzberg, 1966; Herzberg, Mausner & Snyderman, 1959). Herzberg states that job satisfaction and job dissatisfaction are not opposite ends of the same continuum; rather, they are two different continua. The factors that lead to no job satisfaction are quite different from those that lead to no job dissatisfaction, and the resulting behaviors from these two states are also quite different.

Herzberg regards the lack of such extrinsic factors as satisfactory pay, adequate technical supervision, enlightened company policies and administration, good working conditions, and job security as job dissatisfiers. He suggests that employees need the presence of most, if not all, of these extrinsic, or *hygiene,* factors not to experience job dissatisfaction. Dissatisfied employees are more likely to be absent, file grievances, or quit the job. Herzberg likens hygiene factors to a water filtration plant. Not having one will very likely result in illness, but drinking purified water will not necessarily keep one from becoming sick.

The presence of hygiene factors results in employees who come to work, but they will not create job satisfaction or motivation. Rather, satisfaction and motivation result from such intrinsic on-the-job factors as a sense of achievement for performing a task successfully, recognition and praise, responsibility for one's own or another's work, and advancement or changing status through promotion. To the extent that these intrinsic, or *motivating,* factors are present, an employee is assumed to experience job satisfaction and hence will be highly motivated to perform the job effectively.

Herzberg's results, however, appear to be quite specific to the research methodology he used. Other researchers have found little or no relationship between satisfaction and motivation. Thus, while Herzberg's hygiene factors (generally lower order needs) and satisfiers (generally higher order needs) have enjoyed a popularity among managers second only to Maslow's need hierarchy, the weight of research evidence indicates that it, too, is an inadequate tool for managing employee motivation.

◆ PROCESS THEORIES OF MOTIVATION

For all their popularity, content theories only explain why a person behaves in a particular way. In contrast, *process theories* do much more than just *explain* behavior; they assist in *understanding* the processes involved in why people behave as they do. This increased level of understanding results in increased ability to predict what an employee is likely to do on the job, which implies the ability to influence that behavior toward desired organizational goals.

REINFORCEMENT THEORY

One process approach to motivation is *reinforcement theory,* which views motivation as learning (Skinner, 1953). According to this theory, behavior is learned through a process called *operant conditioning,* in which a behavior becomes associated with a particular consequence. In operant conditioning, the response-consequence connection is strengthened over time—that is, it is learned. The behavior is called an operant behavior because the individual is seen as operating on his or her environment to obtain a desired consequence.

To produce a desired behavior with operant conditioning, a manager must be able to control or manipulate the consequences of that behavior. Consider a nursing student who correctly administers an intramuscular injection. The patient remarks, "It didn't hurt at all," and the instructor says, "Well done!" In this instance, the praise of both patient and instructor are desired consequences that occur only when the behavior (giving the injection) is properly performed. Each time this behavior-consequence sequence occurs, the behavior is strengthened or better learned.

The focus on desirable consequences (e.g., praise, money, favored task assignments) refers to *positive reinforcement*. A positive reinforcer is a consequence that strengthens the likelihood of an operant response. Behavior that does not lead to positive consequences tends not to be re-peated. Obviously, both processes are important in an organization. We wish employees would do things that they are not currently doing and we also wish employees would not do things that reflect ineffective performance.

Reinforcement increases the frequency or magnitude of a behavior. This is shown in the left column of Figure 8-1 which indicates that the frequency or magnitude of a behavior may be increased by either positive or negative reinforcement. In the former, some positive consequence or reinforcer (e.g., praise) is applied for the express purpose of increasing a desired behavior. However, behavior may also be increased by removing something from the environment, as shown in the lower left quadrant of Figure 8-1. This is known as *negative reinforcement* and is sometimes called escape or avoidance learning. If the individual's performance can terminate a noxious or undesirable consequence, it is called escape learning. When behav-

FIGURE 8-1 TYPES OF REINFORCEMENT

Desired behavioral response

		Increase behavior	Decrease behavior
Action of reinforcing agency	Add consequences	Positive reinforcement	Punishment
	Remove consequences	Negative reinforcement	Extinction

ior can prevent the onset of a noxious consequence, this is called avoidance learning. Both are types of negative reinforcement.

A simple example should make the difference between positive and negative reinforcement quite clear. Suppose a staff nurse does a complete job of charting which is reinforced by the nurse manager with praise. This is positive reinforcement. In contrast, negative reinforcement occurs when a staff member stops engaging in an undesirable behavior to avoid a reprimand. For example, a nurse who has been tardy repeatedly arrives for work on time and, therefore, is not reprimanded for tardiness. In this case, the staff member has engaged in avoidance learning by increasing effective or desirable performance.

As shown in the right column in Figure 8–1, there are different ways to decrease the frequency or magnitude of a behavior as well. In the second example, the nurse manager wishes to stop a behavior (e.g., coming to work late) incompatible with effective job performance. Pressure applied to reduce the occurrence of a behavior is known as *punishment*. However, when a reinforcer is simply removed from a situation to reduce the occurrence of a given behavior, the procedure is known as *extinction*. Punishment is an active managerial response, while ignoring the behavior is a passive response.

Nurse managers should emphasize positive reinforcement since repeated studies have demonstrated that this is the best way to change behavior. This is not to say that other reinforcement procedures are inappropriate. To be sure, punishment, especially if severe enough, will produce an immediate and drastic change in behavior which is why it is used so much. However, research has shown that the cessation of

undesirable behavior because of punishment is generally not permanent. The undesirable behavior will be suppressed only as long as the manager is monitoring the situation and the threat of punishment is present. Punishment is negative in character and may lead an employee not only to avoid behaving appropriately but also to avoid the manager and the job as well. In short, reliance upon punishment as a primary means of changing behavior is likely to result in lower job satisfaction, less cooperation with management, and perhaps greater absenteeism and turnover without necessarily producing better performance.

Extinction means that there is no consequence at all for a behavior. With extinction, the behavior eventually stops. This is a relatively inefficient way to go about changing employee behavior because it may take a long time. The most efficient way to change behavior is to ignore (i.e., extinguish) undesirable behavior *and* simultaneously to positively reinforce desirable or appropriate behavior when it occurs. For example, the manager should ignore lateness and praise punctuality. This is much easier for the employee to understand and much more effective. After all, only rarely do we want individuals to do nothing; rather, we want them to do something different. That something must be appropriate and constructive in terms of job performance.

The problem with operant conditioning for many managers is that there is no sure way to elicit the desired behavior so that it can be reinforced. The manager must wait for the employee to perform in the desired manner before a positive reinforcer (consequence) can be administered. However, one can simply *tell* employees what they should be doing (e.g., set a goal) and what they should not be doing. In most cases, this is sufficient to elicit the desired behavior which then should be positively reinforced.

Sometimes, however, this procedure is not sufficient. Consider the case of Mrs. Armstrong, a nursing assistant, who never came to work less than 20 minutes late. Her uniform was always wrinkled and sometimes soiled, her personal hygiene left something to be desired, and her general attitude was quite unpleasant. The nurse manager decided a procedure called *shaping* would be the most appropriate remedy. Shaping involves selectively reinforcing behaviors that are successively closer approximations to the desired behavior. For Mrs. Armstrong, it was not a matter of not knowing what to do; she had been reprimanded and counseled innumerable times on appropriate job behavior. Her problem did not appear to be lack of knowledge, but a simple lack of motivation.

The nurse manager, Ms. Ernest, tried for a week to find a single, positive behavior to reinforce. The following week, she found occasion to praise Mrs. Armstrong several times. One day, for example, Mrs. Armstrong came to work only 10 minutes late and her relative punctuality was promptly reinforced. Similarly, she seemed to have made at least an attempt to comb her hair, so she was positively reinforced for her improved appearance. On every occasion, however, Ms. Ernest was met with a low grunt and an occasional icy glare from Mrs. Armstrong, who continued about her own business. After a few weeks, however, she seemed to respond more favorably to the praise and increased interest (rewards) of the nurse manager. Her comb appeared to have wandered through her hair at least twice on most days and, while wrinkled, her uniform was relatively clean.

Within a period of approximately two months, Mrs. Armstrong's performance, although not perfect, was substantially improved,

and she had ceased to be an embarrassment to her colleagues and the hospital. Moreover, her disposition had improved and she had actually begun to develop some friendships with other members of the staff. Her appearance and hygiene were, for the most part, quite acceptable, although her punctuality had improved only slightly. While she was clearly no superstar, she had come to be regarded as a valuable and necessary member of the staff.

The main point of this actual story is that behavior modification via the principles of positive reinforcement may take some time especially when shaping procedures must be implemented. Each successively closer approximation to the desired behavior is reinforced and well established before progressive reinforcement is given only to closer approximations of the desired behavior. When people become clearly aware that desirable rewards are contingent upon a specific behavior, their behavior will eventually change.

Behavior modification works quite well provided: (a) rewards can be found that, in fact, are seen as positive reinforcers by employees and (b) supervisory personnel can control such rewards or make them contingent upon performance. This does not mean that all rewards work equally well or that the same rewards will continue to function effectively over a long time. Were a nursing manager to praise someone four or five times a day every day, the praise would soon begin to wear thin; it would cease to be a positive reinforcer. Care must be taken not to overdo a good thing. For this reason, a *continuous schedule* of reinforcement—reinforcement every time a desired behavior occurs—may result in the reinforcer losing its effectiveness over time (see Table 8–1).

Partial schedules of reinforcement, however—reinforcing the behavior upon every second or third occurrence, for example—may be quite useful. This *fixed ratio schedule* of reinforcement requires very close monitoring by the nurse manager to reinforce *every nth* response and is obviously not very practical. However, reinforcing on a fairly regular basis, labeled a *variable ratio schedule,* is much more feasible. In this instance, every second or third response *on the average* over a period of time is positively reinforced. It is also common in organizations to use a *fixed interval schedule* of reinforcement, as

with the distribution of weekly or monthly paychecks.

Some rather interesting research findings have emerged over the years on continuous and partial schedules of reinforcement. For example, we know that a continuous schedule of reinforcement (i.e., every response is reinforced) is the fastest method of establishing or learning a new behavior, while any kind of partial schedule of reinforcement is much slower. On the other

TABLE 8-1 EFFECTS OF DIFFERENT REINFORCEMENT SCHEDULES

Arrangement of reinforcement contingencies	Schedules of reinforcement contingencies	Effect on behavior when applied	Effect on behavior when removed
Positive reinforcement	Continuous reinforcement	Fastest method to establish a new behavior	Fastest method to extinguish a new behavior
	Partial reinforcement	Slowest method to establish a new behavior	Slowest method to extinguish a new behavior
	Variable partial reinforcement	More consistent response frequencies	Slower extinction rate
	Fixed partial reinforcement	Less consistent response frequencies	Faster extinction rate
Avoidance reinforcement		Increased frequency over preconditioning level	Return to preconditioning level
Punishment extinction		Decreased frequency over preconditioning level	Return to preconditioning level

Adapted from Behling; O., Schreisheim, C., & Tolliver, J. Present theories and new directions in theories of work effort. *Journal Supplement Abstract Service* of the American Psychological Corporation.

hand, behaviors learned under a continuous schedule also extinguish very quickly once reinforcement stops. Behavior learned on a partial schedule continues for a much longer time without being reinforced. In addition, continuous schedules of reinforcement are probably better when money is used rather than other reinforcers such as praise.

Although reinforcement definitely changes behavior, there is nothing to indicate what is reinforcing to a given individual or why; a reinforcer is effective only if it is a reward for *that* individual. Most people are motivated by different kinds and amounts of rewards, but reinforcement theory does not explain such individual differences in response to reinforcers and punishment.

EXPECTANCY THEORY

Victor Vroom introduced expectancy theory in 1964 to explain work motivation. In contrast to behavior modification, which focuses strictly on observable behaviors, expectancy theory suggests that people's thoughts about and evaluation of the environment and events (i.e., their expectations) are important in determining behavior. The major difference between expectancy theory and behavior modification is that expectancy theory regards people as reacting consciously and actively to their environment, while behavior modification suggests that people react passively to reinforcement contingencies in their environment. Expectancy theory is concerned with conscious choice behavior, while behavior modification focuses on learned response–consequence bonds that are formed as a result of positive reinforcement. Both theories, however, strongly emphasize the role of rewards and their relationship to the performance of desired behaviors.

Expectancy theory asserts that individuals are motivated by their expectancies (beliefs) about future outcomes (consequences of behavior) and by the value they place on those outcomes (Mitchell, 1974; Vroom, 1964). To predict what a person chooses to do and how much effort the person will put forth in doing it, three components are important: expectancy, instrumentality, and valence. *Expectancy (E)* is the perceived probability that effort will lead to a specific performance level or behavior. This variable reflects the degree to which people expect they "can do" something. *Instrumentality (I)* is the belief that a given performance level or behavior will lead to some outcome (reward or punishment). This variable receives its name from the degree to which an individual believes performance is instrumental to receiving outcomes. *Valence* is the perceived value (attractiveness or unattractiveness) of an outcome.

Some examples should help you to understand how these three building blocks are combined to form the basis of expectancy theory. Let's examine the decision processes that a nursing student might go through in determining what course grade she intends to work toward and how much effort she will expend in trying to attain that grade. Table 8–2 helps you follow this process. The first example, the *behavioral choice model,* illustrates how a student might choose a grade goal in a given course.

First, we must consider the potential outcomes that a student nurse might expect from receiving a grade in a course. These are the same things that reinforcement theory considers to be reinforcers and punishers. In this example, we assume a scale of attractiveness with values from −7 (very unattractive) to +7 (very attractive). This student regards such things as completing a required course (+5) and losing scholarship eligibility (-5) to be important (i.e., valent) outcomes. Of course, what is attractive to one student is not necessarily attractive to another. We should measure the valences of outcomes that each individual student regards as

relevant; however, it is likely there will be a fairly common core of such relevant outcomes for most students. Relevant outcomes can be identified through informal discussions and by asking individuals to add their own unique

---

TABLE 8-2 BEHAVIORAL CHOICE MODEL, $\Sigma(IV)$
EXAMPLE OF A STUDENT CHOOSING A COURSE GRADE GOAL

		Performance level alternative					
	Outcome	Grade of A		Grade of B		Grade of C	
Performance contingent outcome	valence	I	I x V	I	I x V	I	I x V
a. Completing a required course	5	1.0	5.0	1.0	5.0	.7	3.5
b. Feelings of competence	5	1.0	5.0	.8	4.0	.2	1.0
c. Being reprimanded by instructor	-2	0.0	0.0	0.0	0.0	.2	$-.4$
d. Receiving praise from family	4	1.0	4.0	.8	3.2	0.0	0.0
e. Losing scholarship eligibility	-5	.2	-1.0	.4	-2.0	.8	-4.0
f. Time for recreational activities	7	0.0	0.0	.4	2.8	.7	4.9

Attractiveness of grade (performance choice) = $\Sigma(IV)$ 13.0   13.0   5.0
Conclusion: The student finds a grade of "B" equally attractive as a grade of "A."

TABLE 8-2 EFFORT MODEL, $\Sigma[Ex\Sigma(IV)]$
EXAMPLE OF A STUDENT CHOOSING EFFORT IN CLASS

		Effort level alternative					
	Performance	Studying 12 hours/week		Studying 12 hours/week		Studying 12 hours/week	
Performance level	attractiveness	E ×	Ex$\Sigma(IV)$	E ×	Ex$\Sigma(IV)$	E ×	Ex$\Sigma(IV)$
a. Course grade of "A"	13	.5	6.5	.5	6.5	.1	1.3
b. Course grade of "B"	13	.8	10.4	.7	9.1	.5	6.5
c. Course grade of "C"	5	.1	.5	.5	2.5	.9	4.5

Choice of effort level (studying) = $\Sigma[E \times \Sigma(IV)]$ 17.4   18.1   12.3
Conclusion: The student will maximize outcomes and minimize effort by choosing to study 8 hours per week

items to their personal list of outcomes. We should note that any number of scale points will do for measurement purposes (e.g., +10 to −10).

Second, we must define different performance levels. For simplicity, we consider only the performance levels of "A," "B," and "C" grades in the course. Each performance level has a different likelihood (instrumentality, or I) of yielding each outcome. In this example, the student believes that receiving praise from family has a probability of 1.0 if she earns an "A," a probability of .8 if she earns a "B," and a probability of 0.0 if she earns a "C" in the course.

Next, the instrumentality of each grade for receiving each outcome is multiplied by the valence of the respective outcome ($I \times V$). Finally, these products are summed for each performance or grade level, written as $\Sigma(IV)$. This results in values of 13.0, 13.0, and 5.0 for grades of "A," "B," and "C," respectively. Thus, while the student finds either an "A" or a "B" more attractive than a grade of "C," she perceives no difference in incentive value between an "A" and a "B" grade, as a grade of "A" is no different from "B" for receiving outcomes that the student values.

In the second example, we consider the student's choice of how much effort to expend (the *effort model,* measured as the number of hours spent studying each week). Again, for simplicity, we consider effort as having only three levels: high effort (studying 12 hours/week), medium effort (studying 8 hours/week), and low effort (studying 4 hours/week). Obviously, each level of effort might lead to a different level of performance and each performance level might be more or less attractive or desirable. The behavioral choice model gives us the desirability of each performance level as $\Sigma(IV)$. These values are listed in the performance attractiveness col-

umn in the effort model example and are taken directly from the results of the behavioral choice model in the top half of Table 8–2.

The attractiveness of each performance level is then multiplied by the expectancy (E) that a given level of effort will, in fact, produce that performance level. After the products are summed, the level of effort (e.g., low, medium, high) that the student will choose to expend is that with the largest $\Sigma[E \times \Sigma(IV)]$ value. This minimizes the amount of effort expended while maximizing the rewards received for performance.

Referring again to Table 8–2, the student believes there is a 50 percent chance (.50 probability) that high effort will result in an "A" grade and an 80 percent chance that it will produce a "B." This student also seems to believe that studying only 8 hours/week is just as likely to produce an "A" as is studying 12 hours/week. Apparently this student believes that something besides high effort is very important in getting a high grade (e.g., exam difficulty, luck). After multiplying a grade's attractiveness by each expectancy term and summing the values for each level of effort, we see that the largest sum is obtained for studying 8 hours/week, or a moderate level of effort. Thus, the student in the example is really indifferent between earning a grade of "A" or "B" and has chosen to work moderately hard in the course. She believes working harder isn't really worth it and working less hard will likely result in a less desirable "C" grade. Expectancy theory becomes more complex in a situation involving multiple outcomes, multiple levels of performance, and multiple levels of effort.

Keep in mind that expectancy theory is specifically designed to predict an individual's conscious choice of performance level or behavior and choice of *effort* (rather than performance level actually achieved). An important factor in expectancy theory is that such decisions are not based on "objective" reality but on psychological reality. It is the person's *perception* of expectancies and instrumentalities in combination with the *perceived* value of various rewards and punishments that determines an individual's choices. Thus, a manager must determine an individual's beliefs regarding her expectancy that work will yield achievement (expectancy), that achievement will yield rewards (instrumentality), and how the rewards are valued (valence).

The net effect of these rather complicated mental calculations is that the three components are multiplied together ($E \times I \times V$) to determine the amount of effort an individual will exert. Thus, when *any one* component is drastically reduced, so is motivation (effort). If staff members do not believe that they are capable of performing a task (expectancy), *or* if they believe there is little chance of reward for their work (instrumentality), *or* if the value of the outcome (valence) is low, motivation is reduced. In fact, multiplication of these components indicates that a zero value for *any one* of them results in zero motivation.

Expectancy theory also considers multiple outcomes. Consider the possibility of a promotion to nurse manager. Even though a staff nurse believes such a promotion is positive and is a desirable reward for competent performance in patient care, the nurse also realizes that there are possibly some negative outcomes (e.g., working longer hours, losing the close camaraderie enjoyed with other staff members). Therefore, when considering rewards, the nurse manager must always ask: What is the likelihood that this individual can accomplish a task successfully (expectancy), the probability that successful task performance will lead to outcomes (instrumentality), and the desirability of those outcomes (valence)?

Expectancy theory is very useful because of its clear managerial implications. First, expectancies can be maximized by assigning tasks to employees that they are capable of performing or by providing them necessary training. In addition, removing obstacles (inadequate resources, lack of information or cooperation from others) increases employees' expectancies. Second, instrumentalities can be maximized by making certain that rewards (and punishment) are made contingent on performance. Obviously, reinforcement theory provides considerable detail on how to accomplish this. Finally, rewards must be perceived as desirable enough to make the effort toward high performance worthwhile. Similarly, punishment must be regarded as sufficiently undesirable to act as a successful deterrent to inappropriate job behavior.

EQUITY THEORY

Equity theory suggests that effort and job satisfaction depend upon the degree of equity or perceived fairness in the work situation (Adams, 1963; 1965). Equity simply means that a person perceives that one's contribution to the job is rewarded in the same proportion that another person's contribution is rewarded. Since contributions may differ, rewards may differ. Contributions may include such things as ability, education, experience, and effort, while rewards may include job satisfaction, pay, prestige, and any other outcomes an employee regards as relevant. Thus, equity theory is concerned with the conditions under which employees perceive their contributions to the job and the rewards obtained therefrom as fair and equitable. Equity does not in any way imply equality; rather, it suggests that those employees who bring more to the job deserve greater rewards.

As long as one's perceived *ratio* of outcomes to input is approximately equal to that of a relevant comparison person, a state of equity is said to exist. For example, most employees understand that the registered nurse and the nursing assistant have different and unequal salaries, but most also understand that each brings different and unequal education and experience to the job. Therefore, perceived equity in their assigned duties and in their salaries usually exists. Inequity occurs when an employee's outcome/input ratio is perceived to be disproportional to that of a relevant comparison person. The comparison person may be a co-worker, a person doing a similar job for a different employer, or an "ideal worker," or it may actually be the person at some other time or in some other job situation.

Inequity motivates a change in behavior that may either increase or decrease actual effort and job performance. Perceived equity simply motivates the status quo. The nurse who sees the nursing assistants' salaries raised while staff nurses' salaries are not may be motivated to reduce effort to restore perceived equity. Equal percentage salary increases are likely to motivate continued effort at the same level. Again, one must be aware of the difference between behavior and performance. Reducing inequity may or may not change performance.

Employees can try to restore what they perceive as equity in a variety of ways. First, they can increase or decrease actual contributions, especially effort. Nurses can attempt to increase their status by assuming more patient care assignments, spending more time on charting, or exhibiting other behaviors reflecting additional effort. Second, they may attempt to persuade the comparison person(s) to increase or decrease their inputs—persuading the nursing assistants to work less, for instance. Third, they may attempt to persuade the organization to change either their own rewards or those of the comparison persons (e.g., salary changes or perquisites). Fourth, they may psychologically distort the perceived importance and value of their own contributions and rewards ("How could they run this unit without me?"). Fifth, they may distort the perceived importance and value of the comparison persons' contributions or rewards ("What can you expect of assistants?").

Psychologically distorting perceptions of a comparison person's outcomes or inputs are probably the easiest ways to restore equity without actually changing one's effort. Alternatively, the staff member may select a different comparison person, someone who is seen as more relevant for the comparison being made, such as the nurse manager. Finally, the individual may actually leave the organization.

It is very difficult to predict exactly what a given individual will do in response to perceived inequity. However, some basic principles may help in predicting reactions. First, it is assumed that people try to maximize rewards and minimize increasing contributions. Second, they are more resistant to changing their ideas about their own rewards and contributions than to distorting their perceptions of the contributions and rewards of the comparison person. Moreover, perceived contributions and rewards central to an individual's self-esteem and self-concept are more resistant to change than those that are less central to these concepts. In the previous example, if nurses perceive that the increased salaries of the nursing assistants imply a loss of their own status, they are more apt to attempt some type of change to restore perceived equity. Changing a person's reactions to the comparison person also is more difficult once this comparison has stabilized over time. In other words, a nurse must act to restore equity when the salary increase is announced or a change is unlikely to occur. Finally, it is least likely that an individual will leave the situation. Usually this occurs only after all other attempts to restore perceived equity have failed and the individual perceives a great deal of inequity.

The most extensively researched aspect of equity theory is the use of pay as a reward. Pay is an important reward to most people. If we assume that altering job effort is easier than other reactions to inequity, we can make certain predictions regarding pay inequity. Predictions of employee effort vary according to perceived underpayment inequity or overpayment inequity. Most of the research has focused on overpayment inequity, probably because it is more controversial. Equity theory suggests that any kind of inequity, either underpayment or overpayment, will motivate changes in behavior. It is easy to understand why individuals might change their behavior if they feel they are being cheated or underpaid, but it seems less likely that they should change their behavior (i.e., increase effort) when they feel they are being inequitably overpaid. In general, research results support common sense: People are much more likely to experience perceived inequity when they are relatively underpaid than when they are relatively overpaid.

The concept of equity may be seen as one of several potential social norms that operate in groups, particularly with respect to the distribution of rewards. Table 8–3 contrasts some distribution rules regarding allocation of rewards in small groups (Leventhal, 1976). The appropriate distribution rule (equity versus equality) depends on the goal of reward allocation. When the goal is to maximize individual productivity in a group, rewards should be distributed equitably, which means they should be based on individual expertise and contributions. If the goal is to maximize harmony and minimize conflict in a group, however, then rewards

should be more equally distributed to all participants regardless of their contribution.

The degree of cooperation and coordination required for task performance is another important factor in the distribution of rewards. If tasks are essentially individual in nature—if staff members carry out tasks on their own without a great deal of cooperation required—then equity should be the rule for allocating organizational rewards. On the other hand, if a high degree of cooperation and coordination is required for effective task performance (e.g., group or team tasks), then rewards should be distributed equally among group members.

In other words, it is important to differentiate between rewarding individual performance versus group performance. If the nurse manager wants individual staff members to perform individual tasks (e.g., patient care, record keeping) competently and productively, then rewards should be individualized. If the task is essentially a group task (e.g., a surgical nursing team), however, then performance will be maximized when staff members are rewarded for group rather than individual performance.

The important point is that perceived fairness of rewards affects the manner in which individuals view their jobs and the organization and can affect the amount of effort they expend toward task accomplishment. Moreover, the research evidence seems to indicate that inequitable rewards, especially underpayment inequity, lead to increased psychological tension and lower job satisfaction and may have an adverse impact on job performance. In times of economic retrenchment, when no one receives a salary increase, people may perceive the situation as equitable if they believed it to be equitable prior to the retrenchment. In this case, job satisfaction may not be adversely affected. Similar to Herzberg's notion of hygiene factors, pay equity is important to keep a good motivational situation from going sour. However, simply distributing rewards equitably does not necessarily improve an otherwise poor motivational environment.

GOAL SETTING THEORY

There are three basic propositions in goal setting (Locke, 1968). The first is that specific goals lead to higher performance than do general goals such as "Do your best." The second proposition states that specific, difficult goals lead to higher performance than specific, easy goals, provided the goals are accepted. Finally, incentives such as money, knowledge of results, praise and reproof, participation, competition, and time limits affect behavior only if they cause individuals to change their goals or to accept goals that have been assigned to them. Thus, unlike expectancy theory and equity theory, goal setting suggests that it is not the rewards or outcomes of task performance per se that cause effort expenditure, but rather the task goal itself. The only functions of rewards are to help ensure

TABLE 8–3 DISTRIBUTION RULES FOR ALLOCATING REWARDS

Distribution rule	Situations where distribution rule is likely to be used	Factors affecting use of distribution rule
Equity/contributions (outcomes should match contributions)	1. Goal is to maximize group productivity 2. A low degree of cooperation is required for task performance	1. What receiver is expected to do 2. What others receive 3. Outcomes and contributions of person allocating rewards 4. Task difficulty and perceived ability 5. Personal characteristics of person allocating rewards and person performing
Equality (equal outcomes given to all participants)	1. Goal is to maximize harmony, minimize conflict in group 2. Task of judging performer's needs or contribution is difficult 3. Person allocating rewards has a low cognitive capacity 4. A high degree of cooperation is required for task performance 5. Allocator anticipates future interactions with low-input member	1. Sex of person allocating rewards (females more likely to allocate rewards equally than males) 2. Nature of task

Adapted from Leventhal, G. S. Fairness in social relationships. In J. Thibaut, J. Spence, & R. Carson (Eds.), *Contemporary Topics in Social Psychology*, Morristown, N.J.: General Learning Press, 1976. © 1976 John Thibaut. Reprinted by permission of John Thibaut.

the acceptance of an assigned goal or to induce an individual to set a more specific, difficult personal goal. The specificity and difficulty of the goal mobilize energy and direct behavior toward goal accomplishment.

Studies indicate that setting specific goals produces higher levels of performance than does the use of general goals or no goals (Locke et al., 1981). Moreover, the higher the goal, the higher the performance, even when the goal is not always attained. The relationship between goal difficulty and performance typically predicts 50–75 percent of the differences in individual performance levels. Of course, all of this is useful only to the extent that individuals accept performance goals. In practice, employees working at their normal job duties rarely completely reject their performance goals. The legitimacy of the nurse manager/staff nurse relationship is readily accepted by most nurses. If tasks and duties are seen as reasonable, specific, difficult goals are very likely to produce higher performance as long as such performance is rewarded and the individual is held accountable for task accomplishment. There is also some evidence that the continuing presence of supervision helps to ensure goal acceptance. Supervisors who are frequently absent or not available for large periods of the working day are likely to have employees with substantially lower productivity than those of supervisors who are on the job with their employees (Ronan, Latham & Kinney, 1973).

Specific, difficult goals are likely to produce higher levels of job performance regardless of whether the nursing staff participates in every decision in setting performance standards. In some health care institutions and with some nurse managers, participation is a natural and encouraged form of management; with others, less emphasis may be placed on participative

management. Either method is likely to be appropriate and productive, provided the manager is supportive of employees. Support and encouragement, particularly in the face of difficult or undesirable tasks, go a long way toward engendering acceptance of high performance goals and subsequent high levels of performance.

♦ SUMMARY OF MOTIVATIONAL THEORIES

It is obvious that no single approach to motivating staff members is likely to maximize staff performance and satisfaction. Some methods may work better than others with different people or in different settings. However, each theory of work motivation contributes something to our understanding of and, ultimately, our ability to influence employee motivation. All of the motivational theories can be integrated to some extent by recognizing the *need basis* in every theory, including the process theories. For example, reinforcement theory does not specify what is a reinforcer or why it works. However, it seems reasonable that reinforcers are effective in changing behaviors because they lead to the fulfillment of some underlying need. Similarly, in expectancy theory there is nothing to say why an outcome has a strong positive or negative valence. One simply measures valences and assumes that some outcomes are more motivating than others.

It may well be that self-competency, or self-efficacy, a need to cope successfully with the environment, can be used to integrate the various motivational perspectives (Bandura, 1977; 1982; deCharms, 1968; Locke & Schweiger, 1979). Viewed in this way all of the theories, both content and process, are linked by this common human need. While it may be most useful to specify particular processes (e.g., reinforcement, equity, expectancy) to describe human motivational behavior more precisely, recognizing a common basis such as self-competency explains why potential utility may be gained from a variety of theoretical approaches.

Practical utility is especially important for managers in organizations. The content theories recognize that people do have particular needs and that to some degree these needs must be fulfilled. People have needs for money, or at least the things that money can buy, and to some extent they have other needs (e.g., esteem, self-actualization) than can be fulfilled through proper job design and assignment of tasks (e.g., professionalism, altruism). Content theories indicate that people have needs but do not say much about how to satisfy those needs. In contrast, the process theories focus specifically on techniques and methods to improve performance and satisfaction even though these are not phrased in the terminology of need fulfillment. Nevertheless, to the degree that all motivational theories are based upon an underlying need such as self-competency, the techniques and methods of the process theories represent useful means for providing need fulfillment.

The question still remains: How does one motivate staff? Figure 8–2 shows a simple model of how the various motivational theories are related. First, there is a task to be accomplished. If this task is expressed in terms of a specific, difficult goal that is accepted by the staff member, a relatively high degree of performance may realistically be expected in most situations. How does this happen? Goals, perceived ability, and perceived situational constraints all combine to form the perceived likelihood that effort will lead to a given level of performance or goal accomplishment. This expectancy, when combined with the belief that valued rewards will follow from goal attainment (instrumentality), prompts the expenditure of effort (motivation). Thus, goal setting and expectancy theory suggest not only that staff members should know exactly what they should be doing but also that they should perceive rewards as contingent upon performance of their assigned tasks.

Figure 8–2 shows that actual ability and situational constraints combine with effort to produce performance levels. Actual ability levels may be used by the nurse manager to assign tasks that are commensurate with the nurse's aptitudes, education, and experience. Performance may also be enhanced by removing situational constraints such as rotating shifts or providing assistance in overcoming constraints (e.g., assignment to the same shift for more consecutive days). Careful management of these factors by the nurse manager helps ensure that staff members' effort or motivation is actually translated into effective job performance.

Expectancy theory focuses on anticipated rewards. If these rewards are not received (performance is not reinforced), then subsequent instrumentalities are lowered. Performance should also lead to valued rewards that are perceived as being fair or equitable by staff members. Extrinsic rewards or reinforcers help to satisfy lower order needs while intrinsic rewards or reinforcers are more likely to satisfy higher order needs. For example, pay helps to satisfy the need for food, clothing, and shelter, while praise helps satisfy esteem needs.

In terms of future performance, rewards that are contingent on performance and are perceived as being equitable do a great deal to increase motivation. Thus, the effective management of staff motivation relies upon a combination of approaches, taking into consideration individual needs. Such an approach is far more likely than any single method or technique to produce effective job performance. The key to effective motivation is really the nurse manager's attitude that it can be done with a little thought and effort. Motivation of staff members is not always easy, but it is certainly one of the most important parts of the nurse manager's job. With practice and a little ingenuity, most managers find that far more can be done than they had initially realized to motivate their staff to high levels of performance.

FIGURE 8–2 INTEGRATED MODEL OF THE MOTIVATIONAL PROCESS

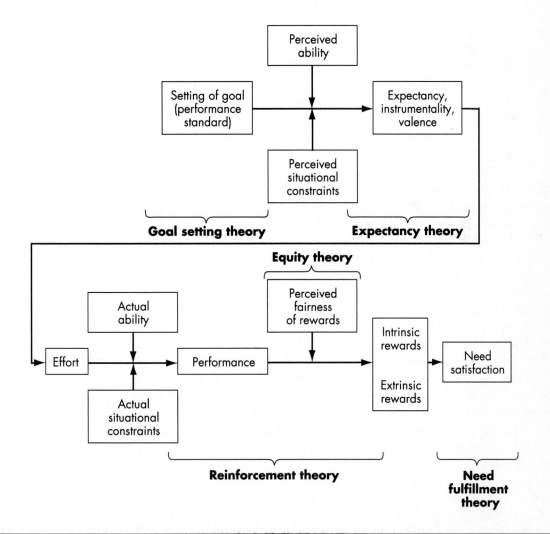

♦ MANAGING CHANGE

UNDESIRABLE JOBS

All organizations have undesirable jobs that someone must perform from time to time. There is a strong tendency to assign these "bad" jobs to the best employee simply because this increases the likelihood that the job will be done properly. This practice, however, may give the high-performing staff member the impression that the rewards of high performance are disagreeable tasks. While the staff member may accept such jobs in the short run as a necessary evil, this practice serves only to lower that person's motivation and decrease job satisfaction in the long run. Assigning desirable tasks or, better yet, allowing the staff members a choice of tasks as a reward for high performance is much more motivating.

Insofar as possible, serious consideration should be given to assigning undesirable tasks contingent upon poor performance (due to low motivation rather than low ability or exceptionally heavy workload). However, there should be few, if any, staff members who are doing an exceptionally poor job. The assignment of undesirable tasks can damage the existing motivation of individuals who are performing at the peak of their capacity. As always, caution and good judgment must be exercised when applying punishment.

If staff members are performing at approximately the same level of performance above some minimal standard, equity and positive reinforcement become critical issues. If the same people always get the undesirable jobs simply because they do them well, feelings of inequity mount rapidly. However, if everyone understands that the undesirable job is regularly rotated so that no one is unduly penalized by having to perform it repeatedly, inequity is less likely to occur. An even better strategy is to provide some incentive for completion of undesirable tasks in a timely and professional fashion. This may be accomplished by allowing the staff member a choice of favored tasks contingent upon completion of the undesirable job.

Individual preferences are important and cannot always be anticipated by the nurse manager. What is desirable or undesirable to one person may be viewed quite differently by another. The nurse manager who knows individual preferences among potential incentives has a powerful tool for motivating employees and fostering their job satisfaction. Task assignment is only one of many potential incentives or reinforcers, but it can be a very powerful incentive when properly used.

JOB DESIGN

The early history of job design was characterized by increasing specialization and fragmentation. Well before the advent of the Industrial Revolution, general craftsmanship was plagued by problems of inefficiency because the craftsman performed each and every job task. This led to the gradual specialization of jobs to increase efficiency and production. Because more workers were now needed to accomplish all the tasks, labor costs rose and completion of products was delayed because of the increased necessity for coordination among specialists. With the advent of the Industrial Revolution and mass production, increased efficiency was brought about by further fragmenting the work into highly specialized movements that were repeated over and over during the course of the workday. Increased worker monotony produced lower job satisfaction and increased absenteeism. The managerial reaction to this problem was an increased emphasis on discipline.

Thus, the scope of jobs has decreased steadily through specialization and fragmentation of the total work effort. In the early days of nursing, nurses assumed all the duties involved in caring for patients, including cleaning the room (see "Job Description of a Floor Nurse"). The recent trend in specialized nursing has somewhat fragmented job duties, so that we now have an IV nurse or an ICU nurse, for instance.

One problem with the specialization of professionals is that their unique preparation does not allow them to change emphasis or specialties easily within a professional career field. After several years, many highly talented nurses become bored with extreme specialization and the monotony of doing the same things over and over or dealing with the same types of patients day after day. The problem in industry was simply that the work remained unchanged; the solution to this was job redesign. In health care there is a corresponding trend back toward more general versus highly specialized health care professionals. The concept of "holistic health" and a concern for the psychological as well as the physical patient have become increasingly important within the past decade. Consider also the trend from team to primary nursing. Thus, the movement is away from job simplification toward job enlargement.

Job enlargement and job enrichment describe two attempts to reduce the negative effects of specialization. *Job enlargement* may be defined as the addition of tasks to increase the variety of skills and talents that staff members must use in the performance of their jobs. This not only increases variety on the job but also provides a sense of completion by allowing an individual to do a larger, and thus more identifiable, piece of the entire task. The problem with job enlargement, however, is that it is frequently just "more work," rather than "better work" or work that

entails greater responsibility and a higher level or different kind of professional skills. Intrinsic, higher order needs are particularly strong among professionals and simply giving them more work as opposed to better work does little to satisfy these needs or to stimulate outstanding job performance.

In contrast to job enlargement, *job enrichment* focuses on closing the gap between the doing and the controlling aspects of a job. In job enrichment, employees are given greater latitude in selecting work methods, evaluating their work, or participating in decisions affecting either their job or the organization as a whole. Thus, job enrichment is characterized by greater responsibility and control over the job as opposed to simply adding more mundane tasks to be accomplished.

The purpose of job redesign is to create jobs that provide a high degree of internal work motivation, a high quality of work performance, high satisfaction with the work, and low absenteeism and turnover (Hackman & Oldham, 1980). These results are more apt to occur in individuals who experience the following psychological states: (a) greater meaningfulness in their work, (b) a sense of responsibility for the results of their work, and (c) feedback regarding the effectiveness of their work (see Figure 8–3).

One might assume that professional employees, such as nurses, would naturally experience these psychological rewards as a result of their work. However, if motivation, absenteeism, and turnover were not problems among professional staff, there would be no need for this chapter. Clearly, motivational systems must be developed and implemented to retain highly talented and productive nurses in jobs where their services are particularly needed. Job redesign is a way to increase the degree to which an individual experiences meaningfulness, responsibility,

---

**BOX 8–1
JOB DESCRIPTION
OF A FLOOR NURSE**

Developed in 1887 and published in a magazine of Cleveland Lutheran Hospital.

In addition to caring for your 50 patients,
each nurse will follow these regulations:

1. Daily sweep and mop the floors of your ward, dust the patients's furniture and window sills.
2. Maintain an even temperature in your ward by bringing in a scuttle of coal for the day's business.
3. Light is important to observe the patient's condition. Therefore, each day fill kerosene lamps, clean chimneys, and trim wicks. Wash windows once a week.
4. The nurse's notes are important to aiding the physician's work. Make your pens carefully. You may whittle nibs to your individual taste.
5. Each Nurse on day duty will report every day at 7 a.m. and leave at 8 p.m., except on the Sabbath, on which you will be off from 12 noon to 2 p.m.

6. Graduate Nurses in good standing with the Director of Nurses will be given an evening off each week for courting purposes, or two evenings a week if you go regularly to church.
7. Each nurse should lay aside from each pay a goodly sum of her earnings for her benefits during her declining years, so that she will not become a burden. For example, if you earn $30 a month you should set aside $15.
8. Any nurse who smokes, uses liquor in any form, gets her hair done at a beauty shop or frequents dance halls will give the Director of Nurses good reason to suspect her worth, intentions and integrity.
9. The nurse who performs her labor, serves her patients and doctors faithfully and without fault for a period of five years will be given an increase by the hospital administration of five cents a day providing there are no hospital debts that are outstanding.

---

and effective feedback. These psychological states should lead to high quality performance and high job satisfaction and are created through a specific set of core job dimensions.

CORE JOB DIMENSIONS. According to job redesign theory, five core job dimensions (Figure 8–3) activate the critical psychological states (Hackman & Oldham, 1980). The first core job dimension is *skill variety,* the degree to which a job provides activities that involve the use of different skills and abilities. The second is *task identity,* the degree to which a job requires com-

pletion of a whole and identifiable piece of work. This entails doing a complete task from beginning to end. These two dimensions generally represent job enlargement. However, job enrichment adds three additional core job dimensions that are important for creating the desired psychological states. In particular, *task significance* is the degree to which a job has importance for the lives and work of other people both inside and outside the organization. The dimension of *autonomy* is important in that an enriched job provides considerable freedom, independence, and discretion to the staff member in scheduling the work to be accomplished and choosing the procedures to be used. Finally, *feedback* is the degree to which individuals are able to obtain clear information regarding the effectiveness of their performance. This may be apparent from the task itself or may be available from other individuals—particularly patients, other nurses, and the nurse manager.

Several principles guide the redesign of jobs to enhance these five core job dimensions. The first principle is to form natural work units combining tasks that logically fit together. This

helps staff members to see the significance of specific tasks and to feel a greater sense of responsibility for the results of what they do. A second and related principle is to combine tasks, which helps to increase perceptions of skill variety and task identity. If tasks are carefully combined, natural work units may be formed, and both principles become available for motivating and satisfying staff members.

A third principle is to establish client relationships. To some extent, this already exists in nursing, where the nurse/client relationship is a

FIGURE 8-3 JOB CHARACTERISTICS MODEL OF WORK DESIGN

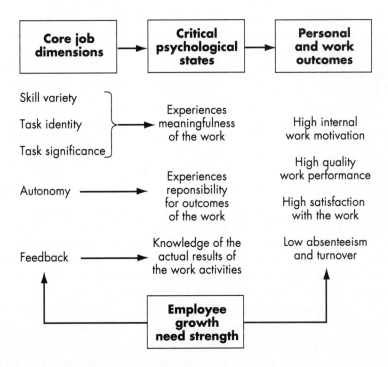

J. R. Hackman & G. R. Oldham, "Motivation through the Design of Work: Test of a Theory," *Organizational Behavior and Human Performance*, 16 (1976): 250-279.

prerequisite to providing care. But the patient does not "hire" the nurse directly. Consequently, additional steps might be taken to encourage clients to provide direct feedback to the nurse on their perception of the nurse's work. For example, the "clients" in a team environment may include a nurse's co-workers. Providing a means of feedback from such "clients" can significantly improve coordination, cooperation, and communication, all prerequisites for effective teamwork. In addition, client relationships increase skill variety because the nurse must practice the interpersonal skills necessary for effective communication with different patients. Finally, client relationships affect autonomy in that the nurse must decide how to manage the relationships with both patients and co-workers in the unit.

The fourth principle is to add control over one's work. Again, allowing staff nurses to participate in decision making, select work methods, and evaluate their own work increases the amount of autonomy experienced from the job.

The fifth principle is to open feedback channels. This involves essentially two things, the first being feedback from the nurse manager regarding job performance, a topic discussed in Chapter 16. However, feedback coming from the job itself (including patients) is even more important in that it is both immediate and specific. For example, staff nurses may be given responsibility for evaluating their own performance, such as patients' responses to their care. In this case, nurses are continually reminded of performance quality without the potential interpersonal problems inherent when negative feedback is provided by the supervisor. Proponents of primary nursing have argued that staff who work in such units have greater satisfaction as a result of these principles being implemented.

BARRIERS TO JOB REDESIGN. The nurse manager should be aware of some common problems in the redesign of jobs. For example, the nurse manager's role may change from leader and director of unit staff to that of coordinator of staff activities. Somehow, the notion of "coordinator" seems inconsistent with our cultural stereotypes of "leadership." We usually think of a leader as the person in charge, or "the boss." That stereotype of leadership tends to include the unilateral and unquestioned use of power, with objectives, strategies, and evaluation defined strictly from the leader's perspective. Some authors treat this issue as a matter of "leadership style" and tend to regard it as a personality characteristic. This particular barrier, however, is one over which the nurse manager can exercise direct and explicit control.

A number of factors are involved in effective leadership other than the power afforded by virtue of job title and reporting relationships. Effective leadership is accepted leadership, and there are many ways to foster acceptance of the nurse manager's legitimate organizational power (see Chapter 9). The strategies and techniques described in this chapter, however, are tools meant to help in achieving both individual and unit effectiveness through the management of staff motivation. If effectiveness means being a coordinator as opposed to being "the boss," then those strategies and techniques are what the nurse manager should use.

Another barrier to job redesign is that the values implicit in job redesign may be at odds with those of the institution's administration. The notion of providing autonomy, feedback, and greater responsibility and self-direction in the performance of jobs may not be in tune with the philosophy and the history of the institutional hierarchy—matters that are not under the nurse manager's immediate discretion or control. However, different management areas afford different degrees of responsibility, and there may be a good deal of flexibility within the limits of the institution's rules. Job redesign is just another tool to use within the limits of the situation at hand.

In some cases, staff members are reluctant to engage in job redesign or other motivational efforts because they fear that increased productivity may have implications for their job security. They are concerned that if productivity increases sufficiently, some people may lose their jobs because they are no longer needed to accomplish the work within the unit. One must remember, however, that most nursing units are chronically understaffed. Increased productivity not only eases the workload but also, if properly managed (e.g., rewarded), it is likely to result in greater satisfaction and organizational commitment and less absenteeism and turnover. Second, there is a tendency to focus on quantity and ignore the quality of work as a separate but equally important dimension. Fears regarding job security usually focus solely on the quantity issue and ignore quality. Effective motivation of staff members involves both of these dimensions, but job enrichment most consistently increases job satisfaction and work quality rather than the quantity of work produced.

The fourth major barrier to job redesign is that not everyone desires change or "growth" in the job. Some people prefer to have their work very clearly prescribed, unvarying in its content or procedure, and highly predictable from day to day. Job redesign is only appropriate for staff members whose jobs are too highly structured to suit their needs.

Still another major barrier to job redesign is the frequent lack of predetermined goals, or exact specifications of what is to be accomplished by redesigning an individual's job. Expectancy theory tells us that people should know exactly what it is they should do to make a given level of performance as high as possible. Thus, in implementing any job redesign measures, clear goals and objectives, planning with respect to how these goals can and should be attained, and periodic monitoring of progress to identify needed changes in strategies or objectives are essential. Job redesign may seem somewhat complex, but it is simply another technique that encompasses a variety of motivational strategies with an eye toward overall nursing effectiveness.

CLIMATE AND MORALE

Climates are clusters of employee perceptions of an organization's events, practices, and procedures. When taken together, these perceptions are useful in characterizing the organization or subunit. There are many climates in an organization. For example, one can identify a productivity climate, a climate for safety, a climate for patient care, and so on. One must specify the climate to which one is referring. Thus, a nursing unit is characterized as having a climate for high productivity to the extent that the work is usually completed at the end of each shift and that patient satisfaction is generally good. When such a climate exists, nurse managers may be reasonably sure that their managerial efforts have been relatively effective in motivating staff to high standards of performance.

Just as climate refers to group versus individual perceptions, morale refers to the combined attitudes of all work group members versus individual job satisfaction. Morale is essentially a matter of "group spirit" or cohesiveness. It is important because cohesiveness reflects the attractiveness of group members to the group and indicates the degree to which group values and expectations (norms) are adopted by individual members.

High morale can aid in pursuing both productivity and effectiveness goals. In contrast, low or negative morale may lead to active resistance efforts by group members to a nurse manager's leadership and motivational efforts. For example, there may be a norm to restrict productivity, a low standard for a "fair day's work" that is enforced by subtle group pressures. This is not uncommon in some nursing units. High morale can, however, be used as a positive force for productivity under more favorable conditions. Again, the feeling of "togetherness" or group cooperation is the strongest determinant. A second factor is agreement on goals. Third, there must be progress toward attaining those goals, and, finally, each group member should have specific and meaningful tasks necessary for goal achievement. While not all of these factors are absolutely essential to bring about group cohesiveness and commitment to organizational objectives, they can all be fostered by careful planning, inclusion of staff members in diagnosing problems, developing action plans for solving problems, and carefully managing performance based on the principles and techniques outlined in this chapter. In short, morale can be a significant factor in either helping or hindering the nurse manager's efforts to motivate staff members.

SUMMARY

♦ Content theories of motivation define motivation primarily in terms of need satisfaction.

♦ Process motivation theories describe how motivational processes operate and prescribe specific actions for implementation by the nurse manager.

♦ Content and process theories provide different perspectives on what mobilizes, directs, and sustains effort (motivation).

♦ Reinforcement theory views motivation as a process of learning in which specific behaviors lead to outcomes which are either unrewarded or punished. Positive reinforcement (reward) is more effective in changing behavior (motivation) than is punishment.

♦ Expectancy theory regards conscious choice as the determinant of motivation, either in what a nurse will do or in how much effort will be exerted on a given task. Three components are necessary: the perception that the nurse can actually perform the task (expectancy), the perception that task performance will actually result in some outcomes (instrumentality), and the perceived value of the outcomes (valence, i.e., reward or punishment value).

♦ Equity theory deals with the perceived fairness of an employee's ratio of outcomes/inputs relative to the same perceived ratio for a comparison person. Either underpayment or overpayment inequity may occur and motivates an individual to do something to restore perceived equity.

♦ Goal setting theory has shown that specific, difficult goals produce higher performance levels than either general goals or specific, easy goals.

♦ No motivation theory provides a complete description of the motivational process; each theory/technique brings a different perspective and contribution to understanding and influencing motivation. Effective staff motivation is best accomplished by judiciously combining the theories and techniques so that their effects are complementary.

♦ Job design includes job enlargement and job enrichment, both of which may be used by the nurse manager to increase employee motivation and satisfaction.

♦ Barriers to job design include stereotyped perceptions of the nurse manager as the "boss" rather than as a "leader" of a professional staff, organizational policies and values, fear of change, job insecurity, personal characteristics, and a lack of predetermined goals.

♦ Group cohesiveness fosters teamwork and can lead to either effective or ineffective individual and unit performance, depending on the behavior expectations (norms) the group holds for its members.

BIBLIOGRAPHY

Adams, J. S. (1963). "Toward an Understanding of Inequity." *Journal of Abnormal and Social Psychology,* 67: 422.

Adams, J. S. (1965). "Injustice in Social Exchange." In: *Advances in Experimental Social Psychology.* Vol. 2. Berkowitz, L. (editor). New York: Academic Press.

Alderfer, C. P. (1969). "A New Theory of Human Needs." *Organizational Behavior and Human Performance,* 4: 142.

Alderfer, C. P. (1972). *Existence, Relatedness, and Growth.* New York: Free Press.

American Academy of Nursing, Task Force on Nursing Practice in Hospitals. (1983). *Magnet Hospitals: Attraction and Retention of Professional Nurses.* Kansas City, MO: ANA Publications.

Bandura, A. (1977). "Self-Efficacy: Toward a Unifying Theory of Behavioral Change." *Psychological Review,* 84: 191.

Bandura, A. (1982). "Self-Efficacy Mechanism in Human Agency." *American Psychologist,* 37: 122.

deCharms, R. (1968). *Personal Causation: The Internal Affective Determinants of Behavior.* New York: Academic Press.

Floyd, G. J., and Smith, B. D. (1983). "Job Enrichment." *Nursing Management,* 14(5): 22.

Freud, S. (1949). "The Unconscious." In: *Collected Papers of Sigmund Freud.* Riviere, J. (translator). London: Hogarth Press. (Original edition, 1915.)

Hackman, J. R., and Oldham, G. R. (1980). *Work Redesign.* Reading, MA: Addison-Wesley.

Herzberg, F. (1966). *Work and the Nature of Man.* Cleveland, OH: World.

Herzberg, F., Mausner, B., and Snyderman, B. (1959). *The Motivation to Work.* New York: Wiley.

Leventhal, G. S. (1976). "Fairness in Social Relationships." In: *Contemporary Topics in Social Psychology.* Thibaut, J., Spence, J., and Carson, R. (editors). Morristown, NJ: General Learning Press.

Locke, E. A. (1968). "Toward a Theory of Task Motives and Incentives." *Organizational Behavior and Human Performance,* 3: 157.

Locke, E. A., and Schweiger, D. M. (1979). "Participation in Decision Making: One More Look." In: *Research in Organizational Behavior.* Vol. 1. Staw, B. (editor). Greenwich, CT: JAI Press.

Locke, E. A., Shaw, K. N., Saari, L. M., and Latham, G. P. (1981). "Goal Setting and Task Performance: 1969–1980." *Psychological Bulletin,* 90: 125.

Maslow, A. H. (1943). "A Theory of Human Motivation." *Psychological Review,* 50: 370.

Maslow, A. H. (1954). *Motivation and Personality.* New York: Harper.

Miner, J. B. (1980). *Theories of Organizational Behavior.* Hinsdale, IL: Dryden Press.

Mitchell, T. R. (1974). "Expectancy Models of Job Satisfaction, Occupational Preference, and Effort: A Theoretical, Methodological and Empirical Appraisal." *Psychological Bulletin,* 81: 1096.

Mitchell, T. R., and Larson, J. R., Jr. (1987). *People in Organizations.* 3d ed. New York: McGraw-Hill.

Ronan, W. W., Latham, G. P., and Kinney, S. B. (1973). "Effects of Goal Setting and Supervision on Worker Behavior in an Industrial Situation." *Journal of Applied Psychology,* 58: 302.

Skinner, B. F. (1953). *Science and Human Behavior.* New York: Free Press.

Steers, R. M., and Porter, L. W. (1979). *Motivation and Work Behavior.* 2d ed. New York: McGraw-Hill.

Vroom, V. H. (1964). *Work and Motivation.* New York: Wiley.

C H A P T E R 9

LEADERSHIP SKILLS

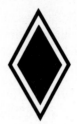

A nurse manager position brings with it new rights, privileges, and responsibilities. Among the last, for instance, are managing the health care of patients, directing the work and activities of employees, implementing and controlling a budget, serving as a vital link in the organizational chain of communication and control, and managing the functions that keep the unit running. The nurse manager's position demands effective leadership—the exercise of power and influence through interpersonal interaction processes—for the execution of these tasks.

Some people use the term *leadership* as a synonym for *management,* but the two terms do not have the same meaning. *Leadership* is an interpersonal relationship in which the leader employs specific behaviors and strategies to influence individuals and groups toward setting goals and attaining them in specific situations. The leader is a group member who influences and directs the contributions of other members toward individual or group achievement. *Management,* in contrast, refers to the coordination and integration of resources through planning, organizing, directing, and controlling to accomplish specific institutional goals and objectives. Thus, the manager is primarily concerned with scheduling and coordinating resources (including staff) and tasks. An implicit prerequisite for effective management is to establish effective leadership to achieve the objectives of management activities.

Supervision, too, is often confused with leadership. *Supervision* is the coordination of the basic work activities of an organizational unit in accordance with plans and procedures. It involves overseeing the work activities of others and directly concerns supervisor/subordinate interaction. It is possible for either a manager or supervisor to also be a leader. However, there

are managers with little or no leadership ability and supervisors with limited management skills. Management refers to certain task-oriented activities in a job. Leadership is the effective combination of management and supervision in a manner that invites or even inspires people to strive to attain organizational goals. In this chapter, the processes and behaviors of effective leadership are developed.

◆ LEADERSHIP DEFINED

Leadership is the use of one's skills to influence others to perform to the best of their ability. Although everyone has a different potential for leadership, the skills can be identified and learned, thereby improving the leader's performance. Historically, the nurse manager has been identified as the person who oversees all activities on the unit, including making patient care assignments, scheduling staff time, and planning inservice education. How effectively nurse managers accomplish these activities depends upon the degree to which they have developed their leadership skills.

Leadership is an interpersonal process of influencing the activities of an organized group toward goal setting and goal achievement (Moloney, 1979; Stogdill, 1974). Thus, leadership requires the presence of other people (followers) and is the relationship between those people and the person who is leading. Mere appointment to a leadership position does not ensure that a person will be accepted by the group or that the person is capable of providing leadership. An effective leader must be able to make people want to accomplish something. Leadership does not mean domination; it is the leader's job to get work done *through* other people. The nurse manager who accurately identifies a personality conflict between two staff members and is still able to achieve agreement between them regarding a vacation schedule is using effective leadership skills.

Leadership can be formal or informal, regardless of the hierarchical position or status of the nursing staff involved. Leadership is *informal* when practiced by a team member who is not designated as the nurse in charge. Whenever one nurse exerts more influence than another in accomplishing the work of the unit, that nurse is exercising leadership. This action can be complementary or contradictory to the goals of the unit or the hospital. Leadership is *formal* when practiced by the designated nurse in charge of the unit.

♦ BASES OF POWER

What resources can the leader bring to bear in a leadership situation? Studies of power have identified six bases of social power common in organizations (French & Raven, 1960; Mitchell & Larson, 1987):

1. *Reward power* is based upon the incentives the leader can provide for group members and upon the degree to which the group members value those incentives. For example, a nurse manager may have considerable influence in determining the salary or vacation time of a staff nurse. Reward power is often used in relation to a leader's formal job responsibilities.

2. *Punishment,* or *coercive power,* is based upon the negative things a leader might do to individual group members or the group as a whole. For example, the nurse manager might give a staff nurse very undesirable job assignments or a formal reprimand, recom-

mend that her or his pay be docked, or even recommend that she or he be fired.

3. *Information power* is based upon "who knows what" in an organization and the degree to which they can control access to that information by other individuals. The nurse manager, for instance, is frequently privy to information obtained at meetings with the nurse supervisor or through other informal channels of communication that either are not available to or are unknown to members of the nursing staff. Information can be either formally or informally gathered and distributed.

4. *Legitimate power* stems from the group members' perception that the nurse manager has a legitimate right to make a request; this power is based on the authority delegated to the nurse manager by virtue of her job and position within the management hierarchy.

5. *Expert power* is based upon particular knowledge and skill not possessed by staff members. Nurse managers, by virtue of their experience and, possibly, advanced education, frequently qualify as the persons who know best what to do in a given situation. For example, newly graduated nurses might look to the nurse manager for advice regarding particular procedures or for help in using equipment on the unit.

6. *Referent power* is based upon admiration and respect for an individual as a person. For example, a new graduate might ask the advice of the nurse manager regarding career planning. Referent power is largely a function of the leader's personal qualities.

This is a fairly impressive list of power bases that are potentially available to the nurse manager. Moreover, it indicates that power and influence may be derived from a number of sources. Rewards and punishment are largely determined by the organization while information power and legitimacy are primarily based upon the nurse manager's position within the organization. Referent power and expertise are derived from the leader's personal characteristics. While all of these sources of power are used at one time or another, the most effective combination seems to depend upon the situation at hand and the people involved.

Some general principles undergird the use of power (Mitchell & Larson, 1987). For example, managers seem to prefer using expert and legitimate power rather than punishment or appeals to friendship. By the same token, subordinates are more likely to comply with legitimate, expert, and referent power than they are with reward and coercive power. Fortunately, there is considerable agreement between what managers prefer to use and what subordinates prefer their managers to use. Nevertheless, there are some important differences, both in individuals and in organizations. For example, some managers are characteristically more authoritarian while others are more participative. The latter tend to rely more on expertise and referent power or peer pressure to get things done. More formally structured organizations often tend to emphasize a greater degree of autocratic control in their management systems.

Table 9–1 analyzes the likelihood of different power bases resulting in staff members' genuine commitment to the nurse manager's requests or to unit objectives, minimal compliance with requests and objectives, or active or passive rejection of the nurse manager's leadership. It is important to note that genuine commitment is far more likely to result from technical and managerial competence and from the nurse manager's

interpersonal behavior than from the use of rewards and punishment, which are readily available because of the manager's position in the organizational flow of communication and authority.

◆ LEADERSHIP: PERSONALITY, BEHAVIOR, OR STYLE?

The search for effective leadership characteristics as personality traits or personal attributes has not been productive. For every example of a great leader with certain characteristics, ten examples of leadership failure on the part of individuals possessing those same characteristics can easily be found. By the early 1950s, it had become clear that the situation itself is a major determinant of the extent to which leadership characteristics have any influence at all in determining leadership effectiveness (Stogdill, 1974).

At about this same time, several researchers began to focus more on what leaders do rather than on what personal characteristics they possess. Thus, leadership behavior research in laboratories at Harvard University found "activity," "task ability," and "likability" leadership behaviors. Studies at Ohio State University were conducted in field settings where subordinates were asked to describe the behaviors exhibited by their leaders. Two major dimensions were identified from the behaviors, one called "consideration" and the other, "initiating structure." Researchers at the University of Michigan also conducted research in the field but asked leaders themselves to describe what they did. This effort produced two major dimensions of leadership behavior: "job-centered behavior" and "employee-centered behavior."

Similarities across these research efforts are remarkably consistent. In each case, concern for the task was identified as a major aspect of leadership behavior (task ability, initiating structure, job-centered behavior), as was a second major dimension dealing with interpersonal relationships (likability, consideration, employee-centered behavior).

Specifically, *initiating structure* refers to behavior in which the nurse manager organizes

TABLE 9-1 EFFECTS OF MANAGERIAL POWER

Power type	Outcome		
	Commitment	**Compliance**	**Resistance**
Legitimate power	Possible–if request is polite and very appropriate	Likely–if request is seen as legitimate	Possible–if arrogant demands are made or request appears improper
Reward power	Possible–if used in a subtle, personal way	Likely–if used in a mechanical, impersonal way	Possible–if used in a manipulative, arrogant way
Information power	Unlikely–usually seen as inappropriate unless combined with expert or legitimate power	Likely–usually seen as inappropriate but recipients often have little counter-power	Possible–usually seen as inappropriate and arbitrary
Coercive power	Very unlikely	Possible–if used in a helpful, nonpunitive way	Likely–if used in a hostile or manipulative way
Expert power	Likely–if request is persuasive and subordinates share leader's task goals	Possible–if request is persuasive but subordinates are apathetic about task goals	Possible–if leader is arrogant and insulting or subordinates oppose task goals
Referent power	Likely–if request is believed to be important to the leader	Possible–if request is perceived to be unimportant to the leader	Possible–if request is for something that will bring harm to leader

Commitment: Subordinates accept leader's goals as their personal intention and exert maximum effort to accomplish them.

Compliance: Subordinates go along with the leader's requests without necessarily accepting the leader's goals. They are not enthusiatic and are likely to exert only the minimally acceptable level of effort in carrying out such requests.

Resistance: Subordinates reject the leader's goals and may pretend to comply but intentionally delay or sabotage the task.

Adapted from G. A. Yukl, *Leadership in Organizations*, 2nd ed. (Englewood Cliffs, NJ: Prentice-Hall, 1989).

and defines the work to be accomplished and establishes well-defined, routine work patterns, channels of communication, and methods of getting the job done. For example, management provides a detailed manual of job descriptions, personnel policies, and procedures for requesting time off on certain holidays. *Consideration,* on the other hand, refers to behavior that conveys mutual trust, respect, friendship, warmth, and rapport between the nurse manager and staff members. In this situation, the employee learns to expect that the nurse manager will hear a complaint openly without any reprisal.

Focusing on nurse manager behaviors to improve staff performance is supported by Jenkins and Henderson (1984), who examined how staff nurses, who perform the bulk of patient care, perceived the behaviors of charge nurses. Nurse manager behaviors that recognized the staff nurse's need for belonging, love, social activity, self-respect, status within the organization, recognition, dignity, and appreciation were viewed as essential for motivation as well as for quality patient care.

In general, the consistency of research on leader behavior has been encouraging, but the relationship of leader behaviors to leader effectiveness has proved to be puzzling. Neither increases in task behavior nor interpersonal behavior necessarily increased leadership effectiveness or employee job performance. Nevertheless, this earlier focus on leadership behavior has been a significant advance in understanding leadership effectiveness. The search for leadership styles or clusters of leadership behaviors began in an attempt to identify particular patterns or styles of leadership that would be most effective in most situations.

With the realization that different combinations of leader behaviors might produce different effects, some researchers began studying ways in which successful leadership is accomplished, or how leaders delegate tasks and how they communicate with their staff members. Thus, leadership styles are clusters of behaviors that characterize the manner in which a nurse manager uses interpersonal behaviors to influence the accomplishment of unit goals and the kinds of social power used. While the number of "leadership styles" one can find in the management literature almost rivals the number of personality traits once thought to be critical to leadership effectiveness, four general styles of leadership have frequently been identified. Typical leadership styles and their effects are briefly outlined in the following list, which is adapted from material by Ruth Jenkins.

Authoritarian or autocratic style

Primarily concerned with task accomplishment rather than relationships.

Primarily uses directive leadership behaviors.

Tends to make decisions alone.

Expects respect and obedience of staff.

May lack group support generated by participation.

Frequently exercises power with coercion.

Useful (even necessary) in crisis situations.

Democratic or participative style

Primarily concerned with human relations and teamwork.

Communication is open and usually goes both ways.

Spirit of collaboration and joint effort results in staff satisfaction.

Participation promotes acceptance of goals and goal commitment.

Permissive or laissez-faire style

Tends to have few established goals or policies; abstains from leading.

Not generally useful in highly structured organizations (e.g., health care institutions).

Bureaucratic style

Insecure leader finds security in following established policies.

Power exercised by fixed, relatively inflexible rules.

Tends to relate impersonally to staff.

Avoids decision making without standards or norms for guidance.

Similar to the research results for leadership behaviors, specific leadership styles appear to be more or less effective depending upon the situation (e.g., nature of tasks, organizational structure, subordinate characteristics). However, one result of research has been the recognition that, unlike traits or other specific characteristics, leadership behaviors and styles can be learned. The fact that a leader's personality or past experience helps form her preferred or "natural" style does not mean that leadership style is unchangeable or that a nurse manager always uses the same style of leadership. Leadership styles range from very authoritarian to very permissive and frequently change according to the situation. A nurse manager may use one style (e.g., authoritarian) when responding to an emergency situation such as a cardiac arrest. Another style (e.g., participation) may be used to encourage creative problem solving in developing a team strategy to care for a multi-problem patient or to generate ideas for use of a new procedure. The most effective leadership style for a nurse manager is the one that best complements

the organizational environment, the tasks to be accomplished, and the personal characteristics of the people involved in each situation.

However, focusing on leadership styles does not explain which style will be most effective under which circumstances, nor do any of these approaches consider the specific and systematic effects of the leadership situation. This recurrent deficiency in leadership research eventually led to the development of several contingency theories of leadership that attempt to integrate leadership traits, leadership behaviors, and leadership situations in a unified theoretical framework. This framework helps us not only to understand more about effective leadership but also to predict what kinds of leader behaviors will be most effective in different circumstances.

♦ CONTINGENCY THEORIES OF LEADERSHIP

FIEDLER'S CONTINGENCY MODEL

In the mid-1960s, Fiedler articulated a contingency model of leadership effectiveness, which suggests that a manager's leadership style must be matched with the requirements of the situation to be effective (Fiedler, 1967). In Fiedler's theory, effectiveness is very carefully defined as the performance of the group itself, rather than a rating of the leader's effectiveness.

Fiedler differentiates two leadership styles, which he calls relationship-oriented and task-oriented leadership. These leadership styles are assessed with a questionnaire called the Least-Preferred Co-worker scale (LPC). The leader rates her least preferred co-worker on a set of 17 bipolar scales anchored at either end by adjectives (e.g., efficient–inefficient, friendly–rejecting). If the leader's least preferred co-worker is described in relatively positive terms, the leader is said to have an underlying relationship-oriented leadership style. If the least preferred co-worker is described in relatively unfavorable terms, then the individual is said to be basically a task-oriented leader.

Since Fiedler (1967) defines leadership as a process of influence, the leadership situation is described on a dimension that represents the relative ease or difficulty with which the leader can influence group members. This dimension, called situation favorability, has three components. The first is *leader-member relations,* the degree to which the leader enjoys the loyalty and support of subordinates. Second, *task structure* is the degree to which the task or finished product is clearly described and/or there are standard operating procedures that guarantee successful completion of the task and make it easy for the leader to determine how well the work has been performed. Finally, *position power* is the degree

to which the leader is able to administer rewards and punishment by virtue of his or her position (i.e., legitimate power).

When leader-member relations are relatively good, when the task is highly structured, and when the leader has high position power, it is relatively easy for the leader to influence the group toward the accomplishment of organizational objectives. Fiedler states that the leader-member relations component is the most important; task structure, the next most important; and the leader's formal position power, the least important determinant of situation favorability.

Figure 9–1 illustrates the preferred leadership styles given different combinations of situational characteristics. According to Fiedler, a leader is most effective when the leadership style and the situation are matched, and he suggests that leaders should attempt to seek situations in which their predominant style is most appropri-

FIGURE 9–1 PREDICTIONS FROM FIEDLER'S CONTINGENCY THEORY OF LEADERSHIP

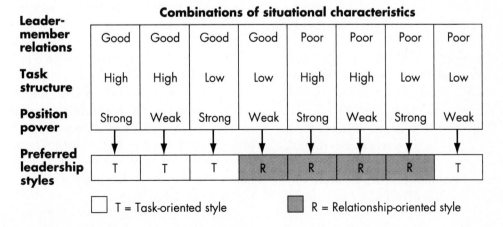

Combinations of situational characteristics

Leader-member relations	Good	Good	Good	Good	Poor	Poor	Poor	Poor
Task structure	High	High	Low	Low	High	High	Low	Low
Position power	Strong	Weak	Strong	Weak	Strong	Weak	Strong	Weak
Preferred leadership styles	T	T	T	R	R	R	R	T

T = Task-oriented style   R = Relationship-oriented style

John R. Schermerhorn, Jr., James G. Hunt, and Richard N. Osborn, *Managing Organizational Behavior.* (New York: John Wiley & Sons, 1982). Used by permission.

ate. Should a mismatch occur, Fiedler suggests that the leader should either attempt to change characteristics or the situation.

PATH-GOAL THEORY

Path-goal theory is an effort to apply a theory of human motivation and task performance to the realm of leadership effectiveness (House & Mitchell, 1974). A primary function of leadership is to motivate group members toward the attainment of organizational objectives. Path-goal theory suggests that this motivational function is carried out through leadership behaviors that remove obstacles to goal attainment and that make personal rewards for employees contingent upon attainment of those goals. Thus, a leader's function is to coach, guide, and provide performance incentives to ensure high work performance. Furthermore, the theory suggests that leader behavior directly affects group members' job satisfaction to the extent that the leader makes rewards available and that the leader's behavior itself is a source of satisfaction to subordinates.

The motivational functions of leadership are built directly on the expectancy theory of work motivation (see Chapter 8). Briefly, employees are likely to work for rewards that they find attractive and that are likely to be awarded for successful performance. However, expectancy theory also suggests that expectancies (the perceived probability that effort will lead to high performance) must be strong before employees will be highly motivated. In this case, the nurse manager's role is to clarify the nature of the task (the performance objective), to facilitate the staff member's attainment of that objective by providing the necessary resources and training, and to ensure the coordination and cooperation of other individuals required for successful task accomplishment.

To accomplish these ends, path-goal theory specifies four leader behaviors: *Supportive leadership* includes behaviors that consider the needs of subordinates, display concern for their well-being, and create a friendly climate in the work unit. *Directive leadership* involves letting subordinates know what they are expected to do, giving specific guidance, asking them to follow rules and procedures, and scheduling and coordinating work efforts. *Achievement-oriented leadership* includes setting challenging goals, seeking performance improvements, emphasizing excellence in performance, and showing confidence that subordinates will attain high levels of performance. In *participative leadership* the manager consults with subordinates and takes their opinions and suggestions into account when making decisions.

Staff members interpret and respond to leader behavior in different ways depending upon such situational factors as subordinate characteristics, and characteristics of the task and environment. Specifically, subordinates' needs for achievement, affiliation, and autonomy; their ability to do the task (i.e., their job skills, knowledge, experience); and their personality traits (e.g., self-esteem) form a background or context within which leader behavior functions. Task and environmental characteristics also form a part of the background and include task structure (defined the same as in Fiedler's contingency model) and the degree of formalization imposed by the organization (e.g., written job descriptions, rules, standard operating procedures, performance standards). The effect of leadership behavior on subordinate satisfaction and effort depends upon the situation in which the leadership behavior occurs.

Supportive leadership behavior should be especially effective when subordinates perceive the job as boring, frustrating, stressful, or otherwise unpleasant. By trying to make the job more tolerable, the nurse manager can directly affect employee satisfaction and perhaps even increase the desirability of the intrinsically motivating aspects of the work. Of course, when the work is perceived as interesting and enjoyable, supportive behavior does not necessarily increase either job satisfaction or motivation. When a nurse has relatively high self-esteem or little fear of failure, supportive leadership may have little or no effect on motivation.

Provided staff nurses do not already know what to do in a particular situation, directive leadership reduces role ambiguity (increasing expectancies) and increases the nurse's satisfaction. When the nurse manager explains the relationship between performance and rewards, instrumentalities should increase. In addition, directive leadership can influence the desirability of outcomes for task success by changing the size or amount of rewards and punishment. However, these effects will be successful only to the extent that the nurse manager actually has control over specific rewards and punishment. As noted in Chapter 8, money is not the only (and often is not the best) incentive that can be used to successfully motivate staff members. Of course, the situation determines whether the directive nurse manager is likely to increase staff motivation and satisfaction.

Achievement-oriented leadership behaviors increase subordinates' confidence in their ability to achieve challenging goals. As noted in the discussion of goal setting theory in Chapter 8, the higher the goal, the higher the performance, even when the goal is not always attained. Thus, the simple act of setting a goal, in addition to the expression of confidence in a staff member's ability, positively influences motivation. Of course, this is more effective when the task is fairly ambiguous and nonrepetitive, meaning it

is relatively unstructured. Setting a specific goal not only clarifies what is to be done, but it also stimulates the development of strategies and plans for goal attainment, thus adding structure to an ambiguous task.

Participative leadership behavior also has its greatest effect with unstructured tasks. Participation gives staff members an opportunity to learn more about an unfamiliar task, and helping to develop both goals and strategies or plans to attain them directly affects employees' understanding of what has to be done and how they must go about accomplishing it. Staff members who have high achievement or autonomy needs respond more favorably to participative leadership behavior than those who have lower needs for achievement and autonomy or who prefer structured tasks with little responsibility for decision making. In fact, the latter may find participation threatening and demanding, leading to less satisfaction with the nurse manager. The effect of specific leadership behaviors on staff satisfaction and motivation depends directly upon the situation (particularly the degree of task structure) and employee characteristics.

Many nursing tasks are highly routinized and structured. However, many aspects of nursing (e.g., patient relationships, orienting new staff members, special projects) are relatively unstructured. Thus, it is not always easy to prescribe a given leadership behavior that would be most effective for a particular task and employee combination. There is no substitute for good common sense and the judicious application of motivation and leadership principles. No formula exists that will work in every situation with every staff member or that can be applied across the board by anyone.

The task of leadership is complex and requires continuous problem solving. To use the path-goal theory of leadership effectively, the nurse manager needs to engage constantly in diagnosing and predicting employee responses to given leadership acts. Path-goal theory provides a framework that casts some light on the effects of specific leadership behaviors and the types of situations in which such behaviors are or are not appropriate. It can be a very useful leadership tool for nurse managers who regard their leadership responsibilities realistically.

THE NORMATIVE MODEL OF DECISION PARTICIPATION

Vroom and Yetton (1973) provide a normative, or prescriptive, model for determining the amount of participation in decision making to be used in different situations. In essence, their model helps managers decide "how to make a decision."

Vroom and Yetton's model suggests that managerial decisions can be made with varying degrees of subordinate participation and that the amount of participation that should be al-

lowed depends upon whether the manager has all of the information needed to make the decision and whether staff members' acceptance of the decision is required to implement it effectively. As Figure 9–2 shows, these factors combine to form a two-by-two table that can be used to help nurse managers decide when to allow their staff to participate in decision making and to what degree staff participation is appropriate.

Participation is not simply present or absent; it varies in amount, as represented by different leadership styles. A nurse manager may (a) delegate all decision authority to a group meeting of staff and agree to live with their decision (delegate); (b) delegate to a staff meeting but participate in the meeting as an "equal" member (join); (c) consult with the staff individually or in a group, make the decision, and then inform the staff (consult); (d) make the decision and then "sell" it to the staff by providing information or other arguments (sell); or (e) simply decide (tell).

FIGURE 9–2 VARIABLES AFFECTING USE OF PARTICIPATION IN LEADERSHIP

		Manager has all of the information needed to make the decision	
		Yes	No
Acceptance of subordinates needed to effectively implement?	Yes	Use some participation	Participation absolutely required
	No	Need no participation	Use some participation

It makes sense that the effectiveness of each of these styles differs according to the type of decision. Figure 9–3 is a decision tree designed to help nurse managers decide when to use each style of decision making.

The nurse manager needs to consider only three questions: (1) Do I have all the information needed to make the decision, (2) is acceptance of subordinates required for effective implementation, and (3) if I delegate, will sub-

ordinates make a decision that I can live with? Figure 9–3 also indicates the time consideration in using each style. Less participative styles usually take less of the manager's (and staff's) time per decision.

Consider the following example: Ms. Jones, nurse manager of the cardiac intensive care unit, is interested in changing her unit from traditional management to shared governance. She has the support of the administration who

FIGURE 9–3 USE OF PARTICIPATIVE LEADERSHIP STYLES

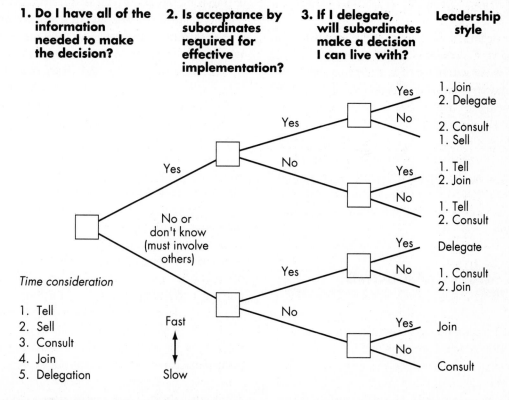

Developed by Phillip J. Decker and James Breaugh. Used by permission.

would like her unit to pilot the model. She now must consider her staff's reactions. Using Figure 9–3, she asks the following questions:

1. Do I have all the information needed to make the decision? Ms. Jones decides "no." She needs to know, for example, how much the staff know about shared governance and how they feel about it.

2. Is acceptance by subordinates required for effective implementation? In this case, the answer is obviously "yes."

3. If I delegate, will subordinates make a decision I can live with? Ms. Jones decides "no," that she is ultimately responsible for the outcome of such a major change and, therefore, must make the final decision.

According to Figure 9–3, the leadership style to use in this case is either join or consult. Ms. Jones could join her staff in a meeting to discuss the hindrances and benefits that would be likely in moving to shared governance. Alternatively, she could discuss the pros and cons of implementing shared governance with the staff; gather information on staff nurse time for decision making, potential costs, and other possible consequences to the unit and ask for staff recommendations; and then make a decision (consult).

♦ A SOCIAL LEARNING APPROACH TO LEADERSHIP

Social learning theory recognizes that although education is one way human beings learn what to do in various situations, most of what people learn throughout life does not come from formal classroom training or even on-the-job coaching. Indeed, the average child of two or three has learned an incredible array of behaviors, most of them without the aid of formal parental training. Rather, the child's behaviors are learned vicariously by observing models (e.g., parents, siblings, television) and then rehearsing these behaviors either covertly or overtly until they are well practiced. The expression, "Out of the mouths of babes . . ." largely reflects instances in which children practice new behaviors without having yet learned fully why they are done or when to display them. The point is that social learning processes begin at a very early age and continue throughout our lives. Although such behaviors are learned, they cannot be effectively performed without some kind of practice.

For example, reading this book on how to be a nurse manager, or, more specifically, this chapter on using leadership skills, will not make you an effective nurse manager. You may know what to do and even to some extent how to do it, but without practice and experience, your learning will be minimal. On the other hand, you can learn a great deal about being a nurse manager (both effective and ineffective) by observing nurse managers for whom you have worked and nurse managers in other units. While this book should provide you with considerable information about being a nurse manager, none of it will truly be yours until you actually put it into practice and make it a part of your personal experience.

So what does social learning theory have to offer you in managing and supervising your nursing staff? Simply this: As a nurse manager you are a very visible and important role model for the staff members whom you lead. If you think it is important for them to accomplish some particular task, then use your expertise as a knowledgeable model. Demonstrate the appropriate behaviors (the right way to do the task), pointing out the pitfalls and potential problem areas along the way. Once you have demonstrated the correct procedure several times, ask the staff nurse to perform the task, giving appropriate feedback and guidance as the task is done. To the extent that you can involve other staff nurses in such training (especially in providing feedback and social support for task accomplishment), the more effective training becomes. (See Chapter 14 for more detail on staff development.)

What about non-training situations? What about the nursing behaviors that, although not technical, are critical to successful nursing performance? What about being at work on time or even a few minutes early to allow time for necessary reports without inconveniencing the departing shift? What about displaying cooperation, sensitivity, and tact with other nurses, doctors, and patients? Remember that your behavior as a role model always serves as a guide for the behavior of others. By becoming more consciously aware of what you do, how you do it, and when you do it, you can more easily begin to diagnose the successes and failures of your staff.

When nurses on your unit do not perform their jobs in accordance with your expectations, first ask yourself whether you have provided the appropriate behaviors as a role model. If you are certain that you have, simply draw their attention to the appropriate behaviors (without necessarily holding yourself up as an example). Gently remind them of what they should be doing and reinforce them with praise when they do the right things. If, on the other hand, your analysis shows that your behavior as role model is deficient, acknowledge your own deficiency to your staff and explain the importance of behaving in the appropriate manner and your intention to do so in the future. This requires courage. If you can do it and, in fact, change your own behavior, your new behavior will be noticed and probably emulated.

PYGMALION EFFECT

The Pygmalion effect, named after George Bernard Shaw's play by that name that was popularized on Broadway as *My Fair Lady* (Patton & Giffin, 1981), refers to self-fulfilling prophecy: An individual or a situation becomes what one expects it to be. In *My Fair Lady,* the professor envisioned the poor, illiterate flower girl as an erudite princess, which she, in fact, eventually became. A fairy tale, perhaps, but its effect is demonstrably both subtle and profound.

For example, elementary school children were tested at the beginning of the school year and matched in terms of their measured intelligence quotients (IQs). Within each "same IQ" pair, one child was randomly assigned to the "high expectation" group, while the other was randomly assigned to the "low expectation" group. Only the researchers knew that the children in each pair had identical IQs; their classroom teachers were given the expectation of high or low performance for each student in the coming school year. The teachers tried to treat each child as an individual, giving each one the particular attention and encouragement required for his or her own development on the basis of their expectations about each child's potential for improvement.

At the end of the school year, each child's intelligence was again tested. The children who had been placed in the "high expectation" group increased their measured IQs significantly above those children who were placed in the "low expectation" group, in spite of the fact that their initial IQs were essentially identical. How and in what subtle ways the teachers' expectations were reflected in intelligence scores at the end of the school year is unknown, but the fact is that the teachers' expectations produced differences in the children's test-taking behavior.

It is fairly easy to understand how a self-fulfilling prophecy can affect human beings who have a high capacity for perceiving and interpreting the responses of others around them. The power of this effect, however, becomes even more apparent in a study in which graduate students who were conducting research with laboratory rats were given expectations about how well particular rats learned. The rats had presumably been bred for effective learning (smart rats) or slower learning (stupid rats). In fact, the rats were litter mates, born of the same mother and reared in exactly the same environment. The only difference lay in the expectations given the graduate students.

The students trained the rats to learn a sequence of left and right turns in a standard laboratory maze. The rats in the "stupid group" were given the same number of trials to learn the maze as those in the "smart group." At the end of the study the "smart" rats were found to have learned the correct sequence of turns significantly faster than the rats in the "stupid group."

How the graduate students conveyed their expectations to the rats is unknown. Obviously, the behavior of the researchers was very subtle and could not have involved formal language as cues or hints regarding their expectations. Nevertheless, the behavior of the rats was distinctly different, illustrating the very potent effect that our expectations of other individuals actually have.

The Pygmalion effect is closely related to social learning, the focus of which is that behaviors are observed and learned vicariously. The Pygmalion effect demonstrates that not only modeled behaviors but also attitudes, particularly attitudes toward the performer, are learned as well. If these attitudes are so easily learned by rats, then how easily can expectations expressed in subtle behaviors be perceived and responded to by staff nurses?

How do the nurse manager's expectations show up in the motivation and performance of a staff nurse? Consider the motivation theories discussed in Chapter 8. Why should a staff nurse be expected to perform well if he or she perceives that the nurse manager has little confidence that he or she can actually accomplish the task? It is very difficult for most people to hide their true feelings and expectations. If the nurse manager really does not think the staff nurse can accomplish the task, then perhaps the task is really too difficult. The key is to have *realistic expectations* about an individual's ability, to expect a performance that is demanding but attainable for that individual. Managerial expectations must be expressed with a "can do" attitude, the kind of behavior that conveys to the staff nurse, "I expect you to be what you *can* be."

Chapter 8 discussed the shaping of behavior, which is positively reinforcing approximations to the behavior that is desired. A key factor in shaping, as in the Pygmalion effect, is to have realistic expectations regarding the degree of approximate behavior to be achieved while maintaining conscious efforts to develop the behavior that is actually desired. In short, do not accept "close" as "good enough"; only "acceptable or better" is "good enough." Of course, "good enough" today may not be "good enough" two weeks from now; a realistic expectation can, and often does, change. However, realistic expectations are never impossible to achieve. Realistic expectations or goals should be challenging and should be supported by the nurse manager's coaching and expressions of confidence and pleasure with staff members' successes.

How does this occur? Achievement-oriented leadership behavior, for example, stresses the attainment of challenging goals. Directive and/or participative leadership behaviors should help to clarify not only what the staff nurse should do but also how to do it. Again, modeling is an excellent way to facilitate this kind of learning. Finally, supportive leadership behavior can be employed to express confidence in the staff nurse's ability to do the job and to express pleasure with the subordinate's success.

The subordinate's success is ultimately the leader's success. If the nurse manager takes pride in the staff nurse's success and does everything in his or her power to bring about that kind of success, then the nurse manager will, indeed, be an effective leader. The important point is that our attitudes are expressed very subtly in our behaviors. Realistic expectations and genuine help in trying to develop employee performance will go a long way toward achieving that end.

◆ BUILDING A TEAM WITH LEADERSHIP

Nursing is an interactive group task requiring continuous problem solving and a great deal of teamwork (see Chapter 5). Unfortunately, research shows that many managers have considerable difficulty building an effective team. In fact, most managers treat a few subordinates as members of a trusted cadre, or "in group," while others are relegated to the "out group" comprising the rest of the staff. In-group employees enjoy more frequent communication with the manager, are more likely to be "in-the-

know" about organizational plans and activities, and are far more likely to be consulted when decisions regarding the department or unit are made. Not surprisingly, these individuals have higher job satisfaction and are generally given higher performance ratings than out-group employees (Dansereau, Graen & Haga, 1975). It should not be surprising that close teamwork is very difficult to develop when managers "play favorites" with some staff members.

Because staff nurses work in close proximity and frequently depend upon each other to accomplish their jobs, the character or climate of leadership and group interaction is extremely important. An effective group atmosphere is one in which staff members feel free to talk about what concerns them, to critique and offer suggestions, and to experiment with new behaviors without threat. Such an atmosphere can only be maintained in a work group that is warm and supportive and is relatively unhindered by interpersonal conflicts, favoritism, and political infighting. Maintaining such an atmosphere or climate is a difficult leadership task.

One of the best ways to develop a supportive climate is to foster a feeling of group cohesiveness. Cohesiveness is the degree of attraction that each group member feels toward the group. Strong group cohesiveness leads to a feeling of "we" as being more important than self-centered "I" feelings and ensures a higher degree of cooperation and interpersonal support among group members. The "catch-22" in group cohesiveness is whether the group norms, the informal or often unstated rules and expectations regarding appropriate behavior for group members, support or subvert organizational objectives. High group cohesiveness fosters either higher or lower individual performance, depending upon group norms.

Groups lacking cohesiveness have difficulty getting much accomplished because members' efforts are more likely to go in scattered directions than to be focused toward the attainment of goals and outcomes valued by the group. Fortunately for the nurse manager, the nursing profession supports high standards of patient care, and nursing education induces values and patterns of behavior that encourage those high standards. However, this is true only to a degree; some work units are more successful than others in providing patient care because of differences in group cohesiveness.

The nurse manager can foster high group cohesiveness primarily through managing group interaction patterns. Cohesiveness is a process of interpersonal attraction, and this attraction is influenced by a number of characteristics (Mitchell & Larson, 1987). For example, the physical proximity of some group members makes it likely that they will develop a friendship. Furthermore, the frequency of interaction and the expectation of future interaction increase the likelihood that individuals will be attracted to those who are physically nearby.

Of particular importance is managing communication processes to facilitate unit effectiveness. The nurse manager who maintains a high degree of information power, for instance, controls not only what information is received but who receives it, funneling it down to specific, individual staff nurses. This represents a highly centralized communication structure in contrast to one in which the nurse manager encourages a high degree of participative group problem solving. In participative groups, each individual has the opportunity, and is encouraged, to communicate frequently with anyone and everyone in the group.

The relative effectiveness of centralized versus decentralized communication networks depends upon the structure of the task (defined in Fiedler's contingency model and in path-goal theory). For very complex and unstructured problems, a decentralized communication structure produces solutions in less time and with fewer errors and enhances member satisfaction more than a highly centralized structure. For rather simple problems or tasks that are more structured, a centralized communication network may yield faster results and have fewer errors than a decentralized structure.

In addition, members of groups who have a history of success with a task are attracted to each other more than if they have not been successful: Success breeds attraction. When group members have a common goal, there is higher attraction than when they have different goals. A common goal provides a bond around which interaction and friendships develop. In addition, the ability to influence group decision processes increases attraction to the group. Nurse managers can influence all of these factors through task design, work assignments, and the decision-making/leadership processes they implement in the unit.

The greatest contributions to interpersonal attraction come from the personal characteristics of group members. People are attracted to those whom they perceive to be similar to themselves. Similarities in race, education, background, attitudes, and values all increase the interpersonal attractiveness of group members. People seem to like each other because they have common goals, because other people can be rewarding in a variety of ways, or because they are similar on a number of important dimensions. This increased attraction influences group processes and results.

In general, the greater the attraction, the greater the influence. In job satisfaction research, results are quite clear: Increased attraction (cohesiveness) leads to increased satisfaction. However, performance is increased only if the norms and goals of the group support the organization's objectives. Cohesive groups can make or break the nurse manager's leadership efforts and should always be taken into account as part of the leadership situation. In particular, communication networks (who talks to whom) have considerable implication for both performance and job satisfaction.

◆ PUTTING IT ALL TOGETHER

At the outset of this chapter leadership was defined as the exercise of power and influence by an individual over the members of a group. Staff members learn very quickly how a nurse manager "operates" and decide whether they will commit to the unit, their work group, and the manager; simply comply with minimum standards of performance; or resist organizational and managerial efforts to influence their job behavior. Ultimately, what you *do* (i.e., your behavior) as a manager can make the task of managing individual and group performance either extremely difficult or pleasant and relatively easy. The contingency theories of leadership can be helpful in suggesting effective leadership behavior in given situations, but it will take considerable practice before you will be comfortable in knowing what to do and when to do it. In any event, how you display leadership behavior is just as critical as what behavior you choose; how you exercise power, in any social relationship, entails the development of skill that can only be attained through careful planning and practice.

Box 9–1 provides some guidelines to help you use your power resources effectively. While the guidelines suggest specific points for each type of power, common themes are applicable to all of them. First, always plan what you are going to do before you do it; never "shoot from the hip" or exercise your power carelessly. Second, always act to maintain or enhance the other person's self-esteem. This is critical and is very easy to remember if you simply get in the habit of putting yourself in the other person's shoes and treating them exactly as you would want to be treated. Finally, keep the exercise of your leadership power impartial and impersonal, regardless of whether you are persuading, rewarding, or punishing a staff member's behavior. Focus on the job-related, professional *behavior* of a staff nurse.

Friendship is personal and should not influence your judicious choice of appropriate leadership behavior. Truly professional staff nurses expect and appreciate professional leadership behavior appropriate to the situation, irrespective of personal considerations. Fairness and impartiality as a manager go a long way in enhancing your referent and expert power, and these go a long way in helping to build genuine commitment to the nursing unit and to you as a nurse manager.

SUMMARY

◆ One of the responsibilities of a nurse manager is leadership—the employment of specific behaviors and strategies to influence individuals and groups toward goal attainment in specific situations.

◆ Leadership differs from management, which is a more global term encompassing processes of planning, organizing, directing (supervising), and controlling.

BOX 9-1
GUIDELINES FOR THE USE
OF POWER IN ORGANIZATIONS

Using authority

1. Make polite requests, not arrogant demands.
2. Make requests in clear, simple language; check for staff understanding.
3. Explain reasons for requests.
4. Follow up to check for compliance.

Using rewards

1. Don't overemphasize incentives; staff will expect rewards for every request. Emphasize mutual loyalty and teamwork.
2. Rewards are unlikely to produce commitment.
3. Reinforce past behavior; don't bribe for future performance.
4. The size of rewards should reflect total performance.
5. Money is not the only (and is often the least effective) reward.
6. Avoid appearing manipulative at all costs.

Using coercive power

1. Avoid coercion and punishment except when absolutey necessary.
2. Punish only to deter extremely detrimental behavior.
3. Try to determine genuine fault before criticizing.
4. Discipline promptly and consistently without favoritism. Fit the punishment to the seriousness of the infraction.
5. State warnings without hostility; remain calm and express desire to help subordinate comply with requirements and avoid punishment.
6. Invite subordinate to share in responsibility for

correcting disciplinary problems; set improvement goals and develop improvement plans.
7. Warn before punishing; don't issue idle or exaggerated warnings you are not prepared to carry out.

Using expert power

1. Preserve credibility by avoiding careless statements and rash decisions.
2. Keep informed about technical developments affecting the group's work.
3. In a crisis, remain calm; act confidently and decisively.
4. Avoid arrogance or "talking down" to staff; show respect for staff ideas and suggestions and incorporate them whenever feasible.
5. Do not threaten subordinates' self-esteem.
6. Recognize subordinates' concerns; explain why a proposed plan of action is best and, what steps will be taken to minimize risk to them.

Using referent power

1. Be considerate, show concern for staff needs and feelings, treat them fairly, and defend their interests to superiors and outsiders.
2. Avoid expressing hostility, distrust, rejection, or indifference toward subordinates. Actions speak louder than words.
3. Explain the personal importance of requests and your reliance on staff support and cooperation.
4. Don't make requests too often; make requests reasonable.
5. Be a good role model.

Adapted from G. A. Yukl and T. Tabor, "The Effective Use of Managerial Power," *Personnel* (March-April 1983).

♦ Leadership behavior can be learned.

♦ Leadership is the exercise of power. Power can come from several sources: control over rewards, control over sanctions, control of

information, authority given by the institution, personal expertise, and referent power.

♦ The exercise of social power through leadership behavior can be important in determining whether staff members are genuinely committed to, passively accept, or actively resist organizational goals and managerial requests.

♦ The search for leadership characteristics has focused on personality traits, leader behaviors, and leadership styles. None of these approaches has adequately defined successful leadership.

♦ Leadership behaviors and styles are not fixed; they can be learned and different behaviors/styles are frequently displayed as the situation requires.

♦ Fiedler took leadership beyond identifying styles/behaviors with his contingency model. He said that successful leadership was an interaction of leadership style and the situation.

♦ House and Mitchell's path-goal theory says a leader is effective to the extent that he or she helps subordinates identify goals and the paths to attaining those goals.

♦ Vroom and Yetton provide a prescriptive model of participative leadership—it tells the nurse manager how much participation to use in different situations.

♦ Nurse managers must pay attention to the examples they provide staff and to their expectations of staff members, as both influence staff behavior.

♦ Providing nursing care is a team effort. The nurse manager must develop an understanding of group communication and interpersonal attraction processes and use that understanding to develop a supportive climate to foster group cohesiveness.

♦ Building an effective team in a nursing unit involves carefully planned and carefully exerted power through leadership behavior. How the nurse manager accomplishes this is just as important as choosing the most appropriate leadership behavior in a given situation.

BIBLIOGRAPHY

Dansereau, F., Jr., Graen, G., and Haga, W. J. (1975). "A Vertical Dyad Linkage Approach to Leadership within Formal Organizations: A Longitudinal Investigation of the Role Making Process." *Organizational Behavior and Human Performance,* 13: 46.

Fiedler, F. E. (1967). *A Theory of Leadership Effectiveness.* New York: McGraw-Hill.

French, J. R. P., and Raven, B. (1960). "The Bases of Social Power." In: *Group Dynamics.* 2d ed. Cartwright, D., and Zander, A. (editors). Evanston, IL: Row, Peterson.

House, R. J., and Mitchell, T. R. (1974). "Path-Goal Theory of Leadership." *Journal of Contemporary Business,* 3: 81.

Jenkins, R. L., and Henderson, R. L. (1984). "Motivating the Staff: What Nurses Expect from Their Supervisors." *Nursing Management,* 15(2): 13.

Mitchell, T. R., and Larson, J. R., Jr. (1987). *People in Organizations.* 3d ed. New York: McGraw-Hill.

Moloney, M. M. (1979). *Leadership in Nursing: Theory, Strategies, Action.* St. Louis, MO: Mosby.

Patton, B. R., and Giffin, K. (1981). *Interpersonal Communication in Action.* 3d ed. New York: Harper & Row.

Stogdill, R. M. (1974). *Handbook of Leadership: A Survey of the Literature.* New York: Free Press.

Vroom, V. H. (1976). "Leadership." In: *Handbook of Industrial and Organizational Psychology.* Dunnette, M. D. (editor). Chicago: Rand McNally.

Vroom, V. H., and Yetton, P. W. (1973). *Leadership and Decision Making.* Pittsburgh, PA: University of Pittsburgh Press.

Yukl, G. A. (1989). *Leadership in Organizations.* 2d ed. Englewood Cliffs, NJ: Prentice-Hall.

Yukl, G. A., and Taber, T. (1983). "The Effective Use of Managerial Power." *Personnel* (March–April): 60(2):37.

C H A P T E R 10

STRESS
AND TIME
MANAGEMENT

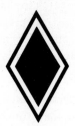

Consider the following scenario. Sue is a medical nurse with 10 years of experience. She is married and has two children under the age of six who attend preschool while Sue is at work. As a nursing clinical director, Sue has 24-hour responsibility for supervision of two 30-bed medical units. She frequently receives calls from the unit nurses during the evenings and nights, and approximately once a week has to return to the unit to intervene in a situation or to replace a nurse or nurses who are absent. Sue is responsible for scheduling all nurses on the units and is not approved for the use of agency nurses, in spite of a 20 percent vacancy rate. Additionally, Sue serves on four departmental committees and the hospital task force on consumer relations. She consistently takes work home, including performance appraisals, quality assessment reports, and professional journals. Although provided with an office, Sue has little opportunity to use it, due to interruptions from nurses, physicians, other departmental leaders, and her supervisor. Recently, Sue saw her family physician, due to persistent headaches, weight loss, and a feeling of constant fatigue. After a complete diagnostic workup, Sue was found to have a slightly elevated blood pressure, with a resting pulse of 100. Her physician prescribed an exercise program, and she was advised to lighten her workload, take a vacation, and reduce her stress.

Steers (1984) defines stress as the reaction of individuals to demands from the environment that pose a threat. Two or more incompatible demands on the body cause a conflict that results in stress. Selye (1978), recognized as the pioneer of stress research, suggests that the body's wear and tear results from its response to normal stressors. The rate and intensity of damage is increased when an organism experiences greater stress than it is capable of accommodating.

Selye maintains that response to stress is the same whether the stressor is positive or negative. The stress associated with negative events, such as job loss, is easily envisioned. However, stress also may be experienced during positive events. For example, John was the director of nursing for critical care in a 400-bed hospital. He was offered the opportunity to develop a specialty unit for ventilator-dependent patients. In assuming the additional responsibility, John began putting in long hours and working weekends. As the project progressed, John became unable to sleep and gained 10 pounds. After the unit opened, John's sleep pattern and weight returned to normal. Clearly, John displayed emotional and physical signs of stress although experiencing a "positive" promotion and career opportunity.

A certain amount of stress is essential to sustain life, and moderate amounts serve as stimuli to performance. But overpowering stress causes one to respond in a maladaptive physiological or psychological manner.

◆ THE NATURE OF STRESS

Stress and the capability to handle it must be balanced. Figure 10–1 depicts this. When the degree of stress is equal to the degree of ability to accommodate it, the organism is in a state of equilibrium and job performance and personal satisfaction tend to be high. Normal wear and tear occur, but sustained damage does not. When the degree of stress is greater than the ability to accommodate it, increased pressure is applied. The situation is often described metaphorically through such statements as "carrying a load on one's shoulders" or "bearing a heavy burden." This often leads to physiological and psychological problems for the person and poor performance for the organization. When the degree of stress is less than the ability to accommodate it, little pressure is applied to the person (either internal or external), and lack of interest, apathy, boredom, low motivation, low performance, and absenteeism may occur.

The stress experience is subjective and individualized. One person's stressful event is another's challenge. One individual can experience an event, positive or negative, that would prove overwhelming for someone else. Even a slight change in institutional policy may cause some individuals to experience stress. On one 36-bed orthopedic unit, the evening charge nurse changed patient assignment criteria. Although the change appeared logical and in the best interests of quality patient care, two nurses complained to the nursing administrator, and one resigned.

FIGURE 10–1 STRESS BALANCE

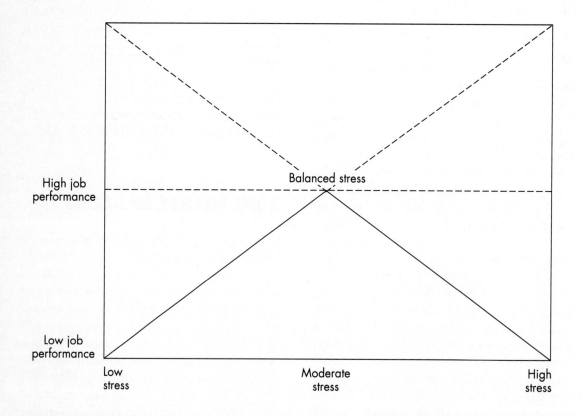

Stress in the workplace and, specifically, for the nurse, can develop from several sources. Figure 10–2 shows a model and includes the antecedents of stress, the intervening variables of role ambiguity and role conflict, and the consequences of stress.

ANTECEDENTS OF STRESS

Stress resulting from *job tasks* and the *physical environment* develops from such conditions as task overload, conflicting tasks, inability to do the tasks assigned due to lack of preparation or experience, or unclear or insufficient information regarding the assignment. Lack of education or experience can contribute to role ambiguity and result in stress. Nurses' jobs are often performed in life-or-death situations. There may be periods of extreme overload caused by emergencies that are potentially stressful. Likewise, nurses who are asked to implement procedures or orders for which they are not educationally prepared experience stress. Such is the frequent complaint of nurses who are required to "float" from one unit to another. Nurse managers need

---

FIGURE 10–2 STRESS MODEL

ANTECEDENTS	INTERVENING CONSTRUCTS	CONSEQUENCES
Organizational factors		**Negative**
Job tasks		Stress
Physical environment		Health problems
Supervisor behavior		Marital problems/divorce
Institutional factors		Alcoholism/drug abuse
Changing environment		Lower performance
Societal/nursing traditions		Lower job satisfaction
Self-worth		Lower self-esteem
Intraprofessional divisiveness		Absenteeism/turnover
	Role ambiguity	Career dissatisfaction/change
Interpersonal factors		**Positive coping**
Role messages		Role redefinition
Trust/respect for senders		Share roles
Multiple roles		Integrate roles
(nurse, manager, parent, spouse)		Confront role senders
	Role conflict	Redefine role
Individual factors		Personal reorientation
Rate of "life change"		Reactive coping
Ability to perform roles		Increased performance
Self-esteem/self-perception		Increased efficiency
Tolerance for ambiguity		Prioritize tasks/goals
Other personality traits		

Phillip J. Decker and Eleanor J. Sullivan. Used by permission.

to recognize such common causes of stress and identify methods of reducing such pressure, through education, orientation, and supervisory support.

The *supervisor's behavior* can be a factor in stress. Close, punitive, and/or authoritarian supervisory behavior is closely related to stress. Participative management, which has been studied since the Depression, has been found to be associated with reduced job stress (Porter-O'Grady, 1986).

Institutional factors that can lead to stress include institutional norms and expectations that conflict with an individual's needs (e.g., understaffing or high vacancies). Multiple and conflicting supervisors are a potential source of stress, especially where satisfying the requests of one makes it impossible to satisfy those of the other.

The rapidly *changing environment* of health care institutions has also been a contributor to stress in nursing. Rapid changes in technology, increased pressures from patients and third-party payers for service, liability issues, increased pressures for efficiency due to competition, and pressure from agencies such as Medicare have made the role of nurses more difficult, conflicting, and stressful.

INTERPERSONAL FACTORS

To add to the pressures created by employment settings, nurses must contend with strained interpersonal relationships. Frequently, nurses perceive divisiveness within the nursing profession itself. Debate begins with conflict regarding educational preparation (i.e., associate degree versus baccalaureate). Nursing relationships may be stressed by questions over whether a supervisor is functioning effectively or a co-worker is performing a fair share of the workload.

Interdisciplinary difficulties may precipitate tension. An example in rehabilitation illustrates this. In one setting, the therapists expect the patients to be bathed, to have eaten breakfast, and to be dressed by 8:30 A.M., when they are ready to start therapy. This expectation places undue stress on rehabilitation nurses, who must motivate patients who complain that they have had far too little sleep. Another example of interdisciplinary conflict is the stress created by the radiology technician who responds to a 9:00 P.M. page for a chest x-ray and informs the registered nurse that the nurse will have to bring the patient down to x-ray because the radiology department is understaffed.

Physician relations often are not conducive to open communication with nurses. Most nurses have experienced an irate response from a physician who is awakened during the night for something the physician thinks should have been handled earlier or might have waited till morning. In one small community hospital, an internist was well known for his outbursts during middle-of-the-night calls. One experienced nurse dealt with necessary calls to him by stating when he answered the phone, "This is Jane from St. Matthew's. I have two important things to tell you about Mrs. Smith." Although nursing leaders may not be able to alter communication patterns of physicians socialized over decades, they must provide support and an opportunity to vent frustration for nurses encountering such situations. Top nursing administrators are responsible, however, for affecting the environment so that staff nurses are treated with respect and courtesy.

Multiple roles are a source of stress. Home-job conflict is a potential source of stress to nurses. Nurses perform a number of roles that often include spouse and parent. Adding to this is the shift and weekend work required by most nursing jobs. Inpatient health care institutions must be staffed 24 hours a day, seven days a week. Individuals who work on evening or night shifts experience interpersonal problems if their spouse and children are on different schedules. This is especially a problem if the nurse rotates shifts. Studies have demonstrated that it takes several weeks to adjust physiologically to a change in shifts (Levi, 1981). Most rotation patterns require the nurse to change shifts several times a month; however, nurse managers must recognize the stress created through shift rotation. The physiological pressure of rotating shifts can be reduced through ensuring adequate rest and work breaks and with patterns requiring rotating only between two shifts and never "doubling back" (working eight hours, off eight hours, working eight hours).

Conflict between the role of a nurse manager and the role of a nurse can be a source of stress. Doing and directing others are different jobs. Directing others is stressful, and it may be tempting for the nurse manager to believe that it will be faster to complete a task by doing it independently.

INDIVIDUAL FACTORS

Stress can result from *individual factors*. One of these factors is the rate of life change. The rate of life change generates cumulative stress that, in turn, leads to the onset of disease or illness (Holmes & Rahe, 1967). These researchers assigned points for various life events based on the event's contribution to the amount of stress (see Figure 10–3). If an individual accumulated more than 150 points within a year's time, he or she had a 50 percent chance of developing serious illness the following year. Individuals who scored 300 or more points had at least a 70 percent chance of contracting a major illness the following year.

Stress often results from incongruence between one's expectations for one's performance and one's perception of the resulting performance. Past experience in coping with stress reflects an individual's expectations for successful coping in current experiences. People tend to repeat coping behaviors in similar situations, regardless of whether the initial behavior reduced stress. Also, an individual's low self-esteem might make it difficult to cope with role conflict or role ambiguity. Individuals with high tolerances for ambiguity can deal better with the strains that come from role ambiguity and, therefore, are likely to be able to cope with this strain and perceive less stress from a given situation. Individuals who perceive the locus of causality for factors in their life as being external to themselves may perceive less stress in a given situation. They are less likely to react negatively when they are controlled by surrounding events. Those who perceive factors as being internal react more negatively to situations that are beyond their control. But when individuals with an internal locus of control have to react to situations within their control, they are more likely to be proactive and engage in positive coping behaviors to change the environment and reduce stresses on themselves (Lazarus & Folkman, 1984).

ROLE CONFLICT AND ROLE AMBIGUITY

These antecedents manifest themselves in the *role-based stress* that results from role conflict and ambiguity. *Role conflict* occurs when the role messages a person receives are incompatible; *role ambiguity* occurs when there is a lack of clear, consistent information about the activities that must be performed and/or the goals to be pursued. Examples of role-based stress are conflict between the role of the professional and the person or conflict between manager and staff member roles.

Role conflict may be the most significant condition causing stress for nurses. A number of factors combine to create this situation. Exter-

nal factors such as strife within the profession, differences in nurses' educational preparation, the structure of practice settings, and the role of labor and professional organizations contribute to the environment in which nurses must func-

---

FIGURE 10-3 SOCIAL READJUSTMENT RATING SCALE

Forty-two common life changes are listed in the order in which Holmes and Rahne found them to be important precursors of illness. Total scores predict your chances of suffering serious illness within the next two years. If you score less than 150 within a year, you have only a 37 percent chance of getting sick within the next two years. But up your score to 150-300 and your chances increase to 51 percent. Hit 300 and you are, according to the doctors, in serious danger. Says Holmes, "If you have more than 300 life-change units and get sick, the probability is you will have cancer, a heart attack or manic-depressive psychosis rather than warts and menstrual irregularities." On the other hand, he adds, "There are worse things in life than illness. It is worse to go on in an intolerable, dull, or demeaning situation."

Life event	Your value score	Life event	Your value score
1. Death of spouse	100 ____	23. Son or daughter leaving home	29 ____
2. Divorce	73 ____	24. Trouble with in-laws	29 ____
3. Marital separation	65 ____	25. Outstanding personal achievement	28 ____
4. Jail term	63 ____	26. Spouse begins or stops work	26 ____
5. Death of a close family member	63 ____	27. Starting or finishing school	26 ____
6. Personal injury or illness	53 ____	28. Change in living conditions	25 ____
7. Marriage	50 ____	29. Revision of personal habits	24 ____
8. Fired at work	47 ____	30. Trouble with boss	23 ____
9. Marital reconciliation	45 ____	31. Change in work hours, conditions	20 ____
10. Retirement	45 ____	32. Change in residence	20 ____
11. Change in family member's health	44 ____	33. Change in schools	20 ____
12. Pregnancy	40 ____	34. Change in recreation	19 ____
13. Sex difficulties	39 ____	35. Change in church activities	19 ____
14. Addition to family	39 ____	36. Change in social activities	18 ____
15. Business readjustment	39 ____	37. Mortgage or loan under $10,000	17 ____
16. Change in financial state	38 ____	38. Change in sleeping habits	16 ____
17. Death of close friend	37 ____	39. Change in number of family get-togethers	15 ____
18. Change to different line of work	36 ____	40. Change in eating habits	15 ____
19. Change in number of arguments with spouse	35 ____	41. Vacation	13 ____
20. Mortgage over $10,000	31 ____	42. Christmas	12 ____
21. Foreclosure of mortgage or loan	30 ____	43. Minor violation of law	11 ____
22. Change in work responsibilities	29 ____	Total ____	

Thomas H. Holmes and Richard H. Rahe, "The Social Readjustment Rating Scale," *Journal of Psychosomatic Research*, 11(1967): 213-218, gives complete wording of the items. Reprinted with permission from Pergamon Press, Ltd. copyright 1967.

tion. Within practice settings, relationships among various groups, such as physicians, patients, staff, and management, add varied expectations and role perceptions to the nurse's job.

Other types of role conflicts occur when an individual has two competing roles, such as when a nurse manager assumes a patient care assignment and is confronted with the need to attend a leadership meeting. Another example is the conflict between nurses' personal roles as parents or spouses versus their roles as professional nurses.

Individual role conflict is the result of incompatibility between the individual's perception of the role and its actual requirements. Novice nurse managers experience this type of conflict when they find that administration expects primary loyalty to the organization and its goals, while the staff expects the nurse manager's first loyalty to be to their needs.

Role conflict within the profession places nursing at a distinct disadvantage in its relationship with other health care workers. This conflict has its roots in a perceived poor regard for nurses. The felt lack of worth is complicated by the divisiveness within the profession and the image nursing presents to others.

Role underload and under-utilization can also occur. Being under-utilized or not having much responsibility may be very stressful to someone who has high self-esteem and/or high achievement needs and can lead to apathy, low productivity, and job dissatisfaction.

CONSEQUENCES OF STRESS

What happens to a person when stress overload occurs? Both physiological and psychological responses occur that can cause structural or functional changes or both. Warning signs of too much stress are (a) *undue, prolonged anxiety,* or a persistent state of fear or free-floating anxiety that seems to have many alternating causes; (b) *depression,* which causes people to withdraw from family and friends, to be unable to experience emotions, and to feel helpless to change the situation; (c) *abrupt changes in mood and behavior,* which may be exhibited as erratic behavior; (d) *perfectionism,* which is the setting of unreasonably high standards for oneself and thereby being under constant stress; and (e) *physical illnesses,* such as peptic ulcer, arthritis, colitis, hypertension, myocardial infarction, and migraine headaches. Psychological disorders attributable to stress include anxiety reactions, depression, and phobias.

Ineffective coping methods for reducing stress include excessive use of alcohol and other mood-altering substances, which can result in chemical dependence. Some people become "workaholics" in an attempt to cope with real or imagined demands. The overused term *burnout* refers to the perception that an individual has used up all available energy to perform the job and feels that insufficient energy remains for task completion. The result of such a perception may be that the individual reduces hours worked or changes to another profession. One director of nursing at a 120-bed nursing home stated that she could no longer handle the overwhelming needs of the patients; the ever-present shortage of qualified, caring nurses; and consistently dwindling resources. When a for-profit chain purchased the home and further reduced economic resources, the director of nursing left nursing altogether and went back to college to become a court reporter.

The results of employee stress are increased absenteeism and turnover, and thus reduced quality of care. Although there are various causes of absenteeism and turnover (see Chapter 17), both may result when the individual attempts to withdraw from a stressful situation.

Job performance suffers during high stress times; so much energy and attention are needed to reduce the stress that little energy is available for performance. Such a situation may be financially costly in industry but may be more costly in human health and recovery in a health care institution.

Positive coping responses to stressful situations include role redefinition. Individuals share their role expectations with others, clarifying these roles and attempting to integrate or tie together the various roles they have to play. Confronting role senders by pointing out the conflicting role messages is also a positive means of coping. Requesting additional information regarding these roles from the role sender can reduce role ambiguity. Recognizing one's own tolerance for ambiguity and keeping out of conflicting situations is also an adaptive coping response. Finally, increasing one's performance, being more efficient, and practicing good time-management techniques by prioritizing tasks and goals are other positive coping responses to stress.

♦ MANAGING STRESS

It is obvious that stress must be resolved if people are to pursue productive lives. A number of individual and organizational strategies can be used to reduce work-related stress (Steers, 1984). Nurse managers can use these strategies to help deal with their own stress, to help manage their unit, and to help staff.

What can nurse managers do about their own stress?

1. Increase self-awareness. Nurses tend to think they can be "all things to all people." One way to develop self-awareness is to respond to the questionnaire shown in Figure 10–4.

2. Develop outside interests, such as hobbies, social groups, and recreational activities, that provide diversion, relaxation, and enjoyment.

3. Maintain a program of regular physical exercise. Exercise has been shown to reduce stress.

4. Take regular vacations. A change of scene, even to the backyard, is essential.

5. Learn how to relax. For a person in a high stress job, this is not easy. Healthy methods for relaxing include listening to music, reading, and socializing with friends.

What can nurse managers do to decrease their subordinates' stress?

1. Identify whether subordinates are under, adequately, or overly stressed. If subordinates are not adequately stressed, they may be undermotivated.

2. If subordinates appear to be under a great deal of stress, the nurse manager must identify the source(s) of the stress and decide how these can be reduced or eliminated.

3. Is role ambiguity or role conflict creating the stress? Can the nurse manager clarify the role(s) of the subordinate, thereby reducing this conflict or ambiguity?

4. Is the nurse manager using the appropriate leadership style? (See Chapter 9.) Does the nurse manager need to clarify subordinates' goals and eliminate barriers that are interfering with goal (task) attainment? Involving subordinates in decision making is an excellent way to reduce stress.

5. Does the subordinate need counseling? Is it appropriate for the nurse manager to fill this need, or are counseling services available in

FIGURE 10–4 STRESS DIAGNOSTIC SURVEY

I. PURPOSE
The following questionnaire is designed to provide you with an indication of the extent to which various individual level stressors are sources of stress to you.

II. INSTRUCTIONS
For each item, indicate the frequency with which the condition described is a source of stress. Next to each item write the appropriate number (1–7) that best describes how frequently the condition described is a source of stress.

- ◆ Write 1 if the condition described is never a source of stress
- ◆ Write 2 if it is rarely a source of stress
- ◆ Write 3 if it is occasionally a source of stress
- ◆ Write 4 if it is sometimes a source of stress
- ◆ Write 5 if it is often a source of stress
- ◆ Write 6 if it is usually a source of stress
- ◆ Write 7 if it is always a source of stress

III. STRESS DIAGNOSTIC SURVEY
_____ 1. My job duties and work objectives are unclear to me.
_____ 2. I work on unnecessary tasks or projects.
_____ 3. I have to take work home in the evenings or on weekends to stay caught up.
_____ 4. The demands for work quality made upon me are unreasonable.
_____ 5. I lack the proper opportunities to advance in this organization.
_____ 6. I am held accountable for the development of other employees.
_____ 7. I am unclear about whom I report to and/or who reports to me.
_____ 8. I get caught in the middle between my supervisors and my subordinates.
_____ 9. I spend too much time in unimportant meetings that take me away from my work.
_____10. My assigned tasks are sometimes too difficult and/or complex.
_____11. If I want to get promoted I have to look for a job with another organization.
_____12. I am responsible for counseling with my subordinates and/or helping them solve their problems.
_____13. I lack the authority to carry out my job responsibilities.
_____14. A formal chain of command is not adhered to.
_____15. I am responsible for an almost unmanageable number of projects or assignments at the same time.
_____16. Tasks seem to be getting more and more complex.
_____17. I am hurting my career progress by staying with this organization.
_____18. I take action or make decisions that affect the safety or well-being of others.
_____19. I do not fully understand what is expected of me.
_____20. I do things on the job that are accepted by one person and not by others.
_____21. I simply have more work to do than can be done in an ordinary day.
_____22. The organization expects more of me than my skills and/or abilities provide.
_____23. I have few opportunities to grow and learn new knowledge and skills in my job.
_____24. My responsibilities in this organization are more for people than for things.
_____25. I do not understand the part my job plays in meeting overall organizational objectives.
_____26. I receive conflicting requests from two or more people.
_____27. I feel that I just don't have time to take an occasional break.
_____28. I have insufficient training and/or experience to discharge my duties properly.
_____29. I feel that I am at a standstill in my career.
_____30. I have responsibility for the future (careers) of others.

John M. Ivancevich and Michael T. Matteson, _Stress and Work_ (Glenview, IL: Scott, Foresman and Company, 1980), pp. 118–119.

the organization that could help the subordinate? Would additional training or education help reduce the stress?

6. Is the stress due to feelings of low self-worth? Can the subordinate be positively reinforced (see Chapter 8)? Can other sources of support, such as the work group, help the subordinate deal with the stress?

7. The nurse manager could suggest that the subordinate deal with personal stress by using some of the techniques suggested above for the nurse manager.

What can health care administrators do to help their employees manage stress? Institutional strategies can be developed to reduce stress for employees. The nurse manager may be able to initiate a few of them or to encourage their adoption. Some institutional strategies include:

1. Attempt to match the job with the applicant during the selection and placement process (see Chapter 13).

2. Increase skills training, even for experienced personnel. Although costly, it pays in reduced stress, less turnover, and better performance (see Chapter 14).

3. Develop a program of job enrichment matched to the individual's goals and desires. Job enrichment may include increased autonomy and participation or a restructuring of assigned tasks across the unit (see Chapter 8).

4. Allow greater participation in decision making. Participation in decisions affecting work increases job involvement and commitment, thereby reducing stress.

5. Encourage a network of social support. Team building is one way to encourage staff to build a network of support with others in their professional field.

6. Keep communication channels open both upward and downward. As discussed in Chapter 7, the grapevine is especially susceptible to misinformation. Keeping personnel informed about what is going on in the organization helps reduce suspicion and rumor.

7. Develop policies that reduce the stress from shift work. These include reducing the number of hours in the night shift, increasing rest time, and providing adequate meal times. Fair policies should be set dealing with the assignment to weekend and/or holiday work (Levi, 1981).

Like external conflict resolution, internal conflict resolution takes planning, time, and energy. But the benefits in better health, a more enjoyable lifestyle, and increased sense of self-esteem are well worth the effort.

◆ TIME MANAGEMENT

Much of the stress experienced by nurse managers results from the perception that staff, patient, and unit needs must be met expeditiously. A common perception is the need to "slow down" and "get off the train." A notable method of coping with and reducing time stress is through time management, because we are not *on* a train, we *are* the train. We determine how, where, and when our time is used. This section discusses the nature of time and time management, time wasters and time management principles, where time goes, and methods to help a nurse manager more effectively manage time and the time of others, both colleagues and superiors.

According to Benjamin Franklin (Bliss, 1976), "Time is the stuff of which life is made." So, time is the essence of living, and it is the scarcest resource. Since the nurse manager has a limited amount of time, it is essential for goal attainment that time be used expeditiously. One lost hour a day every day for a year results in 260 hours of waste, or 6.5 *weeks* of missed opportunity annually.

Time management is a misnomer. No one manages time: What is managed is how time is used. Figure 10–5 shows some of the constraints on individuals' ability to manage time effectively. These patterns of behavior must be un-derstood and dealt with to achieve effective time management.

In addition to these patterns of behavior, certain time wasters prevent the nurse manager from effectively managing time. A time waster is something that prevents a person from accomplishing the job or achieving goals. Common time wasters include:

1. Interruptions such as telephone calls and drop-in visitors

2. Meetings, both scheduled and unscheduled

3. Lack of clear-cut goals, objectives, and priorities

4. Lack of daily and/or weekly plans

FIGURE 10–5 POTENTIAL CONSTRAINTS ON THE ABILITY TO MANAGE TIME EFFECTIVELY

- We do what we like to do before we do what we don't like to do.
- We do the things we know how to do faster than the things we do not know how to do.
- We do the things that are easiest before things that are difficult.
- We do things that require a little time before things that require a lot of time.
- We do things for which resources are available.
- We do things that are scheduled (for example, meetings) before nonscheduled things.
- We sometimes do things that are planned before things that are unplanned.
- We respond to demands from others before demands from ourselves.
- We do things that are urgent before things that are important.
- We readily respond to crises and emergencies.
- We do interesting things before uninteresting things.
- We do things that advance our personal objectives or that are politically expedient.
- We wait until a deadline approaches before we really get moving.
- We do things that provide the most immediate closure.
- We respond on the basis of who wants it.
- We respond on the basis of the consequences to us of doing or not doing something.
- We tackle small jobs before large jobs.
- We work on things in the order of their arrival.
- We work on the basis of the squeaky-wheel principle (the squeaky wheel gets the grease).
- We work on the basis of consequences to the group.

5. Lack of personal organization and self-discipline

6. Lack of knowledge on how one spends one's time

7. Failure to delegate, working on routine tasks

8. Ineffective communication

9. Waiting for others, not using transition time effectively

10. Inability to say no

To deal with these time management constraints and time wasters one must understand the principles of time management. These principles are summarized in Table 10–1.

GOAL SETTING

Nurses are always setting long- and short-range goals, although typically such goals are stated in

TABLE 10-1 PRINCIPLES OF TIME MANAGEMENT

Principle	Discussion/illustration
Goal setting	Annual determination of unit, department, and institutional goals. The nurse manager also sets long– and short–range personal goals.
Time analysis	Conducting a survey of the way the nurse manager spends the day, in 30– to 60–minute increments. Reviewing the daily schedule and keeping it accurate may demonstrate how time is used. A schedule with no "available" time is as problematic as one in which all time is "available."
Priority determination	Time frames for achievement of goals are identified by the nurse manager. The "to–do" list should be prioritized, by classifying activities as "A" or "1" for urgent, "B" or "2" for non-urgent but important, and "C" or "3" for non-urgent, less important.
Daily planning	To–do lists and scheduling constitute the bulk of daily planning devices.
Delegation	A variety of activities may be delegated by the nurse manager. For example, the nurse manager may delegate responsibility for the QA program.
Interruption control	Identify causes of interruptions, and plan to reduce them. The nurse manager might find that consistent interruptions come from a particular physician. To keep this from being an interruption, meeting with the physician could become a planned and scheduled activity, with an alternative time identified for office work.
Evaluation	The nurse manager should make at least a weekly assessment of how effectively time has been used. A good time to complete this review is while identifying priorities for the next week.

Adapted from R. Adcock, and J. Lee, "Time, One More Time," *California Management Review*, 1971, 14 (2): 28–32.

terms of what patients will accomplish rather than what the nurse will achieve. A critical component of time management is establishing one's own goals and time frames. Goals provide direction and vision for actions as well as provide a timeline in which activities will be accomplished. Defining goals and time frames helps with stress reduction by preventing the panic that nurse managers often feel when confronted with multiple demands. Although time frames may not be as fast as the nurse manager would like (the tendency is to expect change yesterday), at least the nurse manager can identify actions to be taken.

The existence of individual or organizational goals is useful in that it encourages thinking about the future and what might happen. Goal setting helps to relate current behavior, activities, or operations to the organization's or individual's long-range goals. Without this future orientation, activities may not lead to the outcomes that will help achieve the goals and meet the ideals of the individual or organization. The focus should be to develop measurable, realistic, and achievable goals. Specific goal setting theory is discussed more extensively in Chapter 8.

It is useful to think of individual or personal goals in categories as shown in Table 10–2. This partial listing is a guide to stimulate thinking about goals. In considering individual goals, it is useful to think about both long-term and lifetime goals and short-term goals. These should be divided into job-related goals and personal goals. Job-related goals may revolve around unit or departmental changes, whereas personal goals may include personal life and community involvement. Short-term goals should be set for the next six to 12 months but need to be related to long-term goals. Five major questions about these goals must be answered if the nurse manager is to manage time effectively:

1. What specific unit objectives are to be achieved?

2. What specific activities are necessary to achieve these objectives?

3. How much time is required for each activity?

4. Which activities can be planned and scheduled for concurrent action and which must be planned and scheduled sequentially?

5. Which activities can be delegated to staff?

TIME ANALYSIS

The second principle of time management is time analysis. Time analysis includes, first, analyzing the duties of the nurse manager as specified in the job description and, second, keeping a time log showing how the nurse manager actually spends time. Using time logs, typically kept in intervals of 30 to 60 minutes, to analyze the actual time spent on various activities is useful. These logs can be reviewed to determine which activities are essential to the nurse manager's job and which activities can be delegated to others or eliminated. The nurse manager's schedule book also may be used to review patterns of time use, rather than a separate log.

A significant difficulty in moving from a staff nurse position to a leadership position is the need to develop different time management and organizational skills. In a staff nurse role, the registered nurse has little, if any, free or uncommitted time. Almost every minute of the shift is assigned to a task. For example, at 6:45 A.M., report is taken; at 7:00 A.M., insulin is administered; at 7:15 A.M., breakfast trays are passed; from 8:00 A.M. to 10:30 A.M., morning care is administered; etc. No planning is required because every minute is taken. In contrast, when the nurse changes to a leadership position, he or she is responsible for defining how time will be spent. Such a change can be frustrating initially unless effective time management strategies are implemented.

SETTING PRIORITIES

Priorities should be established for activities. These priorities should take into consideration both the short- and long-term goals of the nurse manager and should also take into account both the importance and urgency of activities. Table 10–3 is a chart with examples of five types of activities. According to Bliss (1976), activities are (a) urgent and important, (b) important but not urgent, (c) urgent but not important, (d) busy work, or (e) wasted time. Activities that are

TABLE 10-2 INDIVIDUAL GOALS

Goal category	Examples
Department accomplishments	To become involved in one hospital-wide task force by second quarter.
Interpersonal relationships	To develop a solid working relationship with the chief financial officer by third quarter.
Professional growth	To publish one article in a referred journal by fourth quarter.
Education/personal growth	To complete one continuing education course in human resources by third quarter.
Financial security	To identify financial plan for graduate school by second quarter.
Status	To become a member of the school board of directors by fourth quarter.
Family/personal relations	To remember all birthdays and significant events.
Use of free time	To visit Hawaii by fourth quarter.
Physical well-being	To lose 20 pounds by the fourth quarter.
Lifestyle	To work no more than 45 hours a week and no more than one weekend day a month.
Social commitment	To join the Sierra Club by first quarter.
Spiritual growth	To become a member of the church attended by third quarter.

Adapted from H. Knudson, R. Woodworth, and C. Bell, *Management: An Experimental Approach* (New York: McGraw-Hill, 1973); and J. Kotter, *Power and Influence* (New York: Free Press, 1985).

both urgent and important must be completed, such as with the example identified in Table 10–3. Activities that are important but not urgent may be those that make the difference between career progression or maintaining the status quo. Urgent but not important activities must be completed immediately but are not considered important or significant. Busy work and wasted time are self-explanatory.

DAILY PLANNING AND SCHEDULING

Once goals and priorities have been established, the nurse manager can concentrate on scheduling activities. A "to-do" list should be prepared each day, either after work hours the previous day or early before work on the same day. The list is typically planned by workday or workweek. As nurse managers combine many responsibilities, a weekly to-do list may be more effective. Flexibility must be a major consideration in this plan; the nurse manager should leave some time uncommitted to deal with the unexpected emergencies and crises that are sure to

happen. In building this plan, each activity should be prioritized. The focus is not on activities and events, but rather on the outcomes that can be achieved in the time available.

A system to keep track of regularly scheduled meetings (staff meetings), regular events (annual or quarterly report due dates), and appointments is also necessary. This system should be used when establishing the to-do list; it should include both a calendar and files. The calendar might include information on the purpose of the meeting, who will be attending, and the time and place, while a file might contain correspondence or reports related to the meeting. This file can be arranged by date so that it is readily available at the time needed.

A calendar is essential for planning. Several commercial planning systems are available, including Day Runner®, DayTimer®, and Filofax®. Any such system includes a daily, weekly, or monthly calendar; a to-do section; a memo or note section; and an address component. It is useful to have a calendar that is small enough to be taken to meetings or home.

TABLE 10-3 IMPORTANCE-URGENCY CHART

Category of time use	Examples
Important and urgent	Replacing two call-offs and insuring sufficient staffing for the upcoming shift.
Important, not urgent	Drafting an educational program for nurses on the changes in Medicare reimbursement
Urgent, not important	Completing and submitting the "beds available" list for a disaster drill.
Busy work	Compiling new charts for future patient admissions.
Wasted time	Sitting by the phone waiting for return calls.

◆ DELEGATION

According to Roberts (1990), every rider who plans to get back on a horse after dismounting requires a horse holder. In his text, *Leadership Secrets of Attila the Hun,* Roberts notes that even Attila would have failed in his conquest without the ability to find loyal chieftains to whom he could delegate national unification responsibilities for his growing force. Delegation is the process by which responsibility and authority for performing tasks (functions, activities, or decisions) is assigned to individuals.

Delegation involves assigning tasks, determining expected results, and granting authority to the individual to accomplish these tasks. It means conveying *rights* and *obligations* to a subordinate. Delegation includes stating the ends to be achieved and providing the means (authority) to the subordinate to achieve these ends. It is not the same as direction which is telling someone specifically what to do. Delegation is perhaps the most difficult leadership skill for nurses to acquire. Student nurses learn clinical skills by giving direct patient care to small groups of patients but few undergraduate programs provide actual leadership experiences. Most nurses do not encounter the difficulties of delegation until after graduation. It is not unusual for an experienced nursing assistant to attempt to tell the new registered nurse "how things work in *this* hospital." One example is Cindy, who graduated from a baccalaureate program in June, completed state boards in July, and anxiously began clinical practice in August. Cindy was team leading for 15 patients on the evening shift and had three nursing assistants working with her. She consistently found herself working from 3:00 P.M. until 1:00 A.M., while the nursing assistants were ready to leave at 10:00 P.M. Cindy thought her problem in overtime was disorganization until she realized that ineffective and insufficient delegation was the culprit.

Cindy's experience is typical of novice nurses who must delegate tasks to nursing assistants with decades more experience. One reason total patient care is more effective and easier to implement than team nursing is that the need to delegate is reduced when the registered nurse is responsible for all clinical needs of a small group of patients. When overtime is overused, nurse managers need to assess the staff's delegation practices. Nurse managers who find themselves working too many hours, too many days, and weekends should question their delegation effectiveness.

Concepts related to delegation include responsibility and accountability (Davis, 1951). *Responsibility* means that the subordinate has an obligation to carry out the activities needed to accomplish the assigned task. *Accountability* is being held answerable for the results. The nurse manager may delegate tasks to another individual, but the manager is still accountable for the performance of these tasks; accountability for delegated tasks cannot be relinquished.

THE DELEGATION PROCESS

The five stages in the delegation process are (1) analyzing the delegator's job to determine what could be delegated, (2) analyzing the subordinate's job strengths and weaknesses to determine which tasks could be delegated to the subordinate, (3) determining the specific tasks to be delegated and the authority and level of delegation, (4) delegating appropriate tasks to the subordinate, and (5) providing feedback to subordinates and following up to see if the tasks have been accomplished.

STEP 1. When analyzing their job and the activities that need to be performed, nurse managers should determine which responsibilities can be or should be delegated to others. In addition, personal characteristics that prevent the manager from delegating should be analyzed. Many attitudes—some valid, some not—can lead to under-delegation. Risk factors, time constraints, feelings about subordinates' capabilities, and a strong need to prove oneself are some of the attitudes commonly expressed by nurse managers to explain why they do not delegate more. Poteet (1984) identifies the following obstacles to delegation:

1. Ignorance about the delegation process

2. Incomplete transition from staff nurse to nurse manager

3. Anxiety over prospect of losing technical competence

4. Fear of losing control

5. Crisis management orientation

6. Failure to set goals and timetables

7. Job confusion

8. Desire to control upward communication

9. Competition for managerial positions

10. Personal job insecurity

11. Poor time management

12. Lack of commitment to employee development process

13. Lack of confidence in subordinate's abilities

14. Fear of managerial incompetence

STEP 2. The second step in the delegation process is to analyze subordinates' jobs to see how much time is available for them to perform delegated tasks, evaluating their capability to perform some of the nurse manager's tasks, and determining the subordinates' characteristics that prevent them from accepting responsibility. These forces include the following, identified by Newman (1956):

1. It is easier to ask the supervisor.

2. Subordinates fear criticism.

3. Subordinates lack information and/or resources to perform the task.

4. Subordinates have more work than they have time to do.

5. Subordinates lack self-confidence.

6. Positive incentives are inadequate to ensure task performance.

STEP 3. Step three is deciding what tasks or responsibilities should be delegated and how much authority should be given to the subordinate to achieve these tasks.

Just as a nurse manager cannot do everything that must be done, so many functions and activities cannot be delegated. Responsibilities for nurse managers vary from one institution to another, but some responsibilities should never be delegated. These include disciplining an immediate subordinate, handling morale problems within the unit, and responsibilities for which the nurse manager has legal accountability. Additionally, it is a mistake for a nurse manager to consistently delegate less-than-desirable tasks. Nurse managers who fail to roll up their sleeves and participate in care generally are not well respected. The staff to whom such nurse managers delegate perceive the nurse manager as "too good" to become involved. In contrast, nurse managers who make a point of answering patient call lights and assisting with direct patient care as needed are more likely to be viewed by the nursing staff as a member and leader of the team.

When authority is delegated, two decisions must be made. First, what areas of authority, or what resources, must the person control to achieve the expected results? Second, what are the limits, boundaries, or parameters for each area of authority or resource to be used? A unit manager who is responsible for maintaining adequate supplies needs budget authority. The authority to spend money on supplies, however, may be limited to a specific amount for specific supplies or may be allocated to supplies in general.

In addition, each task that is delegated has a level of responsibility attached to it; thus the manager must provide the subordinate with clear guidelines on how much responsibility he or she has. According to Whetten and Cameron (1984), the five levels of task delegation are:

1. Gather information for the manager so he or she can decide what needs to be done.

2. Determine alternative courses of action from which the manager may choose.

3. Perform one part of the task at a time after obtaining approval for each new step.

4. Outline an entire course of action for accomplishing the whole task and have it approved.

5. Perform the whole task using any preferred method and report only results.

STEP 4.   This step requires an understanding of the communication process and how tasks

should be assigned. If the subordinate lacks the knowledge or ability to perform a task, then he or she must receive training and/or coaching. Key behaviors in delegating tasks include:

1. Give your attention to the person.

2. Maintain appropriate nonverbal behaviors—use open body language, be straight and square to the person, lean toward her, and maintain eye contact.

3. Use an "I" statement to request, such as "I would like . . ."

4. Explain the specific task to be delegated, the level of delegation, the amount of authority, and the expected completion time.

5. Explain briefly why the task is important.

6. Ask for suggestions.

7. Provide the subordinate with any additional information or resources that might be needed.

8. Ask the subordinate to confirm his or her understanding of the task, the level and authority to be delegated, and the completion time (get feedback).

9. Obtain agreement to do the task.

STEP 5.   The purpose of this step is to provide a feedback and control system to ensure that the delegated tasks are carried out. Decide if written reports are necessary or if brief oral reports are sufficient. If written reports are required, indicate whether tables, charts, or other graphics are necessary. Be specific about reporting times. Identify critical events or milestones that might be reached and brought to the nurse manager's attention. The nurse manager has to decide how closely the assignment will be supervised. However, controls should never be so tight that they limit subordinates' opportunity to grow. Control should be thought through when objectives are established, not as an afterthought. For example, a nurse is responsible for administering medications and therefore is given authority to access drugs, draw up medications, and administer doses to patients. The nurse is held accountable by several controls which might include the narcotics key control, end-of-shift drug counts, review of patients' records, medication charts, and shift reports.

GROUPING ACTIVITIES AND MINIMIZING ROUTINE WORK

Work items similar in nature and requiring similar environmental surroundings and resources for their accomplishment should be grouped within divisions of the work shift. Routine tasks, especially those that are not important or urgent and contribute little to overall objectives, should be minimized. If you insist on doing them, group them together and do them in your least productive time. List a few 5- to 10-minute discretionary tasks. This helps to use the small bits of time that become available. Set aside blocks of uninterrupted time for the really important tasks. If a person is having difficulty completing important tasks and is highly stressed, routine tasks can be beneficial in reducing this stress. Pick a task that can be successfully completed and save it for the end of the day. Reaching closure on even a routine task at the end of the day can reduce the sense of overload and stress.

CONTROLLING INTERRUPTIONS

An interruption occurs any time the nurse manager is stopped in the middle of one activity to give attention to something else. Interruptions can be an essential part of the nurse manager's job or they can be a time waster. An interruption

that is more important and urgent than the activity in which the nurse manager is involved is a positive interruption; it deserves immediate attention. An emergency or crisis, for instance, may cause the nurse manager to interrupt daily rounds. Some interruptions interfere with achieving the nurse manager's job and are less important and urgent than the nurse manager's current activities. These interruptions should be limited.

Keeping an interruption log on an occasional basis may help. The log should show who interrupted, the nature of the interruption, when it occurred, how long it lasted, what topics were discussed, the importance of the topics, and time-saving actions to be taken. Analysis of these data may identify patterns that can be used to plan ways to reduce the frequency and duration of interruptions. These patterns may indicate that certain staff members are the most frequent interrupters and greatest source of distraction.

TELEPHONE CALLS

Telephone calls are a major source of interruption, and the interruption log will provide considerable insight for the nurse manager regarding the nature of telephone calls received. Though it is not possible to function today without a telephone, some people do not use the telephone effectively. A ringing telephone is highly compelling; few people can allow it to go unanswered. The nurse manager has many telephone calls, some of them time wasters. Handling telephones effectively is a must.

MINIMIZE SOCIALIZING AND SMALL TALK. If you answer the phone with, "Hello, what can I do for you?" rather than, "Hello, how are you?" the receiver is encouraged to get to business first. Be warm, friendly, and courteous, but do not allow others to waste time with inappropriate or extensive small talk. Calls placed and returned just prior to lunchtime, at the end of the day, and on Friday afternoons tend to result in more business and less socializing.

PLAN CALLS.   The manager who plans telephone calls does not waste anyone's time including that of the person called. A small pad or note paper kept by the telephone is essential. Topics to be discussed are written down before the call is made. This prevents the need for additional calls to inform the other party of an important point or ask a forgotten question.

SET A TIME FOR CALLS.   The nurse manager may have a number of calls to return as well as calls to initiate. It is best to set aside a time to handle routine phone calls, especially during "downtime." An attempt should be made not to interrupt what is being done at the moment. If an answer is necessary before a project can be continued, then phone; if not, phone for the information at a later time.

STATE AND ASK FOR PREFERRED CALL TIMES AND THE PURPOSE OF THE CALL. If a party is not available, it is essential to state the purpose of the call and provide several time frames when you will be available for a return call. Have those accepting messages ask for the same information. This makes it easier for the call responder to be prepared for the call and helps to prevent "telephone tag" or "trading pink slips" (Mayer, 1990).

DROP-IN VISITORS

Although often friendly and seemingly harmless, the typical "got-a-minute" drop-in visit lasts 10 minutes (Mackenzie, 1990). Rather than eliminate drop-in visits, the nurse manager should skillfully direct the visit by identifying the issue or question, arranging an alternate meeting, referring the visitor to someone else, or redirecting the visitor's problem-solving efforts. An additional strategy is to stand up to greet the visitor and remain standing. It appears gracious yet is uncomfortable and tends to speed the visit.

The nurse manager who is fortunate enough to have an office will find that open doors are open invitations for interruption. While it is essential that nurse managers be available and accessible, concentration time also is necessary. It can be achieved by informing the staff that time will be available to address issues during a specific block of time (a few hours at most).

Interruptions can also be controlled by the arrangement of furniture. The nurse manager whose desk is arranged so that immediate eye contact is made with passers-by or drop-in visitors is asking for interruptions. A desk turned 90 or even 180 degrees from the door minimizes potential eye contact.

Encouraging appointments to deal with routine matters also reduces interruptions. Regularly scheduled meetings with those who need to see the nurse manager allow them to hold routine matters for those appointments. Holding such meetings in the other person's office places the nurse manager in charge of keeping the time. It is easier to leave someone's office than to remove an individual from yours.

PLAN IMPLEMENTATION ANALYSIS

Implementation of the daily plan and daily follow-up is essential to time management. In addition, time analysis should be repeated at least semiannually to see how well you are managing your time and whether your job or the environment has changed, which requires changes in your planning activities. This can help preclude reverting to poor time management habits.

PERSONAL ORGANIZATION AND SELF-DISCIPLINE

Some other time wasters that have not been discussed are lack of personal organization and self-discipline, including the inability to say no, waiting for others, and excessive or ineffective paperwork.

Personal organization results from clearly defined priorities based upon well-defined, measurable, and achievable objectives. Since the nurse manager does not work alone, priorities and objectives are often related to those of many other professionals, as well as to objectives of patients and their families. How time is used is often a matter of resolving conflicts among competing needs. It is possible for the nurse manager to become overloaded with responsibilities, with more to do than should be expected in the time available. This is typical. There is never sufficient time for all the activities, situations, and events in which the nurse manager might like to become involved. To be effective, the nurse manager must be personally well organized and possess self-discipline. This often includes the ability to say no. Taking on too much work can lead to overload and stress. Being realistic in the amount of work to which you commit is an indication of effective time management. If a superior is overloading you, make sure the person understands the consequences of additional assignments. Be assertive in communicating your own needs to others.

Lack of personal self-discipline also includes a cluttered desk, working on too many tasks at one time, and failing to set aside blocks of uninterrupted time to do important tasks. Clean your desk, get out the materials needed for your highest priority task, and start working on it immediately. Focus on one task at a time making sure to start with a high priority task.

TRANSITION TIME

Much time is spent in transition or waiting. Using this time effectively can increase the time available. Commuting time can be used for self-development or planning work activities. We all have to wait sometimes, whether it is waiting for a meeting to start or waiting to talk to someone. Bring along materials to read or work on in case you are kept waiting. View waiting/transition time as an opportunity.

PAPERWORK

Hospitals cannot function effectively without good information systems. In addition to telephone calls and face-to-face conversations, nurse managers spend considerable time writing and reading communications. Increasing government regulations, avoidance of legal action, new treatments and medications, data processing, work processing, and electronics place pressure on the nurse manager to cope with increasing paperwork. Some basic principles can help the nurse manager process information while reducing it as a waster of time.

PLAN AND SCHEDULE PAPERWORK.

Writing and reading reports, forms, letters, and memoranda are essential elements of the nurse manager's job. They cannot be ignored. They will, however, become a major source of frustration if their processing is not planned and scheduled as an integral part of the nurse manager's daily activities. Nurse managers should learn the institution's information system and requirements immediately, analyze the paperwork requirements of their position, and make significant progress on that part of the job daily.

SORT PAPERWORK FOR EFFECTIVE PROCESSING.

A system of file folders or trays in which to sort mail can be very helpful. For instance, all paperwork requiring action is placed in the file labeled "A"; it can then be handled according to its relative importance and urgency. All paperwork that is informational in nature and related to present work is placed in a file labeled "I." Other reading material, such as professional journals, technical reports, and other items to read that do not relate directly to the immediate work, is placed in a file labeled "R." The "I" file contains things that must be read immediately, whereas the "R" file materials are not as urgent and can be postponed.

Do not be afraid to throw things away or erase them from the memory of your electronic information system. When they no longer have value, do not let them become clutter. Every nurse manager needs a wastebasket. Have a big one and fill it often.

SHARE PAPERWORK RESPONSIBILITIES.

Delegate both routine and non-routine paperwork functions. Teaching staff members to process paperwork effectively strengthens a unit's capacity to handle this important element of its responsibilities.

WRITE EFFECTIVELY.

Handwrite less and dictate more. The person with average dictation skills can dictate on a machine at least five times as quickly as he or she can write or type. Dictate all letters, memos, and reports. The keys to successful dictation are outlining, good grammar, and clear enunciation. If dictating equipment and secretarial support are unavailable, learn to use the computer and electronic mail. Improved typing skills are essential for using the computer effectively.

ANALYZE PAPERWORK FREQUENTLY.

Review filing policies and rules regularly, and purge files at least once each year. All standard forms, reports, and memos should be reviewed annually. Each should justify its continued existence and its present format. Do not be afraid to recommend changes and, when possible, initiate those changes.

DO NOT BE A PAPER SHUFFLER.

"Handle a piece of paper only once." This is often impossible if taken literally. It really means that each time a piece of paper is handled, some action is taken to further the processing of that paper. Paper shufflers are those who continually move things around on their desks. They unreasonably delay action; the paper problem mounts. A desktop is a working surface; it is not for files and piles.

RESPECTING TIME

The key to using time management techniques is to respect one's own time as well as that of others. Nurse managers who respect their time are likely to find others respecting it also. The same values and attitudes indicate respect for one's own time and for that of others. Using the above suggestions regarding time management communicates to those who interact with the nurse manager that respect for time is demanded. The nurse manager, however, must reciprocate by respecting the time needs of others. For example, if the nurse manager needs to talk to someone, it is appropriate to arrange an appointment, particularly for routine matters. The nurse manager should continually ask, "What is the best use of my time right now?" and should answer in three ways: (1) for myself and my goals, (2) for my subordinates and their goals, and (3) for the organization and its goals.

SUMMARY

♦ Stress is the reaction of the individual to demands from the environment that pose a threat.

♦ Some antecedents of stress come from job and organizational factors, from interpersonal factors, and from individual factors.

♦ Stress in nursing often results specifically from the nature of the work, from role conflict and role ambiguity, and from problems of self-worth and divisiveness within the profession.

♦ The consequences of stress are physiological and psychological problems for the individual, poor job performance, low job satisfaction, and high absenteeism.

♦ Strategies to help individuals, as well as institutions, reduce stress include clarifying goals and roles; providing support, including training and education on stress management; using participative management techniques; and practicing personal stress management techniques.

♦ Nurse managers must use time wisely to accomplish everything that is expected of them. This takes planning. Without time management, only more time will help.

♦ The nurse manager's work shift is subject to many interruptions. An interruption log helps identify patterns that can be used to plan ways to reduce unnecessary interruptions.

♦ Telephone calls are a major source of interruption. They can be controlled by minimizing small talk, planning calls, using a timer, and stating preferred call times.

♦ Drop-in visitors are also a source of interruption. One should meet visitors outside the office, keep visits short, encourage appointments, keep staff informed, and arrange furniture to discourage unscheduled visitors.

♦ Nurse managers who respect their own time are likely to find others respecting it also.

♦ Written communication can also cause interruptions. These can be minimized by planning and scheduling paperwork, sorting, delegating, writing effectively, and using an effective filing system.

♦ Delegation is a major tool in time management. The nurse manager must understand his or her role and the staff's abilities to effectively delegate. When authority is delegated, the nurse manager must set the limits of responsibility. Assignments must be given clearly and precisely.

♦ Several steps can be taken to ensure effective delegation: plan before delegating, define responsibility in terms of results, define authority limits, don't complete subordinates' assignments, hold subordinates accountable, and select subordinates who are capable.

♦ Three things should never be delegated: disciplining immediate subordinates, handling morale problems within the unit, and responsibilities for which the manager has legal accountability.

BIBLIOGRAPHY

Adcock, R., and Lee, J. (1971). "Time, One More Time." *California Management Review,* 14(2): 28–32.
Albanese, B. (1981). *Managing: Toward Accountability for Performance.* Homewood, IL: Irwin.

Bliss, E. (1976). *Getting Things Done.* New York: Bantam Books.

Brooten, D., Hayman, L., and Naylors, M. (1978). *Leadership for Change: A Guide for the Frustrated Nurse.* Philadelphia: J. B. Lippincott.

Davis, R. (1951). *The Fundamentals of Top Management.* New York: Harper & Row.

Douglass, L. (1983). *The Effective Nurse: Leader and Manager.* 2d ed. St. Louis, MO: C. V. Mosby.

Gustafson, D. (1983). "Practical Tips on Time Management." *Plant Services,* 4(7): 66–67.

Holmes, T., and Rahe, R. (1967). "The Social Readjustment Rating Scale." *Journal of Psychosomatic Research,* 11: 213.

Ivancevich, J., and Matteson, M. (1980). *Stress and Work.* Glenview, IL: Scott, Foresman.

Ivancevich, J., and Matteson, M. (1987). *Organizational Behavior and Management.* Plano, TX: Business Publications.

Klein, S., and Ritti, R. (1984). *Understanding Organizational Behavior.* 2d ed. Boston: Kent.

Knudson, H., Woodworth, R., and Bell, C. (1973). *Management: An Experimental Approach.* New York: McGraw-Hill.

Kotter, J. (1985). *Power and Influence.* New York: Free Press.

Lakein, A. (1973). *How to Get Control of Your Time and Your Life.* New York: Signet.

Lazarus, R., and Folkman, S. (1984). *Stress, Appraisal and Coping.* New York: Springer.

Levi, L. (1981). *Preventing Work Stress.* Reading, MA: Addison-Wesley.

Locke, E., and Latham, G. (1984). *Goal Setting: A Motivational Technique That Works!* Englewood Cliffs, NJ: Prentice-Hall.

Mackenzie, A. (1990). *The Time Trap.* New York: American Management Association.

Marriner, A. (1979). "Conflict Theory." *Supervisor Nurse,* 10(4): 12.

Matteson, M., and Ivancevich, J. (1979). "Organizational Stressors and Heart Disease." *Academic Management and Research,* 4: 347–357.

Mayer, J. (1990). *If You Haven't Got the Time to Do It Right, When Will You Have the Time to Do It Over?* New York: Simon and Schuster.

Newman, W. (1956). "Overcoming Obstacles to Effective Delegation." *Management Review,* 45(1): 36–41.

Porter-O'Grady, T. (1986). *Creative Nursing Administration: Participative Management into the 21st Century.* Gaithersburg, MD: Aspen.

Poteet, G. (1984). "Delegation Strategies: A Must for the Nurse Executive." *Journal of Nursing Administration,* 14(9): 18–21.

Roberts, W. (1990). *Leadership Secrets of Attila the Hun.* New York: Warner Books.

Selye, H. (1978). *The Stress of Life.* 2d ed. New York: McGraw-Hill.

Steers, R. (1984). *Introduction to Organizational Behavior.* 2d ed. Santa Monica, CA: Goodyear.

Thomas, K. (1976). "Conflict and Conflict Management." In: *Handbook of Industrial and Organizational Psychology.* Dunnette, M. (editor). Chicago: Rand McNally. Pp. 889–935.

Whetten, D., and Cameron, K. (1984). *Developing Management Skills.* Glenwood, IL: Scott, Foresman.

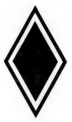

C H A P T E R 11

CRITICAL THINKING

PROBLEM SOLVING
    Problem-Solving Methods
    Problem-Solving Process

DECISION MAKING
    Decision-Making Strategies
    Decision-Making Conditions
    Decision-Making Process
    Stumbling Blocks

CREATIVITY IN DECISION MAKING
    Characteristics of Creative Persons
    Managing Creativity in Health Care
      Settings

ritical thinking is the process of examining underlying assumptions about current evidence and interpreting and evaluating arguments for the purpose of reaching a conclusion from a new perspective. The conclusion reached is a critical thinking outcome. Critical thinking is a higher level cognitive process that includes creativity, problem solving, and decision making (Figure 11–1).

Nurse managers are expected to use knowledge from various disciplines to solve problems with patients, staff, and the organization, as well as problems in their own personal and professional lives. They also are constantly faced with the necessity of making decisions in dynamic situations. Do the advantages of the primary nursing care delivery system outweigh costs and recruitment difficulties during a nursing shortage? Would a new model of differentiated practice be more useful? Is the present "floating" policy adequate for both patients and nurses? Which is the best staffing pattern to pre-

FIGURE 11-1 MODEL OF CRITICAL THINKING

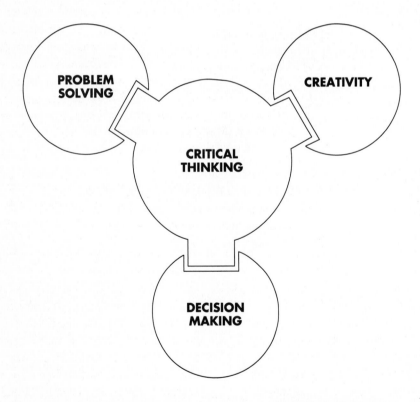

vent turnover and assure standards of patient care? Critical thinking helps nurse managers see all sides of an issue and look for different and exciting ways to solve old problems.

The critical thinking process seems abstract unless it can be related to practical experiences. One way to develop this process is to consider a series of questions when examining a specific problem or making a decision. The following questions are suggested.

1. What are the underlying assumptions?

   Underlying assumptions are beliefs that influence an individual's reasoning. They are perceptions that may or may not be grounded in reality. For example, some people believe the AIDS epidemic is punishment for homosexual behavior. This attitude toward persons with AIDS could alter ones approach to care for an AIDS patient.

2. How is evidence interpreted?

   Interpretation of the information can also be value laden. Is the evidence presented clearly? Can the facts be substantiated? Are the persons presenting the evidence using emotional or biased information? Are there any errors in reasoning?

3. How are the arguments to be evaluated?

   Is there objective evidence to support the arguments? Have all value preferences been determined? Is there a good chance the arguments will be accepted? Are there enough persons to support it? Health care institutions decided to move to a smoke-free environment when it was found that passive smoking was injurious to individuals' health. In addition, the value system of society favored non-smokers and a strong majority supported the movement.

Critical thinking thus far is defined as open inquiry, ability to question, examining underlying assumptions, and interpreting and evaluating arguments. Critical thinking includes and depends upon decision-making and problem-solving skills, which draw upon creative abilities and are discussed later in this chapter.

The label *problem solving* is used inconsistently and often interchangeably with *decision making* in organizational literature. While the two processes appear similar and may in some instances depend on one another, they are not synonymous. Solving a problem may involve a set of decisions; conversely, a major decision may have involved the solving of several related problems. However, some decisions are not of a problem-solving nature, such as a decision about scheduling, equipment, inservices, or other matters that have no immediate bearing on selecting future courses of action. By contrast, some problems do not involve decision making as a deliberate process. Habitual action may be a mode of problem solving, such as holding onto a wall when walking down a wet hospital corridor or stopping a patient from pulling out an IV.

Most of the time, however, decision making is a subset of problem solving. Decision making within problem solving results when a dynamic situation is recognized, a problem is identified, and a solution or reaction is needed. The main distinctions between problem solving and decision making are: (1) problem solving involves diagnosing a problem and solving it, which may or may not entail deciding on the one correct solution, and (2) decision making may or may not involve a problem but it always involves selecting an alternative from among several, each of which could be appropriate under certain circumstances.

♦ PROBLEM SOLVING

Critical thinking skills can be used to rationally resolve problems. Identifying, analyzing, and questioning the evidence and implications of each problem stimulate and illuminate critical thought processes. *Problem solving* can be defined as a process used when a gap is perceived between an existing state (what is going on) and a desired state (what should be going on). It involves searching for information, which clarifies the nature of the problem and suggests alternative solutions. These solutions are carefully evaluated and the best is chosen for implementation. The implemented solution is then maintained over time to assure its immediate and continued effectiveness. If difficulties are encountered, some or all of the process is repeated.

PROBLEM-SOLVING METHODS

A variety of methods can be used to solve problems. Managers with little management experience, for instance, tend to use *trial and error,* applying one solution after another until the problem is solved or appears to be improving. These managers are unable to judge from past experience and have little time for research.

For example, in a step-down unit showing an increasing incidence of medication errors, Nancy Anderson, the nurse manager, uses various strategies to decrease the errors, such as asking nurses to use calculators, having the charge nurse check medications, and posting dosage and medication charts in the unit. After a few months, when none of the methods has worked, it occurs to Ms. Anderson that perhaps making individuals responsible for their actions would be more effective. A point system for medication errors is developed. When nurses accumulate a certain amount of points they are required to take a medication test in which repeated failure

may eventually lead to termination. Ms. Anderson's solution is effective and a low level of medication errors is restored. As this example shows, a trial-and-error process can be more time-consuming than is desirable and may even be detrimental. Although some learning can occur, the nurse manager risks being perceived as a poor problem solver who has wasted time and money on ineffective solutions.

Experimentation, another type of problem solving, is more rigorous than trial and error. Pilot projects or limited trials are examples of experimentation. It involves having a theory (hypothesis) or hunch that produces knowledge, understanding, or prediction. A project or study is carried out in either a controlled or an uncontrolled setting using a group of people on whom the theory is tested. Data are collected and results interpreted to determine if a solution exists and has practical usefulness for the problem encountered. For example, a nurse manager of a pediatric floor has received many complaints from mothers of children who think the nurses are short-tempered with them. The manager has a hunch that 12-hour shifts recently implemented on her floor are contributing to the problem. She can test her theory that nurses who must interact frequently with families perform better on eight-hour shifts by setting up a small study examining the two staffing patterns and patient satisfaction.

Experimentation may be creative and effective or uninspired and ineffective, depending on how it is used. As a major method of problem solving, it may be inefficient due to the amount of time involved. However, if all previous methods of problem solving have failed, experimentation may be beneficial. For example, if a nurse manager and staff nurse disagree about management decisions, the staff nurse may continually undermine the authority of the nurse manager in these matters. Constant trouble brews among staff due to this staff nurse's inappropriate comments and criticism. Counseling, confrontation, and threats fail to bring about the manager's desired goals of mutual alliance, improved morale, and productivity. In this situation the nurse manager may wish to experiment. Rather than being terminated, the staff nurse might be assigned to a special project requiring initiative and the assumption of a particular responsibility for a defined time. The effectiveness of this strategy is noted before a second solution is attempted. One of the two attempts might prove to be innovative, solve the problem, and salvage an employee.

Still another problem-solving technique is reliance on *past experience*. Everyone has various and countless experiences. Individuals build a repertoire of these experiences and base future actions on what were considered successful resolutions in the past. If a particular course of action consistently resulted in positive outcomes, it will be tried again when similar circumstances occur. In some instances, an individual's past experience can determine how much risk will be taken in any present circumstance. The nature and frequency of the experience also contribute significantly to effectiveness of this problem-solving method. How much has been learned from these experiences, positive or negative, can affect the current viewpoint and can result in either subjective and narrow judgments or very wise ones. This is especially true in human relation problems. A nurse manager who has an unfortunate experience with a nurse recovering from chemical dependency may be biased and, in the future, may judge negatively the performance of all nurses with acknowledged chemical dependency problems.

Some problems are *self-solving*: If permitted to run a natural course they are solved by those personally involved. This is not to say that a uniform laissez-faire style solves all problems. The nurse manager must not ignore managerial responsibilities, but often difficult situations become more manageable when participants are allowed to discover their own solutions. This typically happens, for example, when a newly graduated BSN joins a unit where most of the staff are diploma RNs with many years of experience. The new graduate may be defensive and overly assertive in his or her role, while the diploma RNs may resent her level of education as well as her lack of experience. If the nurse manager intervenes, a problem that might have been worked out by the staff becomes an ongoing source of conflict. The great skill required here is knowing when to do nothing! Chapters 7 and 22 discuss this issue.

PROBLEM-SOLVING PROCESS

The nurse manager may not always be able to go to the library to research a problem since nursing problems usually require immediate action. Nurse managers simply may not have time for formalized processes. Therefore, learning an organized method for problem solving and enlarging problem-solving skills that come from critical thinking are needed to select the best solutions. One practical method for problem solving is the seven-step process shown below.

1. Define the problem.

2. Gather information.

3. Analyze the information.

4. Develop solutions.

5. Make a decision.

6. Implement the decision.

7. Evaluate the solution.

DEFINE THE PROBLEM. The most important part of problem solving is defining the problem. The problems nurse managers perceive determine the solutions or changes they implement. For our purposes, a problem can be identified as a departure from a desirable state of affairs as perceived by the nurse manager who is responsible for dealing foresightedly with the situation.

Suppose a nurse manager reluctantly implements a self-scheduling process on her floor and finds evenings and some weekend shifts not adequately covered each time the schedule is posted. She might identify the problem as the immaturity of nurses to function under democratic leadership. The causes may have been lack of interest in group decision making, minimal concern over providing adequate patient coverage, or, perhaps more correctly, a few nurses who do not understand the process. The definition of a problem should be a descriptive statement of the state of affairs, not a judgment or conclusion. If one begins the statement of a problem with a judgment, the solution may be equally judgmental and could overlook critical descriptive elements. If the nurse manager defines the above problem as immaturity and reverts to making out the schedules herself without further fact finding, a minor problem could develop into a full-blown crisis.

Premature interpretation can alter one's ability to deal with facts objectively. Are there other explanations for the apparent behavior without negative assumptions about maturity of the staff? Accurate assessment of the scope of the problem also determines if a lasting solution needs to be sought or just a stopgap measure. Is this just a situational problem requiring only intervention with a simple explanation, or is it more complex, involving the leadership style of the manager? Problems must be defined and classified for action to be taken.

In defining a problem, the nurse manager should determine the area it covers and ask: Do I have the authority to do anything about this myself? Do I have all the information? the time? Could I get someone else to do it? What benefits could be expected? A list of potential benefits provides the basis for comparison and choice of solutions. The list also serves as a means for evaluating the solution.

GATHER INFORMATION. Problem solving begins with collecting a set of facts. This information gathering initiates a search for additional facts that provide clues to the scope and solution of the problem. A search that is careful, systematic, and complete facilitates accomplishment of goals and evaluation of the effects of the solution. Information gathered will probably be a combination of facts and feelings. Relevant, valid, accurate, detailed descriptions should be obtained from appropriate persons or sources, and the information should be put in writing. This encourages people to report facts accurately. The nurse manager may choose to have everyone involved provide information. While this may not always provide objective information, it may reduce misinformation, and it allows everyone an opportunity to tell what he or she thinks is wrong with a situation. Lack of time, of course, may prevent gathering written data.

Experience is another source of information—the nurse manager's own experience as well as the experience of other nurse managers and staff. Everyone involved usually has ideas on what should be done about a problem and many of these ideas represent good information and valuable suggestions. Yet, information gathered may never be complete. Some data will be useless, some inaccurate, but some will be useful to develop innovative ideas worth pursuing.

ANALYZE THE INFORMATION. The information should be analyzed only when all of it has been sorted into some orderly arrangement. The following is suggested:

Categorize information in order of reliability.

List information from most important to least important.

Set information into a time sequence. What happened first? next? What came before what? What were the concurrent circumstances?

Set information up in terms of cause and effect. Is A causing B or vice versa?

Classify information into categories: human factors such as personality, maturity, education, age, relationships among people, problems outside the institution; technical factors such as nursing skills or the type of unit; and temporal factors such as length of service, overtime, type of shift, and double shifts. Also ask, "How long has this been going on?" Consider policy factors, such as hospital procedures or rules applying to the problem.

Since no amount of information is ever comprehensive, critical thinking skills are important to examine the assumptions, evidence, and potential value conflicts.

DEVELOP SOLUTIONS. As the nurse manager analyzes information, numerous possible solutions will suggest themselves. These should be written down and the nurse manager should immediately start developing the best of them. It is not good to limit oneself only to simple solutions, because doing so may constrain creative thinking and cause over-concentration on detail. Developing alternative solutions makes it possible to combine the best parts of several solutions into one superior one. Also, alternatives are valuable in case the first-order solutions prove impossible to implement.

When exploring a variety of solutions, it is important to maintain an uncritical attitude toward the way the problem has been previously handled. Some problems have a long-standing history before they reach the nurse manager and attempts may have been made to resolve them over a long period of time.

Past experience may not always supply an answer but can aid the critical thinking process and help prepare for future problem solving. For assistance with future problem solving, nurse managers can review the literature, attend relevant seminars, and brainstorm with others. Sometimes others have solved similar problems and those methods can be applied to a comparable problem.

MAKE A DECISION. After the nurse manager has reviewed the list of potential solutions, the one most feasible and satisfactory that has the fewest undesirable consequences is selected. Some solutions have to be put into effect quickly: Matters of discipline or compromises in patient care delivery need immediate intervention. Nurse managers should have, in advance, authority to act in an emergency and know the penalties to be imposed for various infractions.

If the problem is a technical one, however, and the solution to it brings about a change in the method of doing work (or using new equipment), there may be resistance. All people become disturbed by changes that reorder their habit patterns and threaten personal security or status. Many solutions fail because the manager does not recognize the change process that must be set in motion before solutions can be implemented. If the solution involves change, those who will be affected by it should be fully informed of the process. (See Chapter 20 for a complete discussion of the change process.)

IMPLEMENT THE DECISION. Implementation follows the decision on the best course of action. If new problems, previously not considered, emerge after implementation, these impediments must be evaluated as carefully as any other problem. The nurse manager must be very careful, however, not to abandon a workable solution just because a few individuals object. A minority always will. If the previous steps in the problem-solving process have been followed, the solution has been carefully thought out, and potential problems have been addressed, implementation should move forward. The nurse manager must remember that no solution is perfect and all change is stressful.

It is worthwhile to mention here what Chester Barnard refers to as the "zone of acceptance" in executive problem solving (Barnard, 1937). Most employees cooperate only with directives (solutions) that fit into their "zone of acceptance." Some solutions are clearly unacceptable, some are neutral, others are barely acceptable, and some are fully acceptable. This last group lies within the zone of acceptance. Thus, if a solution is chosen that the nurse manager knows will not be accepted, steps must be taken to educate or motivate the staff to comply with it. For example, the nurse manager may decide that when the census is low, nurses will "float" to other units. The unit's own staff, however, has negative ideas about floating and does not wish to cooperate. If the nurse manager cannot educate or motivate staff to see floating as an acceptable solution to fluctuating census problems, the solution, no matter how good, will fail because it is not within the staff's zone of acceptance. For a discussion on using staff participation to avoid these problems, see Chapter 9.

EVALUATE THE SOLUTION. After the solution has been implemented, the nurse manager should review the plan instituted and compare the actual results and benefits to those of the idealized solution. Individuals tend to fall back into old patterns of habit or give lip service to change when actually the same old behavior is taking place. The nurse manager must ask, "Is the solution being implemented? If so, are the results better or worse than expected? If they are better, what changes may have contributed to the success?" Such a periodic checkup gives the nurse manager valuable insight and experience to use in other situations and keeps the problem-solving process on course.

The outcome of the solution should be studied somewhat as a football coach studies videotapes of a football game. Where were mistakes made? How can they be avoided in the future? What decisions were successes? Why? Many ineffective solutions are never challenged once they are implemented. If the nurse manager evaluates the outcome to ensure problem resolution has indeed occurred and builds upon the experience, problem solving becomes an expert skill that can be used throughout a management career.

◆ DECISION MAKING

Considering all the practice individuals get in making decisions, it would seem they might become very good at it: The more IVs a nurse starts successfully, the better he or she becomes. But the number of decisions made have nothing to do with skills at making them or results obtained. The assumption is that decision making comes naturally, like learning to breathe. It does not! The decision-making process described in this chapter provides nurse managers with a system for making decisions that is applicable to any decision. *Decision making* can be defined as the process of establishing criteria by which alternative courses of action are developed and selected. It is a useful procedure for making practical decisions. Phases of the seven-step process may proceed concurrently and be repeated. However, thinking critically throughout the process of completing all the steps is the best assurance of a sound alternative.

DECISION-MAKING STRATEGIES

Satisficing is not a misspelled word; it is a decision-making strategy whereby the individual chooses an alternative that is not ideal but either is good enough (suffices) under existing circumstances to meet minimum standards of acceptance or is the first acceptable alternative. An *optimizing* approach, by contrast, first identifies all possible outcomes, examines the probability of each available alternative, and then takes the action that yields the highest probability of achieving the most desirable outcome.

Nursing management situations present a multitude of problems that are ineffectively solved with satisficing strategies. For example, Sue Goodwin, a nurse manager in charge of a busy neurosurgical floor with high turnover rates and high patient acuity levels uses a satisficing alternative when hiring replacement staff. She hires all nurse applicants in order of application until no positions are open. Instead, Ms. Goodwin should optimize by replacing staff with nurse applicants who possess skills and attitudes important to neurosurgical nursing regardless of the number of applicants or desire for immediate action. She should also develop a plan to promote job satisfaction, the lack of which is the real reason for the vacancies.

Nurse managers who solve problems using satisficing usually lack specific training in prob-

lem solving and decision making. They view their units or floors as drastically simplified models of the real world and are content with this simplification because it allows them to make decisions with relatively simple rules of thumb or from force of habit. Optimizing techniques, however, make demands on their willingness and ability to collect information, analyze it, and choose the best alternatives.

DECISION-MAKING CONDITIONS

The question is often asked whether decision making is an individual or an organizational process: Do nurse managers or organizations make decisions? In this chapter, managerial decision making is treated essentially as an individual process that occurs in an organizational context. Even though decision making is basically individual, the conditions surrounding it can change dramatically. Within the organization, nurse managers make decisions under conditions of *certainty, risk,* or *uncertainty.*

DECISION MAKING UNDER CERTAINTY.

When nurse managers know the alternatives and the conditions surrounding each alternative, a state of *certainty* is said to exist. Suppose a nurse manager on a unit with acutely ill patients wants to decrease the number of skin entries a patient experiences when an IV is started as well as reduce costs resulting from failed venipunctures. Three alternatives exist: (1) establish an IV team on all shifts, which is known to minimize IV attempts and reduce cost; (2) establish a reciprocal relationship with the anesthesia department to start IVs when nurses experience difficulty, which results in multiple venipunctures and increased costs; and (3) set a standard of two insertion attempts per nurse per patient. While this last method reduces the number of times an IV is started, equipment costs are not substantially lowered. The manager, however, knows the alternatives (IV team, anesthesia department, standards) and the conditions associated with each (reduced costs, assistance with starting IVs, minimum attempts, some cost reduction). A condition of certainty is said to exist, and the decision can be made with full knowledge of what the payoff will be.

DECISION MAKING UNDER CONDITIONS OF RISK. In organizational settings few decisions are made under certainty. The complexity of health care problems makes such situations rare. The more common decision-making condition is that of *risk*. The nurse manager does not always know the state of the situation. If the weather forecaster predicts a 40 percent chance of snow, the nurse manager is operating in a situation of risk when trying to decide how to staff the unit for the next 24 hours. In a risk situation, availability of each alternative, potential successes, and costs are all associated with probability estimates. *Probability* is the likelihood, expressed as a percentage, that an event will or will not occur. If something is certain to happen, its probability is 1.00. If it is certain not to happen, its probability is 0. If there is a 50-50 chance, its probability is .50.

Suppose a nurse manager decides to use agency nurses to staff a unit during heavy vacation periods. Two agencies look attractive and the manager must decide between them. Agency A has had modest growth over the last 10 years and offers the manager a three-month contract freezing wages during that time. In addition, the unit will have first choice of available nurses. Agency B is much more dynamic and charges more but explains that the reason they have had an increased rate of growth is because their nurses are the highest paid in the area. The nurse manager can choose the first alternative, provid-

ing a safe, constant supply of nursing personnel, or the second alternative, which may or may not deliver the needed nurses and at higher costs. After careful consideration one might decide that the first agency is better, but one must examine the risks involved. When staffing the unit, the nurse manager will need to decide how much risk the hospital is willing to assume for the cost of full coverage.

The key element in decision making under conditions of risk is to accurately determine the probabilities of each alternative. The nurse manager can use a probability analysis whereby expected risk is calculated or estimated. In the above example of the two agencies, Table 11–1 illustrates the probability analysis. From this calculation it appears as though Agency A offers the best outcome. However, if the second agency had a 90 percent chance of filling shifts and a 50 percent chance of fixing costs, a completely different situation would exist. The nurse manager might decide the potential for increased costs was a small tradeoff for having the unit fully staffed during vacation periods.

DECISION MAKING UNDER CONDITIONS OF UNCERTAINTY. Most critical decision making in organizations is done under the con-

TABLE 11-1 DECISION MAKING UNDER RISK

	Probability Analysis
Agency A	60% Filling shifts 100% Fixed wages
Agency B	50% Filling shifts 70% Fixed wages

dition of *uncertainty*. The individual making the decision does not know all the alternatives, attendant risks, or likely consequences of each. Uncertainty originates with the complex and dynamic nature of health care organizations. Consider the problem of increased technology in health care. John Jackson, a nurse manager of a specialized cardiac intensive care unit, faces the task of recruiting scarce and highly skilled nurses to care for coronary bypass patients. The obvious alternative is to offer a salary and benefit package that rivals that of all other institutions in the area. However, this means the nurse manager will have costly specialized nursing personnel in his budget who are not easily absorbed by other units in the institution. The probability that coronary bypass procedures will become obsolete in the future and will no longer be used by surgeons is unknown. In addition, other factors (e.g., increased competition, government regulations regarding reimbursement) may contribute to conditions of uncertainty.

The nurse manager may use three approaches in situations of uncertainty. First is to select an alternative whose best possible outcome is the best possible outcome for all alternatives. This optimistic approach is often called the *maximax* approach. In the example described above, the nurse manager would recruit the best nurses he could find based on the assumption that coronary bypass procedures would continue to be desirable.

A second approach is to compare the worst possible outcome for each alternative and choose the one that seems the least objectionable. This pessimistic approach is called the *maximin* approach. In the coronary bypass example, Mr. Jackson would not try to recruit highly skilled nurses based on the assumptions that the procedure is likely to become obsolete

or that competition will limit the number of admissions.

The last approach is to choose the alternative with the least variation among its possible outcomes. This *risk-averting approach* makes for more effective planning. If Mr. Jackson decides not to recruit any nurses, the outcome can vary from having patients and no highly skilled nurses to having few patients and no highly skilled nurses. A risk-averting approach might be to recruit a few highly skilled nurses who could prepare other nurses to work in the unit and who could be successfully absorbed in other settings if a decrease in admissions occurs. The key to effective decision making under uncertainty is to gather as much relevant information as possible using a logical and rational perspective and to rely on past experience. Highly developed critical thinking skills also play a major role in decision making under uncertainty.

There are other types of quantitative approaches, decision trees, inventory models, and payoff matrices that are beyond the scope of this chapter. They are more likely to be considered by top level administrators rather than first line nurse managers. They are used when highly statistical methods are needed to make decisions under conditions of uncertainty and at high risk. A short description of each is presented in the following section.

Decision trees allow administrators to follow results of alternatives over time. The institution's nurse executive might decide to completely change the delivery system of patient care in the institution, which would then involve a decision based on the high or low probability of available nurses. The possible alternatives and their consequences are laid out in a branching tree manner so the nurse administrator can study consequences more carefully. Again, probabilities are applied to determine the expected value along each branch of the tree, and the one with the highest value is selected (Everett & Ebert, 1986).

Inventory models have been developed to deal with almost all types of inventory problems. An inventory model helps the nurse manager plan the optimal level of inventory to carry. For example, ordering large quantities of supplies decreases the chances that supplies will run out but increases costs and the need for storage. Having fewer supplies reduces costs and demand for storage but increases the chances of running out and having nurses take time to order and pick up supplies. An inventory model can help with estimating just how many supplies should be stocked (Lapin, 1978).

A *payoff matrix* involves alternatives, conditions under which the alternatives will occur, and probabilities associated with each. Consider an administrator who is selecting a management information system for the institution. There is one probability that the least expensive system will have a poor service record and another probability that it will be sufficient. Given the probabilities and the payoffs of the purchase, the nurse administrator can determine the expected value for each alternative (least expensive, poor service record or least expensive, adequate service record) and select the one with the greatest payoff.

DECISION-MAKING PROCESS

The policies and administration of many health care systems are often delegated implicitly to nurse managers. Therefore, the quality of care and overall administration can depend on the ability of this key person to make and implement decisions and provide managerial guidelines that complement the organization.

Much of the management literature describes decisions as discrete events made by an individual manager or a group using an orderly, rational process. Yukl (1989) found this picture sharply contradicted by the descriptive research on managerial work and related research on managerial decision making (Cohen & March, 1974; McCall, Kaplan & Gerlach, 1982; Schweiger, Anderson & Locke, 1985; Simon, 1987). Managers seldom make major decisions at a single point in time and often are unable to recall when a decision was finally reached. Some major decisions are the result of many small actions or incremental choices taken without regarding larger strategic issues. In addition, decision processes are likely to be characterized more by confusion, disorder, and emotionality than by rationality. For these reasons it is essential that the nurse manager develop appropriate technical skills and the capacity to find a good balance between lengthy processes and quick, decisive action.

The decision-making process begins when the nurse manager perceives a gap between what is actually happening and what should be happening, and it ends with action that will narrow this gap or close it. The simplest way to learn decision-making skills is to integrate a model into one's thinking by breaking the components down into individual steps. The seven steps of the decision-making process are described in Table 11–2 and are as applicable to personal problems as they are to nursing management problems. Each step is elaborated by pertinent questions clarifying the statements, and they should be followed in the order in which they are presented.

Consider an example of the decision-making process at work in a clinical situation. A step-down unit in a busy 900-bed hospital is normally 100 percent occupied. Mary Andrews is the nurse manager. Most patients have multiple systems compromised and depend on some form of ventilatory support. Mr. G, an 85-year-old man with sleep apnea, has been in the unit for nine months. Six feet tall and 225 pounds, he is ventilator dependent, with chronic sepsis, a tracheostomy, feeding tube, Foley catheter, IV lines, and early decubitus skin changes from constant diarrhea. He has expressed a "wish to die," has made several attempts to disable the ventilator, has grown progressively more abusive of nurses, and has generally brought on nurses' transfers, threats of resignation, or refusal to render care.

Complicating this is his status as a major benefactor of the hospital. Ms. Andrews' first attempt was to allow nurses to make out their own assignments. As a result, Mr. G had a different nurse each shift and received no continuity of care. The second attempt was a patient care plan meeting attended by Mr. G's physicians, nurses, and personnel from physical therapy, social services, psychiatry, occupational therapy, pastoral care, and the employee assistance program. As a result, some 32 suggested orders were written. All were designed with the best of intentions to alleviate the suffering on both sides. Some included talking books to keep Mr. G occupied and a portable punching bag to

---

TABLE 11-2 STEPS IN THE DECISION MAKING PROCESS

1. Identify the purpose: Why is a decision necessary? What needs to be determined? State the issue in the broadest possible terms.

2. Set the criteria: What needs to be achieved, preserved, and avoided by whatever decision is made? The answers to these questions are the standards by which solutions will be evaluated.

3. Weight the criteria: A simple methodology is presented. Each criterion is ranked on a scale of values from 1 (totally unimportant) to 10 (extrememly important).

4. Seek alternatives: List all possible courses of action. Is one alternative more significant than another? Does one alternative have weaknesses in some areas? Can these be overcome? Can two alternatives or features of many alternatives be combined?

5. Test alternatives: First, using the same methodology as in Step 3, rank each alternative on a 10–high scale. Second, multiply the weight of each criteria by the rating of each alternative. Third, add the scores and compare the results.

6. Troubleshoot: What could go wrong? How can you plan? Can the choice be improved?

7. Evaluate the action: Is the solution being implemented? Is it effective? Is it costly?

allow him to vent his hostility. However, 10 days later none of the orders were being implemented. Nurses and other health care personnel functioned as before and morale on the unit eroded further.

Ms. Andrews decided a situation so difficult and frustrating required a highly systematic approach to enable them all to make better decisions. The seven-step decision-making process was instituted.

In the first step *(identify the purpose)* the need for a decision assumes the existence of an issue (or problem). The nurse manager must have complete understanding of the issue. The means for getting that type of understanding is to ask, "Why is a decision necessary? What needs to be determined? What is the purpose of the decision?" In the case of Mr. G, a decision is necessary because if nothing is done, a strong possibility exists that, given the strain under which the nurses are working, quality of care will suffer and resignations may occur. The purpose of any decision is to reduce, remove, or prevent adverse consequences or to accept desirable ones. Is the primary purpose in this example to wean Mr. G from the ventilator or to assure continuity of care? Many times the purpose is identified in narrow, restrictive terms. When defining the purpose it is important to avoid statements that elicit just black and white answers. For example, should the nurses plan a weaning schedule for Mr. G? If the purpose is formulated to include all or most opportunities, a wider range of alternatives is generated. If just weaning was chosen and it was unsuccessful, the nurses would be back where they started. Ms. Andrews knows it is important for Mr. G's condition to improve so he can be transferred to a long-term facility. If Mr. G's condition becomes chronic, he will no longer be eligible for an acute

care bed. Ms. Andrews knows several excellent long-term facilities in the area that will accept ventilator patients but not a septic patient with a decubitus ulcer and IV lines. In the best possible terms, she finally defines the purpose as, "Determine the best way to discharge Mr. G to a long-term facility."

With the purpose clearly formulated, Ms. Andrews brings the statement to a staff meeting and asks for help to *set the criteria,* the second step. Answers to three standard questions become the criteria by which alternatives are selected and evaluated: What is to be achieved? What is to be preserved? What is to be avoided? Most of the time individuals making decisions have certain criteria by which they are bound, but if they make decisions before examining the criteria, standards that would have encouraged the widest range of possible alternatives are missed. It is important to let the criteria suggest alternatives, not vice versa. A decision based on premature alternatives is made less likely when one determines what needs to be achieved, preserved, and avoided. Table 11–3 indicates criteria generated by the nurse manager and staff that they thought most appropriate for Mr. G's discharge.

In the third step, *weight the criteria,* a simple methodology is presented. This is a priority-setting exercise. The aim is to produce a list of activities or services that are ranked in order of preference. The nurse manager rates each criterion according to its place on a scale of values from 1 point (totally unimportant) to 10 points (extremely important). Those criteria that receive a value of 10 become the standards by which less important objectives are measured. For example, if she chooses a criterion that seems just as likely to prove unimportant as important it might receive a value of 5. The numerical values become part of the weighting system by which the choices are evaluated and alternatives selected. There is no right or wrong weighting order, as rankings reflect individual needs and values. As numerical values are assigned to the criteria, certain compromises may become evident. Some criteria may emerge as less important than originally thought, may have been duplicated, or may be combined with other criteria. Twelve of the original criteria established by the group remain on the list in Table 11–4.

"Job satisfaction" and "resignations" were eliminated by merger with "preserving morale." The "suicide" criterion was also omitted, assuming that if Mr. G's cognitive function improved, he would be less inclined to remove himself from the ventilator. Other items were excluded as she determined they were outside the staff's ability to influence an outcome (e.g., health of spouse) or the criterion was not grounded in reality (e.g., independent ADL). Medical prognosis was clearly against Mr. G's return to independence in activities of daily living.

To *seek alternatives* is the fourth step. The first question to ask is, "What are the possible ways to fulfill each criterion?" It is also possible to combine the best features of many alternatives or modify them to fit the criteria. Ms. Andrews examined all options that appeared to address the criteria. Several alternatives were combined and others omitted before the final list was compiled. The four tentative alternatives identified are as follows: (1) up in a chair each shift for 30 minutes to one hour, as tolerated, with tracheostomy plugged, tube feedings instituted, and schedules posted and checked by all personnel on the unit; (2) private duty nurses to be employed by the patient on the day and evening shifts; (3) visits by a psychologist, occu-

---

TABLE 11–3 SETTING CRITERIA

Purpose Determine the best way to discharge Mr. G. to a long-term facility.

Criteria		
Achieve	**Preserve**	**Avoid**
Wean from the ventilator	Staff morale	Respiratory distress
Bowel and bladder training	Job satisfaction	Decubitus ulcers
Removal of IV lines	Mr. G's cognitive function	Suicide
Continuity of care	Health of spouse	Diarrhea
Support systems	Financial independence	Resignations
G-tube function		Condition worsening
Asepsis		
Independent ADL		
Weight gain		
Ambulatory		

pational therapist, physical therapist, social service personnel as needed; and (4) institute primary nursing for Mr. G.

The fifth step, *test alternatives,* is done to reduce biased thinking. Table 11–5 indicates how Ms. Andrews tested the alternatives. She rated the alternatives from 1 to 10 on desirability and multiplied the rating and the criteria weight. The best alternative is usually the one scoring the highest on the most desirable criteria (10 points) and at least 15 percent higher than other alternatives. Testing alternatives allows her to make objective decisions based on a standard of comparison. By assigning numerical values to the criteria and alternatives, beliefs and values are submitted to critical appraisal. If two or more alternatives are close, it is important to reevaluate steps to determine if values assigned to criteria clearly demonstrate priorities. When Ms. Andrews examined the four possible solutions, it appeared as though she had given Alter-

native A higher ratings because she simply preferred that alternative. However, examining the evidence showed that a clear rationale had been identified for each rating. She realized that getting Mr. G up in a chair three times a day would benefit respiratory, gastrointestinal, and circulatory function and contribute to homeostasis and possible discharge.

Troubleshooting is an extremely important step but seldom is given enough attention. Here Ms. Andrews should ask what could go wrong and anticipate the possible adverse repercussions of the actions to be taken. She should lay plans to prevent, minimize, or overcome problems. Three actions are helpful when troubleshooting any decision:

1. List all possible problems that could occur with the alternative selected.

2. List the likelihood of each problem occurring (high, medium, or low).

3. List preventive measures for each potential problem.

In the example with Mr. G, one problem that could develop with the decision to get him up in a chair three times a day is failure of personnel to adhere to the schedule. The likelihood of this happening was rated as high by Ms. Andrews. As a troubleshooting measure, the charge nurse on each shift was asked to post an assignment list with initials identifying one person responsible for this task and to check a box showing task "accomplished" or "not accomplished/reasons." With this strategy in place, compliance was high.

When asked about failure to troubleshoot, nurse managers often respond that it focuses on failures, would upset morale, or would erode consensus. For similar reasons, staff may be reluctant to tell a nurse manager what could go

TABLE 11–4 WEIGHTING THE CRITERIA

Purpose Determine the best way to discharge Mr. G. to a long-term facility.

Criteria	Value
Asepsis	10
No decubitus ulcers	10
G-tube function	10
No diarrhea	10
No IV lines	9
Wean from ventilator	9
Preserve staff morale	9
Stable finances	6
Cognitive function	6
Respiratory distress	3
Ambulatory	2
Continuity of care	1

TABLE 11–5 TESTING THE ALTERNATIVES

Title / Criteria	Weight*	Alternative A — Up in chair 30 to 60 minutes/trach plugged/ tubefeedings/ schedules posted		Alternative B — Private duty nurses on day/ evening shifts		Alternative C — Visits by psychologist/ other disciplines		Alternative D — Primary nursing for Mr. G.	
		Rate*	Score	Rate*	Score	Rate*	Score	Rate*	Score
Asepsis	10	10	100	5	50	0	0	5	50
No decubitus	10	10	100	10	100	5	50	10	100
G-tube function	10	10	100	10	100	5	50	5	50
No IV lines	10	9	90	5	50	5	50	5	50
No diarrhea	9	5	45	3	27	3	27	3	27
Wean from ventilator	9	5	45	5	45	5	45	5	45
Preserve staff morale	9	10	90	10	90	10	90	10	90
Avoid financial crisis	6	10	60	5	30	5	30	5	30
Maintain cognitive function	6	5	30	10	60	10	60	5	30
Prevent respiratory distress	3	5	15	5	15	5	15	5	15
Ambulatory	2	3	6	5	10	3	6	1	2
Continuity of care	1	10	10	10	10	0	0	10	10
Totals			691		587		423		499

*Weight x rate = score

wrong. It is all the more important to remember and to remind others that more time is spent doing things over than doing them right the first time. Troubleshooting is the extra effort that can avoid this added frustration.

The last step is to *evaluate the action*. The aim is formally to determine if the selected alternative is effective and has accomplished the desired result. In the initial analysis, it was deemed highly important for Mr. G to be discharged within a reasonable period of time. The alternative chosen to address this goal was "up in a chair three times a day." If Mr. G is successfully discharged Ms. Andrews can assume the most effective alternative was chosen and the situation has been corrected. On the other hand, if the day of discharge seems not to be getting any closer, she will realize the first alternative is not working and new action is necessary. In this example, Mr. G was discharged within six weeks, largely due to the nurse manager's persistence and application of decision-making techniques.

STUMBLING BLOCKS

Personality traits, inexperience, lack of adaptability, and preconceived ideas are several obstacles to problem solving and decision making experienced by nurse managers. They are discussed in the following section.

PERSONALITY. The nurse manager's personality can and often does affect how and why certain decisions are made. Many nurse managers are selected because of their expert clinical, not management, skills. They often start out insecure and resort to various unproductive activities. A nurse manager who is insecure may make decisions primarily on an approval-seeking basis. When a truly difficult situation arises, rather than lose face with the staff, he or she

makes a decision that will placate people rather than one that will achieve the larger goals of the institution. On the other hand, a nurse manager who demonstrates an authoritative type of personality might make unreasonable demands on the staff, not rewarding staff for long hours because of her "workaholic" attitude or giving the staff no control over patient care activities. Similarly, a lazy manager may cause a unit to flounder because any new ideas or solutions to problems may demand action he or she is not inclined to take.

RIGIDITY. Rigidity, an inflexible management style, is another obstacle to problem solving. It may result from ineffective trial-and-error solutions or fear of risk taking or may be an inherent personality trait. As discussed previously, ineffective trial-and-error problem solving can be avoided if the nurse manager gathers sufficient information and determines a means for early correction of wrong or inadequate decisions. Also, to minimize risk in problem solving, the goal is to know and understand alternative risks and expectations. Personality traits are difficult to change, but awareness inventories from management seminars or evaluations from staff may indicate to an individual that her or his attitudes are not conducive to effective leadership.

The nurse manager who uses a rigid style in problem solving easily develops tunnel vision—the tendency to look at new things in old ways and from established frames of reference. It then becomes very difficult to see things from another perspective, and problem solving becomes a process whereby one person makes all of the decisions with little information or data from other sources. In the current dynamic, changing health care setting, rigidity can at times be a nurse manager's greatest barrier to effective problem solving.

BOX 11-1

A recent study examined nursing administration research from 1980 to 1989 and found only 4 % of the studies included variables reflecting effective management of the services nurses offered or the impact of leadership models on the delivery of care. Organizational processes such as decision making, problem solving, and critical thinking were studied slightly or not at all. Half of the research focused on descriptions of nursing work patterns (hours, performance, retention, and turnover).

Some (22 %) investigated attitudes of nurses' work patterns (job satisfaction, commitment, and perception of working conditions). Another category (13 %) looked at patient factors (length of stay, patient classifications, and cost of care). Thus, the emphasis of research was on nurses, patients, and consumers rather than on organizational processes contributing to effective management.

C. McDaniel, "Nursing Administration Research as a Paradigm Reflection," Nursing & Health Care, 11: 184-189

PRECONCEIVED IDEAS. Effective nurse managers do not start out with the preconceived idea that one proposed course of action is right and all others wrong. Nor do they assume that only one opinion can be voiced and others will be silent. In short, they start out with a commitment to find out why staff members disagree, not necessarily with any preconceived idea about who has the right answers. If the staff sees a different reality or even a different problem, nurse managers need to integrate this information into a database to develop additional problem-solving alternatives.

Most people have preconceived ideas about the nature of problems and their solutions. Those who are certain that only their perception is accurate may never accept the final decision reached and possibly the whole argument process. Nurse managers, however, have formal responsibility for problem solving and decision making and must put personal ideas on hold until they have gathered enough information to view the situation objectively and in the widest possible perspective.

◆ CREATIVITY IN DECISION MAKING

A realistic approach, good management climate, and an environment conducive to hard thinking and evaluation are all important. What turns a mediocre problem-solving team into an excellent one is the quality and originality of thinking. Creativity is an essential part of the critical thinking process. *Creativity*, simply defined, is the ability to develop and implement new and better solutions. Maintaining a certain level of creativity is the only way to keep an organization alive. One that functions by rule only stifles creativity, is inflexible, and is on the road to oblivion.

Wallas (1945) writes that creativity has four stages: preparation, incubation, insight, and verification (Figure 11-2). Some persons may be naturally more creative than others, but Wallas's model provides a way for all to be creative, even those who think themselves less gifted. First, the individual must acquire information necessary to understand the situation. Anyone can do this through hard work and observation. Consider Ms. Elliott who has been promoted to manage a unit and has identified the foremost problems on her new unit to be that care plans do not accurately reflect patients' needs or problems. She gathers information about lack of documentation; reviews the literature on motivation, incentives, etc.; and discusses the issue with other nurse managers *(preparation)*. She continues to manage the unit thinking about the information she has gathered but does not consciously make a decision or close off new ideas *(incubation)*. When working on a new problem, self-scheduling, she realizes a connection between the old and new problems. Many nurses complain that by the time they receive the schedule the desirable shifts are filled. The nurse manager states that she will review the care plans, and those nurses whose care plans are updated

and provide an accurate assessment of patient needs will receive a "perk": They will be allowed, on a rotating basis, first choice at selecting the schedule they want to work (this is the *insight* stage). She discusses the plan with the staff and proposes a two-month trial period to determine whether the solution is effective *(verification)*.

Campbell, Daft & Hulin (1982) found, in a survey of organizational scientists, that the first three stages of the creative process were most important. Results indicated that significant exposure to the topic as well as intuition and chance were main contributors to creativity. The more knowledge, skill, and ability the individual acquires about a potential problem or issue, the more likely it is that a creative solution will result.

CHARACTERISTICS OF CREATIVE PERSONS

Steiner (1965) found general agreement among top managers regarding many of the intellectual and personality characteristics of creative persons. In general, they are people who:

1. Generate ideas rapidly

2. Are flexible, can discard one frame of reference for another, and/or can change approaches spontaneously

3. Have a tendency to provide original solutions to problems

4. Prefer complex thought processes to simple and easily understood ones

5. Are independent in judgment and more able to believe in themselves, even under pressure

6. Exhibit distinct individualistic characteristics, seeing themselves as different from their peers

FIGURE 11–2 CREATIVE PROCESS

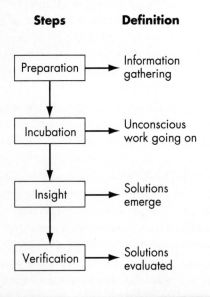

Steps	Definition
Preparation	Information gathering
Incubation	Unconscious work going on
Insight	Solutions emerge
Verification	Solutions evaluated

7. View authority as conventional rather than absolute, which means they accept authority as a matter of expedience rather than personal allegiance or moral obligation

8. Are willing to entertain and express personal whims or impulses, exhibit a more diverse "fantasy life" on clinical tests, and inject humor into situations

Creative people are likely to view authority as not absolute, make few black-and-white distinctions, have a less dogmatic view of life, show more independence of judgment and less conformity, be willing to give consideration to their own impulses, have a sense of humor, and be less rigid and freer but less effectively controlled.

MANAGING CREATIVITY IN HEALTH CARE SETTINGS

For creativity to be of value to the nurse manager, it must be useful in problem solving, decision making, and other health care activities. Creative processes must be focused on health care problems. Two widely used techniques for channeling creativity are brainstorming and synectics. *Brainstorming* (Osborn, 1953) is the use of one's brain to "storm" a creative problem in a group meeting and to do so in rapid fashion, with each "stormer" audaciously attacking the same objective. To obtain maximum creativity from a group with the brainstorming technique, four basic rules must be fully understood and adhered to:

1. Judgment is ruled out. Criticism of ideas must be withheld until later.

2. Free-wheeling is welcomed. The wilder the idea, the better; it is easier to tame down ideas than to think them up.

3. Quantity is the goal; the greater the number

of ideas, the more likelihood that some are winners.

4. Imagination and improvement are sought. In addition to contributing their own ideas, participants should suggest how two or more ideas can be joined into still a third (Osborn, 1953).

While the ideas may be wild, they may also lead to some creative solutions. Some criticisms of this approach have been the high cost factor, the time consumed, and the superficiality of many solutions.

A second method for stimulating creativity is *synectics* (Gordon, 1968). Through careful selection, a group of nurse managers is formed who have demonstrated skills in solving health care problems. While brainstorming concentrates on generating a greater number of ideas, synectics tries to identify one different new idea. To avoid eliciting obvious or common solutions, the group leader does not provide the group with a detailed analysis of the problem. Instead the leader tries to be as general as possible in giving background information. Four methods based on analogies are used in group discussions. The first is *personal analogy,* which asks group members to identify with the problem. For example, a group of staff nurses who constantly feel the nurse manager should help with "hands-on" patient care might imagine themselves as managers and determine how they might accomplish all their managerial tasks in addition to patient care. *Direct analogy* is the second method, in which comparisons are made with parallel concepts such as the human brain and a computer. The third method is *symbolic analogy,* which attempts to describe the problem using impersonal images. Pain, for example, has been described in color equivalents like red or orange. The final method is *fantasy.* Members break conventional thinking patterns and suspend judgment to evoke highly fanciful and imaginative ideas. For example, an assignment for a group of health care managers might be to identify a new concept in outpatient surgery. The leader may have the group discuss patient needs when anticipating surgery, such as proximity to parking, ease with transfer to a car after surgery, or efficient use of time. One solution that might emerge is the "drive-through" concept. In fact, this concept was used as a solution to make outpatient surgery more marketable at a major medical center.

While brainstorming and synectics are useful to promote creativity in organizations, nurse managers seldom use these techniques. Nurse managers should assess their own beliefs and make sure they subscribe to creative management. There is no substitute for a day-to-day role model. The attitude on the unit also must be favorable to giving new ideas a fair and proper hearing to reduce the tendency to destroy all creative processes within the individual or group.

The purpose of this section is to present a rational approach for encouraging creativity. The following steps can help stimulate the generation of new ideas.

STEP 1. A carefully designed planning program is essential. For example, creativity conferences can be planned around questioning all work methods. A method of work simplification, built on the premise that most people can increase productivity not by working harder but by eliminating certain steps and creating a new service or solutions, can be used at these conferences. Some organizations have instituted such conferences on a monthly or bimonthly basis, involving all employees. The focus is on prob-

lems any member of the group chooses to bring up that are creating difficulties for the unit or individual. This is not a gripe session, but problem solving in a creative manner. To facilitate progress at these conferences, one should (a) pick a specific task to improve, (b) gather relevant facts, (c) challenge every detail, (d) develop preferred solutions, and (e) implement improvements.

STEP 2. The nurse manager also needs to meet with new employees routinely as part of the orientation process, at which time information about solutions to problems is sought. New employees are not encumbered with details of accepted practices and can offer suggestions based on their prior experiences or insights before they get set in their ways or have their innovative ideas "turned off." The advantages offered by new employees should be explored, for all staff on the unit gain from such use of human resources.

STEP 3. Most nurse managers are employed in bureaucratic settings that do not foster creativity. Control is exercised over staff and rigid adherence to formal channels of communication jeopardizes innovation. In addition, there is no room for failures, and when they do occur they are not tolerated very well. When staff are afraid of the consequences of failure, creativity is inhibited and innovation does not take place. It has been suggested that if risk cannot be accepted, special ground rules need to be established that permit innovative managers and staff to function without fear of reprisals or termination if they fail. In addition, nurse managers must realize, as other organizations do, that innovative people may not fit the organizational mold. They generally avoid highly structured and controlling situations. At times they appear disorganized, lackadaisical, and even obnoxious. The challenge for nurse managers is to know when, for whom, and to what extent control is appropriate. If creativity does have a priority in the health care setting, then the reward system should be geared to and commensurate with that priority. Those whose creativity is prized should not be promoted into situations whereby they lose their creativity. Advancement and status should be provided within the area of creativity.

STEP 4. Creativity demands a certain amount of exposure to outside contacts, receptivity to new and seemingly strange ideas, proper research assistance, a certain amount of freedom, and some permissive management. The climate must promote the survival of potentially useful ideas. Many good new ideas go unused because they arise in an environment grown cold to creativity. A new idea is extremely perishable and its creator is likely to be its sole supporter, after which it may have none, since the usual reaction is either to ignore it or to look for its defects. The nurse manager can build an attitude favorable to giving new ideas a fair and proper hearing and thereby reduce the tendency to destroy the creative process within individuals and groups. The major limitation on creativity stems from the initial cost. The greater the creativity sought and the greater the departure from present practice, the greater the investment will be. In the long run, however, creative ideas may be highly cost-effective. The challenge is to determine if and when they are important, how important they are, and to encourage creative exchange of such ideas broadly among other units so there is a visible effect of the nurse manager's lead-

ership, measurable in enhanced vitality and productivity.

SUMMARY

- Critical thinking requires examining underlying assumptions about current evidence, interpreting information, and evaluating the arguments presented to reach a new and exciting conclusion.

- Critical thinking is a higher level process that includes creativity, problem solving, and decision making.

- Problem-solving and decision-making processes require nurse managers to develop critical thinking skills.

- There are two main distinctions between problem solving and decision making. Problem solving involves selecting the one correct solution to a problem, while decision making may or may not involve a problem and requires selection of one alternative from several, each of which could be appropriate in certain circumstances.

- Problem solving involves (1) defining the problem, (2) gathering information, (3) analyzing information, (4) developing solutions, (5) making a decision, (6) implementing the decision, and (7) evaluating the solution.

- Various methods of problem solving include trial and error, experimentation, past experience, tradition, and knowing when problems are self-solving.

- Stumbling blocks to problem solving and decision making are personality characteristics, rigidity, and preconceptions.

♦ Two strategies used for managerial decision making are a satisficing strategy, which identifies acceptable but not ideal alternatives, and an optimizing strategy, which identifies all alternatives and opts for the most desirable outcome.

♦ Decisions may be made under conditions of certainty, risk, or uncertainty.

♦ The decision-making process involves seven steps: (1) identify the purpose, (2) set the criteria, (3) weight the criteria, (4) seek alternatives, (5) test alternatives, (6) troubleshoot, and (7) evaluate the action.

♦ Creativity is an important concept in decision making. The creative process involves preparation, incubation, insight, and verification.

♦ Creative decision making is important, and a supportive management climate is necessary to turn mediocre problem solvers into ones who develop innovative solutions.

BIBLIOGRAPHY

Barnard, C. (1937). *Functions of the Executive.* Cambridge, MA: Harvard University Press.

Campbell, J. P., Daft, R. L., and Hulin, C. L. (1982). *What to Study: Generating and Developing Research Questions.* Beverly Hills, CA: Sage Publications.

Cohen, M. D., and March, J. G. (1974). *Leadership and Ambiguity.* New York: McGraw-Hill.

Everett, A., and Ebert, R. (1986). *Production and Operations Management.* 3d ed. Englewood Cliffs, NJ: Prentice-Hall.

Gordon, W. J. (1968). *Synectics.* New York: Collier Books.

Lapin, L. (1978). *Statistics for Modern Business Decisions.* New York: Harcourt Brace Jovanovich.

McCall, M. W., Jr., Kaplan, R. E., and Gerlach, M. L. (1982). *Caught in the Act: Decision Makers at Work.* Technical Report no. 20. Greensboro, NC: Center for Creative Leadership.

Osborn, A. F. (1953). *Applied Imagination.* New York: Charles Scribner's Sons.

Schweiger, D. M., Anderson, C. R., and Locke, E. A. (1985). "Complex Decision Making: A Longitudinal Study of Process and Performance." *Organizational Behavior and Human Decision Processes,* 36: 245–272.

Simon, H. (1987). "Making Managerial Decisions: The Role of Intuition and Emotion." *Academy of Management Executive,* 1: 57–64.

Steiner, G. (1965). *The Creative Organization.* Chicago: University of Chicago Press.

Wallas, G. (1945). *The Art of Thought.* London: C. A. Watts.

Yukl, G. (1989). *Leadership in Organizations.* 2d ed. Englewood Cliffs, NJ: Prentice-Hall.

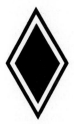

C H A P T E R   12

MANAGING GROUPS

The development of groups is an inevitable part of human activity and, therefore, groups are a fact of life in all organizations. Because staff nurses work in close proximity and frequently depend upon each other to accomplish their jobs, the character or climate of group interaction is extremely important. A viable atmosphere in which staff members feel free to talk about what concerns them, to critique and offer suggestions, and to experiment with new behaviors without threat can only be maintained in a work group that is warm, supportive, and relatively unhindered by interpersonal conflicts and political infighting. Maintaining such an atmosphere or climate is an important task for nurse managers. Besides meeting with their staff, nurse managers are often in other group settings with nursing administrators and other managers, or in committees and task forces. Understanding the nature of groups and group processes, how groups develop, how they influence organizational performance, how they influence member satisfaction, and how leaders can influence their performance are essential to the effectiveness of a nurse manager.

There are two primary types of groups. *Informal groups* evolve naturally as a result of people's interaction within an organization. They are informal in the sense that they are not part of any organizational design. An example is a group of people who regularly eat lunch together. *Formal groups* are work units developed by the organization either temporarily or permanently to accomplish organizational tasks. Formal groups, such as departmental (or command) groups, task groups (or teams), task forces, committees, and informal organizational groups are discussed in this chapter. Informal groups such as family, social, special interest, and therapy groups are not covered.

◆ DEFINITION OF GROUPS

A group is a collection of individuals who share a common set of norms, who generally have differentiated roles among themselves, and who interact with one another to jointly pursue common goals (Steers, 1984). *Command groups* are organized to achieve organizational goals. The supervisor of the group has line authority over the group members. A *task group* is several persons who work together with or without an assigned leader to perform certain tasks. A task group can also be a command group but usually there are several task groups in a department or there are task groups (teams) that include members from several departments, such as a patient care group that includes a nurse, a physician, a dietitian, and a social worker.

There are also special groups such as *committees or task forces* that are formed to deal with specific issues involving several departments. These could include a committee that is responsible for safety or a task force assigned to develop better procedures. There are many committees used in health care institutions on which nurse managers serve, including nursing education committees, nursing policy and procedures committees, disaster committees, and patient care evaluation committees.

Formal groups can be lateral, vertical, or diagonal: members from the same work group, from different levels in the organization, or from different departments in the organization. Task groups can be vertical, horizontal, or diagonal while command groups are vertical groups. Likert (1961) suggests that an important role of a command group leader such as a nurse manager is to serve as a link with groups higher in the organization. This link facilitates problem solving and communication in the organization.

Groups can be permanent or temporary. Command groups, teams, and committees usually are permanent groups while task forces are often temporary. Each different type of group presents opportunities and difficulties for the nurse manager.

Leadership roles in a group are very important and can be either formal or informal. For example, the nurse manager leads the staff group (formal) but may also serve as a leader in an informal grouping of nurse managers. The leader's influence on group processes and the ability of the group to work together often determines whether the group is effective in accomplishing organizational and personal goals, regardless of the formality of the leader's role. In this chapter we discuss how nurse managers can effectively manage groups by presenting a model of group processes and then discussing group decision making, teams and team building, and the management of committees and task forces.

◆ GROUP PROCESSES

A modified version of George Homans's (1950; 1961) social system conceptual scheme is shown in Figure 12–1. This schematic identifies the background factors that influence the leadership style and the required system, which in turn influence the emergent system, the emergent behavior of the group members, and the group's social structure. These in turn influence the productivity of the group as well as the satisfaction, development, and growth of the group members. This framework distinguishes between those things that are "required," which come from the external system, and those things that "emerge" and are part of the internal system of the group.

The three essential elements of Homans's framework are activities, interactions, and attitudes. *Activities* are the observable behaviors of people. *Interactions* occur when there are exchanges of words or objects among two or more persons. Oral communication is an example of interaction. Interaction can also be nonverbal. For example, a highly skilled surgical team can perform complex operations with a minimum of verbal communication. The third important element is *attitudes*. These are the perceptions, feelings, and values held by individuals, and they can be both positive and negative.

PHASES OF GROUP DEVELOPMENT

Background factors and the required system can affect the development process. Groups typically develop following a set pattern of activities: they *form,* or come together; they *storm,* or develop leaders and roles; they *norm,* or define goals and rules for acceptable behavior; they *perform,* or agree on basic purposes and activities and start working; and they *adjourn or reform* (see Tuckman, 1965, and Tuckman & Jensen, 1977). These phases of group development are true for both formal and informal groups.

In the initial stage, forming, group members are cautious in approaching others, become familiar with each other, and begin to develop an understanding of the requirements of group membership. At this stage the members are often quite dependent on the group leader. As the group begins to develop, the second stage, storming, occurs, where conflict arises among the members of the group on issues that are important to the members. During this stage members often vie for power and status. In the third stage, norming, the group begins to define what are or are not acceptable behaviors and attitudes and becomes organized into an effective unit. In

FIGURE 12–1 BASIC SOCIAL SYSTEM CONCEPTUAL SCHEME

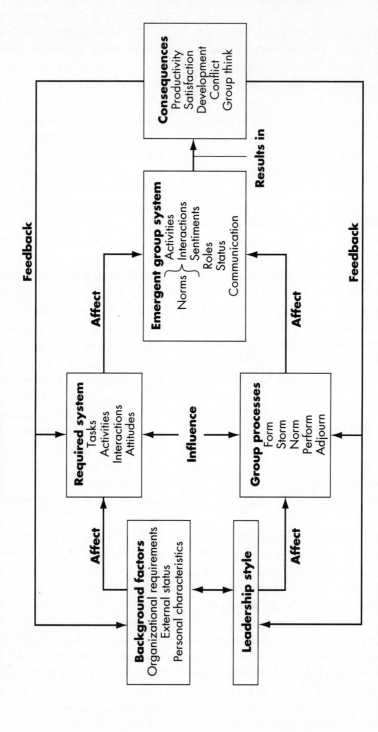

Adapted from G. Homans, *The Human Group* (New York: Harcourt Brace Jovanovich, 1950; and G. Homans): *Social Behavior: Its Elementary Forms* (New York: Harcourt Brace, 1961).

the perform stage the energy of the group members is channeled into the work, good communication occurs among the members, and they have a relaxed atmosphere of sharing. The fifth stage is either adjourning (the group has achieved its purpose) or reforming when some major change takes place in the membership or environment of the group, causing the group to recycle through the previous four stages.

NORMS

Norms are the informal rules of behavior shared and enforced by group members; they emerge whenever humans interact. Nursing groups develop norms that must be adhered to for continued membership in the group. An important norm that groups often establish is how hard a group member should work. Norms for a nursing team member include taking care of no more than nine patients on a medical unit or two in intensive care on a given day, checking for coverage with another team member before leaving the unit, or checking the procedure book before beginning a special task.

According to Feldman (1984), norms are likely to be enforced by a group if they facilitate group survival, if they make predictable what behavior is expected of members, if they help the group avoid embarrassing interpersonal problems, or if they express the central values of the group and clarify what is distinctive about the group's identity. Groups go through several stages in enforcing norms (Leavitt & Bahrami, 1988). First, members use rational argument, presenting reasons for the norms to the deviant nurse. Second, if rational argument doesn't work, members can use seductive techniques, reminding the deviant how important the group is to him or her. The third stage is attack. This can be verbal or physical and can include sabotaging the deviant's work. The final stage is ignoring

the deviant. Leavitt and Bahrami suggest it is increasingly difficult for a deviant to acquiesce with the group as these stages progress: Agreeing to rational argument is easy, but agreeing after attack is very difficult. When the final stage is reached (ignoring), acquiescence may be impossible because nobody listens to the deviant's surrender.

GROUP ROLES

Norms apply to all group members, while roles are specific to positions in the group. A *role* is a set of expected behaviors that fit together into a unified whole and relate to an individual's position within a group. Specific roles in groups include the task leader, the maintenance or social-emotional leader, the friendly helper, and the newcomer. Roles in the group can also be divided into regular group members, deviants, and isolates as to whether they comply with the group's norms. Regular members tend to comply with norms while deviants do not.

Status is the social ranking of individuals relative to others in a group because of the position they occupy in the group. Status comes from factors the group values such as achievement, personal characteristics, the ability to control rewards, or the ability to control information. Status is usually enjoyed by members who most conform to group norms. Higher status members often have more influence than lower status members in group decisions. Status incongruence occurs when the factors contributing to group status are not congruent, such as when a younger, less experienced person is appointed as the group leader. Status incongruence can have disruptive impact on a group. For example, isolates are members who have high external status and different backgrounds from regular group members. They usually produce at acceptable levels but are isolated from the group because they do not fit in. Sometimes this occurs because this person does not need the group's approval (Cohen et al., 1988).

The most important role in a group is the leadership role. Leaders are appointed by the organization for most formal groups such as command groups. Usually someone is appointed by the formal organization to head teams, committees, or task forces. Leaders in informal groups emerge. Some of the factors contributing to emergence of leadership in small groups include the ability to accomplish group goals, group sociability, good communication skills, having confidence in oneself, and having a desire for recognition. Guidelines for performing this leadership role are discussed later in this chapter.

COMMUNICATION IN GROUPS

Groups provide an important channel of communication in organizations, as other group members are often the source of information about what is going on in the organization and usually disseminate this information. Groups that have gone through all the stages of development and have achieved mutual acceptance have members who communicate openly with one another. Effective nurse managers can facilitate communication in groups by maintaining an atmosphere in which staff members feel free to talk about what concerns them, to critique and offer suggestions, and to experiment with new behaviors without threat. An important leadership role that can be beneficial to group communication is the gate-keeping role—attempting to keep communication channels open, facilitating the participation of all group members, and suggesting procedures for discussing group problems.

GROUP CONSEQUENCES

There are many consequences to group behavior. Groups affect the nature and process of communication and engender a degree of competition and political activity much greater than might be expected by examining individual behavior. Groups are greater than the sum of their parts; they can bring out the best and the worst in individuals because group members are aroused by the presence of others. Frequently, this increased arousal is transformed into increased motivation, especially when the individual's contribution to the task is fairly clear or easily measured. On the other hand, groups can lead to greater conformity among group members. They can be tyrannical toward members and ruthless toward nonmembers and thereby contribute to conflict in the organization. Some issues involved in intragroup, intergroup, and intraorganizational conflict are discussed in Chapter 22, while the effect of groups on productivity, satisfaction, and development and growth are discussed here.

GROUP COHESIVENESS AND PRODUCTIVITY

Productivity in a nursing unit includes the extent to which work is completed at the end of each shift and patient care and satisfaction are good. Productivity is influenced by groups, especially cohesive groups. *Cohesiveness* is the degree to which the members are attracted to the group. It includes how much the group members enjoy participating in the group and how much they are willing to contribute to the group. In highly cohesive groups where powerful norms are established on how hard members should work, uniformity exists among group members' productivity. When cohesiveness is low, wide differences can exist in employees' productivity. Groups can restrict productivity, especially when they oppose the organization's leaders.

Cohesiveness is also related to homogeneity of interests, values, attitudes, and background factors. Several propositions on group interaction and cohesiveness are shown in the following list.

1. The greater the opportunity or requirements for interactions, the greater the likelihood of interaction occurring (Homans, 1950; 1961).

2. The more frequent the interaction among people, the greater the likelihood of their developing positive feelings for one another (Homans, 1950; 1961).

3. The greater the positive feelings among people, the more frequently they interact (Homans, 1950; 1961).

4. The more frequent the interactions required by the job, the more likely that social relationships and behavior will develop along with task relationships and behavior (Homans, 1950; 1961).

5. The more attractive the group, the more cohesive it is (Festinger, Schacter & Black, 1950).

6. The more cohesive the group, the more influence it has on its members. The less certain and clear a group's norms and standards are, the less control it has over its members (Festinger, Schacter & Black, 1950; Homans, 1961).

7. The greater the similarity in member attitudes and values brought to the group, the greater the likelihood of cohesion (Homans, 1961).

8. Group cohesion is increased by the existence of a superordinate goal (an overarching goal to which group members subscribe) accepted by the members (Sherif, 1967).

9. Group cohesion is increased by the perceived existence of a common enemy (Blake & Mouton, 1961).

10. Group cohesion is increased by success in achieving the group's goals (Sherif & Sherif, 1953).

11. Group cohesion increases in proportion to the status of the group relative to other groups in the system (Cartwright & Zander, 1968).

12. Group cohesion increases when there is low frequency of required external interactions (Homans, 1950).

13. The more easily and frequently member differences are settled in a way satisfactory to all members, the greater is group cohesion (Deutsch, 1968).

14. Group cohesion increases under conditions of abundant resources (Blake & Mouton, 1961).

15. The more cohesive the group, the more similar is the output of individual members (Homans, 1950).

16. The more cohesive the group, the more it tries to enforce compliance with its norms about productivity (Blake & Mouton, 1961).

17. The greater the cohesion of the group, the higher productivity is if the group supports the organization's goals, and the lower productivity is if the group resists the organization's goals (Zaleznik, Christensen & Roethlisberger, 1958).

18. A cohesive group by definition has a high overall level of satisfaction (Blake & Mouton, 1961).

Cohesive groups are more likely to develop where there are shared values and beliefs, where individuals have similar goals and tasks, where individuals have to interact together to achieve these tasks, where group members work in the same unit and on the same shift, and where group members have specific needs that can be satisfied by the group. Group cohesiveness is also influenced by the formal reward system. Groups whose members are treated equally, have similar pay, and have similar tasks, especially where the tasks require interaction among the members, are cohesive. The characteristics of group members also influence whether a group becomes cohesive. Similarities in educational experiences, social class, sex, age, and ethnicity that lead to similar attitudes strengthen group cohesiveness.

Cohesiveness can lead to social pressure and conformity. Highly cohesive groups can demand and enforce conformity to their norms regardless of their practicality or effectiveness. This makes it more difficult for the nurse manager to influence nurses when the group norms deviate from his or her expectations or goals. In addition, groups can affect absenteeism and turnover. Groups with high levels of cohesiveness exhibit lower turnover and absenteeism than groups with low levels of cohesiveness. Cohesiveness influences member satisfaction and intragroup and intergroup conflict. Cohesiveness can also lead to a phenomenon called "groupthink," which is discussed later in this chapter.

SATISFACTION

Individuals join groups for various reasons.

1. Security—People want protection from threats; groups provide social support.

2. Proximity—People often come together because they are located together.

3. Group goals—People form groups to pursue goals that cannot be accomplished alone.

4. Economics—People often form groups (e.g., collective bargaining organizations) to pursue economic self-interest.

5. Social needs—People often join groups because they want to belong or be needed or because they want to lead.

6. Self-esteem needs—People often join prestigious groups to increase their self-esteem.

DEVELOPMENT AND GROWTH

Groups can also provide learning opportunities by increasing: (a) individual skills or abilities, (b) the range of resources available, or (c) ability to function effectively as a group in changed circumstances (Cohen et al., 1988). The group can help socialize new employees into the organization by showing them "the ropes." The nurse manager must establish an atmosphere that encourages the learning of new skills and knowledge. He or she can help group members to improve these skills and knowledge through training and development. These subjects are covered in depth in Chapter 14.

THE NURSE MANAGER AS LEADER

Influencing group processes toward the attainment of organizational objectives is the direct responsibility of the nurse manager. The nurse manager can do a great deal to facilitate productivity in groups and promote the individual benefits of group membership. For example, through planning work and making assignments, the manager can increase the interdependence of group members. He or she can foster the sharing of common interests and exert considerable control over rewards and punishments for the attainment or nonattainment of work goals. The functions of group membership for individuals operate regardless of whether there is a formal leader, but the nurse manager can do a great deal to foster effective individual and group performance by exercising constructive influence on these functions through leadership behavior. Indeed, this is one of the manager's primary roles in a nursing organization.

The nurse manager also acts as an observer of the direction in which the group is moving. He or she brings the attention of the staff members to the goal, clarifies issues in terms of how they relate to the unit's goals, and periodically evaluates the group's progress toward its goals. This evaluation and the subsequent planning and execution of group goals frequently includes the assistance of staff members. Nurse managers can also use groups for help in making decisions.

♦ GROUP DECISION MAKING

Individual decision making is the traditional, status quo approach: The nurse manager is confronted with a problem and decides how to solve it. Today, both the complexity of problems and the desires of staff for involvement create the need for staff participation in decision making and for group approaches to problem solving. What are the advantages and disadvantages in using groups for decision making? Factors influencing the effectiveness of group decision making include the characteristics of the problem and the characteristics of the people (see Maier, 1967). Since groups possess greater knowledge and information than any of their members individually and are less limited in the approaches used to solve a problem, they can deal with more complex problems than individuals can. Where an individual might continue

using a particular approach, a group is more likely to try several approaches. Rather than suffering from tunnel vision as some individuals do, groups have a greater variety of training and experiences and approach problems from more points of view. Involving numerous personnel may yield more complete, accurate, and less biased information than that obtained from only one person, since it has been clarified through group exposure. Groups more effectively deal with problems crossing group boundaries or presenting procedural change needing the various departments involved in the decision process. Participation in problem solving has additional advantages over individual decision making in that it increases acceptance and understanding of the decision and leads to enhanced cooperation in effective implementation.

GROUP TASK

The group's task can influence its effectiveness. The more people who work on an *additive task* (group performance is the sum of individual performance), the more resources can be used. On a *disjunctive task* (the group succeeds if only one member succeeds), more people provide a greater likelihood that someone in the group will be able to solve the problem. With a *divisible task* (tasks with a division of labor), more people provide a greater opportunity for specialization. However, with a *conjunctive task* (the group succeeds only if all members succeed), more people increase the likelihood that one person can slow up the group. Consequently, group productivity often depends on the group task.

On many divisible tasks, the level of interdependence is important. There are three kinds of interdependence: (a) *pooled,* where each individual contributes but none is dependent on any other member (e.g., a committee discussion);

(b) *sequential,* where members must coordinate their activities with the members on each side or above and below them (e.g., an assembly line); and (c) *reciprocal,* where members must coordinate their activities with every other individual in the group (e.g., health care and nursing) (Thompson, 1967).

Finally, *task uncertainty* plays a role in group effectiveness. Tasks that are highly uncertain require that individuals process more information, identify multiple goal paths, increase effort, and coordinate activities more precisely. Consequently, task uncertainty places more demands on group members.

GROUP SIZE AND COMPOSITION

Groups with five to seven members tend to be the most effective. In larger groups, each member contributes less of his or her potential. Large group size has been found to be associated with low satisfaction, higher absenteeism, and turnover. Groups tend to perform better the higher the abilities of each member. But coordination of effort, proper utilization of abilities, and task strategies must be considered. Furthermore, homogeneous groups tend to function more harmoniously, while heterogeneous groups may experience conflict.

DISADVANTAGES OF GROUP DECISION MAKING

Group decision making also has disadvantages in that it takes time and resources and can lead to conflict among members. Group decision making also can lead to the emergence of benign tyranny within the group. Those members who are less informed or confident may allow stronger members to present all solutions and decisions. This sets the stage for a power struggle between the nurse manager and a few assertive group members. Social loafing and free rid-

ing can also occur in groups (see Harkins, Latane & Williams, 1980). *Social loafing* refers to individuals' tendency to produce below their maximum capabilities in a group. *Free riding* occurs when a loafer receives the full benefits of group membership. Social loafing is more likely to occur as the group becomes larger. Group decision making can also be affected by groupthink.

Groupthink is a negative phenomenon that occurs in cohesive groups. The group members think alike, have similar prejudices and blind spots such as shared stereotypes of outsiders, tend to want to achieve consensus and harmony, and fail to engage in critical thinking. Groupthink occurs when there are shared norms or expectations that (a) the group is invulnerable to outside pressure; (b) the group believes itself to be morally right, which inclines members to ignore the ethical and moral consequences of their decisions; (c) the group rationalizes warnings and other forms of negative feedback; (d) there is direct pressure upon any individual who expresses doubts about the group's shared illusions or who questions the validity of arguments supporting an alternative favored by the majority; (e) there is self-censorship, in which individuals are pressured to conform to the group consensus; and (f) a shared illusion of unanimity exists within the group (Janis, 1982). These norms and expectations interfere with critical thinking and can make group decision making ineffective.

Janis suggests several approaches to prevent groupthink in cohesive groups, which are shown in the following list.

1. The leader of a policy-forming group should assign the role of critical evaluator to each member, encouraging the group to give high priority to airing objections and doubts.

This practice needs to be reinforced by the leader's acceptance of criticism of his or her own judgments to discourage the members from soft-pedaling their disagreements.

2. The leaders in an organization's hierarchy, when assigning a policy-planning mission to a group, should be impartial instead of stating preferences and expectations at the outset.

3. The organization should routinely follow the administrative practice of setting up several independent policy-planning and evaluation groups to work on the same policy question, each carrying out its deliberations under a different leader.

4. The group should from time to time divide into two or more subgroups to meet separately, under different chairpersons, and then come together to hammer out their differences.

5. Each member of the policy-making group should discuss periodically the group's deliberations with trusted associates in his or her own unit of the organization and report back their reactions.

6. One or more outside experts or qualified colleagues within the organization who are not core members of the policy-making group should be invited to each meeting on a staggered basis and should be encouraged to challenge the views of the core members.

7. At every meeting devoted to evaluating policy alternatives, at least one member should be assigned the role of devil's advocate.

8. Whenever the policy issue involves relations with a rival, time should be spent surveying all warning signals from the rivals and con-structing alternative scenarios of the rivals' intentions.

9. After reaching a preliminary consensus about what seems to be the best policy alternative, the policy-making group should hold a "second chance" meeting at which every member is expected to express as vividly as possible all residual doubts and to rethink the entire issue before making a definitive choice (Janis, 1982: 262–271).

Yet, it is important for managers to understand that conflict is not always dysfunctional and dissent must be allowed if good decisions are to be made.

A technique resulting in less groupthink is the use of *dialectical inquiry*. Dialectical inquiry uses a formal debate between advocates of a plan and others who propose a counterplan. This technique formalizes conflict by allowing disagreement, encourages the exploration of alternative solutions, and reduces the emotional aspects of conflict (Cosier & Schwenk, 1990). This approach can be used regardless of a manager's feelings. The benefits from this method come from the presentation and debate of the basic assumptions underlying proposed courses of action. Any false or misleading assumptions become apparent, and the process promotes better understanding of problems and leads to higher levels of confidence in decisions. But the method does have some potential drawbacks. It can lead to an emphasis on who won the debate rather than what the best decision is, or it can lead to inappropriate compromise (Cosier & Schwenk, 1990).

RISKY SHIFT

Groups tend to make more risky decisions than individuals, i.e., work groups are more likely to go on record as supporting unusual or unpopular positions than are individuals. They tend to be less conservative than individual decision makers and frequently display more courage and support for unusual or creative solutions to problems. This phenomenon is referred to as *risky shift* (see Napier & Gershenfeld, 1985).

Several factors play a role in this phenomenon. Individuals who lack information about alternatives may choose to select a less risky decision, but after group discussion of the various alternatives they may feel more comfortable about a less secure alternative and agree to that decision. This could be due to persuasive argumentation from others and social comparison (Levine & Moreland, 1990). The group setting also allows for the diffusion of responsibility. If something does go wrong with the decision, others can also be assessed the blame or risk. In addition, leaders may be greater risk takers than individuals and a social value may be attached to risk taking. Risky shift may be less of a problem in health care institutions because society values risk taking less where health is of a concern, but nurse managers should be aware of this phenomenon.

WHEN TO USE GROUPS FOR DECISION MAKING

Vroom and Jago have developed a model for deciding whether to use a group for decision making (Vroom & Jago, 1974; Vroom & Jago, 1988). This model is discussed in Chapter 9. In practice, the degree of participation is determined by several factors: (a) who initiates ideas; (b) the extent that subordinate support is required for implementation of a solution; (c) how completely an employee carries out each phase of decision making—diagnosing, finding alternatives, estimating consequences, and making choices; (d) how much weight the nurse man-

ager attaches to the ideas received; and (e) the amount of knowledge the nurse manager has about the matter. Likert (1961) has found that when individuals are allowed to participate they function more productively, and implementing solutions becomes easier because of the shared problem solving.

Generally groups should be used for decision making when time is available for a group decision but there is a deadline, the problem is complex or unstructured, the group members share the organization's goals, there is need for acceptance of the decision or at least understanding of the decision to implement it properly, and the process will not lead to unacceptable conflict among group members.

TYPES OF DECISION-MAKING GROUPS

The different types of decision-making groups include ordinary interacting groups, nominal group technique, brainstorming groups, statistical aggregation, the Delphi technique, and quality circles (see Levine & Moreland, 1990; Murninghan, 1981; and Ouchi, 1981). Each type of group has advantages and disadvantages in decision making.

Ordinary interacting groups usually have a designated formal leader, but they can be leaderless. Most task groups and committees are this type. They usually begin with a statement of the problem by the group leader followed by an open, unstructured discussion of the problem. Normally the final decision is made by consensus, but the decision can also be by vote of the majority, by vote of a significant minority, by an expert, by the leader, or by some authority figure after the group makes a recommendation. Interacting groups enhance the cohesiveness and esprit de corps among group members. Participants are able to build strong social ties and there will be commitment to the solution decided upon by the group.

Ordinary groups are often dominated by one or a few members. If the group is highly cohesive, its decision-making ability can be affected by groupthink. Excessive time may be spent dealing with social-emotional relationships, reducing the time spent on the problem and making it difficult to come to a consensus. Ordinary groups may reach compromise decisions that may not really satisfy any of the participants. Because of these problems, ordinary groups are very dependent on the skills of the group leader.

Two techniques have been developed to allow input from various individuals while avoiding some of the disadvantages of ordinary groups: the nominal group technique (NGT) and the Delphi technique. The *nominal group technique,* developed by Van de Ven and Delbecq (1974) is a structured group decision-making process and is a group in name only because no social exchange is allowed between members. NGT consists of (a) silently generating ideas in writing, (b) round-robin feedback from group members to record each idea in a terse phrase on a flip chart, (c) discussing each recorded idea for clarification and evaluation, and (d) voting individually on priority ideas, with the group decision being mathematically derived through rank ordering or rating using the group's decision rule.

The second method, which isn't very common in nursing administration, is the *Delphi technique.* Judgments on a particular topic are systematically gathered from participants who are physically separated and do not meet face to face. These are collected through a set of carefully designed sequential questionnaires interspersed with a summary of information and opinions derived from previous questionnaires. The process can include many iterations but normally does not exceed three. This technique can rely on the input of experts widely dispersed geographically. It can be used to evaluate the quality of research proposals or to make predictions about the future based on current scientific knowledge. This technique is useful when expert opinions are needed and the experts are geographically separated, but it is costly and time-consuming.

On fact-finding problems with no known solution, the NGT and the Delphi technique are superior to the ordinary group technique, and satisfaction of group members is highest in NGT (Van de Ven & Delbecq, 1974). Both NGT and the Delphi technique minimize the chances of more vocal and persuasive members influencing the less forceful persons and allow the opportunity to think through ideas independently.

Two other group techniques are statistical aggregation and brainstorming. Like the Delphi technique *statistical aggregation* does not require a group meeting. Individuals are polled regarding a specific problem and their responses are tallied. It is a very efficient technique but it is limited to a narrow range of problems: those for which a quantifiable answer can be readily obtained. One disadvantage of both statistical aggregation and the Delphi technique is that no opportunity exists for group members to strengthen their interpersonal ties.

In *brainstorming,* group members meet together and are encouraged to generate as many diverse ideas as possible without consideration of their practicality or feasibility. A premium is placed on generating lots of ideas as quickly as possible and on coming up with unusual ideas. In addition, and most important, members are asked not to critique the ideas as they are proposed. Evaluation takes place after all the ideas have been generated. Members are encouraged to "piggyback" on each other's ideas. These sessions are very enjoyable, but are often less successful because the members violate the three rules and, as a result, the meetings shift to the ordinary interacting group format. NGT can be used to overcome some of the problems of the brainstorming technique but it is not as exciting to the participants.

Quality circles are another type of group used in participatory decision making. Quality circles, adapted from Ouchi's Theory Z (Ouchi, 1981), have been successful in this country as well as in Japan. This style, which can easily be adapted to nursing, is based on trust and workers' involvement in decisions that affect them. The system emphasizes consensus-based decision making and a strong commitment to the goals of the organization. The desired results are increased job commitment, higher productivity, and lower turnover.

Quality circles have been used in health care situations, but their use requires total organizational decision and commitment. Nurse managers would not ordinarily use this technique unless their institution was using it. However, it may be useful to understand the process.

As an example, nurses on each floor are divided into circles of eight or ten individuals, with a facilitator appointed for each circle. The facilitators form another circle, which interfaces with circles at higher and lower levels, so reciprocal representation exists at all levels. Circles are thoroughly disciplined operations committed to training, group skills, and rigorous step-by-step improvement procedures. There is continuous discussion within the circles whenever a policy or procedural change is made, until a true consensus has been achieved.

Many management decisions are made in circles, and no decision is final until every member has had a part in the decision and agrees with the outcome. This can be a time-consuming process, but once consensus is reached, implementation is instantaneous and the net effect is increased productivity. In other forms of participatory decision making, a majority wins, leaving a dissatisfied, obstinate minority who may sabotage implementation. In consensus-based decision making, everyone feels a part of the process, has a voice in the decision, and is therefore a winner. While research on quality circles in health care is limited, one study has shown improved morale, decreased alienation, and greater incentives for unified productivity when quality circles were introduced (Moore et al., 1982).

Likert's System 4 theory also closely approximates management by consensus. The research he and his colleagues have done supports the conclusion that the more that employees are allowed to participate, the greater the likelihood of superior performance (Likert, 1961). However, the most important limitation to its use is the extent to which it is germane to the Japanese culture, which is quite different from Western culture (Smith, Reinow & Reid, 1984). The work ethic in Japan puts high value on teamwork, while in the United States, independent accomplishment is more highly valued. Thus, group decision making is very workable in Japanese settings and less so in U.S. ones. Another important element is that quality circles may be more useful when members represent various interacting units or disciplines, especially in health care. This model, because of the greater participation it provides and the long-term rewards built into the system, certainly needs to be evaluated in terms of nursing management. It shows potential for use in an area where innovative management is badly needed.

The nurse manager needs to assess the health team members on the unit to determine if a participatory process would enhance decision making. If staff show similar qualifications and work well together, perhaps quality circles could be instituted with success. If the group is extremely diversified and individualistic, however, NGT might be beneficial, or, if creativity is required, brainstorming might be beneficial. If the requisite leadership skills are available, then the ordinary group technique could be used. It is essential to match the decision-making method with the capabilities of the staff.

◆ TEAMS AND TEAM BUILDING

Teams are groups established to perform organizational tasks requiring the diverse skills and the interaction and cooperation of the team members to achieve these tasks. Teams have command or line authority to perform tasks and membership is based on the specific skills the individual can offer to accomplish the team's task. Teams can be lateral, vertical, or diagonal in member composition. They can have a short life or can exist over long periods of time. Not all work groups are teams. For example, co-acting groups, where members perform their tasks independently of each other, are not teams, nor are competing groups, where members compete with each other for resources to perform their tasks or where members compete for recognition. Specific difficulties teams experience include goal confusion, hidden agendas, territoriality, disagreement over procedures, competition among team members, intragroup conflict, intergroup conflict, and a nonsupportive climate.

Team building is a popular organizational development (OD) technique that can be used to overcome some of these difficulties. OD team-building activities include using outside intervention to build team cohesiveness. For example, McGraw-Hill (CRM/McGraw-Hill) has a Task-Oriented Team Development Program designed to be self-administered by the team leader and members themselves. They have also developed an excellent film, *Team Building* (CRM/McGraw-Hill, 1983), which can be used by a facilitator to help improve team performance. The various volumes of *A Handbook of Structured Experiences for Human Relations Training* (J. W. Pfeiffer and J. E. Jones, Iowa City, IA: University Associates) also provide many useful team-building exercises. Intervention strategies are covered in depth in *Team Building: Blueprints for Productivity and Satisfaction* (W. B. Reddy and K. Jamison, eds., Alexandria, VA: NTL Institute for Applied Behavioral Science, 1988). Wilson (1985) provides specific exercises to resolve conflicts in groups, release tensions, promote trust and self-disclosure, and promote cohesion among group members. These are shown in Table 12–1.

To develop effective teams, four conditions are necessary: The group must have mutually agreed objectives; the group members must depend on each other's experiences, abilities, and commitment; group members must be committed to team effort; and the group must be accountable as a unit within the organization (Patten, 1979). Team-building techniques can be used to create these conditions. Team-building activities can also be used to overcome one of the most important difficulties in managing teams (and task forces) in organizations, which

TABLE 12-1 A SAMPLING OF EXPERIENTIAL EXERCISES

Type of exercise	Expected outcome
Warm-ups	
Batting balloons	Become acquainted; move into Child Ego State
Saying "Hello" nonverbally	Prepare for self-disclosure
Saying "Hello" with crayons and paper	Become acquainted
Verbal introductions in dyads	Become acquainted
Sharing nicknames	Become acquainted
Verbal introductions in dyads with roleplay	Become acquainted
Kinetic techniques	
Freeze tag	Awareness of the process of asking for help
Family sculpture	Awareness of one's position in the family system
Breaking into the circle	Awareness of being isolated
Movement techniques	
Fantasies	Awareness of one's immediate feelings
Exploring space	"Letting go" to explore unknown space
Dyad sculpturing	Experiencing the feeling of controlling others or being controlled
Passing on a movement	Experiencing directing or controlling others
Lifting and rocking a member	Experiencing giving up control to others
Improvisation	Awareness of one's immediate feelings
Protective techniques	
Bataca swords	Safe expression of anger
Body bag/punching bag; pillows	Safe expression of anger
Lifting and rocking a member	Reduce tension
Parachute toss	Reduce tension
Behavioral rehearsal	
Roleplaying	Increase repertoire of possible responses to situations
Sociodrama	Expand repertoire of role performance
Psychodrama	Explore individual intrapsychic phenomena within one's role
Group building	
Verbal exchanges in dyads	Increase group cohesion
New games	Increase group cohesion
"Spider web" and yarn	Increase group cohesion
Group mural, collage, poem	Increase group cohesion
Blind walk	Promote trust and self-disclosure
Passing a member around	Promote trust

M. Wilson, *Group Theory/Process for Nursing Practice* (Bowie, MD: Brady Communications Company [Prentice-Hall]), p. 175

is that teams must go through the normal stages of group development (form, storm, norm, perform, and adjourn or reform) quickly and are expected to perform at a high level immediately. Team-building techniques also can be used to intervene in traditional work groups that are experiencing problems or in any other type of group such as quality circles, task forces, and committees.

The first and most important activity in team building is diagnosis. Questions must be asked about the group's climate, including its mission and goals; the group's organization, including group members' roles, group procedures, and decision-making style; the group's interpersonal relationships in the group, including members' feelings about each other; and the group's relations with other groups.

Questions to be asked include:

1. Do the members understand and accept the goals of the group? Is there any goal confusion? Goal confusion occurs when the team is unsure of its goals or there is disagreement over these goals.

2. Do the members have any hidden agendas that interfere with the group's goal attainment? Hidden agendas are members' individual goals that are not shared with the group as a whole and keep the members from being committed and enthusiastic team members.

3. Is the leadership role being handled adequately?

4. Does each member understand and accept his or her role in the group?

5. How does the group make decisions?

6. How does the group handle conflict? Are conflicts dealt with through avoidance, forcing, accommodating, compromising, competing, or collaborating methods?

7. What feelings do members have about each other?

8. Do members trust and respect each other?

9. What is the relationship between the team and other units in the organization?

Only after diagnosing the problems of the team can the team leader take actions to improve team functioning. Survival exercises discussed in the sources listed above are useful for bringing the group together in an unusual setting to learn about itself, its processes, and its decision-making procedures. Survey feedback forms (anonymous surveys asking questions similar to those discussed above) can also be used to improve teams. The results of the survey are discussed by the group and action steps are defined to overcome these problems. After a period of time another survey is taken to see if change has occurred and whether the process needs to be repeated. An outside intervention specialist can be brought in to conduct team-building sessions including holding a confrontation meeting to address team problems.

Argyris (1965) summarizes the characteristics of an effective team:

1. Contributions made within the group are additive.

2. The group moves forward as a unit; there is a sense of team spirit, high involvement.

3. Decisions are made by consensus.

4. Commitment to decisions by most members is strong.

5. The group continually evaluates itself.

6. The group is clear about its goals.

7. Conflict is brought out into the open and handled.

8. Alternative ways of thinking about solutions are generated.

9. Leadership tends to go to the individual best qualified.

10. Feelings are dealt with openly.

♦ MANAGING COMMITTEES AND TASK FORCES

Formal committees are part of the organization and have authority as well as a specific role, while *informal committees* are primarily for discussion and have no delegated authority. *Task forces* are ad hoc committees appointed for a specific purpose and a limited time. They work on problems or projects that cannot be easily handled by the organization through its normal activities and structures. Task forces tend to make recommendations and then are disbanded. Task forces often must deal with problems crossing departmental boundaries. Committees are more permanent in nature and deal with recurring problems. Membership on committees is usually based on organizational position and role. This section presents general guidelines for conducting meetings. In addition, special guidelines for managing task forces and conducting conferences are provided.

GENERAL GUIDELINES FOR CONDUCTING MEETINGS

To conduct a successful meeting, the leader should spend time thinking about the purpose of the meeting; preparing an agenda; determining who should attend; making assignments prior to

group meetings, including determining who should take minutes; and selecting an appropriate time and place for the meeting. An agenda should be established for meetings ahead of time and sent to the participants. The ideal committee size is five to seven persons. Having too few or too many members can limit the effectiveness of a committee or task force. It is helpful to limit membership to persons with similar status, as large status differences among committee members can impede communication.

Meetings should be held in spaces where interruptions can be controlled and at a time when there is some natural time limit to the meeting, such as late in the morning or afternoon when lunch or dinner make natural time barriers. In addition, meetings should start and finish on time. Starting late positively reinforces latecomers while punishing those who arrive on time or early. Locking the door at the appointed time or "fining" latecomers can discourage such behavior. If it is the leader who is late, informing him or her as to the cost of starting meetings late can be effective.

The behavior of each member may be positive, negative, or neutral in relationship to the group's goals. Members may contribute very little or they may use the group to fill personal needs. Some members may assume most of the responsibility for the group action, thereby "helping" the less participative members to be noncontributers. Appropriate behaviors, listed in Table 12–2, can facilitate the group's action.

LEADERSHIP OF MEETINGS

A leader can play an effective role in conducting meetings by ensuring that the 12 leadership roles shown in Table 12–3 are present. Even though a leader's personality and value systems might make it difficult for him or her to perform all of these roles, the leader is still responsible to make sure that these various task and group relations functions do occur, even if they are performed by other members.

A leader can also increase effectiveness by not letting one person dominate discussion; separating idea generation from evaluation; encouraging members to refine and develop the ideas of others (a key to the success of brainstorming); recording problems, ideas, and solutions on a blackboard or flip chart; frequently summarizing information and the group's progress to date and encouraging further discussion; and bringing disagreements out into the open where they may be reconciled. The leader is also responsible for drawing out the members' hidden agendas

(personal needs individuals bring to a group that are not disclosed to the group but influence the members' contributions) so these do not interfere with group decision making.

Summary guidelines for leading group discussions are:

Set a warm, accepting, and nonthreatening climate conducive to participation and cohesiveness.

Define all terms and concepts.

Foster cooperation in the group.

Establish group goals and identify major objectives.

Keep the group focused on the task.

Focus the discussions on one topic at a time.

Allocate time for all decision-making steps.

Encourage participation so that all members have an opportunity to contribute.

Help integrate the material and ideas that have been generated.

Help group members identify the implications of the ideas.

Help the group evaluate the quality of the discussion.

Allow persons with dissenting opinions to explain their point of view.

Summarize discussion and ask the group to arrive at a decision.

Determine the plan of action for implementing the decision.

Request arrangements for follow-up from individual members.

TABLE 12–2 KEY BEHAVIORS FOR GROUP MEETINGS

♦ Come prepared with necessary information.

♦ Listen to others with an open mind.

♦ Contribute information, ideas, and opinions.

♦ Ask other members for ideas and opinions.

♦ Request clarification of information.

♦ Recognize opposing points of view.

♦ Keep remarks on the topic.

♦ Be willing to state disagreement and give rationale.

♦ Volunteer to help with the implementation of decisions, when appropriate.

David P. Gustafson. Used by permission.

TABLE 12–3 THE FUNCTIONS OF A GROUP LEADER

Task functions

Initiating:	Proposing tasks or goals; defining a group problem; suggesting a procedure or ideas for solving a problem.
Information or opinion seeking:	Requesting facts; seeking relevant information about group concern; asking for suggestions or ideas.
Information or opinion giving:	Stating a belief; providing relevant information about group concern; giving suggestions or ideas.
Clarifying:	Elaborating, interpreting, or reflecting ideas and suggestions; clearing up confusions; indicating alternatives and issues before the group; giving examples.
Summarizing:	Pulling together related ideas; restating suggestions after group has discussed them; offering a decision or conclusion for the group to accept or reject.
Consensus testing:	Sending up "trial balloons" to see if group is nearing a conclusion; checking with group to see how much agreement has been reached.

Group relations functions

Encouraging:	Being friendly, warm, and responsive to others; accepting others and their contributions; regarding others by giving them an opportunity for recognition.
Expressing group feelings:	Sensing feelings, moods, relationships within the group; sharing one's own feelings with other members.
Harmonizing:	Attempting to reconcile disagreements; reducing tension; getting people to explore their differences.
Modifying:	When the leader's own idea or status is involved in a conflict, offering to modify this position; admitting error; disciplining themselves to maintain group cohesion.
Gate-keeping:	Attempting to keep communication channels open; facilitating the participation of others; suggesting procedures for sharing opportunity to discuss group problems.
Evaluating:	Evaluating group functioning and production; expressing standards for group to achieve; measuring results; evaluating degree of group commitment.

K. Benne and P. Sheats, "Functional Roles of Group Members," *Journal of Social Issues*, 4, no. 2 (1948): 42-45

GROUP MEETINGS

Thompson and Wood (1980) provide a useful framework that describes a meeting as a play that requires a script, preparation of the actors, and a competent director to ensure a successful performance. They summarize the contributions of the various components as follows:

1. *The director,* known as the chairperson, is responsible for planning the meeting, preparing the agenda, directing the meeting, and the follow-up of plans made.

2. *The script,* known as the agenda, is important in determining the effectiveness of the group's activities. Thompson and Wood (1980) suggest the following guidelines for agenda preparation: (a) if you can put it in a memo, don't put it on the agenda, (b) have a clear purpose behind every meeting you hold and behind every agenda item on the agenda, and (c) every item should require some kind of action by the group.

3. *The actors,* otherwise known as the group members, are not in the audience to be entertained; they are the participants. Their responsibility is to come prepared, respond to others' ideas and comments, and make contributions in a clear, concise, and logical manner.

4. *The stage,* or meeting room. Where the meeting is held and where people sit affect what happens in the meeting and the outcomes. If conflict between participants is expected or if one participant is a great deal more powerful than the other(s), then the site chosen for the meeting should be in neutral territory.

The head of the table is the most powerful position and should usually be occupied by the chairperson. Those who sit on the sidelines may see themselves as of lesser importance to the group's activities or may be antagonists. The seat at the foot of the table may also be selected by an antagonist.

MANAGING TASK FORCES

There are a few critical differences between task forces and formal committees. For example, the members of a task force have less time to build relationships with each other, and, since task forces are temporary in nature, the need for long-term positive relationships might be lacking. Formation of a task force can represent a criticism of the regular organization, leading to tensions among task force members and between the task force and other units in the organization. The various members of a task force usually come from different parts of the organization and, therefore, have different values, goals, and viewpoints. Specific actions a leader can take to deal with these differences and increase the effectiveness of task forces are grouped by Ware (1983) into four categories:

1. Preparation prior to the first meeting

2. Conducting the first meeting

3. Managing subsequent meetings and subgroups

4. Completion of the task force's report

PREPARATION PRIOR TO THE FIRST MEETING. Prior to the task force's first meeting the leader must determine the objectives of the task force, its membership, the task completion date, how often and to whom the task force should report while working on the project, and the group's authority including the task force's budget, availability of information, and ability to make decisions. The task force leader should be in contact with the administrators who commissioned it so its mission can be clarified.

Task force members should be selected on the basis of their knowledge, skills, and personal interest in the task, their time available to work on the task, and their organizational credibility. They should also be selected on the basis of their interpersonal skills. Those who enjoy group activities and won't dominate the group's efforts are especially good members.

CONDUCTING THE FIRST MEETING. According to Ware the goal of the first meeting is to come to a common understanding of the group's task and to define the group's working procedures and relationships. Task forces must rely on the general norms of the organization to function. The task force leader should legitimize the representative nature of participation on a task force and encourage members to discuss the task force's process with other members of the organization.

During the first meeting everyone should be encouraged to participate. The leader should be careful to be neutral and should prevent a premature consensus. Working procedures and relationships among the various members, subgroups, and the rest of the organization need to be established. The frequency and nature of full task force meetings and the number of subgroups must be determined. Ground rules for communicating must be established along with norms for decision making and conflict resolution.

MANAGING SUBSEQUENT MEETINGS AND SUBGROUPS. In running a task force, especially when several subgroups are formed, the leader should hold full task force meetings often enough to keep all members informed of the group's progress. Unless a task force is small,

subgroups are mandatory. The leader must not be aligned too closely with one position or subgroup too early in the deliberations. Interim project deadlines should be established, and the task force and subgroups should be held to these deadlines. The leader must be sensitive to the conflicting loyalties created by belonging to a task force. One of the leader's most important roles is to communicate information to both task force members and the rest of the organization.

COMPLETION OF THE TASK FORCE'S REPORT. In bringing a project to completion, Ware suggests that a written report summarizing the findings and recommendations to the commissioning administrators be prepared, with drafts of this report shared with the full task force prior to presentation to the administrators. A two-meeting approach should be used to present the task force's report. The first meeting is to present the report without making any decisions on it. This gives administrators a chance to read and respond to the report before they have to make a decision on it. It is especially important for the task force leader to personally brief the key administrators prior to presentation of the report to reduce defensive reactions.

NURSING CONFERENCES

The nurse manager also participates in conferences. These are usually one-time affairs, held for a limited time to deal with a specific patient's problem. Table 12–4 shows various types and purposes of conferences; the purpose usually determines the members and the leader. For example, a nurse manager might call a report conference to request an update from staff members regarding the effectiveness of a new staffing procedure.

SUMMARY

◆ Groups influence organizational success, so it is important for nurse managers to understand the nature of groups and group processes and what they can do to influence group effectiveness.

◆ A group is a collection of individuals who share a common set of norms, who generally have differentiated roles among themselves, and who interact with one another to jointly pursue common goals (Steers, 1984).

◆ The types of groups important to nurse managers include formal groups such as command groups, task groups, teams, task forces, and committees, as well as informal organizational groups.

◆ A group's emergent system, including its norms and roles, is influenced by the members' personal systems and external status, the organizational culture, the technology and layout, the reward system, the style of the formal leader, and the required activities, interactions, and sentiments. The emergent system directly influences the productivity and satisfaction of group members and their ability to develop and grow.

◆ Groups develop through the five stages: form, storm, norm, perform, and adjourn or reform.

◆ Cohesive groups establish strong norms that influence the behavior of group members, especially their productivity.

◆ Groups help satisfy member needs of affiliation, security, esteem, reality testing, and task accomplishment.

◆ Groups can be effective in making decisions

TABLE 12–4 TYPES OF NURSING CONFERENCES AND THEIR PURPOSES

Type	Purpose
Direction-giving conference	Give job assignments Specify areas of responsibility Give client care information
Client-centered conference	Analyze one client's problem Discuss alternative solutions Plan for implementing solutions
Content conference	Learn new information related to nursing care
Report conference	Inform leader about member activities
General Problems conference	Discuss communication problems among group members

Adapted from L. M. Douglass and E. O. Bevis Nursing Management and Leadership in Action (St. Louis, MO.: C. V. Mosby, 1983). Used by permission.

especially if they are small, if time is available to use a group technique, and if there is need for member acceptance or understanding of the decision.

♦ There are several different types of decision making groups: ordinary interacting groups, nominal group technique, brainstorming groups, statistical aggregation, the Delphi technique, and quality circles. The nominal group technique tends to be superior to the others because it is effective and cheap and member satisfaction is high.

♦ Group decisions can be affected by groupthink, the tendency for cohesive groups to fail to engage in critical thinking, and risky shift, the tendency for groups to accept more risk than the average member would.

♦ Team-building activities and the OD model can be effectively used to develop teams.

♦ Committees and task forces can be effectively managed by a nurse manager who understands group processes and, in the case of task forces, understands some of the critical stages of task force development.

A group will be effective when:

1. The members are attracted to it.

2. Members trust each other.

3. Norms and goals of the group are congruent with organizational goals.

4. Group size, structure, and heterogeneity match the task to be accomplished.

5. Group members are motivated to communicate openly and cooperate.

6. The group is rewarded for goal attainment.

7. Social loafing is reduced.

BIBLIOGRAPHY

Argyris, C. (1965). *Organization and Innovation.* Homewood, IL: Irwin.

Bartunek, J. M., and Murningham, J. K. (1984). "The Nominal Group Technique: Expanding the Basic Procedure and Underlying Assumptions." *Group and Organization Studies,* 9: 417–432.

Benne, K., and Sheats, P. (1948). "Functional Roles of Group Members." *Journal of Social Issues,* 4(2): 41–49.

Blake, R. R., and Mouton, J. S. (1961). "Reactions to Intergroup Competition under Win-Lose Conditions." *Management Science,* 7(4): 420–425.

Cartwright, D., and Zander, A. (1968). *Group Dynamics: Research and Theory.* New York: Harper & Row.

Cohen, A. R., Fink, S. L., Gadon, H., and Willits, R. D. (1988). *Effective Behavior in Organizations.* Homewood, IL: Irwin.

Cosier, R. A., and Schwenk, C. R. (1990). "Agreement and Thinking Alike: Ingredients for Poor Decisions." *Academic Management Extract,* 4(1): 69–74.

Deutsch, M. (1968). "The Effects of Cooperation and Competition upon Group Process." In: *Group Dynamics: Research and Theory.* Cartwright, D., and Zander, A. (editors). New York: Harper & Row. Pp. 414–448.

Douglass, L. (1980). *The Effective Nurse: Leader and Manager.* St. Louis, MO: C. V. Mosby.

Feldman, D. C. (1984). "The Development and Enforcement of Group Norms." *Academic Management Review,* 9: 47–53.

Festinger, L., Schacter, S., and Black, K. (1950). *Social Pressures in Informal Groups: A Study of a Housing Project.* New York: Harper & Row.

Gilles, D. A. (1989). *Nursing Management: A Systems Approach.* 2d ed. Philadelphia: Saunders. Pp. 188–201.

Gustafson, D. P. (1992). "Dealing with Groups." In: *Nursing Administration.* Decker, P., and Sullivan, E. (editors). Norwalk, CT: Appleton-Lange Publishing.

Harkins, S., Latane, B., and Williams, L. (1980). "Social Loafing: Allocating Effort or 'Taking It Easy.' " *Journal of Experimental Social Psychology,* 16: 457–465.

Homans, G. (1950). *The Human Group.* New York: Harcourt Brace Jovanovich.

Homans, G. (1961). *Social Behavior: Its Elementary Forms.* New York: Harcourt Brace.

Janis, I. L. (1982). *Groupthink: Psychological Studies of*

Some of the material in this chapter was part of Chapters 8, 9, 10, 12, 22, and 25 in the second edition. Acknowledgment of the contributions to this chapter is given to Eleanor J. Sullivan, Dennis L. Dossett, Ruth Launius Jenkins, Phillip J. Decker, Marlene K. Strader, David P. Gustafson, David O. Evans, and Rusti C. Moore. In addition, material from Gustafson (1992) has been used in this chapter.

Policy Decisions and Fiascos. 2d ed. Boston: Houghton Mifflin.

Johnson, D. W., and Johnson, F. P. (1975). *Joining Together.* Englewood Cliffs, NJ: Prentice-Hall.

Leavitt, H. J., and Bahrami, H. (1988). *Managerial Psychology.* 5th ed. Chicago: University of Chicago Press.

Levine, J. M., and Moreland, R. L. (1990). "Progress in Small Group Research." *Annual Review of Psychology,* 41: 585–634.

Likert, R. (1961). *New Patterns of Management.* New York: McGraw-Hill.

Maier, N. R. F. (1967). "Assets and Liabilities in Group Problem Solving: The Need for an Integrative Function." *Psychological Review,* 74(4): 239–249.

Moore, R., et al. (1982). "On the Scene: Quality Circles at Barnes Hospital." *Nursing Administration Quarterly,* 6: 3.

Murninghan, K. (1981). "Group Decision: What Strategies to Use?" *Management Review,* 70: 55–61.

Napier, R. W., and Gershenfeld, M. K. (1985). *Groups: Theory and Experience.* Boston: Houghton Mifflin. Pp. 247–255.

Organ, D. W., and Batemen, T. (1986). *Organizational Behavior.* 3d ed. Plano, TX: Business Publications.

Ouchi, W. (1981). *Theory Z: How American Business Can Meet the Japanese Challenge.* Reading, MA: Addison-Wesley.

Patten, T. H. (1979). "Team Building Part 1: Designing the Intervention." *Personnel,* 56(1): 11–21.

Robey, R. (1986). *Designing Organizations.* 2d ed. Homewood, IL: Irwin. Chapter 8.

Schien, E. H. (1970). *Organizational Psychology.* 2d ed. Englewood Cliffs, NJ: Prentice-Hall.

Sherif, M. (1967). *Group Conflict and Cooperation: Their Social Psychology.* Boston: Routledge & Kegan Paul.

Sherif, M., and Sherif, C. W. (1953). *Groups in Harmony and Tension.* New York: Harper & Row.

Sherif, M., and Sherif, C. W. (1969). *Social Psychology.* New York: Harper & Row.

Sherif, M., Harvey, O. J., White, B. J., Hood, W. R., and Sherif, C. W. (1961). *Intergroup Conflict and Cooperation: The Robbers' Cave Experiment.* Norman, OK: University Book Exchange.

Smith, H. L., Reinow, F. D., and Reid, R. A. (1984). "Japanese Management: Implications for Nursing Administration." *Journal of Nursing Administration* 14(9): 33–39.

Steers, R. M. (1984). *Introduction to Organizational Behavior.* 2d ed. Glenview, IL: Scott, Foresman.

Thompson, A. M., and Wood, M. D. (1980). *Management Strategies for Women.* New York: Simon and Schuster.

Thompson, J. D. (1967). *Organizations in Action.* New York: McGraw-Hill.

Tuckman, B. W. (1965). "Developmental Sequences in Small Groups." *Psychological Bulletin,* 72: 384–399.

Tuckman, B. W., and Jensen, M. A. (1977). "Stages of Small Group Development Revisited." *Group and Organizational Studies,* 2: 419–427.

Van de Ven, A. H., and Delbecq, A. L. (1974). "The Effectiveness of Nominal, Delphi, and Interacting Group Decision Making Processes." *Academic Management Journal,* 17(4): 605–621.

Vroom, V. H., and Jago, A. G. (1974). "Decision Making as a Social Process: Normative and Descriptive Models of Leader Behavior." *Decision Sciences,* 5: 743–769.

Vroom, V. H., and Jago, A. G. (1988). *The New Leadership.* Englewood Cliffs, NJ: Prentice-Hall.

Ware, J. (1983). "Managing a Task Force." In: *Managing Behavior in Organizations.* Schlesinger, L. A., Eccles, R. G., and Gabarro, J. J. (editors). New York: McGraw-Hill. Pp. 116–126.

Wilson, M. (1985). *Group Theory/Process for Nursing Practice.* Bowie, MD: Brady Communications Company (Prentice-Hall).

Zaleznik, A., Christensen, C. R., and Roethlisberger, F. J. (1958). *The Motivation, Productivity and Satisfaction of Workers.* Boston: Harvard University Business School.

P A R T 3

HUMAN RESOURCE MANAGEMENT SKILLS

C H A P T E R 13

RECRUITING AND SELECTING STAFF

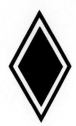

In service or labor-intensive organizations such as health care organizations, the quality of personnel hired and retained determines whether an organization successfully accomplishes its objectives. The cost of improper selection can be high. The visible cost is represented in recruiting, selecting, and training an employee who must later be terminated because of unsatisfactory performance. The hidden costs may be even more expensive and include low quality of work performed by the unmotivated employee, disruption of harmonious working relationships, and patients' ill will and dissatisfaction, which may make patients reluctant to return to the particular unit or institution.

The purpose of the selection process is matching people to jobs. It includes the following elements: job analysis; methods of recruiting applicants; selection technique(s) that measure applicants' skill, ability, and knowledge; and assurance that the selection techniques developed and used conform to legal requirements.

Responsibility for selection of nursing personnel in health care institutions is usually shared by the human resources management (HRM) department (or personnel department) and the nursing department. The first-line nursing managers are the most knowledgeable about job requirements and can best describe the job to applicants, although senior-level managers are aware of the effect of planned changes on job tasks. HRM performs the initial screening and monitors hiring practices to be sure they adhere to legal stipulations.

Figure 13–1 shows a flowchart of the selection process and suggested responsibilities. As indicated in the chart, the selection process is a joint effort among the nurse manager, the nursing department, and the HRM department. The selection process begins with job analysis, which is a careful determination of job duties and requirements by nursing service, with technical assistance from HRM. Based on the job analysis, recruiting plans and selection systems are developed and implemented. In most institutions, HRM monitors the success of these systems. Once an applicant makes contact with the institution her or his application blank is reviewed, and a preliminary interview may be conducted by HRM. If the applicant does not meet the basic needs of the open position or positions, he or she should be so informed. Rejected applicants may be qualified for other positions or may refer friends to the institution and thus should be treated with utmost courtesy.

The next three stages include the selection instruments used: tests, assessment centers, reference checks, and managerial interviews. In most cases, the interview is last, but practices may vary. Even if an applicant does poorly on the selection test or receives poor references, it is prudent to carry out the interview so the applicant is not aware that the test or reference checking led to the negative decision. In addition, applicants may feel they have a right to "tell their story" and may spontaneously provide information that explains poor references. The nurse manager should participate in the interview process because he or she (a) is generally in the best position to assess applicants' technical competency, potential, and overall suitability and (b) is able to answer applicants' technical, work-related questions more realistically. In some institutions, the candidate's future co-workers also participate in the interview process to assess compatibility.

After the managerial interview, the applicant is given a comprehensive medical examination to protect the institution from legal actions. For example, individuals with back problems

FIGURE 13-1 FLOWCHART OF TYPICAL SELECTION PROCESS

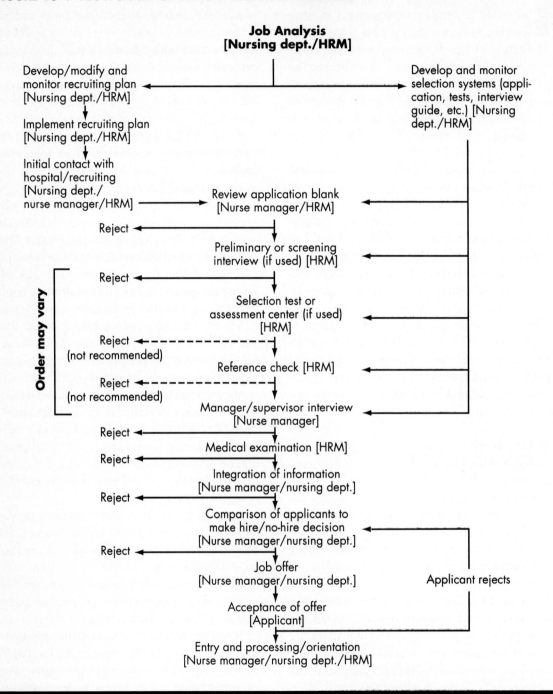

should not be hired to work on a rehabilitation unit, where a great deal of lifting of patients is required. In addition, state boards of health and other regulatory bodies require drug screens, rubella testing, tetanus testing, and tuberculosis testing. The Occupational Safety and Health Administration (OSHA) requires that the hepatitis immune series be offered to health care workers who are non-hepatitis immune.

Once the medical examination has been completed, the nurse manager reviews the information available on each candidate and makes a job offer. The nurse manager must keep others involved in the selection process informed. The nurse manager is usually the first to be aware of potential resignations, requests for transfer, and maternity leaves that require personnel replacement. She or he is also aware of changes in the work area that might necessitate a re-distribution of staff, such as the need for a night nurse instead of a day one. Communicating these needs to the appropriate person promptly and accurately helps ensure effective coordination of the selection process.

♦ JOB ANALYSIS

Before recruiting or selecting new staff, those responsible for hiring should be familiar with the job description and the skills, abilities, and knowledge required to perform the job. Duties and requirements are defined through *job analysis*—a research process that determines (a) the principal duties and responsibilities involved in a particular job, (b) tasks inherent in those duties, and (c) the personal qualifications (skills, abilities, knowledge, and traits) needed for the job. The outcome of a job analysis is a job description.

Almost all human resource functions require an understanding of job requirements. Before nurse managers can orient new staff, they must know the tasks of the job; before they can appraise a person's performance in a position, they must know the performance required. Job analysis provides the means by which this can be accomplished. If no job descriptions currently exist, then the nurse manager, with the assistance of HRM, should develop one for each job on the unit. All staff members (new or existing) need to have an up-to-date copy of their job description.

An important factor in job analysis for the purpose of selection is the job specification, which details the knowledge, skills, and abilities (KSAs) needed, the tasks to be performed, and the behavior required to perform them. While KSAs can be inferred from a description of the tasks to be performed, a description of KSAs does not necessarily permit an inference about tasks and behaviors. Consequently, a job analysis that lists tasks is usually better than one that lists only KSAs. Commercially available instruments listing only KSAs should be avoided unless they were specifically developed for nursing.

Many tools are available for performing job analysis (Cascio, 1987). They vary substantially in complexity and in applicability to different kinds of jobs. Different tools include supervisory conferences, critical incidents, work sampling, observation, interviewing, questionnaires, and checklists.

In a *supervisory conference,* the job analyst brings the supervisors and/or first-line managers together to identify the critical tasks or duties required in a job. The *critical incident* technique also requires the involvement of managers, who keep records of subordinates' behaviors that have contributed to particularly successful or unsuccessful job performance. Both methods are very time-consuming, and the critical incident method does not always give a complete picture of the job because only the very positive or negative behaviors are listed. *Work sampling,* in which the job analyst actually performs the job, is rarely used because it is so time-consuming and requires that the analyst learn the job to be studied.

Observation is one of the most common methods used by job analysts. It is often used for analysis of jobs that consist largely of repetitive, short-cycle, manual operations. *Interviewing,* another common method, relies on staff members providing information to a job analyst about tasks or personal characteristics required for the job. Figure 13–2 is an example of a structured interview guide used for job analysis.

FIGURE 13–2 INTERVIEW GUIDE FOR JOB ANALYSIS

Job Description Questionnaire

Department: _____   **Name:** _____

                                              Position/Title: _____

I. Please briefly describe the main purpose or objective of your job.

II. Respondent's title: _____

Whom do you supervise? _____

Check this box if you do not supervise ☐

Job Title	Number of People
_____	_____
_____	_____

III. Please list, **in order of importance**, the primary reponsibilities of your job. For instance: "insure medications are administered on time"....

A. _____
B. _____
C. _____
D. _____
E. _____

(continued)

FIGURE 13-2 (continued)

IV. Please describe (in the same order) the steps that you go through in order to perform the above stated responsibilities. That is, what duties or tasks must you do to insure fulfillment of your responsibilities? For instance: "Check with Pharmacy to see that medications are delivered on time, check with Xray to see that patients are scheduled as ordered" etc....

A. _____

B. _____

C. _____

D. _____

E. _____

V. Please list, **in order of importance**, any specific duties that you perform periodically.

A. _____

B. _____

C. _____

VI. Whom do you contact on institution-related matters (excluding supervisors and subordinates) both inside and outside of the institution (e.g., Central Supply, Laboratory, Physical Therapy, product representatives)?

A. Inside institution? _____

B. Outside institution? _____

VII. What equipment do you use or need to know how to use to:

A. Perform your job successfully? _____

B. Train others? _____

VIII. Briefly describe the environment in which you do your work (e.g., noise level, traffic area).

IX. If a friend asked you to describe the good and bad points of your job, what would you say? Please be as specific as possible.

X. What is the **absolute minimum** education requirement for this job (none, H.S., some college, etc....)? Why?

XI. What is the **absolute minimum** amount of experience a person would require, in a similar or related area, to perform this job **reasonably** well? Why?

(continued)

FIGURE 13-2 (continued)

XII. What other training or courses, not easily available at school, would be absolutely required to perform your job reasonably well? Why?

_____

What training do you think would be helpful?

_____

XIII. How long should it take someone with the necessary requirements to perform your job reasonably well? Why?

XIV. What are the absolute minimum physical requirements of this job (e.g., weight lifting, energy level, sleep cycle)?

Requirements	**Reason**
_____	_____
_____	_____

XV. What skills, knowledge, or abilities **must** you have to be able to perform your job reasonably well and why (e.g., communication skills, management ability, technical nursing skill)?

Skill, knowledge, ability	**Reason**
_____	_____
_____	_____

XVI. Are there any other details about your job you think need to be stated?

Adapted from a form developed by Douglass Max. Used by permission of Angelica Uniform Co., Director of Personnel & Industrial Relations, St. Louis, MO.

Questionnaires and *checklists* also rely on staff members as a source of information on job requirements. (See Fox and Blue (1988) and Chase (1988) for discussions of the development of job analysis questionnaires for perioperative nursing and orthopedic nursing, respectively.) Questionnaires may be open-ended, whereas checklists tend to be more structured and may consist of 200 or more items for the individual respondent to check off if performed. These data are analyzed to determine the tasks performed by the majority of persons currently in the job. When a checklist is used as the basis for job analysis, a large number of staff members are needed to supply the data because of the statistical analysis techniques used. The nurse manager often needs to participate in developing a job analysis, usually through a supervisory conference, interviewing, or by the use of questionnaires (Bouchard, 1976).

Assuming they are free of error and distortion, job descriptions and specifications can be compared to a photograph in that they represent what the job is at the time the job analysis is performed. The information regarding tasks and duties can be used to construct performance appraisal instruments and training programs. The job specification information can be used to develop selection procedures.

◆ RECRUITMENT

Recruitment links analysis of staffing needs and job analysis with selection. Ideally, the purpose of recruitment is to locate and attract enough qualified applicants to provide a pool from which the required number of individuals can be selected. Even though recruiting is primarily carried out by HRM staff and nurse recruiters, nurse managers play an important role in the process. Recruiting is easier when current employees spread the recruiting message, reducing the need for expensive advertising and bounty methods. To a very large extent, proper management can serve as the best recruiting tool. A nurse manager who is able to create a positive work environment through leadership style and clinical expertise will have a positive impact on efforts to recruit for her or his unit because potential staff members will hear about and be attracted to that unit. In contrast, an autocratic manager is more likely to have a higher turnover rate and is less likely to attract sufficient num-

bers of high-quality nurses to that unit. There are essentially four elements in any recruiting strategy: where to look, how to look, when to look, and how to sell the organization to potential recruits.

WHERE TO LOOK

For most health care institutions, the best place to look is in their own geographic area. When hard pressed to find enough nurses, however, many institutions conduct national searches. This effort is frequently futile, as most nurses look for jobs in their local area. If the hospital is in a major metropolitan area, a search may be relatively easy; if it is located in a rural area, however, recruitment may need to be conducted in the nearest city. In the final analysis, organizations tend to recruit where past efforts have been the most successful. Most institutions adopt an incremental strategy whereby they recruit locally first and then expand to a larger and larger market until a sufficient applicant pool is obtained.

As noted above, proximity to home is a key factor in choosing a job; therefore, recruitment efforts should focus on nurses living near the institution (Decker, Moore & Sullivan, 1982). The state board of nursing can provide the names of registered nurses living in zip code areas surrounding the institution so recruitment efforts can be targeted. Also, personnel officers in large companies or other organizations near the health care institution can be asked to assist in recruiting nurse spouses of newly hired employees.

Students in local schools of nursing are obviously an excellent potential source of employees. The best way to recruit them is to be a clinical training site and treat them *very* well. The nurses who work with the students play a key role in recruitment. Recent graduates of such programs should also be used in recruitment efforts.

HOW TO LOOK— RECRUITING SOURCES

There are many choices in deciding how to look: employee referrals, advertising in newspapers and professional journals, attendance at professional conventions, visits to educational institutions, employment agencies (both private and public), and temporary help agencies. Most applicants are drawn to the institution by some form of advertising, although, in times of nursing shortage, some institutions are offering bonuses to staff members who refer candidates. Direct applications and employee referrals are quick and relatively inexpensive ways of recruiting people, but these methods also tend to perpetuate the current racial or social mix of the workforce. Organizations can benefit from the diversity of a staff comprised of persons from a wide variety of social, experiential, and educational backgrounds.

Advertisements may be placed in the classified sections in local newspapers or journals and in the job listings at professional meetings. Advertising can be an effective recruiting tool, but it tends to be expensive. No matter the cost, "classy" display ads in local newspapers reassure currently employed nurses that the organization is serious about its commitment to provide additional staff. Furthermore, if currently employed nurses are looking at advertisements, a "classy" display ad for their current employer may discourage them from looking elsewhere.

In recruiting, both the medium and the message must be considered. The medium is the agent of contact between the organization and the potential applicant. Obviously, it is desirable to find a medium that gives the widest exposure. Unfortunately, these media tend to be inefficient and low in credibility. The more influential media in terms of selling an organization tend to be the more personal ones: present employees and recruiters. Acquaintances or friends of the recruit have prior credibility and the ability to communicate more subtle aspects of the organization and the job. Also, personal contact tends to be warmer.

Empirical evidence shows that a relationship exists between the recruiting source (e.g., advertisement, employee referral) and subsequent tenure with an organization (Decker & Cornelius, 1979). Nurses referred by informal methods (e.g., recommended by friends, walk-ins, and rehires) tend to remain with an organization longer than those recruited by formal methods (e.g., newspaper and other advertising and employment agencies) and also tend to be more productive (Breaugh & Mann, 1984). The reason for this difference is that nurses coming from informal sources of referral are likely to have more realistic information about the job and the institution and, therefore, their expectations more closely fit reality. Those who come to the job with unrealistic expectations may experience dissatisfaction as the result. In an open labor market, these individuals may leave the organization, creating high turnover. When nursing jobs are less plentiful, dissatisfied staff members may tend to stay in the organization because they need the job, but they are not likely to perform as well as other employees. Consequently, even *where* applicants are sought may have significant consequences later on.

One source of new nurses that is frequently overlooked is the inactive nurse. Survey statistics show that between 27 percent and 40 percent of registered nurses in any geographic area are not working in health care and that, of those nurses, approximately 70 percent would consider returning to nursing, given refresher training, continuing education, etc. (Decker, Moore & Sullivan, 1982). Many inactive nurses would volunteer their time to learn new skills to reenter nursing, although they frequently require an extensive (and costly) orientation to the job. Most of these now inactive nurses would look for the following components in employment (listed by priority): proximity to home, management support, quality of orientation, salary, and opportunity to specialize (Decker, Moore & Sullivan, 1982).

WHEN TO LOOK

The time lag in recruiting has always been a concern in nursing, except for brief periods when an excess supply of nurses was available. Today the shortage of nurses is severe, especially in certain locations and specialties. Careful planning is necessary to ensure that recruitment begins well in advance of anticipated needs. Human resource planning is discussed in more detail in Norton and Crissman (1992).

HOW TO SELL THE ORGANIZATION

The final issue in developing a recruiting strategy is communicating with job candidates. Developing an effective recruiting message is difficult. Sometimes the tendency is to use a shotgun approach, sugarcoat the message, or make it very slick. A more balanced message, which includes honest communication and personal contact, is preferable. Overselling the organization creates unrealistic expectations that may lead to later dissatisfaction and turnover. Realistically presenting the job requirements and rewards improves job satisfaction, in that the new recruit learns what the job is actually like. Promising a nurse every other weekend off and only a 25 percent rotation to nights on a severely understaffed unit and then scheduling him or her off only every third weekend with 75 percent night

rotations is an example of giving unrealistic job information. It is important to represent the situation honestly and describe the steps management is taking to improve situations that the applicant might find undesirable. The candidate can then make an informed decision about the job offer.

◆ THE SELECTION PROCESS

The primary purpose of recruitment activities is to generate a pool of qualified applicants. The primary purpose of any selection process is to assess an applicant's ability and motivation relative to the requirements and rewards of the job so that a matching process can be carried out. To the extent that these matches are made effectively, positive outcomes such as high job satisfaction, low turnover, and high-quality performance can result. Selection techniques include interviewing, tests, and assessment centers.

◆ INTERVIEWING

The most common selection method, the interview, is an information-seeking mechanism between an individual applying for a position and a member of an organization doing the hiring. A candidate's first interview may be an initial screening conducted by the HRM to determine whether an applicant meets the educational and experience criteria for the job. Following the initial screening, the nurse manager usually conducts an interview.

The interview is used to clarify information gathered from the application form and to evaluate the applicant's responses to questions. Additionally, the interviewer should provide information about the job and the institution.

BOX 13-1
THE JOB SEARCH:
EVALUATING EMPLOYERS

These factors are believed to contribute most to the job satisfaction or dissatisfaction of employees at the professional level. They are grouped according to category but are not listed in any priority order. Since people vary greatly in the factors they judge important, you may want to establish your own order of priorities by assigning a value to each factor. Each organization can then be rated according to how satisfactorily it meets that value.

THE JOB
1. Intellectual stimulation
2. Opportunity to learn new skills
3. Opportunity to apply academic training
4. Variety of work assignments
5. Opportunity for individual achievement
6. Exposure to outstanding colleagues
7. Opportunity to work independently
8. Opportunity for travel
9. Frequency of travel
10. Personalities of supervisors and colleagues
11. Social significance of job
12. Physical environment and working conditions
13. Pressure and pace of work

THE INDUSTRY
1. Growth history
2. Future needs for goods and services
3. Dependence on the business cycle
4. Dependence on government policies and programs

THE ORGANIZATION
1. Technologically innovative
2. High investment in R&D
3. Quality of products or services
4. Management style
5. Opportunities for advancement
6. Encouragement of professional growth
7. Reputation and image of company
8. Financial stability
9. Salary and benefits
10. Personnel policies (demands on personal time, required relocations, record of layoffs)
11. Technical people in top-level positions
12. Future directions of organization's growth

THE LOCATION
1. Proximity to graduate schools
2. Opportunities for spouse's career
3. Climate
4. Cost of living
5. Community life
6. Proximity to family

Finally, the interview should create good will toward the employing institution through good "customer relations." Research suggests that decision making is improved if the interviewer postpones reviewing information not needed for the interview itself, such as test scores, until after the interview. The improvement in decision making is due to the fact that reviewing such information before the interview may lead to ignoring data that disconfirms this information (Gatewood & Feild, 1990).

An effective interviewer must learn to solicit information efficiently and to gather relevant data. Interviews typically last for one or one-

and-a-half hours and, as shown in Figure 13–3, include an opening, an information gathering and giving phase, and a closing. The opening is important because it is an attempt to establish rapport with the applicant so she or he will provide relevant information. Gathering information, however, is the core of the interview. Giving information also is important, as the interviewer can create realistic expectations in the applicant and sell the organization, if that is needed. However, this portion of the interview should take place after the information has been gathered, so that the applicant's answers will be as candid as possible. The interviewer should answer any direct questions posed by the candidate. Figure 13–4 is an example of realistic information for applicants. Finally, the closing is intended to provide information on the mechanics of possible employment.

PRINCIPLES FOR EFFECTIVE INTERVIEWING

PREPARING FOR THE INTERVIEW. Most managers do not adequately prepare for the interview, which should be planned just like any business undertaking. All needed materials should be on hand, and the interview site should be quiet and pleasant. If others are to see the applicant, their schedules should be checked to make sure they are available at the proper time. If coffee or other refreshments are to be offered, advance arrangements need to be made. Lack of advance preparation may lead to insufficient interviewing time, interruptions, or failure to gather important information. Other problems include losing focus in the interview because of a desire to be courteous or because a particularly dominant interviewee is encountered. This typically keeps the interviewer from obtaining the needed information.

In general, when time is limited, it is better to use part of it for planning rather than squander all of it on the interview itself. This is preferable to spending more time later trying to correct the performance of a poor employee. Before the interview, the interviewer should review the job requirements, the application blank, and the résumé and write any specific questions to be asked. Planning should be done on the morning

---

FIGURE 13–3 TIME SCHEDULE FOR AN INTERVIEW

	1½ hours	1 hour
Opening	7 minutes	3
Disclosure of interview procedure	3 minutes	2
Interests	5 minutes	5
Educational history	20 minutes	10
Job history	20 minutes	15
Future plans	10 minutes	5
Information about the organization and position	15 minutes	10
Additional questions and answers	5 minutes	2
Closing	5 minutes	3

Adapted from P. J. Decker, *Selection Interviewing Procedures for Healthcare Managers.* Copyright 1983, by Phillip J. Decker, Used by permission.

of the interview or the evening before for an early morning interview. If you are sure that time will be available, planning is best done immediately before an interview or between interviews. Unfortunately, a busy manager may have to deal with minor crises between interviews and may not be able to use the time to plan the next interview.

A cardinal rule is to review the application or résumé before beginning the interview. If the interviewee arrives with the résumé or application in hand, ask him or her to wait for a few minutes while you review the material. In doing a quick review, consider three things. First, are there clear discrepancies between the applicant's qualifications and the job specifications? If the answer is yes, then only a brief interview may be necessary, to explain why the applicant will not be considered. (If a preliminary screening is performed by the HRM, such applicants should not be referred to nurse managers.) Second, look for

specific questions to ask the applicant during the interview. Finally, look for a "rapport builder" (something you have in common with the applicant) to break the ice at the beginning of the interview.

To provide a relaxed, informal atmosphere, the setting is important. Both the interviewer and the applicant should be in comfortable chairs, as close as is comfortably possible. No table or desk should separate them. If an office is used, the interviewer should arrange chairs so that the applicant is at the side of the desk. There should be complete freedom from distracting phone calls and other interruptions. The applicant should not be seated so she or he can look out a window, if the view is distracting.

OPENING THE INTERVIEW. The interviewer should start on time; give a warm, friendly greeting; introduce herself or himself; and ask the applicant his or her preferred name.

FIGURE 13–4 STAFF NURSE POSITION, BURN UNIT: REALISTIC PREVIEW INFORMATION

I. Positive information
- Patients are here for length of time – lots of patient and family teaching
- Critical as well as recovering patients
- Decision-making opportunities
- Bedside nursing
- Learning environment
- Able to assist with research
- Small unit, close knit, dedicated group
- Burns as well as other prior difficulties or concurrent problems to work with
- Children as well as adults

II. Negative information
- Type of patient is sometimes difficult to deal with; i.e., young children or elderly – often alcoholics, psychological difficulties
- Emotionally stressful
- Physically difficult

Adapted from a form used by Barnes Hospital Nursing Service, St. Louis, MO. Used by permission.

The interviewer should try to minimize status, not patronize or dominate. The objective is to establish an open atmosphere so applicants reveal as much as possible about themselves. Rapport should be established and maintained throughout the interview. This can be done by talking about yourself, discussing mutual interests such as hobbies or sports, and using nonverbal cues such as maintaining eye contact. Finally, the interviewer should start the interview by outlining what will be discussed and setting the time limits for the interview.

The interviewer must be very careful not to form hasty first impressions and make equally hasty decisions. Interviewers tend to be influenced by their impressions of a candidate—shaking hands with someone who has a limp, sweaty handshake, for instance—and such judgments often lead to poor decisions. First impressions may degrade the quality of the interview by coloring the search for information; interviewers tend to search for information to justify their first impressions, good or bad. If the first impression is negative and the interviewer decides not to hire a potentially successful candidate, the interviewer has wasted an hour or so and possibly lost a good recruit. If, because of a positive first impression, the interviewer hires an unsuccessful candidate, problems may continue for months. On the other hand, personal characteristics of the interviewer may influence the applicant's decisions. First impressions of the interviewer are created by her or his tone of voice, eye contact, personal appearance, grooming, posture, and gestures.

DEVELOPING STRUCTURED INTERVIEW GUIDES

Unstructured interviews present problems; if interviewers fail to ask the same questions of every candidate, it is often difficult to compare them. With any human skill or trait, no standard or true score exists that can serve as a basis on which to compare applicants. People can only be compared to other people. Consequently, the interview is most effective when the information on the pool of interviewees is as comparable as possible. Comparability is maximized via a structured interview supported by an interview guide. An *interview guide* is a written document containing questions, interviewer directions, and other pertinent information so that the same process is followed and the same basic information is gathered from each applicant. An interview guide ensures that the interviewing process is "content valid," a concept discussed later in this chapter. The guide should be specific to the job, or job category, as shown below.

Do job analysis to determine job tasks

↓

Use tasks to determine required personal characteristics (skills, abilities, knowledge)

↓

Write questions and develop behavioral simulations to tap whether the applicant has the required personal characteristics

↓

Put these questions and ideas in the interview guide format to guide you in the interview

Behavioral simulations differ from tests, in that they capture actual behavior, not what individuals say they would do. They are exercises designed to elicit behavior by placing the person in a controlled situation similar to the job. Examples are typing tests or administering medications. To be legal, simulations must (a) have standardized administration, (b) be administered to all applicants reaching the same level of the selection process, (c) require skills that will not be provided by brief training, (d) be job related, and (e) provide the applicant with appropriate time for preparation.

Figure 13–5 is an interview guide format. This figure can be used to construct your own interview guide, but do not copy the questions verbatim; develop your own questions based on the categories. Figure 13–6 is an example of job-related questions for an oncology unit that could be asked in area 6 of the interview guide. As noted earlier, Figure 13–4 is an example of the type of information that would be presented in area 8, job preview information.

Interview guides reduce interviewer bias, provide relevant and effective questions, reduce leading questions, and facilitate comparison among applicants. Space left between the questions on the guide provides room for note-taking, and the guide also provides a written record of the interview.

Using the structured interview guide, the interviewer should take notes, telling the candidate that this is being done to aid recall and that he or she hopes the candidate does not mind. There are various ways of asking questions, but only one question should be asked at a time and, where possible, open-ended questions should be used, such as, "Please tell me about your most rewarding experience as a nurse." Open-ended questions cannot be answered with a single yes, no, or one-word answer and usually elicit more information about the applicant. Close-ended questions (e.g., what, where, why, when, how many) should only be used to elicit specific information.

Work sample questions are used to determine an applicant's knowledge about work tasks and ability to perform the job. It is easy to ask a nurse if she or he knows how to care for a patient who has a central venous pressure (CVP) line in place. An answer of "yes" does not nec-

FIGURE 13–5 INTERVIEW GUIDE FORMAT

1. **The interviewer should record responses to each question during the interview. Immediately after the interview, indicate your reaction to each answer beneath the response.** Use what is appropriate (e.g., Education questions may not be necessary for a candidate out of school 10 years with extensive work history).

Candidate: _____

Interviewer: _____

Date: _____ Position sought: _____

Review of application form:

Items of interest to you on the application:

(continued)

FIGURE 13-5 (continued)

2. **Open the interview and establish rapport.**

___ Warm friendly greeting.
___ Names are important, yours and the applicant's. (Use first or last name correctly.)
___ Break the ice–talk about his/her trip to_____, hobbies, weather, etc. and/or talk briefly about yourself–position, hobbies, etc.

Outline topics to be covered in the interview.

___ Education
___ Work History
___ Miscellaneous
___ Job Preview

3. Education

I. A. High School Name _____

B. Year Graduated _____

C. Which courses did you like best? _____

D. Which courses did you like least? _____

E. Extracurricular activities you enjoyed the most: _____

II. A. Nursing School (College or Hospital) _____

B. Year Graduated _____

C. Additional College Work _____

D. Additional Degrees _____

E. Which courses did you like best? _____

F. Which courses did you like least? _____

G. If you had the opportunity to start your education all over again knowing what you know now, what would you do differently? _____

H. What were some of the highlights of your years in school? _____

4. Employment history

A. Tell me about your current job. What are your duties? What kind of decisions do you normally make? _____

(continued)

FIGURE 13–5 (continued)

    B. What is there about your present position you like most? _____

    C. The least? _____

    D. What aspects of your work is your supervisor especially pleased with? _____

    E. What areas do you feel you could improve on? _____

    F. What is there in your present job that you would change if you could? _____

    G. What things in a job do you consider to be important? _____

    H. What type of supervisor do you prefer working for? _____

    I. Why are you leaving your present job? _____

5. Self-evaluation

    A. What are the most important ways in which you've changed in the last 5-10 years? _____

    B. What do you see yourself doing in the next 10 years? _____

    C. What are some of the things you can work on to better your chance of getting where you want to go? _____

    D. What do you like to do in your spare time? _____

    E. What do you consider to be your strongest asset? _____

    F. What are other assets? _____

    G. What are 2 or 3 things that you have done in your lifetime of which you are the most proud? _____

    H. What is there in your overall background that you feel would enable you to do a good job in this position? _____

6. Job-related situation: Tell me how you would handle this situation...
(see Figure 13–6)

7. Will you work night/weekend rotations? _____ yes _____ no

(continued)

FIGURE 13-5 (continued)

8. Job preview information

    A. Unit structure (Personnel)
    B. Orientation period
    C. Duties
    D. Available shift
        1. D/E, E, N
        2. 8 hrs, 10 hrs
    E. Tour of unit – Discussion of nursing care in general

9. Closing the interview

    A. Is there anything you would like to add?
    B. Date available to start _____
    C. Follow-up date _____
    D. Thank you

Adapted from guides used by Barnes Hospital Nursing Service, St. Louis, MO, and from P.J. Decker, *Selection Interviewing Procedures for Healthcare Managers.* Copyright 1983, by Phillip J. Decker. Used by permission.

essarily prove the ability, so the interviewer might ask some very specific questions about CVP lines. Leading questions in which the answer is implied by the question should be avoided (e.g., "We have lots of overtime. Do you mind overtime?"). The interviewer may also want to summarize what has been said, use silence to elicit more information, reflect back the applicant's feelings to clarify the issue, or indicate acceptance by urging the applicant to continue.

GIVING INFORMATION. Before reaching the information-giving part of the interview, the interviewer should consider whether the candidate is promising enough to warrant spending time in giving detailed job information. Unless the candidate is clearly unacceptable, the interviewer should be careful not to communicate a negative impression, because the evaluation of the candidate may change when the entire packet of material is reviewed or more promising candidates decline a job offer. The interviewer also must know what information he or she should give and what is to be provided by others. Detailed benefit or compensation questions are usually answered by HRM. If a promising candidate's questions cannot be answered, the interviewer should arrange for someone to contact the candidate later with the desired information.

In closing the interview, the interviewer may want to summarize the applicant's strengths. The interviewer should make sure that the applicant is asked if she or he has anything to add or questions to ask related to the job and the organization. The interviewer also may want to mention the candidate's weaknesses, particularly if they are objective and clearly related to the job, such as lack of experience in a particular field. Mentioning a perception of a subjective weakness, such as poor supervisory skills, may lead to legal problems. Thanking the applicant and completing any notes made during the interview conclude the interview process. Figure 13–7 provides a set of key behaviors for an effective interview. These should be followed in every interview. These key behaviors can also be

---

FIGURE 13–6 ONCOLOGY UNIT JOB-RELATED QUESTIONS

Describe how you would intervene in the following situations:

♦ A patient that you admitted with a diagnosis of lymphoma is going to begin chemotherapy and you are preparing to hang the first dose. When you enter the room she says, "You know I just can't believe that I have cancer. I know it is what the doctor says but it just doesn't seem possible to me."

♦ The wife of a patient overhears some doctors caring for her husband say that the patient has received the incorrect dose of chemotherapy. You are caring for him.

♦ A young man is diagnosed with acute leukemia and expresses anger and frustration in the presence of his wife. You witness the frequent outbursts and become increasingly aware of the sense of hopelessness on the part of both him and his wife.

♦ A leukemia patient has been classified as a no code. On the night shift the patient develops dyspnea, becomes uncomfortable, anxious and screams out periodically. The patient is on 100% O_2 already but his wife insists that something more be done.

♦ A physician making rounds notices a discrepancy in your patient's I&O. The weights indicate that he has gained 10 pounds but the intake records do not show how this could have happened.

♦ You are working nights and caring for an extremely seriously ill man receiving platelets and antibiotic therapy. The patient's blood pressure is continuing to drop. You have talked to the resident on call twice by telephone and he tells you to continue the present orders. The man's condition continues to decline. What would you do?

Adapted from a form used by Barnes Hospital Nursing Service, St. Louis, MO. Used by permission.

typed on a large index card for easy reference while interviewing.

INTEGRATION OF INFORMATION. When comparing candidates: First, weigh the qualities required for the job in order of importance; more emphasis should be placed on the more important elements. Second, weigh the qualities desired on the basis of the reliability of the data. The more consistent the observation of behavior from different elements in the selection system, the more weight should be given that dimension. Third, weigh job dimensions by trainability—consider the amount of education, experience, and additional training the applicant can reasonably be expected to receive, and consider the likelihood that the behavior in that dimension can be improved with training. Dimensions most likely to be learned in training (such as use of a particular piece of equipment) should be given the least weight so that more weight is placed on dimensions less likely to be learned in training (such as being able to work effectively with terminally ill children).

The interviewer should attempt to compare data across individuals in making a decision. It is more accurate to make decisions based on a comparison of several persons than to make a decision for each individual after each interview. Analysis of the entire applicant pool requires good interview records but lessens the impact of early impressions on the hiring decision because the interviewer must consider each job element across the entire pool.

INTERVIEW RELIABILITY AND VALIDITY

Numerous research studies have been performed on the reliability and validity of employment interviews (Arvey and Faley, 1988). In general, agreement between two interviews of the same candidate by the same interviewer (*intra-rater reliability*) is fairly high, agreement between two interviews of the same candidate by several interviewers (*interrater reliability*) is rather low, and the ability to predict job performance (*validity*) of the typical interview is very low. Research also has shown that (a) structured

---

FIGURE 13-7 THE EFFECTIVE INTERVIEW

♦ Give a warm, friendly welcome.
   a. Relax and smile.
   b. Use appropriate name, be consistent and pronounce it correctly.

♦ Talk about yourself to help applicant relax.

♦ Tell applicant the purpose and structure of the interview.

♦ Use your Interview Guide, follow the order and content exactly.

♦ Take brief notes, and inform the applicant that you intend to.

♦ Probe to get details about negative or unclear information.

♦ Listen attentively.

♦ Summarize what you have heard for each main section of the interview.

♦ Give job preview information which is realistic.

♦ Give a friendly goodbye.
   a. Outline the next steps in the selection process.
   b. Ask for any additional comments/questions.
   c. Say goodbye and thank applicant for coming in.

Adapted from P. J. Decker, *Selection Interviewing Procedures for Healthcare Managers.* Copyright 1983, by Phillip J. Decker. Used by permission.

interviews are more reliable and valid; (b) interviewers who are under pressure to hire in a short period of time or meet a recruitment quota are less accurate than other interviewers; (c) interviewers who have detailed information about the job for which they are interviewing exhibit higher interrater reliability and validity; (d) the interviewer's experience does not seem to be related to reliability and validity; (e) there is a decided tendency for interviewers to make quick decisions and therefore be less accurate; (f) interviewers develop stereotypes of ideal applicants against which interviewees are evaluated, and individual interviewers may hold different stereotypes, thus decreasing interrater reliability and validity; and (g) race and sex have been found to influence interviewers' evaluations.

Possibly the greatest weakness in the selection interview is the tendency for the interviewer to try to assess an applicant's "basic character" during the interview (Goodale, 1982). Judgments are made about the applicant's personality characteristics as well as knowledge and skill. Although it is difficult to eliminate such subjectivity, evaluations of applicants are often more subjective than they need to be, particularly when interviewers try to assess personality characteristics. Information collected during an interview should answer three fundamental questions: (a) can the applicant perform the job? (b) will the applicant perform the job, and (c) will the candidate fit in to the culture of the unit and the institution? The best predictor of the applicant's future behavior in these two respects is past performance. Previous work and non-work experience, previous education and training, and current job performance all should be considered, not personality characteristics, which even psychologists cannot measure very accurately.

♦ STAYING WITHIN THE LAW

Equal employment opportunity (EEO) law and succeeding court decisions have had two major impacts on selection procedures. First, organizations have been more careful to use predictors and techniques that can be shown not to discriminate against protected classes. Second, organizations are reducing the use of tests, which may be difficult to defend if they screen out a large number of minority applicants, and are relying more heavily on the interview as a selection device. However, Title VII of the Civil Rights Act of 1964 (43 Fed. Reg., 1978), discussed more extensively later in this chapter, applies to interviews as much as it does to tests. Many interviewers become annoyed with what they perceive as restrictions imposed by EEO legislation, but EEO legislation does not restrict the employer from asking or measuring job-related characteristics. The legislation simply says it is illegal to make a personnel decision based on a person's race, color, sex, religion, national origin, or other characteristics added by state law. Figure 13–8 presents questions that are appropriate to ask in interviews (see also Poteet, 1984). The basic rule of thumb in interviewing is when in doubt about a question's legality, ask yourself how it is related to job performance. If it can be proven that only job-related questions are asked, EEO law will not be violated.

TESTING FOR SELECTION

A *test* is any systematic standardized procedure for obtaining information from individuals. For employment purposes, a test gathers information pertaining to the applicant's abilities, skills, knowledge, or motivation believed to be required to carry out the job. There are aptitude tests, personality and interest tests, and work

FIGURE 13–8 PRE-EMPLOYMENT QUESTIONS

	Appropriate to ask	**Inappropriate to ask**
Name	Applicant's name.	Questions about any name or title that indicate race, color, religion, sex, national origin or ancestry.
Address	Questions concerning place and length of current and previous addresses.	Any specific probes into foreign addresses that would indicate national origin.
Age	Requiring proof of age by birth certificate *after* hiring.	Requiring birth certificate or baptismal record *before* hiring.
Birthplace or national origin		Any question about place of birth of applicant or place of birth of parents, grandparents or spouse.
		Any other question (direct or indirect) about applicant's national origin.
Race or color		Any inquiry that would indicate race or color.
Sex		Any question on an application blank that would indicate sex.
Religion		Any questions to indicate applicant's religious denomination or beliefs.
		Request a recommendation or reference from the applicant's religious denomination.
Citizenship	Question about whether the applicant is a U.S. citizen; if not, whether the applicant intends to become one.	Questions of whether the applicant, his/her parents, or spouse are native born or naturalized.
	Question if applicant's U.S. residence is legal and require proof of citizenship *after* being hired.	Require proof of citizenship *before* being hired.
Photographs	May be required after hiring for identification purposes only.	Request photograph *before* hiring.
Education	Questions concerning any academic, professional, or vocational schools attended.	Questions asking specifically the nationality, racial or religious affiliation of any school attended.
	Inquiry into language skills, such as reading and writing of foreign languages.	Inquiries into the applicant's mother tongue or how any foreign language ability was acquired (unless it is necessary for the job).
Relatives	Ask for the name, relationship and address of a person to be notified in case of an emergency.	Any unlawful inquiry about a relative as specified in this list.

Figure 13.8 (continued)

Organization	Questions about organization memberships and any offices that might be held.	Questions about any organization an applicant belongs to which may indicate the race, color, religion, sex, national origin or ancestry of its members.
Military service	Questions about services rendered in armed forces, the rank attained, and which branch of service.	Questions about military service in any armed forces other than the U.S.
	Require military discharge certificate *after* being hired.	Request of military service records before hiring.
Work schedule	Questions about the applicant's willingness to work required work schedule.	Ask applicant's willingness to work any particular religious holiday.
References	Ask for general and work references not relating to race, color, religion, sex, national origin or ancestry.	Request references specifically from clergymen (as specified above) or any other persons who might reflect race, color, religion, sex, national origin or ancestry of applicant.
Other qualifications	Any question that has direct reflection on the job to be applied for.	Any non-job-related inquiry that may present information permitting unlawful discrimination.

Adapted from a document distributed by the Ohio Civil Rights Commission, 220 S. Parsons Ave., Columbus, OH 43215. Used by permission.

sample tests. *Aptitude tests* measure those individual characteristics that are likely to lead to acquiring knowledge or skill; they therefore indicate what tasks the applicant might be able to perform in the future, given the opportunity and/or training. *Personality and interest inventories* attempt to measure a person's motivation or personality characteristics, but they are not used to any great extent in employee selection. Aptitude tests are more accurate in predicting training success than job performance. In general, neither aptitude tests nor personality and interest inventories are accurate employment predictors.

Work sample tests are quite literally samples

of the work performed on the job, the underlying assumption being that performance of a representative sample of the job predicts performance on the job itself. Work samples can be split into two categories: behavioral and knowledge. *Behavioral* work samples are tests in which a person actually performs some of the tasks involved in the job, such as a typing test. *Job knowledge* tests measure the knowledge required to do the job, such as a medical terminology test for an applicant for a unit secretary position.

Paper-and-pencil testing, such as job knowledge tests, is not done in the typical health care institution because of the costs and effort required in validity studies. If carried out, testing is usually the province of HRM, and the nurse manager seldom becomes involved because of the need to ensure standardized administration policies.

EDUCATION, EXPERIENCE, AND PHYSICAL EXAMS

Education and experience requirements for nurses have long been important screening factors and bear a close relationship to work sample tests. Educational requirements are a type of job knowledge sample since they tend to ensure that applicants have at least a minimal amount of the knowledge necessary to do the job. Experience requirements are very much like behavioral samples because the assumption is that, given a certain number of years of experience, the nurse would have performed most of the tasks required for the job.

References and letters of recommendation also are used to assess the applicant's past job experience but there is little evidence that these have any validity. Since very few persons write unfavorable letters of recommendation, such letters do not really predict job performance. However, in the rare instances when candidates are described in negative terms, it is usually indicative of the potential for problems. Criticisms are likely to be very mild and may be reflected by the lack of positive language. Letters with any criticism should be verified with a telephone call if possible to avoid overreacting to an unusually honest author. To avoid legal problems, some organizations do not allow supervisors to write letters of recommendation. On the other hand, almost every organization will at least verify position title and dates of employment. This helps in detecting the occasional applicant who counterfeits an entire work history. Unfortunately, omission of a position from the work

history is more common than including a position not actually held. The only way to detect such omissions is to ask that candidates list year *and month* of all educational and work experiences. Caution is necessary when asking about time between jobs; be careful not to inquire about marital status.

In almost every selection situation, an applicant fills out an application form that requests information regarding previous experience, education, and references. Most application forms also ask for the applicant's medical history and other personal data. As application forms are reviewed, the critical question to be asked is: "Has this applicant distorted her or his responses, either intentionally or unintentionally?" Studies looking at this question indicate that there is usually little distortion, at least not on the easily verifiable information. Applicants may stretch the truth a bit, but rarely are there any complete falsehoods. Relative to other predictors, the application form may be one of the more valid predictors in a selection process. Its validity parallels that of work sample exercises because it documents actual job performance.

The pre-employment physical exam serves a number of purposes. It screens out applicants who may have major physical or obvious mental impairments that would seriously impede successful job performance. It also identifies applicants with health problems that are likely to lead to poor attendance or excessive claims against health insurance.

ASSESSMENT CENTERS

Many organizations have turned to the use of assessment centers, especially for selecting supervisory/managerial personnel. Although they are a relatively new practice in the health care field, some institutions are now using such centers. An *assessment center* is not a place; it is a process used for identifying individual strengths and weaknesses for a specified purpose such as selection, promotion, or development (Moses & Byham, 1977). Individuals engage in a series of exercises, both individual and group, constructed to simulate critical behaviors related to success on the job. The assessment center method is particularly appealing to organizations because judgments are based on the applicant's overt behavior in the assessment center, which parallels that required on the job. The likelihood of predicting future job performance is enhanced by using multiple assessment techniques, standardizing methods of making inferences, and pooling the judgments of multiple assessors.

Assessment centers are useful when job requirements are quite different from the requirements of the candidates' current positions, such as selection of a staff nurse for the job of nurse manager. It is very difficult to judge how well a staff nurse who is performing mostly clinical skills will perform in a managerial role. The institution may very well end up with a poor manager and lose a good clinician because of an attempt to judge managerial ability by evaluating clinical skills. In this case, an assessment center is an appropriate method because it simulates the job of a manager.

The essential elements of the assessment center process are as follows: (a) relevant job behaviors are analyzed to determine the attributes, characteristics, skills, abilities, or knowledge to be evaluated; (b) the techniques or exercises are designed to provide information to be used in evaluating the candidate on job-related dimensions, skills, or abilities; (c) multiple assessment techniques are used, and at least one is a behavioral simulation; (d) multiple dimensions that describe the relative skills, abilities, and knowledge required to do the job are evaluated; (e)

multiple assessors (nursing managers and directors) receive thorough training to process information in a fair and impartial manner; and (f) judgments resulting in hiring or promotion decisions are based on pooling information from the different assessors and techniques and are made by consensus. Common exercises in assessment centers include interviews, organizational games, in-baskets (assessee working through the typical nurse manager's in-basket material), leaderless group discussions (staff meetings), some kind of presentation, role plays, and occasionally paper-and-pencil tests.

◆ LEGALITY IN HIRING

Staffing activities have been subject to considerable scrutiny regarding discrimination and equal employment opportunity, mainly as a result of Title VII of the Civil Rights Act of 1964, as well as the Equal Pay Act of 1963 and Age Discrimination Act of 1967. Title VII of the Civil Rights Act specifically prohibits discrimination in *any personnel decision* on the basis of race, color, sex, religion, or national origin. "Any personnel decision" includes not only selection but also entrance into training programs, performance appraisal results, termination, promotions, benefits, and so on. The act applies to most employers with more than 15 employees, although there are several exemptions—among them, "bona fide occupational qualification" (BFOQ), "business necessity," and validity of the procedure used to make the personnel decision (as discussed below). Discrimination is allowed on the basis of national origin (citizenship or immigration status), religion, sex, and age, for instance, if that discrimination can be shown to be a "bona fide occupational qualification reasonably necessary for the normal operation of a business." The classic example of a genuine BFOQ is a sperm donor. More realistic examples are a female part in a play, a Sunday school teacher of a certain religion, or a female correctional counselor at a women's prison. Claims of "customer preference" for female flight attendants or gross gender characteristics such as "women cannot lift over 30 pounds" have not been supported as BFOQs.

A *BFOQ* allows an organization to actually exclude members of certain groups (such as all men or all women), if the organization can demonstrate that a selection method is a *business necessity,* despite the fact that members of certain groups are likely to be excluded. Business necessity is likely to withstand legal challenge only in the unusual instances when a selection method that discriminates against a protected group is necessary to ensure the safety of workers or customers. For example, in *Spurlock v. United Airlines,* the court found that a flight time requirement and a college degree requirement were legal in hiring pilot trainees, despite the fact that these requirements discriminated against black applicants. Both requirements were found to be related to flight safety. The fact that hiring members of a particular protected group would lead to an economic loss for the organization is not adequate evidence for business necessity; the validity of the selection method would have to be demonstrated.

Title VII also is a complaint-oriented law: Any person who feels he or she has been discriminated against may file a complaint with the government against an employer. When a complaint is filed, the Equal Employment Opportunity Commission (EEOC) *or* the applicable state agency created to enforce the EEO law sends notice to the employer and initiates an investigation of the complaint. The EEOC has broad investigatory powers and access to all relevant employment records and documents. If it finds there is reasonable cause to believe that illegal discrimination has taken place, it will notify the employer and attempt to settle the complaint through conciliation. If this attempt fails, the EEOC or the individual may file a lawsuit against the company. Any legal action can result in reinstatement and/or back pay of up to two years.

When an individual files a complaint of discrimination, initially he or she need only prove unequal treatment or that fewer members of minority than of non-minority groups are hired. The latter is known as *adverse impact.* The burden of proof then shifts to the organization, which must justify that its decisions were based on some job-relevant predictor and were not related to the individual's race, color, sex, religion, national origin, handicapped status, or other categories that state laws may add. There are two possible methods of justifying this claim: (a) to indicate that the institution did not have the information on race, sex, and so forth in the first place and therefore could not have used it (this is a very difficult claim to make since most applicants are interviewed or are seen in a health care organization before hire) or (b) to prove that the hire/no-hire decision was based on some job-relevant criterion and not on race, sex, color, religion, or national origin.

The EEOC is charged with enforcing and interpreting the Civil Rights Act and has issued Uniform Guidelines on Employee Selection Procedures (43 Fed. Reg., 1978). The guidelines specify the kinds of methods and information required to justify the job relatedness of selection procedures. These guidelines are not described in detail here; however, the methods of selection discussed in this chapter do follow their specifications. Remember that the law *does not say* one cannot hire the best person for the job or that one must hire so many whites and so many blacks, although goals may be established based on the relevant applicant pool. What it says is that race, color, sex, religion, or national origin must not be used as selection criteria. As long as the decision is not made on the basis of minority status, one is complying with U.S. EEO law. Canadian civil rights law generally parallels U.S. law.

♦ VALIDATION

Any selection procedure should include only valid selection predictors; these are instruments (application form, tests, interviews) that are predictive of applicants' future effectiveness as employees on the job. Validity of a predictor cannot be assumed but must be investigated statistically by measuring the connection between a predictor score and some measure of success on the job. Job analysis information helps to develop both the predictor and the measure of success. The use of valid predictors not only is desirable in choosing the best employee but also satisfies legal requirements.

A *validation study* is the procedure used for gathering evidence that a predictor is job related. The outcome of a validation study is information indicating the degree to which the predictor is related to job success. Three major types of validation studies are possible: criterion-related, content, and construct. *Criterion-related* validation is the most vigorous, costly, and time-consuming. However, criterion-related studies may still be cost-effective because they enable the organization to establish the most cost-effective cutoff scores, or scores that applicants must achieve to be hired. *Content* validation is considerably more feasible because it takes the form of a logical argument rather

than an empirical argument, but it may not always make the strongest argument for job relatedness. *Construct* validation is a useful strategy for theoretical research on psychological characteristics, but it is very difficult to apply to the employment setting and is not discussed further.

In criterion-related validation studies, scores on both the predictor and the criterion (job performance) measures are obtained from job applicants or employees. If employees are used in a *concurrent* validation study, both predictor and criterion scores are obtained concurrently (at the same time). *Predictive* validation is a method wherein predictor scores are obtained from a sample of job applicants and selection decisions are then made about those applicants without the predictor being studied. The criterion scores are collected after the applicants have been hired.

Criterion-related validation studies are performed by HRM or by consultants because they are complex and require precise collection of data. Not only does the nurse manager rarely become involved with statistical validity, but also many institutions simply do not do it. Unless adverse impact—under-utilization of a protected class—can be proven, the government will not scrutinize any part of the selection system. Therefore, if the number of minorities in a given job classification such as staff nurse or unit secretary is representative of the community at large, there is no purely legal reason to do validation studies and many institutions do not do them. In any case, content validity (being based on job content) can always be used and should be in most situations, regardless of whether an institution believes there may be adverse impact in given job categories.

Content validity is a logical process demonstrating that the predictor is an actual sample of the tasks and duties required of a job incumbent or reflects an actual part of the job. Content validity is most often used for work sample or job knowledge predictors such as interviews, typing tests, and assessment centers. A content validation study begins with a job analysis to identify the major tasks and KSAs required for the job. Each predictor currently in use must be shown to reflect these tasks or KSAs or must be dropped. Some major tasks or KSAs may not be reflected in an existing predictor. New predictors, such as interview questions, work samples, or paper-and-pencil tests, should be developed or purchased to measure such tasks or KSAs. The preparation of an interview guide, de-

scribed earlier in this chapter, is an example of a content validation study.

Assessing empirical validity is not always easy but most organizations should be able to perform the simple test of validity described below. As applicants are hired, the evaluations used for the hiring decision should be retained by the HRM office, not the applicant's new supervisor. After a suitable period of time, the new hire's job performance should be measured and compared to the hiring evaluation. Figure 13–9 is a graphical depiction of a situation in which 70 applicants were interviewed and hired by a nursing department over the period of a year.

FIGURE 13–9 VALIDATING THE SELECTION INTERVIEW

		Marginal (25)	High (45)
Performance	**High (30)**	5	25
	Moderate (25)	10	15
	Low (15)	10	5

Interview assessment

Taken from J.G. Goodale, *The Fine Art of Interviewing* (Englewood Cliffs, N.J.: Prentice-Hall, 1982). Used by permission.

After they had been employed for at least six months, their performance appraisal forms were collected and grouped into three categories of performance: high, moderate, and low.

These three *performance ratings* are listed on the left side of the table, and the *interview assessments* (whether they were rated high or marginal for future performance) are across the bottom. In this example, 45 of the applicants were assessed to be in the high category and 25 in the marginal one. Of the 45 applicants who rated high, the performance appraisals showed 25 to be performing well, 15 moderately well, and only 5 low. This indicates a fairly good level of selection accuracy. If the same proportion was true for the 25 initially assessed as marginal, this would not indicate high validity. More sophisticated correlational analysis of validity is possible with larger numbers of applicants.

It is important that nursing departments examine the validity of their selection procedures, even if the only procedure is interviewing. Only then can managers be sure that the selection of applicants is being done effectively. Validity and other legal issues regarding selection are discussed in Arvey and Faley (1988) and in Gatewood and Feild (1990).

SUMMARY

♦ The selection of staff is a critical function that requires matching people to jobs. Responsibility for hiring is often shared by HRM and nurse managers.

♦ Selection processes most often include screening application forms, résumés, medical exams, reference checks, and interviews but may also include tests and assessment centers.

♦ Job analysis is fundamental to all selection efforts because it defines the job. Selection procedures are designed to elicit information about the applicant. Then people can be placed in positions for which they are suited.

♦ Recruitment is the process of locating and attracting enough qualified applicants to provide a pool from which the required number of new staff members can be chosen. Poor-quality applicants and/or a small pool will result in poorer matches between jobs and applicants.

♦ Selection interviewing is a complex skill that is intended to obtain information about the applicant and give the applicant information about the institution.

♦ There are several principles of effective interviewing: *plan* and structure the interview, *respond* to the applicant to encourage rapport, *elicit* information through questioning techniques, *give* realistic job information, and *process* the information obtained to make a final placement decision.

♦ Developing a structured interview guide is a critical element in selection interviewing because it establishes the content validity of the interviewing process, is legally sound, helps the interview "stay on track," and provides a mechanism for taking and storing notes that relate the applicant to the job requirements.

♦ Tests and assessment centers are complicated, standardized mechanisms for gathering application data that are sometimes used in selection. The nurse manager is not always involved in the use of these selection techniques. Assessment centers are most often used in hiring managers.

♦ All selection systems should be job related as demonstrated by validation studies. The validity of a selection system provides a defense against charges of discrimination on the basis of race, color, sex, religion, or national origin, which is a requirement of the Civil Rights Act of 1964. Two other, and less common, defenses against charges of discrimination are BFOQ and business necessity.

BIBLIOGRAPHY

Arvey, R. D., and Faley, R. H. (1988). *Fairness in Selecting Employees*. Reading, MA: Addison-Wesley.

Bouchard, T. J., Jr. (1976). "Field Research Methods: Interviewing, Questionnaires, Participant Observation, Systematic Observation, Unobtrusive Measures." In: *Handbook of Industrial and Organizational Psychology*. Dunnette, M. D. (editor). Chicago: Rand McNally.

Breaugh, J. A., and Mann, R. B. (1984). "Recruiting Source Effects: A Test of Two Alternative Explanations." *Journal of Occupational Psychology*, 57: 261–262.

Cascio, W. F. (1987). *Applied Psychology in Personnel Management*. Reston, VA: Reston.

Chase, J. A. (1988). "Certification and Job Analysis." *Orthopaedic Nursing*, 7(2): 26–29.

Decker, P. J., and Cornelius, E. T., III. (1979). "A Note on Recruiting Sources and Job Survival Rates." *Journal of Applied Psychology*, 64: 463.

Decker, P. J., Moore, R. C., and Sullivan, E. (1982). "How Hospitals Can Solve the Nursing Shortage." *Hospital Health Services Administration*, 27(6): 12.

Fox, V., and Blue, Sister M. R. (1988). "Job Analysis, National Certification Board: Perioperative Nursing Inc., Document." *AORN Journal*, 47(5): 1256–1269.

Gatewood, R. D., and Feild, H. S. (1990). *Human Resource Selection*. Chicago: Dryden.

Goodale, J. G. (1982). *The Fine Art of Interviewing*. Englewood Cliffs, NJ: Prentice-Hall.

Moses, J., and Byham, W. (1977). *Applying the Assessment Center Method*. New York: Pergamon Press.

Norton, S. D., and Crissman, S. (1992). "Staffing: Recruiting, Selecting, and Promoting." In: *Nursing Administration*. Decker, P., and Sullivan, E. J. (editors). Norwalk, CT: Appleton & Lange.

Poteet, G. (1984). "The Employment Interview: Avoiding Discriminatory Questioning." *Journal of Nursing Administration*, 14(4): 38–42.

Spurlock v. United Airlines, 475 F.2d 216 (10th Cir. 1972), pp. 218–219.

STAFF DEVELOPMENT AND PATIENT EDUCATION

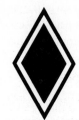

STAFF DEVELOPMENT
Needs Assessment
Planning and Implementation
Learning Principles
Memory Span
Social Learning Theory
Relapse Prevention
Adult Education Theory
Staff Development

EVALUATION

PATIENT EDUCATION
Barriers to Teaching
The Staff Development Department
Record Keeping and Evaluation

Every individual is unique and will, therefore, vary in education, skills, and ability. There are a few common denominators: new staff nurses will have attended nursing school and new unit clerks will have attended high school, trade school, or college. Yet many within each group probably will not have developed all of the skills and knowledge necessary to perform their jobs at the expected level. Further, new nursing practices and technology call for continuing staff education. One of the nursing manager's major responsibilities is to assist subordinates in developing specific job skills, an activity usually referred to as *staff development*.

Most early educational theories were based on the belief that the fundamental purpose of education was the transmission of the totality of human knowledge from one generation to the next. This is a workable assumption provided that the quantity of knowledge is small enough to be collectively managed by the educational system and that the rate of change is small enough to enable the increase of knowledge to be packaged and delivered. Today, however, these conditions do not exist. Instead, we live in a period of knowledge explosion in which cultural and technological change are rapid. This means that we simply cannot pass the totality of human knowledge from one generation to the next. We cannot even keep up year by year. The implications of this are twofold. First, education will no longer be primarily or exclusively directed toward children. We will see much more education of adults, and that education will be specifically formulated for adults. Second, we will see education moved to a partnership between the teacher and the learner so that it occurs every day in an unstructured manner.

The process of education can be considered to operate constantly during conscious human activity and calls for consideration of several issues: how people learn, the content of what they need to learn, the processes of learning, and how to teach. People even need to be taught how to learn so they can do their learning efficiently and are prepared to learn new information as it becomes available.

Every health care institution has specific goals, and their attainment requires trained personnel. Therefore, most institutions have specialized educational personnel, either assigned directly to nursing service or in separate education departments. Such departments administer ongoing employee development programs and often orientation programs, yet the nurse manager, too, often is extensively involved in the instructional process. A new employee, for example, must be taught specific work rules and tasks as well as new nursing or medical practices at the unit level. Nurse managers are also extensively involved in patient education. Trained personnel are the key to success in a unit and in the institution itself. Properly educating employees usually results in higher productivity, fewer accidents or mistakes, better morale, greater pride in work, and better nursing care.

Whether educational activities are planned for staff or patients, the basic model of the staff development function or the basic process of education remains the same. Figure 14–1 shows this process, which is similar to the nursing process and includes assessment, planning, implementation, and evaluation. *Assessment* is the process of investigation that provides knowledge about the learner's readiness to learn and her or his specific learning needs, such as skill, ability, or knowledge. *Planning* entails obtaining learning resources to present to the learner and the matching of educational needs and methods. *Implementation* is the gathering together of the educators, the learners, and all of the materials and methods needed for the educational program(s). *Evaluation* is an investigative process in which one determines whether the education was cost-effective, whether the objective was achieved, and whether the learning was transferred from the learning site to actual use on the job.

♦ STAFF DEVELOPMENT

NEEDS ASSESSMENT

The first step in staff development is to determine that a need for an educational program exists. An institution should commit its resources to an educational activity only if, in the best judgment of its nurse managers, the education can be expected to achieve some organizational goal such as better patient care, reduced operating cost, or more efficient or satisfied personnel. Only educational institutions can legitimately view education as an end in itself.

This naturally leads to a question: On what should education resources be spent? This decision must be based on the best available data. In hospitals, these data can come from staff development specialists, other knowledgeable managers in the organization, and continuous systematic and accurate analysis of the personnel's educational needs. In educational institutions,

the decision comes from monitoring the needs and resources of the community and the kinds of behaviors that are useful in the sites that employ the institution's graduates.

A health care institution seeks behavioral change or increased knowledge as a means toward some organizational goal. For the educational institution, the process is fairly simple: determine what behaviors are needed by the employees and then teach those new behaviors. To the extent that the employees change their behavior to that which is desired, the education is successful. For the health care institution, the problem is more complex. First, those activities that can be made more effective by educational efforts that change behavior must be identified. Also, a great deal of maintenance-type instruction is always going on in any organization. This type of instruction is used with both new employees and current employees who are promoted. A certain amount of staff development resources must be assigned to such instruction. The remaining resources should be aimed at specific activities that will increase the effectiveness of the organization.

Too often, staff development programs are initiated simply because they have been well advertised and marketed or because other organizations have found them useful; however, it

---

FIGURE 14-1 STAFF DEVELOPMENT MODEL

Assessment ⟶ **Planning** ⟶ **Implementation** ⟶ **Evaluation**

Assessment	Planning	Implementation	Evaluation
Learner's readiness to learn	Finding resources	Learners	Cost-effective
Learning needs	Matching needs and methods	Educators	Achievement
Skill/ability/knowledge		Materials	Transfer of learning
		Methods	

BOX 14–1
CASE: EDUCATION IS
NOT ALWAYS THE ANSWER

A sales representative for a medical equipment company was concerned that not enough blood tubing was being used in the institution considering the amount of blood being utilized from the blood bank. This representative felt that nurses did not understand the advantages of using the special blood tubing. He made plans to fly in two of the company educators to hold round the clock classes for personnel in the 30+ units in the hospital. This effort would have taken several days and would have been very costly. The assistant director for staff development investigated the problem to make sure that the planned intervention was necessary and had the potential to solve the problem. This investigation revealed that the new blood tubing

was stocked at the pharmacy. The blood bank still issued the old tubing when filling blood requests. A simple phone call to the pharmacy and blood bank resulted in the pharmacy issuing the tubing to the blood bank, which now stocks both types of tubing and issues the appropriate set for each patient/nursing unit. Information for staff was provided in the regular inservice education settings instead of in the costly special classes that originally had been planned. A nine-month follow-up revealed that correct tubing was being used. This management problem was corrected by the staff development director's initiative and subsequently, a simple change in availability of the equipment.

---

does not make sense for an organization to adopt an expensive staff development effort simply because other organizations are doing it. Such a faddish practice can be reduced by systematically determining educational needs and using them as a base for developing very specific content. In this way, organizations use staff development programs only for people and situations where needed.

PLANNING AND IMPLEMENTATION

After the needs have been determined, the next step is to plan the staff development program. Nurse managers usually are involved in educating their staffs and patients, but they don't necessarily have to do it themselves. They can routinely delegate it to other staff members or to a staff nurse who becomes a preceptor (a staff member who supervises the instruction of an

employee). It can be done through the closed-circuit television system in the institution, by educational specialists assigned to either nursing service or an education department. Thus, the nurse manager has many resources for staff development at her or his disposal.

Wexley and Latham (1981) suggest three main questions to be considered in assessment and planning: Is the individual educable? How should the staff development program be arranged to facilitate learning? What can be done to ensure that what is learned will be transferred to the job? There are no well-developed and tested theories of learning to answer these questions, so educators must rely on simple principles of learning and basic knowledge about educational methods to develop instructional interventions. Also, theories of motivation (see Chapter 9) can help ensure that the learner has a desire to learn and to apply any skills or concepts that are taught.

LEARNING PRINCIPLES

Two sets of principles guide learning activities. One set has been found to facilitate learning and another to determine the degree of transfer of learning from the educational context to the job.

READINESS TO LEARN.   Before the learner can benefit from any formal education, he or she must be ready to learn. Readiness refers to both the maturational and experiential factors in the learner's background that are critical for further learning. Students do not take algebra, for instance, before they take basic math, and after algebra they take geometry, trigonometry, and calculus, in that order. The logic is that learner readiness at any stage is primarily due to previous learning in particular subjects. Educational programs fail if the prerequisite skills and knowledge are not considered, since it is very difficult to learn a new sequence of behaviors if the component behaviors have not been previously learned. Maturational factors also relate to readiness to learn. There are limits to the amount of information a person can acquire and retain at any one time.

MOTIVATION TO LEARN.   Most researchers agree that motivation affects performance through an energizing function: A motivated individual works harder to achieve a consequence. Motivation has been studied in two ways: (a) the process, which seeks to explain *how* behavior is energized, directed, sustained, and stopped; and (b) the content, which considers which specific things motivate specific people. In education, motivation exercises its influence in two areas: (a) motivation to attend to the ed-

ucational content and (b) reinforced motivation, in the form of anticipated benefits, for accurate behavioral rehearsal and practice. If learners are informed in advance about the benefits that will result from learning the content and adopting the modeled behavior, it strengthens their motivation. Furthermore, anticipated benefits can strengthen retention of what has been learned observationally by motivating people to encode and rehearse modeled behavior that they value. Motivation, of course, is only one of the things that commands attention. It is difficult *not* to hear compelling sounds or to look at captivating visual displays.

The learner's first attempt to reproduce the target behavior may not always be successful; reinforcement from teachers and other learners helps the behavior to endure. When individuals try to reproduce learning demonstrations, they compare their attempt with the symbolic representation they have retained. Through practice, they correct their reproduction attempts until the reproduction matches the symbolic representation. This is *self-reinforcement*. Furthermore, maintenance of behavior can be influenced by external reinforcement (i.e., rewards or benefits) on the job.

CONDITIONS FOR PRACTICE.   Learning theory research has shown that when a complex task is to be learned, it should be broken down into its parts and each part should be learned separately, starting with the simplest and going on to the most difficult. However, *part learning* should be combined with *whole learning*—that is, learners should be shown the whole performance so they know what their goal is and where they are going. The educational content should then be broken down into integrated parts, and each part should be learned in practice until it is retained intact and can be recalled accurately. Then a learner should be allowed to put all of the parts together and practice the whole performance.

It has also been determined that spaced practice is more effective than massed practice, especially for motor skills. If the learner has to concentrate for long periods of time without some rest, learning and retention suffer. It's a little like cramming for an examination: the test scores are usually relatively high, but rapid forgetting sets in very soon. Consequently, spaced practice seems to be more productive for long-term retention and for transfer of learning to the work setting.

Overlearning, or practicing beyond the point of first accurate recall/reproduction, can be critical in both acquisition and transfer of knowledge and skills. Overlearning is desirable in a program when the task to be learned is not likely to be immediately practiced in the work situation and also when performance must be maintained during periods of emergency and stress. Consequently, in any learning situation, practice should be encouraged to the point of overlearning.

TRANSFER OF LEARNING. The ultimate goal of any educational program, especially in organizational staff development, is that the learning be transferred into the context in which it will be used. Ellis has made the following suggestions for maximizing transfer. First, maximize the similarity between the educational context and the job (ultimate transfer) context; the instruction should look as much like the job, or like the situation where the behavior is to be used, as possible. Adequate practice—in fact, overlearning—is recommended.

Second, transfer does not occur until the learning has become part of long-term memory. The practice should include a variety of stimulus situations so that learners learn to generalize their knowledge. Third, transfer occurs more readily when the important features of the content to be learned can be labeled or identified to distinguish the major steps involved. Finally, the general principles underlying the specific content or behavior to be learned should be understood or coded along with the physical behavior. This can be done by asking the learner to apply the general principles in a variety of situations and by supplying her or him with a written description of the rules that underlie the behavior across contexts (Ellis, 1965).

MEMORY SPAN

The ability to retain what has been learned is obviously relevant to the effectiveness of a staff development program; yet generally speaking, the better the memory, the more effective the learning. There are two types of memory: short-term and long-term. *Short-term memory* is a system that stores information for current attention and where actual information processing is carried out. The amount of energy or capacity available to short-term memory is limited; thus, only a few storage or processing activities can be carried out simultaneously. *Long-term memory,* in contrast, represents the products of an individual's experience that have been processed through short-term memory and then stored for long-term use. Products in the long-term memory range from individual letter or word codes to more general things such as strategies for processing and maintaining information.

Many factors have been found to increase memory span. *Rehearsal* is perhaps the simplest strategy that can be used to process and store things for long-term memory. Rehearsal is generally viewed as an interactive process. It maintains information in short-term memory by ensuring a sufficiently high level of activation and it facilitates the transfer of information to long-term memory. Adults have the capacity to rehearse several different items at the same time, while children under nine years old usually do not. The more rehearsal a person experiences, the better will be the performance in recall tasks.

Grouping of items or activities to be learned also tends to increase memory span. Groups of no more than three or four are best when items are presented orally; more items (four to six) can be included in a group when sequences are presented visually. Adults tend to group spontaneously to enhance memory. Recall is also enhanced when grouping is prompted by an experimenter.

A third facilitator of memory span is *"chunking,"* which refers to the recording of two or more nominally independent items of information into a single familiar unit. Thus, only familiar sequences can be chunked, and the more familiar the sequence, the greater the ease with which it can be chunked. Short-term memory has only limited capacity to chunk, but the amount of information that can be stored and processed through short-term memory increases in direct proportion to the size of the chunk. Consequently, any time a given amount of information can be recoded and represented in a smaller space, memory is enhanced.

Organization also enhances memory span. With increasing maturity, people become increasingly able to package material so that it is organizationally consistent with already stored material. The more organized the material presented, the more likely it is to be learned.

SOCIAL LEARNING THEORY

Social learning theory attempts to integrate much of what we know about how people learn. It suggests that a person can observe her or his own behavior and that of others and use this observation to plan future action. How a person behaves over time influences what that person becomes. People think about *when* to use behavior and try to use certain behaviors to increase the likelihood of positive consequences. If these positive consequences occur, the response will probably be more use of the behavior.

Social learning theory is a behavioral theory and it builds on principles of reinforcement theory. Bandura (1977) explains that, except for elementary reflexes, people are not equipped with an inborn repertoire of behavior. Instead, new response patterns are acquired either by direct experience or by observation.

Positive and negative results affect the actions of people in their day-to-day functioning. Some behaviors are successful (rewarded or satisfying) and some are not; some actually result in punishing consequences. Through this process of differential reinforcement, successful behaviors

---

FIGURE 14–2 REINFORCEMENT PROCESS

Positive Reinforcement (reward)

Stimulus ⟶ Behavior ⟶ Positive consequences (behavior will increase)

Negative Reinforcement (punishment)

Stimulus ⟶ Behavior ⟶ Adverse consequences (behavior will diminish)

Adapted from P. J. Decker, *Health Care Management Microtraining*, St. Louis: Decker & Associates, 1983. Used by permission.

are retained and behavior that leads to no consequence or a punishing consequence is no longer used. This is shown in Figure 14–2. In a given situation, a behavior that leads to a positive consequence (reward) is repeated (positive reinforcement). If the consequence is negative (punishment), the behavior is not repeated. If we learned everything in this trial-and-error way, though, it would be impossible to explain the quickness of human learning, learning that occurs without evidence of behavior change (no-trial learning), and how the human species has survived.

In the social learning analysis of behavior, information about oneself and the nature of the environment is developed and verified through four different processes. First, people derive much of their knowledge from direct experience of the effects produced by their actions. Second, information about the environment is frequently extracted from vicarious experience: observation of the effects produced by someone else's actions. Third, when vicarious experience is limited, people can develop and evaluate their conceptions about the environment in terms of the judgment voiced by others. Last, people can use the information gained from active, vicarious, and social sources of verification (all of which rely on external influences or sources) as a basis for logical determination of the nature of the environment. After people acquire rules of inference based on active, vicarious, or social sources, they can evaluate the soundness of their reasoning through logical processes, either inductive or deductive.

Social learning theory suggests that anticipation of reinforcement is one of several factors that influence what is observed and what goes unnoticed (see Figure 14–3). Knowing that a given person's (the *model*) behavior effectively

FIGURE 14–3 SOCIAL LEARNING THEORY

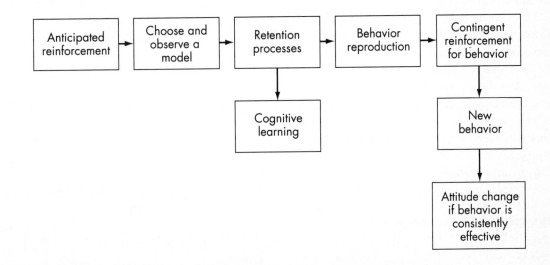

produces valued outcomes or avoids punishing ones increases the observer's attentiveness to the model's actions. This suggests, furthermore, that observational learning is more effective when observers are informed in advance about the benefits of adopting a model's behavior; this is preferable to waiting until the observers produce imitative behavior and then rewarding them.

However, attending to a model's behavior is insufficient unless several retention processes are used so that the behavior is actually learned and retained. According to social learning theory, behavior is learned symbolically through cognitive processes before it is performed. Then, after these cognitive processes have been completed, a person tries out the behavior. If it leads to positive consequences, it will be used in the future. This is the motivational process that maintains the new behavior. By observing the model, an individual forms an idea of how and in what sequence response components must be combined to produce a desired new behavior. People guide their actions by prior notions rather than relying on the outcomes to tell them what they must do.

Modeling transmits information to observers about new responses and how these responses can be combined into new patterns. This information can be conveyed by physical demonstration, pictorial representation, or verbal description. Much social learning occurs on the basis of casual observation of the behavior of others. However, people also learn desired behaviors through written descriptions of how to behave and from different media sources such as television.

RELAPSE PREVENTION

Marx (1982) presents a model to increase the long-term maintenance of newly learned behaviors. This model emphasizes the learning of a set of self-control and coping strategies (see Figure 14–4).

The first step is to make learners aware of the relapse process itself. Most staff development programs are presented as being quite successful. Awareness of what may make the program vulnerable is neglected and learners consequently may not be able to avoid situations in which the educational content will be unsuccessful. Learners are asked to pinpoint situations that are likely to sabotage their efforts. Learners can then be (a) taught to anticipate high-risk situations, (b) taught coping strategies for avoiding high-risk situations, and (c) taught that slight slips or relapses are predictable outcomes of any educational paradigm and need not become full-blown relapses. These techniques should increase learners' self-efficacy (feelings of control over the situation requiring use of the content).

The importance of this model is in showing that learners' exposure to possible failure situations enables them to expect and prepare for such situations in advance. This advance mental preparation for trying situations decreases the probability of small relapses turning into absolute failure due to the "*abstinence violation effect*." The effect occurs when guilt over a small violation of the instructional content leads a learner through cognitive dissonance to deny the possible effectiveness of the content. Such denial almost guarantees that a small slip will end up as a total relapse or non-use of the content. Again, the keys are (a) awareness of the relapse process, (b) identification of high-risk situations, and (c) the development of coping responses. The learner should not be afraid to discuss possible failure situations and ways to cope with them. Better yet, learners should practice such situations using the content in the neutral environment of education. In this way the learners prepare themselves for the difficult situations. But, the learners will not be motivated to prepare for the difficult situations unless they know about the relapse process.

ADULT EDUCATION THEORY

Thirty years ago, the only educational concepts and techniques available were those developed for the education of children. It was assumed that anybody who knew anything about basic education and was reasonably good at managing the development and logistics of educational programs could be a good teacher of adults. However, in the last 10 to 20 years, varying techniques for helping adults to learn have been developed, and one of the primary discoveries is that adults as learners are very different from children. Knowles suggests there are no funda-

mental differences in the ways adults and children learn, but he does point to significant differences that come from the situations surrounding adult and child learning. He suggests four basic concepts (see Figure 14–5) on which differences in adult and child education can be shown (Knowles, 1970).

The first is the individual's *self-concept*. Children see themselves as dependent persons but, as they move toward adulthood, they become increasingly aware of themselves and their own decision making and they become very capable in self-direction. This change in self-concept from dependency to independent autonomy characterizes maturity. Adults tend to resent being in situations where they are treated with a lack of respect, talked down to, judged, or oth-

FIGURE 14–4 A MODEL OF THE EDUCATIONAL RELAPSE PROCESS

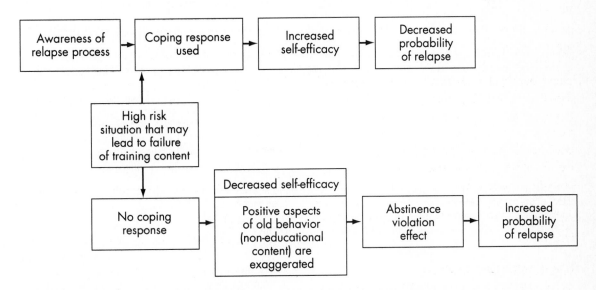

Adapted from R.D. Marx, "Relapse Prevention for Managerial Training: A Model for Maintenance of Behavior Change," *Academy of Management Review.* 7(3): 433-441. Used by permission.

erwise treated like children. Thus, adult educators should be facilitators rather than dominant teachers and the adult learner should have some input into what is taught.

The second concept is *experience*. Adults have accumulated vast quantities of experience whereas children have not, and that experience can lead adults to make choices about what is

FIGURE 14-5 CHARACTERISTICS OF ADULT LEARNERS AND EDUCATIONAL IMPLICATIONS

Characteristics of Adult Learners	Implications for Adult Learning
Self-concept: The adult learner sees himself as capable of self-direction and desires others to see him the same way. In fact, one definition of maturity is the capability to be self-directing.	A climate of openness and respect is helpful in identifying what the learners want and need to learn.
	Adults enjoy planning and carrying out their own learning exercises.
	Adults need to be involved in evaluating their own progress toward self-chosen goals.
Experience: Adults bring a lifetime of experience to the learning situation. Youths tend to regard experience as something that has happened to them, while to an adult, his experience is him. The adult defines who he is in terms of his experience.	Less use is made of transmittal techniques; more of experiential techniques.
	Discovery of how to learn from experience is key to self-actualization.
	Mistakes are opportunities for learning.
	To reject adult experience is to reject the adult.
Readiness to learn: Adult developmental tasks increasingly move toward social and occupational role competence and away from the more physical developmental tasks of childhood.	Adults need opportunities to identify the competency requirements of their occupational and social roles.
	Adult readiness-to-learn and teachable moments peak at those points where a learning opportunity is coordinated with a recognition of the need-to-know.
	Adults can best identify their own readiness-to-learn and teachable moments.
A problem-centered time perspective: Youth thinks of education as the accumulation of knowledge for use in the future. Adults tend to think of learning as a way to be more effective in problem solving today.	Adult education needs to be problem-centered rather than theoretically oriented.
	Formal curriculum development is less valuable than finding out what the learners need to learn.
	Adults need the opportunity to apply and try out learning quickly.

Taken from Knowles, M.S. *The Modern Practice of Adult Education.* (New York: Association Press, 1970). Used by permission.

taught and in what format. In adult education, this should be valued because the teacher can use theory to integrate and formalize it. The educator knows the theory, but the learners have the experience. In contrast to child education, which is oriented toward one-way communication, assigned readings, and audiovisual presentations, adult education should therefore include experiential learning, two-way and multidirectional communication such as group discussions, role playing, teamwork exercises, and skill practice sessions. This way, the experience of all participants can be brought out and focused on the problem being discussed.

The third concept is *readiness to learn*. The main task of child education is to sequence the learning activities in a way that fits the developmental steps of the content. Adults, however, have already completed their basic education in reading, writing, speech, and so on, and their developmental tasks increasingly relate to the social roles that form their immediate concerns: working, living, family, recreational activities, and the like. In child education, the teacher decides on both the content to be learned and how and in what sequence learning will take place. In adult education, the learners themselves can help to identify what they wish to learn and the sequence of learning. The teacher of adults acts as a resource person to help learners form interest groups to diagnose their learning needs.

The last concept is the *time perspective*. Education has been considered in terms of preparation for the future rather than preparation for the present. Thus, child education is the business of having students store up information for use on some far-off day; teachers present information neatly packaged so students can use it later. But in adult education, learning is problem-centered rather than subject-centered. Adult education is a process for defining problems and solving them for the present.

STAFF DEVELOPMENT

Education in hospitals includes programs for patients, their families, staff, and members of the general community. Education can be divided into two areas: staff development and patient education. *Inservice education* refers to the continuing education that seeks to improve staff members' knowledge of or ability to perform job-related tasks. Sometimes this is referred to as staff development, although the latter usually includes management training and other areas of staff enrichment such as assertiveness, counseling skills, and group process skills. Much of this staff development is done by the education department, but in this chapter, the focus is primarily on on-the-job instructional techniques and orientation. Patient education follows.

ORIENTATION. Getting an employee started in the right way is important. Among other things, a well-planned orientation reduces the anxiety that new employees feel when beginning the job. In addition, socialization into the workplace contributes to unit effectiveness by reducing dissatisfaction, absenteeism, and turnover (see Chapters 13 and 16).

Orientation is a joint responsibility of both the institution's staff development personnel and the nursing manager. In most institutions the new staff nurse completes the hospital orientation program, followed by an onsite orientation by the nurse manager or someone appointed to do this. There should be a clear understanding of the specific responsibilities of development and unit staff so nothing is left to chance. The development staff should provide information involving matters that are organization-wide in nature and relevant to all new employees, such as information regarding such things as the cafeteria, benefits, parking, or work hours. The nursing manager concentrates on those items unique to the employee's specific job.

New employees, as discussed in Chapter 13, often have unrealistically high expectations about the amount of challenge and responsibility they will find in their first job. Then, if they are assigned fairly undemanding, entry-level tasks, they feel discouraged and disillusioned. The result is job dissatisfaction, turnover, and low productivity, so one function of orientation is to correct any unrealistic expectations. The nurse manager needs to outline very specifically what is expected of new employees and assure them that they will eventually be able to progress to more challenging tasks. Such *realistic job previews* should cover the informal or non-concrete aspects of the job about which an employee could possibly have more unrealistic expectations than such concrete areas as the pay scale or hours.

Socialization of new employees can sometimes be very difficult because of the anxiety people feel when they first come on the job. They simply do not hear all of the information they are given, they spend a lot of energy attempting to integrate and interpret the information, and they consequently miss some information. One company experimented with incorporating a six-hour anxiety reduction session into its normal orientation period. The group did not have to work that first day but were allowed to relax, sit back, and use that time to get acquainted with the organization and their new co-workers. This increased the learning rate of the new employees, increased productivity, and lowered absenteeism and tardiness (Knowles, 1970).

Since nurse managers are an extremely important part of the socialization process, everything that they expect of the new employee should be discussed openly and specifically. The new employee adapts more rapidly to the new

unit if this is done. Everything from standards of performance, attendance, and how to treat the patients to what to expect as far as feedback in performance appraisal should be discussed.

One method of orientation is to use the *preceptor model* to assist the new employee and the staff nurse. The preceptor model provides a means for orientation and socialization of the new nurse as well as providing a mechanism to recognize exceptionally competent staff nurses (May, 1980). Staff nurses who serve as preceptors are selected based on their clinical competence, organizational skills, ability to guide and direct others, and concern for the effective orientation of new nurses. The primary goal is for the preceptor to assist the new nurse to acquire the necessary knowledge and skills so that he or she can function effectively on the division.

Preceptorships offer new nurses the advantage of an on-the-job instruction program tailored specifically to their needs. Staff nurses (preceptors) benefit by having an opportunity to sharpen their clinical skills, increasing their personal and professional satisfaction. The new nurse will work closely with the preceptor for approximately three weeks, although the duration of the preceptorship may vary depending on the nurse's individual learning needs or the hospital's policies.

The preceptor's role is that of orientor, teacher, resource person, counselor, role model, and evaluator (Murphy & Hammerstad, 1981). The primary function of the preceptor is to orient the new nurse to the unit. This includes proper socialization of the new nurse within the group as well as familiarizing her or him with unit functions. The preceptor teaches any unfamiliar procedures and helps the new nurse develop any necessary skills. The preceptor acts as a resource person on matters of division functions as well as policies and procedures.

New nurses may need to utilize their preceptors as counselors as they make their transition to the unit. If new nurses experience discrepancy between their educational preparation or their expectations and the realities of working in the unit, the preceptor's role as counselor can prove invaluable in helping them cope with "reality shock."

The preceptor also serves as a staff nurse role model; the new nurse not only learns actual work-related tasks, but also observes the preceptor to learn how to set priorities, problem solve and make decisions, manage time, delegate tasks, and interact with others (Murphy & Hammerstad, 1981). In addition, the preceptor evaluates the new nurse's performance and provides both verbal and written feedback to encourage development.

The department of education plays an integral role in the preceptor concept. The education staff provide the new nurse an initial orientation, familiarization with the institution and the general policies and procedures before beginning work with the preceptor. The education personnel also provide the necessary education for staff nurses to become preceptors. The department of education's function is to teach the staff nurse the role of a preceptor, the principles of adult education applicable to educational needs, how to teach necessary skills, how to plan as well as evaluate teaching and learning objectives, and how to provide both formal and informal feedback. Thus, the education department assists the staff nurse in acquiring the necessary knowledge and skills to effectively educate new nurses.

STAFF DEVELOPMENT METHODS. Staff development can be divided into internal (on the unit) and external (off the unit) sources. Internal sources include on-the-job instruction, workshops for the unit nurses, and inservice programs. External sources are formal workshops presented by an education department within the hospital and all educational activities done outside the hospital, including college courses, conferences, and continuing education workshops.

It simply is not feasible to discuss the relative merits of the many educational methods available, but, based on the concepts of social learning theory, a model to evaluate the different training programs can be developed. For effective adult education, we need at minimum (a) presentation of the material, (b) practice of the material, and (c) feedback about that practice.

There must be opportunity for practice of the desired terminal behaviors and feedback about it. For instance, reading about or listening to a lecture about some clinical skill represents presentation of material, but it does not include practice of that skill. Or, if workers are shown how to perform a skill, practice it, and then walk away, there is no feedback. All three elements are essential.

The most widely used educational method is *on-the-job instruction*. This often includes assigning new employees to experienced nurses, preceptors, or the nurse manager. The learner is expected to learn the job by observing the experienced employee (preceptor) and by performing the actual tasks under supervision.

On-the-job instruction has several positive features, one of which is its cost-effectiveness. Learners learn effectively while providing some of the necessary nursing services. Moreover, it reduces the need for outside instructional facilities and reliance on professional educators. Transfer of learning is not an issue because the learning occurs on the actual job. However, on-the-job instruction often fails because it has not been formalized, and the on-the-job instructor does not know how to utilize learning theory. As a result, presentation, practice, or feedback may be neglected.

On-the-job instruction fulfills a very important function specifically because of the positive features listed above. However, staff members assigned to conduct on-the-job instruction may not view it as having equal value to more standardized and formal classroom instruction. Therefore, care should be taken to emphasize to both instructors and learners the positive nature of this kind of instruction. Assignments should be formalized so on-the-job instruction is not viewed as happenstance or second-class instruction.

Wexley and Latham make several suggestions for implementing effective on-the-job instruction programs:

1. Employees who function as educators must be convinced that educating new employees in no way jeopardizes their own job security, pay level, seniority, or status.

2. Individuals serving as educators should realize that this added responsibility will be instrumental in attaining other rewards for them.

3. Teachers and learners should be carefully paired to minimize any differences in background, language, personality, attitudes, or age that may inhibit communication and understanding.

4. Teachers should be selected on the basis of their ability to teach and their desire to take on this added responsibility.

5. Staff nurses chosen as teachers should be carefully educated in the proper methods of instruction.

6. It must be made clear to employees serving as teachers that their new assignment is by no means a chance to get away from their own jobs or "take a vacation."

7. Learners should be rotated to different teachers to compensate for weaker instruction by some teachers and to expose each learner to the specific know-how of various staff nurses or education department teachers.

8. The nurse manager must realize that the efficiency of the unit may be reduced when on-the-job instruction occurs.

9. The teacher and nurse manager must realize the importance of close supervision of the learner to prevent any major mistakes and the learning of incorrect procedures.

10. On-the-job instruction should be used in conjunction with other educational approaches. Obviously, the skill learning derived on the job should include theoretical as well as practice knowledge. For example, a knowledge of fluid and electrolyte balance is essential to nurses administering intravenous fluids (Wexley & Latham, 1981).

Figure 14–6 lists the key behaviors for on-the-job instruction, which include the "basic three" of presenting the material, allowing the employee to practice the skill, and providing feedback about that practice. These behaviors also incorporate most of the elements of learning theory discussed earlier in this chapter. Figure 14–7 shows a form on which the educators can write down the actual steps of the task and any key points to be made about those steps before beginning the staff development.

AUDIOVISUAL TECHNIQUES. With the increased size of health care institutions, rapid technological advances, and the number of people requiring instruction, there is always an attempt to make instructions more efficient and accelerate the learning process. Many organizations have therefore begun to use such audiovisual techniques as films, closed-circuit television, audiotapes, videotape recordings, computer-assisted instruction, and interactive video instruction. These methods allow an instructor's message to be given in a uniform manner on several occasions or at several locations at one time and be reused often. They can enhance the instructor's presentation as well as reduce the need for an instructor to present every detail.

Audiovisual materials can be used in almost every development situation, ranging from orientation to more complex uses. However, a film or videocassette is a teaching aid, not an educational program in itself; there still must be practice and feedback. Audiovisual methods can be effective if they are encompassed within a well-developed program rather than made a substitute for such a program.

Their use should be considered, first, when there is a need to illustrate certain procedures or with any kind of behavioral demonstration; second, when there is a need to expose learners to events not easily demonstrated in live presentations; third, when the education is organization-wide and it is far too costly for the teacher to travel from place to place or assemble everyone in one location; and fourth, when audiovisual instruction is supplemented with live lecture, discussion, and/or practice.

Good audiovisual materials need to be adequately introduced. Viewers need to be told what to look for and what they will be seeing. Follow-up discussion is very important and, if the audiovisual is used as a demonstration, then practice and feedback need to be part of the educational program. Remember, audiovisuals are not intended to stand alone in instruction, even though they are often misused in that manner. They should be carefully selected, adequately introduced, and followed up with adequate discussion, practice, and feedback.

See Wexley and Latham (1981) or Breckon (1982) for further information on educational methods.

♦ EVALUATION

Few issues in the education field create as much controversy or discussion as the word *evalua-*

FIGURE 14–6 KEY BEHAVIORS IN ON-THE-JOB INSTRUCTION

1. In writing, outline each step of the task to be taught.
2. Explain the objectives of the task to the employee.
3. Show the employee how to do it (without talking).
4. Explain key points (write them down if they are complex.)
5. Let the employee watch you do it again.
6. Let the employee do the simple parts of the task (optional).
7. Help the employee do the whole task (watch and give feedback).
8. Let the employee do the whole task (give feedback when task is finished).
9. Praise the employee for doing the task correctly.

Adapted from P. J. Decker, *Health Care Management Microtraining* (St. Louis: Decker & Associates, 1983). Used by permission.

tion. Educators usually agree on the *need* for sound appraisal of educational programs but rarely agree on the best method of evaluation and rarely do empirical evaluation. Typically, a program is reviewed at the corporate level and if it looks good the organization uses it. The same programs are used again and again. Sometimes the learners are asked how they liked it, but the

FIGURE 14-7 JOB BREAKDOWN SHEET FOR EDUCATIONAL PUPOSES

Department ———————————— Job ——————

Breakdown made by ————————————— Date ————

Important Steps (what to do)	**Key Points (how to do it)**
A logical segment of the operation, when something happens to advance the work	Anything that may: make or break the job; injure the worker; make the job easier to do

program continues until someone in a position of authority decides that it is no longer useful or no longer works or, more commonly, attendance decreases. All of this is done on the basis of opinions and judgments. Rarely are staff development programs evaluated to determine whether they have caused a change in behavior or in some organizational variable. Most evaluation is done at the end of the program with questionnaires, which provide very little information on whether the employees learned anything or if they will carry it through to the job. If money and time are put into developing an educational program (and billions of dollars are spent in this area), then money and time should also be put into evaluation to determine whether the program is actually doing what it was intended to do and then to take action based on the evaluations.

This leads to the question, "Why evaluate?" One reason to evaluate is to improve the program, to identify elements of it that need to be improved. Another reason for evaluation is to justify staff and budget allocations. If there are objective data to prove that an educational program does have a positive effect on day-to-day operating problems, rarely will money be cut from the staff development program budget. With effective evaluation of cost-effective staff development, the program will continue to be funded.

Despite its value, evaluation may still remain an absent ingredient. A major reason is the difficulty and cost of designing sound evaluation tools. Another reason is that the educator may not be interested in evaluating; she or he has no vested interest in doing so. Additionally, many educators lack the skills in experimental designs related to field settings that are required for organizational staff development evaluation. In short, unless an organization is committed to truly finding out whether its educational programs work, evaluation is not going to be done. This is regrettable, because it all too often results in the continuation of ineffective programs and the cancellation or misuse of effective ones.

Given the commitment, interest, and skills to do evaluation, however, a program's effectiveness can be evaluated in terms of four criteria: *learner reaction, learning, behavior change,* and/or *organizational impact. Learner reaction* is usually ascertained through a questionnaire completed at the end of a program. The questionnaire may contain questions concerning the program's content, the educator, the educator's objectives, the methods used, physical facilities, meals, and other facilities. The specific reactions that the organization wants to know about should be decided upon before the education and included in any questionnaire; irrelevant data should not be gathered.

Favorable learner reactions to a program do not guarantee that learning has taken place or that behavior has changed as a result of the educational program. Nevertheless, learner reactions are important because (a) reports of positive reactions help ensure organizational support for a program, (b) learner reactions can be used to assess the education, and (c) reaction data indicate whether the learners like the program.

Learning criteria assess the knowledge—the facts and figures—learned in the educational program. Knowledge is typically measured by paper-and-pencil tests that can include true-false, multiple choice, fill-in-the-blank, matching, and essay type questions.

But the acquisition of knowledge is not enough. Was that knowledge converted into *behavioral change*? One of the biggest problems is that instruction does not necessarily transfer from the classroom to the job—often because learners are taught the theory and principles of the technique but never learn how to translate this into behavior on the job. There is a big difference between the two, as evidenced by the many educational programs that teach factual material through lecture. A person going through such an educational program may cognitively remember the material but not have any new behavior to use on the job. A test at the end of such a program may prove that the instruction does, in fact, increase learning; if behavior is not measured after the program (or on the job), however, it is not known if the instructional program affects behavior or if it will help new behavior transfer to the job. The transfer of learning from classroom to job is critical, and measuring behavioral criteria is therefore very important in the business of teaching new skills.

The objectives of many staff development programs can be expressed in terms of some end result for the organization such as reduced turnover, fewer grievances, reduced absenteeism, increased quality of care, and fewer accidents. These are usually expressed in quantified data and can be easily tied to dollars.

It is often difficult to determine whether changes in such areas can be unequivocally attributed to the staff development program or to other variables in the organization such as changes in competitiveness or management, increased pay, new equipment, better selection, or changes of some other kind. In evaluating, particular care must be taken in deciding on the length of data collection, the unit of analysis, randomization, and other experimental design issues to be able to rule out the effect of these variables. The most important criteria for measuring results are those that are closely related to the key training behaviors. Despite all of the difficulties in collecting and analyzing such data, the educator should attempt to collect cost-related measures, as they give evidence to management that educational efforts do affect organizational effectiveness.

Figure 14–8 is an analysis form for assessing the cost-effectiveness of proposed programs. The first two items are simply the program name and description, and the next three look at implementation and predicted outcomes. The fifth item calls for identifiable benefits in terms of dollars. The sixth item is concerned with tangible costs; these are simply subtracted from the benefits to calculate probable net benefit/cost. The next two items consider intangible benefits and economic risks, while the last item covers any assumptions and other considerations that need to be calculated into this analysis. This form can be used to determine the probable dollar benefit to an organization conducting a staff development program; however, one should review Cascio (1982) to examine techniques to calculate human resource outcomes in terms of dollars.

Another consideration in determining cost-effectiveness is the direct meeting costs, especially for offsite meetings. For the most part, offsite meetings are not needed in behavioral training, but they are often used. Cascio discusses a method of calculating these costs, as shown in Figure 14–9 (Cascio, 1982). This form can be used to calculate the cost of off- versus onsite programs. It can also be used to determine how time should be spent during the instructional days and whether increasing or shortening instructional hours will in fact change the cost of the staff development program.

◆ PATIENT EDUCATION

A number of factors have converged to bring health teaching into prominence. The increasing

FIGURE 14–8 COST-EFFECTIVENESS ANALYSIS FORM

1. Program name:

2. Description: Legally required: ☐ yes ☐ no

3. Ease of implementation and any special requirements:

4. Expected economic benefits:

5. Total identifiable benefits:

	Potential revenue impact($) x	Probability of occurrence (0-1.0) =	Probable gross benefit($)
1.			
2.			
3.			
4.			
5.			
Total			

6. Total identifiable costs:

	Potential revenue cost($) x	Probability of use (0-1.0) =	Probable cost($)
1. Teacher time			
2. Instructional time			
3. Instructional facilities			
4. Meals/coffee, snacks			
5. Line personnel time			
6.			
7.			
8.			
Total			

7. Intangible cost and benefits:

8. Economic risks:
Consequences of not acting:

9. Assumptions and other considerations:

FIGURE 14–9 COST BREAKDOWN FOR AN OFFSITE MANAGEMENT MEETING

	Total costs	Cost per Participant per Day
I. Development of programs (figured on an annual basis)		
A. Staff development department overhead		
B. Staff development staff salaries		
C. Use of outside consultants		
D. Equipment and materials for meeting (films, supplies, workbooks)	$100,000	$100[1]
II. Participant cost (figured on an annual basis)		
A. Salaries and benefits of participants (figured for average participant)	$20,000	
B. Capital investment in participants (based on an average of various industries from *Fortune* magazine)	$25,000 $ 45,000	190.68[2]
III. Delivery of one meeting of 20 persons		
A. Facility costs		
1. Sleeping rooms	1,000	
2. Three meals daily	800	
3. Coffee breaks	60	
4. Misc. tips, telephone	200	
5. Reception	200 2,260	56.50[3]
B. Meeting charges		
1. Room rental		
2. A/V rental		
3. Secretarial services		
C. Transportation to the meeting	2,500	62.50[4]

Summary: Total Per Day Per Person Cost

I. Development of programs	$ 100
II. Participant cost	190
III. Delivery of one meeting (hotel and transportation)	119
Total	$ 409

Note: Meeting duration: two full days. Number of attendees: 20 people. These costs do not reflect a figure for the productive time lost of the people in the program. If that cost were added—and it would be realistic to do so—the above cost would increase dramatically.

[1]To determine per day cost, divide $100,000 by number of meeting days held per year (10). Then divide answer ($10,000) by total number of management people (100) attending all programs = $100 per day of a meeting.

[2]To determine per day cost, divide total of $45,000 by 236 (average number of working days in a year) = $190.68 per day of work year.

[3]To determine per day, per person cost, divide group total ($2,260) by number of participants (20) and then divide resulting figure ($133) by number of meeting days (2) = $56.50 per day.

[4]To determine per day, person cost, divide group total ($2,500) by number of people and then divide resulting figure ($125) by number of meeting days (2) = $62.50 per day.

Adapted from W. J. McKeon, "How to Determine Off-Site Meeting Costs" *Training and Development Journal* (May 1981): 117. Reprinted by permission.

effort in recent years to maintain health rather than just treat disease has enlarged the amount of knowledge people need and has demanded a change in attitudes about health and health care systems. Shortened hospital stays with early ambulation require preparation of the patient for convalescence at home. Long-term illnesses and disabilities have also increased, so that both patient and family need additional information to assist them in adjusting to daily life. The increase in malpractice suits has also caused an increase in patient education. (If it can be established that institutions and medical staff did not fully inform patients about what they were consenting to, liability may be established.) Finally, the need to control health care costs has led to an increase in patient teaching. This is especially important in these days of prospective reimbursement.

The Joint Commission for Accreditation of Healthcare Organizations (JCAHO) has detailed the need for patient education, and policy statements from both the American Medical Association and the American Hospital Association (AHA) have indicated hospitals' responsibility for educating patients. The AHA's 1982 statement says:

> A hospital has a responsibility to provide patient education services as an integral part of high quality cost effective care. Patient education services should enable patients and their families and friends when appropriate to make informed decisions about their health; to manage their illness; and to implement follow up care at home. Effective and efficient patient education services require planning and coordination, and responsibility for such planning and coordination should be assigned. The hospital should also provide the necessary staff and financial resources.

Nurse managers have several responsibilities in relation to patient education—first, to ensure that their staffs are prepared to function in this area. Nurse managers must document what is being done by their staffs and assess their quality of teaching, both written and oral. They must also be aware of institution-wide programming to avoid duplication of efforts and must serve on patient education committees, especially in their clinical specialties, to assist with program planning to meet the needs of their specific patients. They must identify both individual and general needs within their units, coordinate the patient education activities therein, and delegate responsibility to others. The staff must be provided with patient teaching skills and educational opportunities for their development.

Nurse managers may either do the patient teaching themselves, have staff nurses do it, ask the education department to assist the staff to develop the necessary skills, or utilize the group classes or video presentations being held on an institution-wide basis. Methods of delivery vary and may be either one-to-one or group teaching. Printed materials are helpful to patient and family, and effective audiovisual materials contribute to patient learning. The latter are most effective when they augment teaching done by individuals. No teaching tool can replace the personal, nurse-patient interaction.

Often staff nurses place a high value on patient teaching yet feel unprepared to teach. Most commonly, they feel they have a lack of content knowledge, teaching experience, skill in teaching techniques, or time. The nurse manager must correct these perceived deficiencies, and a good start would be to suggest that staff nurses read Redman (1980) and Corkadeel and McGlashan (1983). Patient education must go on at all times and at any location where effective learning can take place. It can be done while the nurse is caring for the patient at the bedside, during lab tests, in the hallway, and through watching television. It can be done by anyone in the hospital: any staff nurse, any nurse manager, a patient educator, or a specialized instructor.

BARRIERS TO TEACHING

A patient teaching program, even though it may utilize all of the activities in a learning process, may not always be successful. Certain factors can limit its effectiveness, and appropriate steps must be planned to minimize these barriers.

The first is *lack of priority.* If patient teaching is not given top priority by either the nurses or the institution, then it will probably not take place, even though opportunities for teaching are present. Specific ingredients essential in establishing patient education as a priority are: (a) development of a philosophy for patient education by the organization and by nurses; (b) commitment from hospital administration for support of patient education in terms of allocation of time, budget, and staffing; (c) inclusion of accountability for patient teaching as a component of performance evaluation; (d) rewards for doing it and sanctions for not doing it; and (e) provision of reinforcement and recognition for teaching efforts and accomplishments.

The second barrier is *lack of time.* Most nurses say they do not have enough time for patient teaching, often due to a heavy workload or inadequate staffing. It is important to foster the idea that patient education is not a 30-minute block of time specifically set aside to teach the patient. Questions can be answered and information given at any time the nurse is giving care.

The third barrier is *lack of communication.* Each of the staff members involved in a patient's care needs to know about the latter's learning needs. This can be communicated through documentation of teaching in the patient's chart. The fourth barrier is an individual nurse's *lack of knowledge;* accompanying this is usually *lack*

of confidence in ability to teach a patient. Consequently, content review is important for staff nurses and can be offered through patient education inservice programs or attendance at training sessions, workshops, and other continuing education programs.

The fifth barrier is *lack of training skill:* nurses need to know how to teach to be effective in patient education; with this knowledge, they are also more likely to teach. The skill to teach involves specific skills, including interpersonal sensitivity, the ability to communicate, and specific knowledge about how people learn. Corkadeel and McGlashan identify the specific patient teaching skills required of staff nurses as developing trust and rapport; recognizing and anticipating needs; assessing readiness to learn; developing and implementing teaching strategies; evaluating progress; and documenting and communicating (1983).

The sixth barrier to patient education is *lack of family involvement* in the teaching activities. The seventh barrier is *lack of continuity.* Again, many personnel interact daily with the patient and his or her family and may confuse them with different interpretations of facts and material. It is helpful if a detailed teaching record is maintained. The eighth barrier is *poor motivation,* on the patient's part, to learn. This can come from low self-esteem, a crowded schedule, lack of trust in and rapport with the staff, or fear. The ninth barrier is the *patient's physical condition.* Patients often cannot attend to the learning because they are weak or in pain.

The final barrier is the patient's *psychosocial adaptation to illness,* which may affect her or his motivation to learn. Readiness to learn differs at the various stages of the adaptation process. A major way to promote patient teaching is to assemble a patient education planning group. This should (a) help counteract physician resistance, to the extent that physicians are included in the planning group; (b) help develop a philosophy of patient education; (c) define staff expectations regarding patient teaching; and (d) build staff nurse knowledge of the learning process, including teaching skills as well as role clarification, nurse-patient rapport, content review, learning needs/assessment, assessment of readiness to learn, teaching strategies, and documentation.

THE STAFF DEVELOPMENT DEPARTMENT

An excellent resource for patient education in the institution is the staff development department, whose services can be used to increase the nursing staff's teaching skills and competencies. Such a department can offer courses, workshops, inservice and other patient education programs to improve the quality of patient teaching and promote consistency of information disseminated to patients. Often the patient education coordinator position is located within this department.

Having an institution-wide coordinator of patient education is a national trend. Among the reasons are the need for cost-effective programs; avoidance of duplication of efforts in program development and implementation; and centralization of planning, directing, and evaluating patient education programs. The patient education coordinator should be sought out for information, support, and assistance with any patient education situations or problems arising within the nursing units. Instructors within this department are also educational resources for the nurse manager.

In addition to the involvement in the preceptor program, the department of education interacts with nursing service by providing a variety of continuing education programs for nursing staff. The continuing education process begins

with new employee orientation, by introducing the nurse to institution policy and procedure, basic nursing skills, and CPR certification. Ongoing courses, workshops, and inservices conducted by the department of education provide current knowledge and skills to increase clinical competencies and ensure quality patient care. Department of education instructors provide consultation and facilitation services to each nursing division. The services help to identify and assess specific problems or unmet needs of individual nursing divisions.

RECORD KEEPING AND EVALUATION

All health care institutions and health education programs must keep records of patient education—records that can have a direct impact on any liability suit initiated by patients. Liability is usually based on negligence. Patients' records are written accounts of what happened to them while in the institution. They are admissible in court and can be subpoenaed; therefore, they should be complete and accurate. Entries should be made when teaching occurs, and each entry should be dated and signed. They should never be erased, even if incorrect, because the erasures may look like an attempt at concealment. If these basic procedures are followed, liability can usually be reduced.

A variety of educational records can be kept, including the referral forms used when patients are billed specifically for an educational program. Standing orders for educational programs may also be included in a patient's record. So should an intake interview that may include information about a patient's educational needs. It is important to document what has been taught to patients and their families, including whether comprehension or competency on the patient's part has been demonstrated. This can be ascertained by observing the patient, asking direct questions, and discussing specifics with the patient. However, the ability to verbalize an understanding of a concept is not definitive and does not necessarily indicate that a person has developed a certain skill.

The staff development department must also keep records on educational programs completed by staff in the institution or agency as well as, in some cases, persons who are not employees of the institution. These records are necessary for a number of reasons. Certification of staff's completion of certain educational experiences may be necessary for reports to regulatory and credentialing agencies for the organization. Nurses may use staff development experiences to assist in qualifying for individual professional certifications. Some states have mandatory continuing education requirements for licensure as a registered nurse or licensed practical nurse. In addition, records of completion of educational programs may be useful in supporting an institution's case in a legal action. Care should be taken that these records are maintained in a cost-effective manner that makes information readily accessible.

There have been a number of recent developments relating to patient education and staff development. One is further concentration of interest in the behavioral aspects of health and continuing use of the behavioral sciences. This simply recognizes that lifestyle and behaviors are important determinants of health and illness.

Self-care is also developing as a philosophical position. It aims at giving individuals more tools to manage their health and regulate their bodily processes. From the health care institution's viewpoint, it is a delegation of responsibility to patients and families for kinds of care formerly provided by health care professionals. It is essential, however, that patients and their families are taught the skills and knowledge necessary for such care.

SUMMARY

♦ Staff and patient education are always needed. This education should be based on adult learning principles.

♦ Most institutions have specialized staff development personnel but the nurse manager also has a role in both staff and patient education.

♦ The basic staff development function parallels that of nursing: assessment of educational needs, planning, implementation, and evaluation.

♦ Three questions need to be answered in assessment: (a) can the learner do what is required, (b) if not, is it due to lack of skill or lack of motivation, and (c) if it is lack of skill, is educating a present employee a more cost-effective intervention than hiring a person already prepared with the skill?

♦ Many principles of learning must be built into any staff development program: (a) Is the learner ready to learn? (b) Is the learner motivated to learn? (c) Are practice opportunities properly provided? (d) Is transfer of training facilitated? (e) Is too much material provided to learn at one time? (f) Is feedback provided? (g) Is the program formulated for adults?

♦ Staff development includes orientation, formalized education, and on-the-job instruction.

♦ Although done infrequently, evaluation should be carried out following educational intervention to validate the success of the intervention. Criteria for such evaluation include learner reaction to the program, learning achieved, behavior change, and organizational result.

♦ Patient education has increased because of the emphasis on maintaining health, shortened hospital stays, JCAHO and AHA policy statements, and government funding changes (DRGs).

♦ Barriers to teaching include lack of patient education as a priority, lack of time, lack of communication between caregivers, lack of knowledge, lack of training skill, lack of family involvement, and lack of patient motivation.

♦ Educational records include billing records, standing orders, staff educational records, and results.

BIBLIOGRAPHY

Bandura, A. (1977). *Social Learning Theory.* Englewood Cliffs, NJ: Prentice-Hall.

Breckon, D. J. (1982). *Hospital Health Education.* Rockville, MD: Aspen.

Cascio, W. F. (1982). *Costing Human Resources: The Financial Impact of Behavior in Organizations.* Boston: Kent.

Corkadeel, L., and McGlashan, R. (1983). "A Practical Approach to Patient Teaching." *Journal of Continuing Education in Nursing, 14:* 9–15.

Craig, R. L. (editor). (1976). *Training and Development Handbook.* New York: McGraw-Hill.

Crate, M. A. (1965). "Nursing Functions in Adaptation to Chronic Illness." *American Journal of Nursing, 65:* 72–76.

Decker, P. J., and Nathan, B. (1985). *Behavior Modeling Training: Theory and Applications.* New York: Praeger Scientific Publishing.

Ellis, H. C. (1965). *The Transfer of Learning.* New York: MacMillan.

Goldstein, I. L. (1974). *Training: Program Development and Evaluation.* Monterey, CA: Brooks/Cole.

Hall, D. T. (1976). *Careers in Organizations.* Santa Monica, CA: Goodyear.

Knowles, M. S. (1970). *The Modern Practice of Adult Education.* New York: Association Press.

Marx, R. D. (1982). "Relapse Prevention for Management Training." *Academy of Management Review, 7*(3): 433–441.

May, L. (1980). "Clinical Preceptors for New Nurses." *American Journal of Nursing,* 80: 1824–1826.

Murphy, M. L., and Hammerstad, S. M. (1981). "Preparing a Staff Nurse for Precepting." *Nurse Educator* 6(5): 17–20.

Redman, B. K. (1980). *The Process of Patient Teaching in Nursing.* St. Louis, MO: Mosby.

Shaw, M. E., Corsini, R. J., Blake, R. R., and Mouton, J. S. (1980). *Role Playing.* San Diego: University Associates.

Wexley, K. N., and Latham, G. P. (1981). *Developing and Training Human Resources in Organizations.* Glenview, IL: Scott Foresman.

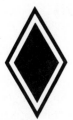

ENHANCING EMPLOYEE PERFORMANCE

A continual and troublesome question facing nurse managers today is why some employees perform better than others. A number of variables have been used to explain performance differences. For example, characteristics such as ability, instinct, and aspiration levels, as well as age, education, and family background explain why some employees perform well and others poorly. Based on these factors, a model that considers motivation and ability as determinants of *job performance* is presented in Figure 15–1.

Since the essence of management is getting things done through other people, skillful nurse managers recognize the importance of directing their energies to enhancing the performance of *all* employees. This chapter discusses the process of diagnosing and remedying performance problems. Strategies for intervention such as day-to-day coaching and dealing with rule violations are presented in some detail. This chapter concludes with chemical dependency as a special performance issue. The philosophical framework for this section is based on the premise that the pursuit of happy and productive employees is considered a cost-effective, worthwhile, although often difficult, endeavor.

♦ A MODEL OF JOB PERFORMANCE

Nurse managers spend considerable time making judgments about the fit among individuals, job tasks, and effectiveness. Such judgments are typically influenced by both the manager's and the employee's characteristics. Making decisions about who performs what tasks in a particular manner without first considering individual behavior can lead to irreversible long-term problems. Each employee is different in many respects. A manager needs to ask how such differences influence the behavior and performance of the job requirements. Ideally this assessment is performed when the new employee is hired. In reality, however, many employees are placed in positions without the manager having adequate knowledge of their abilities and/or interests. This often results in problems with employee

---

FIGURE 15–1 A SIMPLIFIED MODEL OF JOB PERFORMANCE*

Employee Performance	**=**	**f (Motivation**	**and**	**Ability)**
♦ Daily job performance		♦ Compensation		♦ Recruitment
♦ Absenteeism		♦ Benefits		♦ Selection
♦ Lateness		♦ Job design		♦ Training
♦ Rule violations		♦ Supervisory style		♦ Special programs
♦ Accidents		♦ Recruitment and selection		
♦ Theft				

The items listed under the headings of performance, motivation, and ability are not intended to be all inclusive.

*Jim Breaugh.

performance, as well as conflict between employees and managers.

Employee performance literature ultimately reveals two major dimensions as determinants of job performance: motivation and ability (Hershey & Blanchard, 1988). The model presented in Figure 15–1 portrays employee performance as a function of these two dimensions (Decker, 1982). This job performance model identifies six performance categories likely to be viewed as important by the nurse manager. Although there is conceptual overlap in these categories, separate designation of each helps emphasize their importance.

When utilizing this model, the nurse manager should carefully consider several factors. First, a health care institution should establish and communicate clear descriptions of daily job performance so that deviations from expected behaviors can be easily identified and documented. Second, behaviors considered problematic in one department may be acceptable in another department. Finally, some behaviors are viewed as serious only when repeated (e.g., being late to work), while others are classified as problematic following one incident (e.g., medication error with severe consequences).

EMPLOYEE MOTIVATION AS A STIMULUS FOR PERFORMANCE

Motivation describes the forces acting on an employee that initiate and direct behavior (refer to Chapter 8). Because individuals bring to the workplace different needs and goals, the type and intensity of motivators vary among employees. Nurse managers prefer motivated employees because they strive to find the best way to perform their jobs. Motivated employees are interested in producing high-quality products or services; they are more likely to be productive than are non-motivated workers. This is one reason that motivation is an important aspect of enhancing employee performance. Figure 15–1 shows staff motivation influenced primarily by the organization's compensation system, benefits program, job design, style of supervision, and methods of recruitment and selection. Having a performance-based compensation/reward system has been demonstrated to have a direct impact on employee motivation. For example, if staff nurses see their salaries relatively unaffected by their behavior (e.g., across-the-board yearly salary increases) then compensation will not be a strong motivator of performance.

Benefits can also influence employee performance and behavior. Most institutions offer their employees paid sick leave. Typically, institutions offer programs that have the following elements: (1) for every X days worked, employees accrue a specific number of paid sick days; (2) there is a maximum number of sick days that an employee can accumulate; (3) notification of the supervisor is required to be paid for a sick day; and (4) employees who leave the organization without using accumulated sick leave lose these sick days. It is not surprising that these institutions experience relatively high rates of employee absenteeism since there is no reward (motivator) for not using the sick days accumulated. One way to enhance employee performance is to provide options for use of this benefit such as paid time off and/or accumulated vacation time, rather than encouraging employees to "call in sick" to use this benefit (see Chapter 17).

The number of institutions offering wellness programs or fitness centers for employees has increased significantly in the past two decades. Although few data are available, some evidence suggests that these programs do serve as motivators for the staff (Rhodes & Steers, 1990). In addition, employee assistance programs (as a benefit) recognize that alcohol and substance abuse, as well as psychological problems, are behaviors that often lead to lowered productivity and performance problems (McCafferty, 1988).

Another factor over which the nurse manager has some control is job design (see Chapter 8). Challenging and interesting jobs motivate employees (Lawler, 1986); strategies that place nurses in positions that are sufficiently challenging and interesting can increase overall motivation. For example, nurses who are skilled at sharing their expertise with less experienced nurses can be designated as mentors and thus are motivated to continue this role. Not only does this behavior enhance individual employee performance, but it contributes to professionalization of the new graduate as well. Similarly, job enrichment, which is the practice of increasing an individual's discretion to select job activities and outcomes, increases the fulfillment of growth and autonomy needs. This practice increases job depth by providing direct feedback, new learning, participation in scheduling, job uniqueness, control over resources, and an opportunity for employees to be accountable for their jobs (Hershey & Blanchard, 1988).

Nurse managers also can influence the motivation of employees by being sensitive to variations in employee needs, abilities, and goals. The leadership style assumed by the manager reflects a commitment to maximizing each employee's potential. If performance needs to be improved, then managers should intervene to help create an atmosphere that encourages, supports, and sustains improvement. Managers should try to provide employees with jobs that offer equity, task challenge, diversity, and a variety of opportunities for need satisfaction. The manager should also be sensitive to individual differences and consider variations in preferences (*valences*) for rewards among employees. Employees in one study who were encouraged to participate

in practice-related decision making had increased motivation because of this activity (Lawler, 1986). This does not mean *all* employees benefit from increased participation. In fact, some employees prefer to be followers and have decreased performance when placed in independent roles (Kelley, 1988).

Providing realistic job information can increase employee satisfaction and reduce employee turnover. When given accurate information about a position, job candidates can "self-select" out of jobs that are not seen as offering opportunities they value. This is especially important in today's job market for nurses, since high vacancy rates in certain specialty care areas, such as intensive care units, "force" applicants to accept positions they ordinarily would not consider. Methods of screening are recommended to identify prospective employees who are not likely to be motivated by what a position offers (Gatewood & Feild, 1990).

EMPLOYEE ABILITY AS A DETERRENT TO PERFORMANCE

Some employees, even though highly motivated, simply do not have the abilities or skills to perform well. Abilities and skills play a major role in individual behavior and performance. Effective managers are proficient in matching each person's abilities and skills with the job requirement (see Chapter 13). The matching process is important since no amount of leadership, motivation, or organizational resources can make up for deficiencies in abilities or skills. Job analysis is a widely used technique that takes some of the guesswork out of matching. Job analysis is the process of defining and studying a job in terms of tasks or behaviors and specifying the responsibilities, education, and training needed to perform the job successfully (Ivancevich & Glueck, 1986).

Strategies that focus on congruence between ability and job requirements include recruitment efforts directed toward graduates of programs with sound professional curricula, selection methods that identify specific abilities/skills and match them with known employee characteristics, staff development programs that upgrade knowledge and skills of employees as job requirements change, and special programs such as intensive workshops and continuing education. The nurse manager plays a crucial role in ongoing assessment and evaluation of employees, providing opportunities and encouragement for their advancement and maintenance of abilities. In addition, the nurse manager is in the best position to communicate educational needs to the administration so that adequate resources are allocated for this function.

JOB PERFORMANCE = f (MOTIVATION AND ABILITY)

A desired result of any employee's behavior is effective job performance. An important part of the manager's job is to define performance in advance—to state desired results. In organizations, individual and environmental variables affect not only behavior but also performance. Performance-related behaviors are directly associated with job tasks and need to be accomplished to achieve a job's objectives. From a manager's perspective, searching for ways to enhance performance includes such actions as identifying performance problems; planning, organizing, and controlling the work of employees; and creating a motivational climate for subordinates. If employees are not performing well or consistently, managers must investigate the problem. In the next section of this chapter, a model for determining the cause of performance problems is presented.

♦ DIAGNOSING PERFORMANCE PROBLEMS

Job satisfaction has been divided into a number of components: interpersonal relations, achievement, responsibility, advancement, the work itself, recognition, supervision, working conditions, salary, and status. All of these relate in some way to employee productivity. Since managers focus their attention on performance-related behaviors, they search for ways to achieve optimal performance. If employees are not performing well or are performing inconsistently, managers must investigate the problems. Figure 15–2 identifies a model for diagnosing the cause of an employee problem. Included are questions and answers that designate the basis of the performance issue as primarily skill- or motivation-related. The model also specifies that when performance problems are identified, some form of managerial action is required.

The first step in using this model is to begin with accepted standards of performance and an accurate assessment of the current performance of the staff member. This means job descriptions must be current and performance appraisal tools must be written in behavioral terms. It also implies that employee evaluations are regularly carried out and implemented according to recognized guidelines (refer to Chapter 16).

Second, the manager must decide whether the problem demands immediate attention and whether it is a skill-related or motivation-related problem. Once these determinations are made, the manager can proceed to an appropriate plan of action. Skill-related problems can be solved through informal training, such as demonstration and coaching, whereas complex skills require formal training in the form of inservice sessions or workshops. If there are limitations regarding the length of time for an employee to reach the desired level of skill, the manager must determine whether the job could be simplified or whether the better decision would be to terminate or transfer the employee. In any deliberations, the manager must include budgetary considerations in the decision-making process. For example, would it be more cost-effective to hire an experienced nurse at a higher salary rather than to provide the necessary staff development to have the current employee reach a satisfactory performance level? Often, the resources of the organization determine which option the manager is able to exercise.

If the performance problem is motivation rather than ability, the manager must address a different set of questions. Specifically, whether the employee believes the behavior leads to punishment, reward, or inaction must be determined. If the "reward" for conscientiously coming to work on holidays (rather than calling in sick) leads to always being scheduled for holiday work, then good performance is associated with punishment. Only when the employee sees a

strong link between valued outcomes and meeting performance expectations will motivation strategies succeed. The manager plays a role in tailoring motivational efforts to meet the individual needs of the employee. Unfortunately, creating a performance-reward climate does not eliminate all problem behaviors. When the use of rewards proves ineffective, other strategies, such as coaching and discipline, are warranted. These strategies are discussed later in this chapter.

In attempting to differentiate between lack of ability and lack of motivation, an analysis of past performance is useful. If past performance has been acceptable and there has been little change in standards of performance, it is likely that the problem results from a lack of motivation. In contrast, if the nurse has never performed at an acceptable level, the problem may be primarily skill related. Different intervention strategies should be used depending on whether the problem results from a lack of motivation or

---

FIGURE 15–2 KEY BEHAVIORS IN DIAGNOSING AND REMEDYING PERFORMANCE PROBLEMS

- Is the performance deficiency a problem? Will it go away if ignored? (Generally ignore problems that are temporary.)
- Is it due to lack of skill or motivation? How do I know? (Observed in past, used reward/sanction to get performance, tested.)

If Skill:
- Is it a complex skill (formal training) or simple skill (coaching)?
- Is there a cost/time constraint such that selecting a new person is the answer? Can I simplify job? Can I transfer/demote employee?

If Motivation:
- Is desired performance punished? (If so–remove punishment)
- Is desired performance rewarded? (If no–point it out)
- Does the employee value the rewards/see them as equitable? (If not–change them)

P. J. Decker, *Health Care Management Microtraining* (St. Louis, MO: Decker & Associates, 1982), p. 5.

a lack of skill. The objective should be to enhance performance rather than to punish the employee.

Nurse managers may be reluctant to effectively manage problem employees because of claims of discrimination or the feelings of anger and resentment that follow. To ensure that employee civil rights are respected, the nurse manager should work closely with top nursing administration and the human resources department. All employees deserve fair and equitable treatment; however, different responses by employees can lead to claims of discriminatory treatment. It is necessary to document problem behavior and adhere to the guidelines established by valid performance appraisals.

The credibility of the nurse manager influences how well he or she is able to enhance employee performance. How the manager is viewed by employees in the leadership role determines the impact on the performance behavior of employees. If the manager is viewed as fair and genuinely interested in the welfare of each employee as an individual, he or she will facilitate employee motivation. Often the manager

must walk a tightrope between empathy and objectivity in guiding employees to reach their potential.

♦ STRATEGIES FOR INTERVENTION

The specific employee situation, as well as organizational goals and objectives, determine the type of intervention strategies available to assist employee development. Among the most common are coaching, dealing with a rule violation, disciplining, and terminating. The following section considers coaching and dealing with a rule violation as specific intervention strategies. Discipline, termination of employment, and dealing with absenteeism and tardiness are discussed in Chapters 16 and 17.

DAY-TO-DAY COACHING

Before entering into a *coaching* session, the nurse manager (the coach) should spend at least a few minutes preparing for the interaction (see Figure 15–3). The goal of the meeting is to elimi-

---

FIGURE 15–3 KEY BEHAVIORS: COACHING*

- ♦ State the problem in behavioral terms; immediately focus on the problem, do not attack the person.
- ♦ Tie problem to organizational and/or personal consequences.
- ♦ Ask employee why the behavior occurred. Try to bring the reasons for the problem into the open.
- ♦ Ask for suggestions on how to solve the problem. Listen openly. Discuss the employee's ideas or, if none are offered, lead the employee to your own preferred solution by asking if it has been tried.
- ♦ Agree on steps each of you will take to solve the problem. Write them down. If appropriate, ask for employee's commitment to the above steps.
- ♦ Agree on and record a specific follow-up date.

*Always prepare before the meeting

Adapted from P. J. Decker, *Health Care Management Microtraining* (St. Louis, MO: Decker & Associates, 1982). Used by permission.

nate, or at least lessen, a performance problem such as excessive absenteeism or frequent personal phone calls. The manager should try to anticipate how the employee will react (e.g., "Everybody gets personal phone calls") to formulate an appropriate response (e.g., "I am going to talk to each person about this problem"). Problems should be dealt with when they are small or first occur. In general, coaching sessions should last no more than five to 10 minutes.

1. The first key behavior in coaching is to state the problem in behavioral terms: "Mr. Jones's medication was not given on time this morning."

2. Then the supervisor should tie the problem to the functioning of the organization, professional standards, or to the person's self-interest: "The hospital could be sued; you could be terminated." This is an important but often overlooked first step, since it cannot be taken for granted that the employee knows why the behavior is a problem. After all, if persons are expected to act in a specific way, they need to understand why the behavior is important and to be rewarded when it has improved.

3. Having stated the problem behavior, the nurse manager needs to explore the reasons for the problem, never jumping to any conclusions of his or her own but asking the staff nurse what caused the problem behavior. After the staff nurse has explained, the manager decides how to proceed with the coaching session. If the problem was caused by ignorance—for instance, lack of familiarity with institution policy—the manager may simply inform the nurse of the appropriate behavior and end the coaching session.

4. For most problems, however, the nurse manager should ask the employee for his or her suggestions and discuss ideas on how to solve the problem. In many cases, the employee knows best how to solve the problem and is more likely to be committed to the solution if it is his or her own. It is nearly always better to encourage employees to solve their own problems, but this does not mean that managers cannot supplement with their own suggestions for ways to improve. It is essential for managers to listen openly. They need to fully understand their subordinates' perspectives to coach them successfully.

5. How formal should the coaching session be? If the problem is minor and a first-time occurrence, the nurse manager may simply state what actions will be taken to solve the problem and end the meeting. In most cases, however, the nurse manager and staff nurse should agree on steps each will take to solve the problem, and these should be written down for later reference. The steps should be specific and behavioral.

6. Finally, the nurse manager should arrange for a follow-up meeting, at which time the staff nurse will receive performance feedback.

It is possible that a staff nurse may bring up personal problems as a cause of his or her work problems. The coaching session then verges on becoming a counseling session, and the manager must be aware of his or her abilities in this area; most nursing supervisors are not trained in marriage counseling, individual therapy, or drug or alcohol rehabilitation, for instance. Nurse managers must recognize their limitations as counselors. When personal problems are raised, nurse managers should convey their concern and willingness to work with the employee to get help for the problems. In most cases, nurse managers will not be the direct source of the help but rather will seek out other, appropriate sources. It is most important that nurse managers do not themselves delve into potential personal problems (e.g., "Are there problems at home that I should know about?") unless staff nurses raise them. The employee's personal life is not the manager's business.

DEALING WITH A RULE VIOLATION

As with day-to-day coaching, certain key behaviors (Figure 15–4) have been found to be effective for approaching staff members when a rule has been violated. The nurse manager should prepare for the meeting by reviewing the circumstances involved in the rule violation as well as anticipating the reaction of the specific employee to the interaction. Many of the key behaviors involved in coaching are also appropriately applied in this situation.

The first key behavior is to determine if the employee is aware of the rule and if the rule has been consistently enforced. If rules regarding the uniform code are not applied to everyone on a daily basis, efforts to change this behavior in a single employee would predictably be unsuc-

cessful. The nurse manager is better served by identifying rules that are accepted by the majority of the personnel and determining which employee(s) need further direction in compliance.

Second, the nurse manager should describe the behavior that violated the rule in a manner that conveys concern to the employee regarding the outcome. By focusing on the impact of this behavior, the manager avoids making the interaction a personal issue.

The importance of stating the rule that has been violated cannot be overemphasized. It is often helpful to have documenting materials that state the rule in question so interpretation issues can be clarified. If the rule being violated is the requirement that nurses report to a peer when they leave the patient care unit, the nurse manager should have a copy of the job description that lists this as a required behavior.

The next key behavior is to solicit the employee's reason for the behavior (e.g., what is preventing her or him from informing a peer when she or he leaves the patient care unit). Allow sufficient time for the employee to respond while at the same time guarding against the pursuit of extraneous, unrelated issues. In the latter event, redirect the employee's atten-

FIGURE 15–4 KEY BEHAVIORS FOR DEALING WITH A RULE VIOLATION

- ◆ Prepare before the meeting (e.g., is the employee aware of the rule, how will employee react, has the rule been consistently enforced).
- ◆ Without hostility, describe the behavior that violated the rule.
- ◆ State the rule that has been violated.
- ◆ Ask for and listen openly to the employee's reasons for the behavior.
- ◆ Explain why the behavior cannot continue (and offer your help in solving the problem, if you think it would be useful).
- ◆ Set and record a specific follow-up date.

Adapted from P. J. Decker, *Health Care Management Microtraining* (St. Louis, MO: Decker & Associates, 1982).

tion to the rule violation and suggest that any other issues can be dealt with at another time.

The nurse manager must also convey to the employee that she or he cannot continue breaking an established rule. In the previous example, the manager would discuss the effects of the employee's behavior, such as IVs running dry and clients being left unattended, as reasons for requiring staff nurses to follow this rule. It is also beneficial if the manager can respond to the reasons given by the employee for violating the rule and offer alternative solutions so that negative outcomes will be avoided. The leadership style of the manager is important in determining whether the employee perceives he or she is being "told" what to do versus being "sold" on the idea that she or he is an important contributor to the patient care unit. The last step in the process is to set up a reasonable date to follow up with the employee on adherence to the established rule.

While it is not always possible to deal with rule violations in a distinct step-by-step sequence, it is beneficial for the nurse manager to proceed in an orderly manner. Many rule violations require early and decisive interventions and these must be handled in an immediate, forthright manner. However, in other instances positive results will emerge when rule violations are addressed within the context of a formalized plan of action.

◆ CHEMICAL DEPENDENCY: A PERFORMANCE ISSUE

One performance problem, impaired practice, puts the consumer of health services at risk of harm. Also, the employing agency is exposed to greater risk of liability for negligent actions.

Other staff members may also be affected in that they are expected to cover for nurses who are frequently absent and/or not working to capacity. The institution also is responsible for adhering to state licensing laws regarding reporting nurses who are identified as having impaired practice, usually due to alcohol or drug abuse. These laws vary from state to state with exceptions often provided if a diversion program is offered in lieu of disciplinary action. Diversion programs offer referral, assistance, and monitoring of chemically dependent nurses. Identifying and assisting chemically dependent nurses to return to work have been found to be cost-effective (LaGodna & Hendrix, 1989; Sullivan, 1986). The role of the nurse manager varies according to institutional policy. However, early recognition of impaired practice by nurses who may be chemically dependent and prompt referral for treatment are generally recognized as responsibilities of the nurse manager.

IDENTIFYING THE CHEMICALLY DEPENDENT NURSE

It is not easy to identify anyone as possibly chemically dependent. The primary symptom of chemical dependency is denial, which is present in the sufferer as well as in those around him or her. In denial, the person *really* does not believe what seems obvious. Furthermore, alcohol or drug problems in women in general, as well as in nurses in particular, are a stigma in today's society. This stigma, added to the profession's own negativeness regarding the disease, encourages nurses—even those who break through their own denial—to continue to conceal their problem. The result is that chemically dependent nurses go on practicing, endangering both patients' and their own lives. Prior to the development of obvious serious consequences, some general signs and symptoms may become evident as a nurse's chemical dependency progresses (Figures 15–5 and 15–6).

In addition to the signs and symptoms outlined in Figures 15–5 and 15–6, the nurse manager should be alert for frequently incorrect narcotics counts, alteration of narcotics vials, patient reports that pain medications are ineffective, inaccurate recording of pain medication administration, discrepancies in narcotics records, large amounts of narcotic wastage, and marked shift variations in quantity of drugs required on a unit.

If the manager discovers individual signs or symptoms or is aware of the unit changes suggested, he or she should investigate further. Often, with unit discrepancies, that simply means checking the schedule to see who was working when most of the errors occurred. Usually, one or two people emerge as those most likely to have been available during the time of the discrepancies. Further checking and observation may reveal individual behaviors suggesting a person has a chemical abuse problem.

Even if the manager is unsure of his or her perceptions, or if the actions are so vague that the manager has many doubts about the identity of the person, he or she can be certain that the situation will be clarified, nonetheless, in time. Untreated, addiction continues and, as tolerance increases, the person is likely to increase use and become increasingly careless about covering up actions. Thus, the manager will become increasingly more certain about a person's abuse problem. However, the longer the time before identification, the longer time the nurse may be practicing with impaired professional functioning, jeopardizing both patients and himself or herself. Thus, it behooves the manager to carefully assess the information about possible dependency problems but to not wait too long.

FIGURE 15–5 SIGNS OF CHEMICAL DEPENDENCY

- Family history of alcoholism or drug abuse
- Frequent change of work site (same or other institution)
- Prior medical history requiring pain control
- Conscientious worker with recent decrease in performance
- Decreased attention to personal appearance
- Frequent complaints of marital and family problems
- Reports of illness, minor accidents, and emergencies
- Complaints from co-workers
- Mood swings/depression/suicide attempts
- Strong interest in patients' pain control
- Frequent trips to the bathroom
- Increasing isolation (night shift request; eating alone)
- Elaborate excuses for tardiness
- Difficulty in meeting schedules/deadlines
- Inadequate explanation for missing work

E. J. Sullivan, L. Bissell, and E. Williams, *Chemical Dependency in Nursing: The Deadly Diversion* (St. Louis, MO: C. V. Mosby, 1988).

When this decision is made is a matter of judgment, and the manager and his or her supervisors are responsible for making it.

The manager's supervisor should be informed about the situation and should help the manager verify perceptions and clarify procedures. One note of caution: The supervisor may not be well informed about chemical dependency and may need education regarding symptoms and intervention. In that case, higher administration may be able to help. Regardless, the first-line manager should not attempt to handle such a case without at least informing a superior.

STRATEGIES FOR INTERVENTION

Once the manager has identified a nurse with a chemical abuse problem, intervention with that nurse must be planned. With the assistance of a superior, the manager should examine the institution's policies and procedures and prepare for the intervention. Preparation should include collecting all documentation or information about the nurse's behavior that would suggest that an abuse problem exists. This includes collecting records of absenteeism and tardiness (especially recent changes), records of patient complaints about ineffective medications or poor care, staff complaints about job performance, records of controlled substances, and physical signs and symptoms noticed at different times. Dates, times, and behaviors should be carefully noted. Any one behavior means very little; it is the composite pattern that identifies the problem.

Next, the manager should obtain appropriate resources to help the nurse. Internal resources include an employee assistance program (EAP) counselor (if the institution has one) or other nurses identified as recovering from chemical dependency who have offered to help. External resources include the names and phone numbers of treatment center staff and the names and phone numbers of other recovering nurses. It is absolutely essential that several sources be provided so the nurse is able to contact someone who knows how he or she feels and also knows that help is available and how to get it. **This support is so important that it cannot be emphasized enough.** Not having this assistance is like

---

FIGURE 15–6 PHYSICAL SYMPTOMS OF CHEMICAL DEPENDENCY

- Shakiness, tremors of hands, jittery
- Slurred speech
- Watery eyes, dilated or constricted pupils
- Diaphoresis
- Unsteady gait
- Runny nose
- Nausea, vomiting, diarrhea
- Weight loss or gain
- Blackouts (memory losses while conscious)
- Wears long-sleeved clothing continuously

E. J. Sullivan, L. Bissell, and E. Williams, *Chemical Dependency in Nursing: The Deadly Diversion* (St. Louis, MO: C. V. Mosby, 1988).

telling the diabetic he has diabetes and not telling him where he can get insulin.

In addition to assistance for the nurse, the manager should check on health insurance provisions for chemical dependency treatment. Many insurance carriers have recognized that successful treatment reduces the use of other health care facilities and, thus, reduces the cost of health care. Accordingly, they offer coverage for chemical dependency treatment to encourage participants to enter recovery programs. Others, unfortunately, do not. Since many of an institution's employees may be covered under the same health care plan, the manager should check these provisions. If the policy does not cover inpatient care, the nurse may be able to afford outpatient care, which is considerably less expensive. So, the manager should not assume treatment is unavailable even when there is little or no coverage. Alcoholics Anonymous and Narcotics Anonymous are free. However, for the nurse addicted to narcotics, some period of time, even a few days, is needed in a hospital to monitor withdrawal, and most policies do cover this.

Before initiating the intervention, the manager must examine his or her own attitudes about the abuse problem. Probably the chemical abuse has gone on for some time, and both the manager and the staff may have lost patience with the person, whose performance and attendance have forced others to do more than their fair share of the work on the unit. It has likely appeared as though the nurse were shirking duties, and if chemical abuse was suspected, others may have felt that he or she should just "pull himself or herself together," stop "doing it," and, as last resort, he or she should "know better." Once the process is understood, however, it is apparent that none of these behaviors are possible since willpower and education have not prevented others from becoming addicted. The manager will need to deal with staff feelings later, but at this time it is enough to be certain that one's own attitudes will not imperil the intervention. It is important that the message be clearly one of help and hope.

The goal of the intervention is to get the nurse to an appropriate place for an evaluation of the possible problem. Treatment centers or therapists who specialize in chemical dependency are sources recommended for conducting the evaluation. They have the necessary experience for diagnosing and, if indicated, treating the disease.

The manager must also decide, beforehand, what action on the part of the nurse will be acceptable. If the nurse refuses to go for an evaluation, what will be the consequences? Termination? Discipline? Report to the state board of nursing? The institution's policies and the state board of nursing requirements must be met, but, beyond that, the manager must be clear about the consequences and willing to carry them out. Most experts in treating addictions in nurses recommend that the nurse be offered the option of chemical dependency evaluation and, if needed, treatment, and if he or she does not agree to that, then termination and a report to the state board of nursing should follow. Remember, nurses care for very sick patients whose health and safety is in their hands. It is imperative that managers protect both.

Once preparations have been made, the intervention should be scheduled as soon as possible. Others may be asked to join the manager, but the group should be small and restricted to only those involved in past problems or to the manager's supervisor. In some institutions, the top nursing administrator conducts all interventions with chemically dependent nurses and, in that case, the nurse manager must fully inform the administrator of all circumstances leading to the intervention and provide all the documentation needed. Also, the manager should participate in the intervention so that all relevant information is presented and denial is kept to a minimum.

The intervention should be scheduled at a time and place when interruptions can be avoided. It is best to surprise the nurse with a request to come to the office. Denial can build, rationalizations can be developed, and defensiveness can increase when the nurse has time to consider the problem.

The manager should present the nurse with the collected evidence showing that a pattern of behaviors has emerged that suggests an abuse problem *might* be occurring and that an evaluation must be undertaken to know for sure. It is important to focus on the problem behaviors, not on the inadequacy of the person. He or she has already experienced shame and guilt about his or her use, and the manager has an opportunity to help the nurse regain some perspective about chemical dependency. He or she is responsible for doing something about it once it is diagnosed; and the nurse will be better able to accept that a problem exists.

Often, the nurse's response to an intervention is relief at finally being stopped. One nurse said, "Thank God it's over," and this sentiment is expressed frequently. In the best-case scenario, the nurse admits the problem, is grateful to be getting help, and goes willingly to treatment. It is best to go directly to treatment from the worksite if this can be arranged beforehand. A family member or friend can bring a suitcase from home later. The important thing is to move quickly before denial resurfaces.

Other nurses, of course, will continue to deny the obvious, in which case the manager must continue to confront the nurse with the reality of the circumstances. If the nurse refuses to go for an evaluation, the manager must follow the disciplinary process for discharging him or her. If the nurse is using alcohol or drugs at the time, he or she must be removed from the patient care setting immediately. The manager should arrange to have someone (either a family member or another staff member) drive the nurse home whether the nurse is going to treatment or not. Not only do alcohol or drugs make the nurse an unsafe driver, but the stress of the intervention may distract the nurse even more.

If the nurse goes for an evaluation and/or treatment, specific plans must be made for this to occur. It should be clear to all parties (chemically dependent nurse, manager, supervisor) when the nurse will contact the treatment center (the sooner the better even if he or she is not using mood-altering chemicals at this time) and when he or she will report back to the manager the recommended course of action. It is possible to arrange with a treatment facility that reports be made directly to the manager, but federal regulations regarding confidentiality prohibit the staff from reporting a patient's status to anyone without that person's written consent. Since the goal of treatment is recovery, which includes returning to work, most facilities request that the nurse give this consent.

REENTRY

The nurse manager should be involved in planning for reentry to the workplace. It is especially important for the manager and higher administration to recognize the threat to recovery that access to one's drug of addiction poses. Not all treatment staff are familiar enough with nursing to be aware of the danger of putting the nurse in constant, daily contact with these drugs. However, it is vitally important to the nurse's recovery that he or she return to work, preferably in the same setting. This dilemma has often been dealt with in two ways. One method is to reassign the nurse for a period of time (possibly as long as two years) to a job or a unit where few mood-altering drugs are given. Some choices have been the nursery, department of education, rehabilitation, or patient care audits. Although reassignment presents a problem for the institution and is disappointing to the nurse, it is far better to make this accommodation than to jeopardize the nurse's recovery.

Another method is to retain the nurse on the unit but not allow him or her to administer mood-altering medications. This method requires that other staff not only know about the nurse's problem but that they be willing to give pain and sleep medications to that nurse's patients. Since this would require giving the staff an explanation and, thus, possibly disclosing the nurse's addiction, management and staff must decide if this is reasonable to accomplish.

These methods are usually necessary only for the nurse who was addicted to narcotics, but each case should be individually decided based on the amount of stress in the job, the need for rotating shifts, and other factors that may inhibit recovery.

Health care today requires that every employee function at peak efficiency and effectiveness. Health care cannot afford to protect an employee whose professional functioning is impaired by chemical abuse. Discharging the employee and allowing him or her to go to another institution to continue practicing and endangering patients as well as himself or herself cannot be allowed to continue. The nurse manager is the front-line contact with staff. He or she can be alerted to the signs and symptoms of chemical abuse problems, can learn intervention techniques and skills, and can help recovering nurses return to the workplace. The reader is referred to *Chemical Dependency in Nursing* (Sullivan, Bissell & Williams, 1988) for more information.

Concern for patients' safety mandates intervention, and humane concern for nurse colleagues mandates that such assistance be made available.

SUMMARY

♦ A model of job performance suggests that employee performance is determined by motivation and ability.

♦ Motivation factors that influence employee performance are compensation, benefits, job design, supervisory style, and recruitment and selection.

♦ Ability factors that influence employee performance are recruitment, selection, training, and special programs.

♦ Nurse managers can diagnose and remedy performance problems by assessing key behaviors, which differentiate between skill-related and motivation-related issues.

♦ Strategies for intervention that enhance employee performance are day-to-day coaching and dealing with rule violations.

♦ Identifying, intervening, and returning chemically dependent nurses to practice helps the institution, the manager, and the affected nurse.

BIBLIOGRAPHY

Chaney, E. A. (1987). "Nurses and Chemical Dependency: Policy Considerations." *Journal of Pediatric Nursing,* 2(1): 61–63.

Decker, P. J. (1982). *Healthcare Management Microtraining.* St. Louis, MO: Decker and Associates.

Gatewood, R. D., and Feild, H. S. (1990). *Human Resource Selection.* Chicago: Dryden.

Hershey, P., and Blanchard, K. (1988). *Management of Organizational Behavior: Utilizing Human Resources.* 5th ed. Englewood Cliffs, NJ: Prentice-Hall.

Ivancevich, J. M., and Glueck, W. F. (1986). *Foundations of Personnel/Human Resource Management.* 3d ed. Plano, TX: Business Publications.

Kelley, R. E. (1988). "In Praise of Followers." *Harvard Business Review,* 88(6): 142–148.

LaGodna, G. E., and Hendrix, M. J. (1989). "Impaired Nurses: A Cost Analysis." *Journal of Nursing Administration,* 19(9): 13–18.

Lawler, E. E. (1986). *High Involvement Management.* San Francisco, CA: Jossey Bass.

McCafferty, R. M. (1988). *Employee Benefit Programs: A Total Compensation Perspective.* Boston: PWS-Kent.

Rhodes, S. R., and Steers, R. M. (1990). *Managing Employee Absenteeism.* Reading, MA: Addison-Wesley.

Sullivan, E. J. (1986). "Cost savings of retaining chemically-dependent nurses." *Nursing Economics,* 4(4): 179–200.

Sullivan, E. J., Bissell, L., and Williams, E. (1988). *Chemical Dependency in Nursing: The Deadly Diversion.* St. Louis, MO: C. V. Mosby.

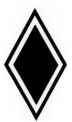

PERFORMANCE APPRAISAL

The performance appraisal process includes day-to-day supervisor-employee interactions (coaching, counseling, disciplining); written documentation (making notes about an employee's behavior, completing the performance appraisal form); the formal appraisal interview; and follow-up sessions that may involve coaching and/or discipline when needed.

When nurse managers are asked what they like least about their jobs, invariably "doing performance appraisals" is near the top of their lists. Among the reasons these nurses give for disliking performance reviews are "You can't evaluate nursing performance," "The form we use is lousy," "Nurses are professionals—they don't need to be evaluated," "If you give someone a low rating, it hurts his or her future performance," "I don't have enough information to rate accurately," and "If I give an employee a low rating, my boss won't back me up." Partly because of such reasons, we find that people who do appraisals generally spend little time on them and tend to give everyone high ratings.

But what about the staff nurse's perspective on performance appraisal? Think back to your own most recent performance review and reflect on three questions: How prepared was the person who did the appraisal? How accurate was the feedback you received? Did the performance feedback session help you improve your performance? If your answers are "not very prepared," "not very accurate," and "didn't help me improve," then your comments are typical.

None of this, however, should be construed as a recommendation to do away with performance appraisals. Instead, this chapter is intended to provide information that will help nurse managers do a better job of appraising their subordinates. Before getting into the specific "nuts and bolts" of doing appraisals, however, we must first understand the numerous factors that affect the way appraisals are done and the assumptions that underlie this chapter.

◆ ASSUMPTIONS

This chapter is based on six underlying assumptions:

1. *A major reason for doing performance reviews is to help employees improve their future performance.* Thus, performance reviews should be future-oriented.

2. *The performance appraisal process is a difficult one, but we can become more skilled at it.* Appraisers can become more accurate in their ratings and more professional in giving constructive feedback.

3. *Very few people like the performance appraisal form they are required to use.* The form "takes too long to complete," "is ambiguous," "requires me to make judgments that I lack data to make," and so on.

4. *To be effective in doing the formal, year-end review, a manager must carry out the day-to-day aspects of the performance appraisal process.*

5. *Supervisors always evaluate their employees' performance.* The question is whether the evaluation is written and shared with the employee.

6. *The prescriptions given in this chapter will not work for approximately 5 percent of your employees.* In fact, nothing works for this 5 percent. Whatever the reason is for this, the focus in this chapter is on the 95 percent of employees for whom these prescriptions will have a positive effect.

◆ USES OF PERFORMANCE APPRAISALS

Performance appraisals often are the basis upon which administrative decisions such as the size of a salary increase or who gets promoted are made (Murphy & Cleveland, 1991). Ideally, accurate appraisal information allows an organization to tie rewards to performance. Performance appraisals are also used for employee development. After a thorough review of an employee's performance, the supervisor and employee may jointly develop action plans to help the individual improve. Such developmental activities may include formal training, academic course work, or simple on-the-job coaching.

A final reason for doing performance reviews concerns fair employment practice law (e.g., Title VII of the 1964 Civil Rights Act, Age Discrimination in Employment Act). Performance appraisals and the decisions, such as layoffs, based on those appraisals are covered by several federal and state laws. In the last two decades, numerous employees have successfully sued their organizations over employment decisions that were based on questionable performance appraisal results.

Regardless of how an organization uses performance appraisals, it is essential that they accurately reflect the employee's actual job performance. If performance ratings are inaccurate, an inferior employee may be promoted, another employee may not receive needed training, or there may not be a tie between performance and rewards (thus lessening employee motivation).

◆ PERFORMANCE APPRAISAL AND THE LAW

Since the passage of Title VII of the Civil Rights Act of 1964, the courts have addressed numerous employment decisions in which performance appraisals have played an important role (Murphy & Cleveland, 1991). In many of these cases, the courts have ruled the employment decisions to be illegal because the organization's appraisal system in some way was unsound. Although you can never be certain that your appraisal system is legally defensible, there are several steps to help ensure that an appraisal system is non-discriminatory.

1. The appraisal should be in writing and carried out at least once a year.

2. The performance appraisal information should be shared with the employee.

3. The employee should have the opportunity to respond in writing to his or her appraisal.

4. Employees should have a mechanism to appeal the results of the performance appraisal.

5. The supervisor should have adequate opportunity to observe the employee's job performance during the course of the evaluation period. If adequate contact is lacking (e.g., the appraiser and the appraisee work different shifts), then appraisal information should be gathered from other sources.

6. Notes (critical incidents) on the employee's performance should be kept during the entire evaluation period. These notes should be shared with the employee during the course of the evaluation period.

7. Evaluators should be trained to carry out the performance appraisal process (e.g., what is reasonable job performance, how to complete the form, how to carry out the feedback interview).

8. Insofar as possible, the performance appraisal should focus on employee behavior

and results rather than on personal traits or characteristics (e.g., initiative, attitude, personality).

♦ PERFORMANCE MEASUREMENT ISSUES

Although nurse managers may not have formal input into the type of appraisal instrument used in their institution, an understanding of some basic issues is important to appreciate the variety of forces that can affect the way appraisals are done. Specifically, it is important to understand the philosophy that underlies the appraisal system as well as the general focus of the system.

EVALUATION PHILOSOPHY
First, one needs to consider whether evaluations are absolute or comparative. Most evaluation systems are based on absolute judgment: In appraising a staff nurse, the nurse manager evaluates the nurse against an internal standard of performance. This internal standard reflects what the manager perceives as reasonable and acceptable performance for a staff nurse. When evaluations are absolute in nature, it is possible for all nurses to be evaluated as exceeding the standard for acceptable performance. Alternatively, it is possible that all nurses are seen as just meeting or as falling below the standard. In other words, the ratings a nurse receives depend entirely on the judgment of the nurse manager.

In contrast, evaluations based on comparative judgment require the nurse manager to rate subordinates by comparing them with one another: How a nurse is evaluated will depend on the level of performance of his or her peers. A teacher who "grades on a curve" is making evaluations based on comparative judgment. Thus, comparative judgments are based on the relative

standing among employees. Because comparative judgment evaluation systems call for the nurse manager to differentiate among those rated (not all nurses can receive high ratings), it is not surprising that most nurse managers prefer to make ratings based on absolute judgment. Examples of rating scales based on absolute judgment and comparative judgment are presented in Figure 16–1.

COMPONENTS TO BE EVALUATED
Nurses engage in a variety of job-related activities. To reflect the multidimensional nature of the nurse's job, the performance appraisal form usually requires a nurse manager to rate on several different performance dimensions such as initiative, job knowledge, and the ability to work with others. In developing an appraisal device, an organization can focus on employee traits, result, behaviors, and/or some combination thereof (Bernardin & Beatty, 1984). The specific focus of the form affects the whole appraisal process.

TRAITS/PERSONAL CHARACTERISTICS.
Most appraisal systems focus on personal traits and characteristics, such as stability or ability to handle stress (Murphy & Cleveland, 1991). Typically, the nurse manager is asked to rate staff nurses on each trait, and she or he does so using an absolute judgment approach. The major reason that most appraisal systems focus on traits is probably cost. Trait-oriented appraisal instruments are inexpensive to develop and can be used for a wide variety of positions.

In recent years, however, there has been a gradual shift away from trait-oriented systems, primarily because of legal problems (minorities often get lower ratings on trait scales than non-minorities) and accreditation pressures. In terms of legal problems, when minorities receive lower

FIGURE 16–1 SAMPLE ITEMS BASED ON ABSOLUTE AND COMPARATIVE JUDGMENT

	Fails to meet performance standard (1)	Does not quite meet performance standard (2)	Meets performance standard (3)	Exceeds performance standard (4)	Far exceeds performance standard (5)
Absolute Judgment Items "Rate each staff nurse based on what you consider satisfactory performance"					
1. Initiative					
2. Dependability					
3. Job knowledge					
4. Adherence to hospital policies					

	Bottom 10% of all staff nurses	Next 20%	Middle 40% of all staff nurses	Next 20%	Top 10% of all staff nurses
Comparative Judgment Items "Rate each staff nurse you supervise by comparing him/her with the others you supervise."					
1. Initiative					
2. Dependability					
3. Appearance					
4. Proper utilization of time					

ratings than non-minorities, the institution should be able to demonstrate the validity (job relatedness) of the appraisal ratings. In most court cases, trait ratings have not been found to be job related (Bernardin & Beatty, 1984). Thus, many organizations have been found guilty of discrimination.

Another reason institutions have moved away from exclusive reliance on trait ratings is their lack of utility for developing employees. In most health care institutions, a major reason for doing performance appraisals is to help employees improve. However, because most trait rating dimensions are somewhat ambiguous (what precisely is meant by "initiative"?), trait-oriented systems do not tell a staff nurse what to do differently in the future.

RESULTS. All organizations, even nonprofit health care institutions, need to be concerned with the so-called bottom line. If a hospital has a 35 percent occupancy rate or a 20 percent employee absenteeism rate, its future is in jeopardy. In recent years, therefore, top management has turned to appraising some employees at least partly on the basis of their results. Although an in-depth discussion of such results-oriented appraisal systems appears later in this chapter, it is important to briefly mention a few of the pros and cons of evaluating health care personnel on the basis of their results.

In theory, a results-oriented appraisal system is ideal. Employees know in advance what results are expected. These objectives are quantifiable, objective, and easily measured. Unfortunately, in practice, it is not easy to identify easily measured, concrete objectives for most health care jobs. For example, some aspects of a staff nurse's job, such as providing quality patient care, are not easily quantified. Other aspects may be easily quantified, such as the average

number of minutes before answering a patient's call button, but not worth the cost of measuring them. In addition, a results-oriented system is of little use for staff development; telling someone that he or she did not accomplish a goal does not tell the person how to accomplish it in the future. Although a results-oriented appraisal system has a number of positive attributes, total reliance on such a system for most health care jobs is often impractical.

BEHAVIORAL CRITERIA. In recent years, many health care institutions have adopted behavior-oriented performance appraisal systems rather than focusing on difficult to measure results or on vague traits that may cause legal problems. Behavior-oriented systems focus on what the employee actually does, as exemplified in Figure 16–2. Such a system gives new employees specific information on how they are expected to behave and is less likely to lead to legal problems, and the behavioral focus facilitates employee development. The major drawbacks of a behavior-oriented appraisal system are that it is relatively time-consuming to develop and that it is tied to only one job or a narrow range of jobs. For example, the behavioral items presented in Figure 16–2 were developed by interviewing a number of staff nurses and their immediate supervisors. Unlike more general trait dimensions (see Figure 16–1), these items would only be applicable to staff nurses.

COMBINING DIFFERENT TYPES OF CRITERIA. As health care institutions have become more concerned with employee productivity in the last few years, some have developed appraisal systems that combine the types of criteria just discussed. In such a system, each employee may have a few major objectives he or she is expected to accomplish. However, in addition to being evaluated on whether these results were attained, individuals are also evaluated in terms of both general personal characteristics and behaviorally specific criteria.

◆ SPECIFIC EVALUATION METHODS

TRADITIONAL RATING SCALES

The most commonly used performance appraisal format is the traditional rating scale that focuses primarily on personal characteristics/traits. According to Heneman et al. (1989), the traditional rating scale has the following characteristics.

1. Several performance dimensions are generated. Normally these dimensions (e.g., dependability) are not based on a job analysis; instead, they are generated arbitrarily.

2. The performance dimensions are general in nature. Thus, they can be applied to a wide variety of jobs. In fact, an organization often uses the same rating scales for all its employees.

3. The performance dimensions are equally weighted in arriving at an overall performance appraisal score. No dimension is seen as more important than any other dimension.

4. Absolute judgment standards are the basis on which ratings are made. Thus, identical behavior on the part of employees may get various appraisal ratings simply because different supervisors have different ideas of what satisfactory performance is.

In filling out a traditional rating scale, the appraiser is required to reflect on the appraisee's performance over the entire evaluation period (usually 12 months) and rate the individual against the rater's internal standard of performance. A common complaint of individuals using trait rating scales is that either the performance dimension (e.g., leadership) is irrelevant to the job in question or that they do not know exactly what is meant by the dimension. Such complaints arise because one appraisal form is being used across a variety of jobs and because the performance dimensions are not tied to concrete behaviors.

ESSAY EVALUATION

With the essay technique, the nurse manager is required to describe the employee's performance over the entire evaluation period by writing a narrative detailing the strengths and weaknesses of the appraisee. If done correctly, this approach can provide a good deal of valuable data for discussion in the appraisal interview. If used alone, however, an essay evaluation is subject to a number of constraints that can limit its effectiveness. For example, essay evaluations can be time-consuming to write, they depend on appraisers' ability to express themselves in prose, and they can be difficult to defend in court because comments made by the manager may not be closely tied to actual job performance. Most organizations have found that essay evaluations are more useful when they are used in combination with other evaluation formats and when they are based on notes taken by the manager during the course of the evaluation period.

FORCED DISTRIBUTION EVALUATION

The forced distribution approach to performance appraisal is similar to grading on a curve. The manager is required to rate employees in a fixed manner (see the comparative judgment items in Figure 16–1). If the rating scale has five categories, the manager may be required to spread employees' ratings equally over the five categories. Since this technique constrains the rater, most evaluators do not like it. One hears such complaints as, "I have two exceptional employees but this system only allows me to put one of them in the highest category," or, "I don't have an employee who deserves to be rated in the lowest category." Because of the general dislike of forced distribution systems, they are not commonly used. In those instances where they are used, forced distribution systems were generally implemented because managers were giving all of their employees high ratings.

FIGURE 16–2 BEHAVIOR-ORIENTED PERFORMANCE APPRAISAL ITEMS FOR THE JOB OF STAFF NURSE

	Outstanding (5)	Above average (4)	Average (3)	Needs improvement (2)	Unacceptable (1)
1. Reorders medication as needed.					
2. Communicates information from physician's rounds to nursing personnel.					
3. Keeps nurse manager or charge nurse informed of changes in patient's condition.					
4. Reports faulty equipment and safety hazards and follows up to see that appropriate action has been taken.					
5. Reviews and clarifies physician's orders before the physician leaves unit.					
6. Communicates pertinent patient information at the change of shift.					

BEHAVIOR-ORIENTED RATING SCALES

As noted earlier, focusing on specific behaviors in appraising performance has tremendous advantages. For example, new employees have specific information on how they should behave. Although there are several varieties of behavior-oriented rating scales, they all share a number of things in common. Behavior-oriented scales are developed as follows:

1. Groups of workers (generally individuals doing the job and their immediate supervisors) who are very familiar with the target job provide written examples (*"critical incidents"*) of superior and inferior job behaviors.

2. Critical incidents that are similar in theme are grouped together and these behavioral groupings (*performance dimensions*) are labeled—for example, "Direct Patient Care," "Nurse-Physician Interactions."

3. Statistical procedures are used to arrive at a subset of the original pool of critical incidents. These procedures eliminate items that do not clearly reflect the performance dimension into which they were grouped, overlap other critical incidents, or are poorly worded.

In view of the way that behavior-oriented rating scales are developed, it is apparent that such behavior-oriented appraisal measures can only be used for one job or a cluster of very similar jobs and that these scales are time consuming and therefore expensive to develop. For these reasons, behavior-oriented systems are generally developed where there are a large number of individuals doing the same job, such as staff nurses. An advantage of these scales is the fact that because job incumbents and their supervi-sors actually develop the appraisal instrument, they have faith in the system and are motivated to use it.

MANAGEMENT BY OBJECTIVES

Whereas the other approaches to performance evaluation focus on an employee's personal characteristics (traits) or behavior, *management by objectives* (MBO) focuses on the results the employee accomplishes. Although there are many variations of this technique, basically MBO involves two steps.

First, a set of work objectives is established at the start of the evaluation period for the employee to accomplish during some future time frame. These objectives can be developed by the employee's supervisor and given to the employee; however, it is better if the supervisor and the subordinate work together and mutually develop a set of objectives for the employee. Each performance objective should be defined in concrete, quantifiable terms and have a specific time frame. For example, one objective may need to be accomplished in one month; another objective may not have to be met for 12 months. In setting objectives, it is important that the employee perceive them as challenging yet attainable. The second step in MBO involves the actual evaluation of the employee's performance. At this time, the supervisor and employee meet and focus on how well the employee has accomplished his or her objectives.

Although an MBO system can be excellent for evaluating some jobs, such a system has not met with much success in hospitals, primarily because it is difficult to set challenging, clear, quantifiable goals for health care jobs, where tasks are based on variable patient needs. For more detail on MBO, see the books by Latham and Wexley (1980) and Carroll and Schneier (1982).

♦ WHO EVALUATES?

In most institutions, an employee's immediate superior is in charge of evaluating her or his performance. In many situations, this makes sense: The superior is familiar with the employee's work and thus is best able to evaluate it. In other situations, however, the immediate supervisor may not have enough information to accurately evaluate a subordinate's performance but completes the evaluation form anyway. Obviously, an appraisal based on inadequate information is likely to be somewhat vague and inaccurate.

Two alternatives are available in this situation. First, the supervisor can informally seek out performance-related information from other sources—the employee's co-workers, patients, or other supervisors, for instance—who are familiar with the person being evaluated. The supervisor weighs this additional information, integrates it with his or her own judgment, and completes the evaluation.

The second alternative involves a more formal use of other sources. In some institutions an employee is formally evaluated by a committee that includes supervisors, peers, and some of the individual's subordinates. To arrive at a final performance rating, the committee also may seek information from the employee (nurse) and his or her clients (patients). Formal use of these nontraditional sources is infrequent, however, and several factors can interfere with the accuracy of such evaluations.

For example, if an employee's peers are used, personal friendships can lead to inflated evaluations. Such inflation is particularly likely if subordinates have input into their supervisors' ratings but are not given total anonymity. To reduce this tendency to inflate ratings, the individuals providing evaluation information should be required to provide several specific examples of the employee's behavior upon which they base their evaluations and their identity must remain anonymous. Not surprisingly, self-evaluations are generally found to be inflated, especially if the rating information is used to determine salary increases or promotion decisions.

♦ POTENTIAL APPRAISAL PROBLEMS

No matter what type of appraisal device is used, problems that lessen the accuracy of the performance rating can arise. This, in turn, limits the usefulness of the performance review. For example, if a performance rating can be shown to be inaccurate, it will be difficult to defend in court.

LENIENCY ERROR
Many nurse managers tend to overrate their staff nurses' performance. This is called *leniency error*. For example, a manager may rate everyone on her or his staff as "above average." Although numerous reasons are given for inflated ratings (e.g., "I want my nurses to like me," "It's difficult to justify giving someone a low rating"), these reasons do not lessen the problems that leniency error can create for both the manager and the health care institution. For example, if you give a mediocre nurse lenient ratings, it is difficult to turn around and take some corrective action such as demoting the person (Boncarosky, 1979).

Leniency error can also be demoralizing to the best staff nurses. This is due to the fact that the best nurses would have received high ratings without leniency. However, with leniency error, these outstanding nurses look less superior compared to their co-workers. Thus, leniency error tends to be welcomed by poorer nurses and disliked by better nurses.

RECENCY ERROR

Another difficulty with most appraisal systems is the length of time over which behavior is evaluated. In most institutions, employees are formally evaluated every 12 months. Evaluating employee performance over such an extended period of time, particularly if one supervises more than two or three individuals, is a difficult cognitive task. Typically, the evaluator recalls recent performance and tends to forget more distant events. Thus, the performance rating reflects what the employee has contributed lately rather than over the entire evaluation period. This tendency is called *recency error;* it can create both legal and motivational problems.

Legally, if a disgruntled employee can demonstrate that an evaluation that supposedly reflects 12 months actually reflects performance over the last two or three months, an institution will have great difficulty defending the validity of its appraisal system. In terms of motivation, recency error demonstrates to all employees that they only need to perform at a high level near the time of their performance review. In such situations, an employee is highly motivated (e.g., asking the supervisor for more work) just prior to her or his appraisal but considerably less motivated as soon as it is completed.

As with leniency error, recency error benefits the poorly performing individual. Nurses who perform well year-round may receive ratings similar to those mediocre nurses who "spurt" as their evaluation time approaches. Fortunately, a simple procedure (recording noteworthy behaviors, discussed later in the chapter) greatly lessens the impact of recency error.

HALO ERROR

Sometimes an appraiser fails to differentiate among the various performance dimensions (e.g., job knowledge, communication skills) when evaluating an employee and assigns ratings on the basis of an overall impression, positive or negative, of the employee. Thus, some employees are rated above average across dimensions, others are rated average, and a few are rated below average on all dimensions. This is referred to as *halo error.*

Sometimes what looks like halo error is actually accuracy. For example, if a nurse is excellent, average, or poor on all performance dimensions, she or he deserves to be rated accordingly. In most instances, however, employees have uneven strengths and weaknesses. Thus, it should be relatively uncommon for an employee to receive the same rating on all performance dimensions. Although halo error is less common and troublesome than leniency and recency error, it still can lead to erroneous feedback (Beer, 1981).

AMBIGUOUS EVALUATION STANDARDS

Most appraisal forms use rating scales that include words such as "outstanding," "above average," "satisfactory," or "needs improvement." But different managers attach different meanings to these words, giving rise to what has been labeled the *ambiguous evaluation standards problem.* Organizations have attempted to address this problem in two ways. One approach is to have a group of nurse managers meet and discuss what each of them sees as outstanding performance, above average performance, and poor performance, on each performance dimension. The goal is to arrive at a consensus on what level of performance is expected on each performance dimension. Thus, the group of nurse managers may decide that to be rated excellent on the dimension of self-development a nurse must attend at least 10 inservice meetings in a year. When agreement is reached on what behavior reflects each level of a performance dimension, this information should be communicated to those being evaluated.

A more formal approach to dealing with the ambiguous evaluation standards problem is to literally develop rating forms that have each gradation along the performance continuum (e.g., excellent, satisfactory) anchored by examples of behavior that is representative of that level of performance. Although a detailed discussion of the process a health care institution would use for developing such performance standards is too complex to go into here (usually a consulting firm works with the institution), simply stated, it involves groups of knowledgeable employees (e.g., job incumbents and their supervisors) meeting to discuss the important performance dimensions (e.g., nurse-physician interactions) for a job and then developing examples of different levels of performance on each performance standard (e.g., a rating of excellent on the dimension of nurse-physician interaction might be anchored by statements such as "have not received one justified complaint from a patient concerning this RN during the last 12 months" or "several times during the year physicians have mentioned to me what an outstanding performer this nurse is").

WRITTEN COMMENTS PROBLEM

Almost all performance appraisal forms provide space for written comments by the appraiser. The wise manager uses the "comments" space to justify in detail the basis for his or her ratings, to discuss developmental activities for the employee in the coming year, to put the ratings in context (e.g., to note that, although the evaluation period is 12 months, the appraiser has only been the nurse's supervisor for the past three months), or to discuss the employee's promotion potential. Unfortunately, few nurse managers use this valuable space appropriately; in fact, the spaces for written comments are often left blank. When there are comments, they tend to be few and general (e.g., "Joan is conscientious"), focus totally on what the individual did wrong, or only reflect recent performance.

The existence of the *written comments problem* should not be surprising. Most nurse managers wait until the end of the evaluation period to identify written comments; thus, the manager is faced with a difficult, time-consuming task. Small wonder, then, that the few comments tend to be vague, negative in tone, and reflect recent events. Fortunately, regular note-taking can lessen the written comments problem.

◆ IMPROVING APPRAISAL ACCURACY

To get maximum benefit from an appraisal, it needs to encompass all facets of job performance and be free from rater error. Although attempting to get totally accurate evaluations is much like the search for the Holy Grail, there are ways to greatly improve the accuracy of appraisals.

APPRAISER ABILITY

Accurately evaluating an employee's performance involves using the job description to identify behaviors required, observing the worker's performance over the course of the evaluation period and recalling it, and knowing how to use the appraisal form accurately (e.g., understanding what is meant by performance dimensions such as "initiative"). To the extent that any of these things are lacking, a manager's ability to rate accurately is limited.

Fortunately, a manager's ability to rate employees can be improved. An institution can develop detailed job descriptions and share them with the rater. Steps can be taken to give the rater greater opportunity to directly or indirectly observe an employee's behavior. For example, other supervisors can provide information on an employee's performance when the immediate supervisor is not present. Managers can be taught to take notes on an employee's behavior to facilitate recall. Last, managers can be made more knowledgeable concerning how to use an appraisal form through formal training.

Formal training programs help to increase appraiser ability by making raters aware of the various types of rating errors (the assumption being that awareness may reduce the error tendency), by improving raters' observational skills and by improving raters' skill in carrying out the performance appraisal interview. More specific information on ways to improve the observational skills and interviewing skills is presented later in this chapter.

APPRAISER MOTIVATION

Although it is often assumed that managers are motivated to accurately appraise their employees, such an assumption is often fallacious (Murphy & Cleveland, 1991). An in-depth discussion of motivation is beyond the scope of this chapter (see Chapter 8), but a brief examination of appraiser motivation is merited here.

Nurse managers have a multitude of tasks to perform, often immediately. Not surprisingly, then, performance appraisals are often viewed as something that can be done "later." Furthermore, many managers do not see doing appraisals as a particularly important task and some question the need for doing them at all. This is especially true if all employees receive the same percentage salary increase. Thus, if nurse managers are to be motivated to do appraisals well, they need to be rewarded for their efforts.

Among the reasons that a nurse manager may spend little time on appraisals are: (a) their institution does not reward the person for doing a good job, (b) the manager's superior spends little time on the nurse manager's own appraisal (thus sending the message that doing appraisals is not important), and (c) if a nurse manager gives low ratings to a poor employee, a superior may overrule him or her and raise the ratings. In short, in many health care institutions, the environment may actually dampen appraiser motivation rather than stimulate it.

Given these reasons for not spending time on appraisals, it is fairly obvious how an institution can enhance appraiser motivation. First, the nurse manager needs to be rewarded for conscientiously doing performance reviews. Second, the nurse manager's superior needs to present a good model of how an appraisal should be carried out. Finally, insofar as possible, the nurse manager should be able to reward those staff nurses he or she rates highly. Pay increases should not be across-the-board, layoffs should not be based on seniority, and promotions should be tied to superior performance.

♦ DOCUMENTING PERFORMANCE

Appraising a subordinate's performance can be a difficult job. A nurse manager is required to reflect on a staff nurse's performance over an extended period of time (usually 12 months) and then accurately evaluate it. Given that many nurse managers have several employees to evaluate, it is not surprising that they frequently forget what an individual did several months ago or that they may actually confuse what one employee did with what another worker did. A useful mechanism for fighting such memory problems is the use of *critical incidents,* which are reports of employee behaviors that are out of the ordinary, in either a positive or a negative direction. These noteworthy behaviors are recorded on a form or an index card with space for four items: name of employee, date and time of incident, a brief description of what occurred, and

the nurse manager's comments on what transpired (see Figure 16–3). Index cards are usually preferred to a page-size form because cards are more easily carried and are less likely to get torn.

Recording noteworthy behavior as it occurs is bound to increase the accuracy of the year-end performance appraisal ratings. Although this type of note-taking may sound simple and straightforward, a nurse manager can still run into problems; for instance, some managers feel sheepish about this kind of record keeping. Many managers are uncomfortable about recording behaviors; they see themselves as spies lurking around the unit attempting to catch someone. What they need to remember is that

FIGURE 16–3 EXAMPLE OF A CRITICAL INCIDENT

1. Name of Employee _____ *Cindy Siegler* _____

2. Date and time of incident _____ *12/2/92   12:30 p.m.* _____

3. Description _____ *I overheard Cindy discussing a patient's lack of personal hygiene in our coffee shop. She referred to the patient by name and spoke loud enough to be heard by people at other tables.*

4. Comments _____ *Her action was unprofessional. She could have caused embarrassment for both the patient and the hospital. I spoke with her concerning this matter.*

this note-taking will enable them to evaluate the employee more accurately. Such note-taking makes recency error much less likely.

The best time to write noteworthy behaviors is just after the behavior occurred. The note should focus on specifically what took place, not on an interpretation of what happened. For example, instead of writing, "Ms. Hudson was rude," write, "Ms. Hudson referred to the patient as a slob." The nurse manager is responsible for deciding what is noteworthy behavior. In some departments, coming to work on time may be noteworthy; in other departments, coming to work late is. Once a noteworthy behavior has been recorded, it should be shared with the employee by the nurse manager in private. If the behavior is positive, this provides a good opportunity for the nurse manager to praise the subordinate; if the behavior is considered in some way undesirable, the manager may need to coach the employee.

Because most nurse managers are extremely busy, they sometimes question whether note-taking is time well spent. In fact, keeping notes is not a time-consuming process. The average note takes less than two minutes to write. If one writes notes during the gaps in the day (e.g., while waiting for a meeting to start), little, if any, productive time is used. In the long run, such note-taking saves time. For example, keeping and sharing notes forces a manager to deal with problems when they are small and thus more quickly addressed. In addition, completing the appraisal form at the end of the evaluation period takes less time when one has notes for reference.

A key factor in effectively using this note-taking approach is how nurse managers introduce the technique to their subordinates. To get maximum value out of note-taking, nurse managers need to keep in mind two important facts: (a) the primary reason for taking notes is to improve the accuracy of the performance review and (b) when something new is introduced, many people react negatively to it. Managers should be open and candid about the first fact, admitting that they cannot remember every event associated with every employee and telling employees that these notes will make more accurate evaluations possible. Even then, employees will still be suspicious about this new procedure. One way to get this note-taking procedure off to a good start is for managers to make the first note they record on an employee a positive one, even if they have to "stretch" a bit to find one. By doing this, each employee's first contact with noteworthy behaviors is positive.

Based on the experience of institutions that have formally introduced the use of noteworthy behaviors, nurse managers tend to make three types of mistakes in using notes. Some managers fail to make them specific and behavior-oriented; rather, they record that a nurse was "careless" or "difficult to supervise." A second mistake concerns the tone of the notes. Some managers only record undesirable behavior. The third error is a nurse manager's failure to give performance feedback to the employee at the time that a note was written.

Each of these errors can undermine the effectiveness of the note-taking process. If the notes are vague, the employee may not know specifically what she or he is doing wrong and therefore does not know how to improve. If only poor performance is documented, employees will resent the system and the nurse manager. If the nurse manager does not share notes as they are written, the employee will often react defensively when confronted with them at the end of the evaluation period. In sum, any nurse manager who is considering using this powerful note-taking procedure needs to take the process seriously and to use it as it is designed.

By increasing the accuracy of the performance review, written notes also diminish the likelihood of lawsuits. Furthermore, if a lawsuit is brought, written notes are very persuasive evidence in court. Sharing the notes with employees throughout the evaluation period also improves the communication flow between the supervisor and the employee. Having written notes also gives the manager considerable confidence when it comes time to complete the evaluation form and to carry out the appraisal interview. The nurse manager will be less prone to leniency and recency error and will feel confident that the appraisal ratings are accurate. Not only does the nurse manager feel professional, but also the staff nurse shares that perception. In fact, it is typically found that with the use of notes, the performance appraisal interview focuses mainly on how the employee can improve next year rather than on how he or she was rated last year. Thus, the tone of the interview is constructive rather than argumentative.

In concluding this section on note-taking, one final issue needs to be addressed. Different employees will react differently to the use of notes. Good employees will react positively. Although the nurse manager will record both what is done well and what is done poorly, good employees will have many more positive than negative notes and therefore will benefit from notes being taken. In contrast, poorer employees do not react well to notes being taken. Whereas once they could rely on the poor memory of the nurse manager as well as on a leniency tendency to produce inflated ratings, note-taking is likely to result in more accurate (i.e., lower) ratings for poor employees. The negative reaction of poor employees, however, tends not to be a lasting

one. Generally, the poor performers either leave the organization or, when they discover that they no longer can get away with mediocre performance, their performance actually improves.

◆ THE PERFORMANCE APPRAISAL INTERVIEW

An accurate evaluation is the first prerequisite for an effective performance appraisal, but a manager should not make the mistake of thinking that when the form is filled out the appraisal process is completed. As noted earlier, a primary reason for doing the appraisal is to help the employee improve. The appraisal interview is a primary vehicle for employee development (Moore & Simendinger, 1976).

PREPARING FOR THE INTERVIEW
In preparing for the performance appraisal interview, the nurse manager must keep in mind what she or he wants to accomplish. If the appraisal ratings are accurate, they are more likely to be perceived as so by the subordinate. This perception should, in turn, make the employee more likely to accept them as a basis for both rewards as well as developmental activities. More specifically, to motivate employees, rewards need to be seen as linked to performance. The performance appraisal interview is the key to this linkage. In the interview, the nurse manager needs to establish that performance has been carefully assessed and that, when merited, rewards will be forthcoming. Developmental activities also need to be derived from an accurate evaluation. If an employee is rated as "needs immediate improvement" on delegation skills, any effort to remedy this deficiency must stem from

the employee's acceptance of the fact that the rating is accurate.

Even though they have tried to fill out the appraisal form accurately, nurse managers should still anticipate disagreement with some of their ratings. Most nurses, just as other employees, tend to see themselves as above-average performers. This tendency to exaggerate one's own performance results from the fact that we tend to forget our mistakes and recall our accomplishments and that we often rationalize away those instances where our performance was substandard (e.g., "I forgot, but with this heavy workload, what do you expect?"). Given this tendency to over-evaluate one's own performance and the fact that most staff nurses previously have had poor experiences with the evaluation process, nurse managers should expect that staff nurses will lack confidence in the whole appraisal process.

A key step for making the appraisal interview go well is proper planning. The performance appraisal interview should be set up in advance; preferably at least two days notice should be given. In setting a meeting time, the manager should allow enough time. Most interviews last 20 to 30 minutes although the time needed will vary considerably depending upon the degree to which the nurse manager and the staff nurse have talked regularly during the year.

In preparing for the appraisal interview, the nurse manager should have specific examples of behavior to support his or her ratings. Such documentation is particularly important for performance areas in which an employee receives low ratings. In addition, the manager should try to anticipate how the staff nurse will react to the appraisal. For example, will the staff nurse challenge the manager's ratings as being too low? By anticipating such a reaction, one can often deal with it effectively, such as by saying, "Before I

made my ratings, I talked with two other head nurses to make sure my standards were reasonable."

The setting should also be considered in planning the meeting. It is critical that the interview take place in a setting that is private and relatively free from interruptions. This allows a frank, in-depth conversation with the employee. Although it is difficult to limit interruptions in a health care setting, choosing the meeting time carefully will help. A nurse manager may be able to schedule the meeting when another manager can cover for her or him or at a time when interruptions are least likely to occur. The most important point to remember is that a poor setting limits the usefulness of the interview. No one wants weaknesses discussed in public. Similarly, interruptions destroy the flow of the feedback session.

THE INTERVIEW

The appraisal interview is most likely to go well if the nurse manager has written and shared noteworthy behaviors throughout the evaluation period. If such feedback has occurred, the staff nurse goes into the interview with a good idea of how she or he is likely to be rated as well as what behaviors led to the rating. If the nurse manager has not kept notes throughout the year, it is very important that she or he recall numerous specific examples of behavior, both positive and negative, to support the ratings given.

The major focus of the feedback interview should be on how the nurse manager and the staff nurse can work together to improve the nurse's performance in the coming year. However, establishing such an improvement-oriented climate is easier said than done. In giving feedback, a manager needs to be aware that every employee has a tolerance level for criticism, beyond which defensiveness sets in. Thus, in reviewing an employee's performance, a manager should emphasize only a few areas—preferably, no more than two—that need immediate improvement. Unfortunately, evaluators often exceed an employee's tolerance level, particularly if her or his performance has been mediocre. Typically, the manager will come up with an extensive list of areas needing improvement. Confronted with such a list, the staff nurse gradually moves from a constructive frame of mind ("I need to work on that") after one or two criticisms are raised to a destructive perspective ("She doesn't like me," "He's nitpicking," "How can I get even?") as the list of criticisms continues.

KEY BEHAVIORS FOR AN APPRAISAL INTERVIEW

The use of a set of key behaviors, which are listed in Figure 16–4, can greatly improve the way appraisal interviews are conducted. Each point is briefly discussed (a paragraph's number corresponds to the number of the key behavior).

1. Many subordinates are nervous at the start of the appraisal interview, especially new employees for whom this is their first evalua-

tion or those who have not received frequent performance feedback from their supervisor over the course of the evaluation period. To facilitate two-way communication during the interview, the nurse manager needs to put the staff nurse at ease. To do this, some managers rely on small talk, such as discussing the weather; others begin the interview by giving an overview of the type of information that was used in making the performance ratings, such as, "In preparing for this review, I relied heavily on the notes I have taken and shared with you throughout the year." Rather than trying to reduce the tension an employee may have at the start of the interview, it is better for a manager to ignore it. In many cases, if the manager has given the employee feedback throughout the evaluation period, the employee will not be nervous at the start of the session.

2. Next, the nurse manager should clearly state the purpose of the appraisal interview to help the employee do the best possible job in the coming year. This improvement-oriented theme should be conveyed at the beginning of the interview.

FIGURE 16–4 KEY BEHAVIORS FOR PERFORMANCE APPRAISALS

1. Put the person at ease.
2. Make it clear that the purpose of the performance review is to help the employee to do the best possible job.
3. Review the ratings with the employee, citing specific examples of behavior that resulted in a particular rating.
4. Ask for the employee's feelings about the ratings and listen, accept, and respond to them.
5. Together decide on specific ways in which performance areas can be strengthened. Write the resulting plans on paper.
6. Set a follow-up date.
7. Express your confidence in the employee.

Adapted from P. J. Decker, *Health Care Management Microtraining.* (St. Louis, MO: Decker and Associates, 1982). Used by permission.

3. Then, the supervisor should go through the ratings one by one with the employee and provide a number of specific examples of behavior that led to each rating. Some nurse managers mistakenly only use behavioral examples to support low ratings and this can cause problems. Subordinates are more likely to become defensive because the entire focus is on problem areas. If no attention is paid to the nurse's good performance in certain areas, she or he pays less attention to these behaviors in the future. In reviewing the ratings, the nurse manager should be careful not to rush. By systematically going through the ratings and providing behavioral examples, the nurse manager projects an image of being prepared and of being a professional. This is important for getting the staff nurse to accept the ratings and act on them.

4. The next step is for the nurse manager to draw out the staff nurse's reactions to the ratings. More specifically, the nurse manager needs to ask for the employee's reaction to the ratings and then listen, accept, and respond to them. Of the seven key behaviors for doing performance reviews, nurse managers have the most difficulty with this one. To effectively carry out this phase of the interview, the nurse manager must have confidence in the accuracy of his or her ratings.

When asked to express their reactions, individuals who have received low ratings will frequently question the rater's judgment ("Don't you think your standards are a little high?"). Not surprisingly, the manager whose judgment has been questioned then tends to get defensive, cutting off the employee's remarks and arguing for the rating in question. Being cut off sends a contradictory message to the employee. He or she was asked for reactions, but when they were given, the supervisor did not want to hear them. The nurse manager should anticipate that his or her ratings will be challenged and must truly want to hear the staff nurse's reaction to them.

After having listened to the employee's reactions, the nurse manager should accept and respond to them in a manner that conveys that the manager has heard what the employee said (e.g., paraphrase some of the comments) and accepts the individual's opinion ("I understand your view"). In addition, the manager may want to clarify what has been said ("I do not understand why you feel your 'initiative' rating is too low. Could you cite specific behavior to justify a higher rating?"). The nurse manager strives for a candid, two-way conversation and wants to know exactly how the subordinate feels.

5. The focus of the interview should now shift to the future. Together the nurse manager and the staff nurse should decide on specific ways in which performance areas can be strengthened and the resulting plans are written down. Because of the possibility of defensiveness, only one or two performance areas needing improvement should be addressed. The nurse manager should choose the area(s) that are most problematic and focus attention on this (these). In arriving at plans for improving performance, the nurse manager should begin by asking the staff nurse for ideas on how her or his performance can be enhanced. After the staff nurse has offered suggestions, the nurse manager can offer additional suggestions. It is critical that such performance plans refer to specific behavior. In some cases, not only will the staff nurse be expected to do things in a different manner (e.g., "I will refer to a patient

as Mr., Mrs., or Ms. unless specifically told otherwise"), but the supervisor may also be expected to change her or his behavior (e.g., "I will post changes in hospital policy before enforcing them").

6. After having agreed on specific ways to strengthen performance in problem areas, the nurse manager should set a follow-up date for a subsequent meeting, usually four to six weeks after the appraisal interview. At this later meeting, the manager provides specific feedback on the nurse's recent performance. This meeting also gives the manager and the nurse the opportunity to discuss any problems they have encountered in attempting to carry out their agreed-upon performance-improvement plans. In most cases, this follow-up session is quite positive. With only one or two areas to work on and a specific date on which feedback will be given, the nurse's performance usually improves dramatically. Thus, the follow-up meeting is one in which the nurse manager has the opportunity to praise the subordinate.

7. The final key behavior—expressing confidence in the employee—is simple but often overlooked. It is nevertheless important that the manager indicate her or his confidence that improvement will be forthcoming.

It has been suggested that no more than two problem areas should be addressed in the appraisal interview; other problem areas are addressed later in the year. If the performance areas targeted for improvement in the appraisal interview improve significantly, in the follow-up meeting the nurse manager praises the employee and encourages him or her to keep it up. However, a week or two after this follow-up session, the manager should meet again with the staff nurse, this time raising an additional area that

needs attention. As before, specific ways to improve the performance deficiency are developed and written down and another follow-up meeting is scheduled. In short, performance deficiencies are not ignored, they are merely temporarily overlooked.

♦ DAY-TO-DAY COACHING

As must be apparent by now, performance appraisals represent a year-round process of recording and sharing noteworthy behaviors. A key element of this process is day-to-day coaching by the nurse manager. As with the appraisal interview, coaching has been found to be quite effective for structuring nurse manager–staff nurse interactions.

Coaching is probably the most difficult task in management. It encompasses needs analysis, staff development, interviewing, decision making, problem solving, analytical thinking, active listening, motivation, and communication skills in one short interaction. Yet, it is a critical skill that, if mastered, usually leads to quality management. Intervening immediately in performance problems on a day-to-day basis usually eliminates small problems before they become large ones and become candidates for discussion in performance appraisal interviews or disciplinary actions. The coaching key behaviors are discussed in Chapter 15.

♦ DISCIPLINING EMPLOYEES

Most managers—including those in nursing—dread having to discipline an employee. Nevertheless, there will be occasions where discipline is necessary (e.g., when a regulation has been violated, thereby jeopardizing patient safety). In viewing the discipline process, the nurse manager must never lose sight of the reason for discipline. The primary function of discipline is not to punish the guilty party but to encourage that person and others to behave appropriately in the future (Boncarosky, 1979).

When faced with a disciplinary situation, the nurse manager should maintain close contact with the institution's human resource department and nursing administration. Before taking any disciplinary action, the manager should discuss the action he or she intends to take and seek approval for it. This close coordination between the nurse manager and the administration is essential to guarantee that any disciplinary action is administered in a fair and legally defensible manner.

To further ensure fairness, rules and regulations must be clearly communicated; a system of progressive penalties must be developed; and an appeals process must be available. To enforce rules or regulations, employees need to be informed of them ahead of time, preferably in writing.

If a rule is violated, penalties should be progressive. For minor violations (e.g., smoking in an unauthorized area), penalties may progress from an oral warning, to written warning placed in the employee's personnel folder, to a suspension, and, ultimately, to termination. For major rule violations (e.g., theft of hospital property) initial penalties should be more severe (e.g., immediate suspension). An appeals process should be built into an institution's disciplinary procedures to ensure that discipline is carried out in a fair, consistent manner. In some institutions, penalties can be appealed to a higher level manager. Other institutions have an appeals board composed of individuals representing a cross-section of jobs in the institution.

Here are some guidelines for effective discipline.

1. Get the facts before acting.

2. Do not act while angry.

3. Do not suddenly tighten your enforcement of rules.

4. Do not apply penalties inconsistently.

5. Discipline in private.

6. Make the offense clear. Specify what is appropriate behavior.

7. Get the other side of the story.

8. Do not let the disciplining become personal.

9. Do not back down when you are right.

10. Stay in touch with personnel.

As with performance appraisal interviewing and coaching, key behaviors have also been developed for disciplining employees (see Figure 16–5). Inasmuch as these closely parallel the key behaviors for coaching found in Chapter 15, they are not discussed here.

♦ RULES OF THUMB

To this point, several techniques and guidelines for doing successful appraisals have been systematically set forth, but there remain some additional suggestions, or "rules of thumb," that derive from practical experience.

Go beyond the form. Too often people doing evaluations use a "poor" form as an excuse for doing a poor job of evaluating their subordinates. No matter how inadequate an appraisal form is, managers can go beyond it. They can focus on behavior even if the form does not require it. They can set goals even if other supervisors do not. They can use noteworthy behaviors. In short, nurse managers should do the best job of managing that they can and not let the form handicap them.

Postpone the appraisal interview if necessary. Once the appraisal interview begins, there appears to be some natural law of management that the session must be completed in the time allotted, whether the session is going well or has degenerated into name calling. Managers forget the goal of the appraisal interview is not merely to get an employee's signature on the form but also to get the employee to improve her or his performance in the coming year. Therefore, if the interview is not going well, a manager should discontinue it until a later time. Such a postponement allows both the manager and the subordinate some time to reflect on what has transpired as well as some time to calm down.

In postponing the meeting, the manager should not assign blame (e.g., "if you're going to act like a child, let's postpone the meeting") but should adopt a more positive approach (e.g., "This meeting isn't going as I hoped it would; I'd like to postpone it to give us some time to collect our thoughts"). Most managers who have used this technique find the second session, which generally takes place a day or two later, goes much better.

Don't be afraid to change an inaccurate rating. New managers often ask: "Should I change a rating if an employee challenges it?" They fear that by changing a rating they will be admitting an error. They also fear that changing a rating will lead to other ratings being challenged. A practical rule of thumb for this situation is: If the rating is inaccurate, change it, but *never* change it during the appraisal interview. Rather, if an employee challenges a rating and the manager believes she or he has a case, the manager should tell the person that he or she wants some time to think about the rating and will get back to the employee.

The logic behind this rule of thumb is as follows. If a manager does a careful job of evaluating performance, he or she should make few inaccurate ratings. But, no one is perfect, and on rare occasions, managers will err. When such an error occurs, it should be corrected. Most employees respect a manager who admits a mistake and corrects it. By allowing for some time to reflect on the ratings, a manager eliminates the pressure to make a snap judgment.

FIGURE 16–5 KEY BEHAVIORS IN DISCIPLINE*

1. Define the problem in terms of lack of improvement since the previous discussion.
2. Ask for and openly listen to reasons for the continued behavior.
3. Explain why the behavior cannot continue.
4. If disciplinary action is called for, indicate what action you must take and why.
5. Agree on specific steps to be taken to solve problem (write them down).
6. Set a follow-up date and outline further steps to be taken if the problem is not corrected.
7. Assure the employee of your interest in helping him/her to succeed.

*Always prepare before the meeting.

Adapted from P. J. Decker, *Health Care Management Microtraining.* (St. Louis, MO: Decker and Associates, 1982). Used by permission.

SUMMARY

♦ Doing performance appraisals is one of the most difficult and most important management activities.

♦ Accurate appraisals provide a sound basis for both administrative decisions (e.g., salary increases) and employee development activities.

♦ Poorly done performance reviews can result in legal problems.

♦ There are a variety of different performance evaluation methods. It is possible to do an effective job of evaluating employees no matter what system or method is used.

♦ Most supervisors are subject to leniency and recency errors.

♦ To improve the accuracy of evaluations, the evaluator's ability and motivation to rate accurately must be improved.

♦ Keeping a record of noteworthy behaviors can greatly improve the quality of performance reviews.

♦ Preparation is essential for doing effective appraisal interviews.

♦ Using appraisal interview key behaviors will enhance the value of the feedback session.

♦ Day-to-day coaching is a critical component of the appraisal process.

♦ If disciplining an employee is necessary, following established guidelines and key behaviors increases managerial effectiveness.

BIBLIOGRAPHY

Beer, M. (1981). "Performance Appraisal: Dilemmas and Possibilities." *Organizational Dynamics,* 10 (Spring): 24–36.

Boncarosky, L. D. (1979). "Guidelines to Corrective Discipline." *Personnel Journal,* 58 (October): 698.

Carroll, S. J., and Schneier, C. E. (1982). *Performance Appraisal and Review Systems.* Glenview, IL: Scott, Foresman and Company.

Heneman, H. G., Schwab, D. P., Fossum, J. A., and Dyer, L. D. (1989). *Personnel/Human Resource Management.* Homewood, IL: Richard D. Irwin.

Klasson, C. R., Thompson, D. E., and Luben, G. L. (1980). "How Defensible Is Your Performance Appraisal System?" *Personnel Administrator,* 25 (December): 77–83.

Latham, G. P., and Wexley, K. N. (1980). *Increasing Productivity through Performance Appraisal.* Reading, MA: Addison-Wesley.

Moore, T., and Simendinger, E. (1976). "Evaluation As a Two-Way Street." *Supervisor Nurse,* 7(6): 58–59.

Murphy, K. R., and Cleveland, J. N. (1991). *Performance Appraisal.* Boston: Allyn and Bacon.

Rakich, J., Longest, B. B., and O'Donovan, T. (1977). *Managing Health Care Organizations.* Philadelphia: Saunders.

Rowland, H. S., and Rowland, B. L. (editors). (1985). *Nursing Administration Handbook. 2nd ed.* Rockville, MD: Aspen Systems Corporation.

UNDERSTANDING AND MANAGING NURSE ABSENTEEISM AND TURNOVER

Historically, health care institutions have had serious problems with excessive employee absenteeism and turnover. This chapter examines the reasons that these two so-called *withdrawal* behaviors occur and discusses their possible effects. Because many of the causes of absenteeism are quite different from those of turnover, these two withdrawal behaviors are examined separately. This chapter also offers suggestions for increasing employee attendance and retention, the counterparts of absenteeism and turnover. This chapter has a "proactive" (action-oriented) emphasis. Rather than merely trying to live with absenteeism and shortage problems, nurse managers can utilize a variety of strategies for managing these behaviors.

♦ ABSENTEEISM

To provide high-quality, reasonably priced patient care, sufficient staff must be available. If staff nurses are absent, the patient suffers either directly or indirectly. For example, a staff shortage can lead to patient care being rushed and, therefore, of poorer quality. Or, if a nurse works a double shift to cover for an absent co-worker, the added cost of the overtime is ultimately passed on to the patient. Dealing with such staff absenteeism is an important aspect of a nurse manager's job.

Although it is difficult to determine the extent or the cost of nurse absenteeism, it is well established that absenteeism in health care institutions is both pervasive and expensive (e.g., Bureau of National Affairs, 1988; Taunton, Krampitz & Woods, 1989). However, the costs of absenteeism go beyond its effects on patient care and dollar costs. Absenteeism can have a detrimental effect on the work lives of the other staff nurses. In some cases, they may have to work shorthanded; they are expected to cover the unit despite their missing colleagues. Working shorthanded, especially for an extended period of time, can create both physical and mental strain. These nurses may be forced to skip breaks, hurry through meals, work extended hours, abbreviate their interactions with patients, cancel scheduled nonwork activities, and so on. Even if temporary replacements are called in, the work flow of the unit will still be disrupted. For example, standard institutional procedure may need to be explained to replacement nurses.

Given the undesirable effects of absenteeism, it is not surprising that absenteeism has drawn a good deal of attention in the health care field. For the nurse manager, the question is: "What can I do to lessen our recurrent absenteeism problem?" But, before considering ways to "manage" absenteeism, we must understand its causes. In the following section, a useful model for understanding nurse absenteeism or, conversely, nurse attendance is presented.

A MODEL OF EMPLOYEE ATTENDANCE

To understand employee absenteeism, it is important to distinguish between *voluntary* and *involuntary* absenteeism. For example, not coming to work in order to finish one's income taxes would be seen as voluntary absenteeism (i.e., absenteeism that is under the employee's control). In contrast, taking a sick day because of food poisoning would be considered involuntary absenteeism (i.e., largely outside of the employee's control). Although this voluntary/involuntary distinction seems reasonable in theory, in practice it is often difficult to distinguish between these two categories due to a lack of accurate information (few employees will admit to abusing sick leave).

Some organizations try to distinguish between voluntary and involuntary absenteeism by the way they measure absenteeism. Traditionally, health care institutions have measured absenteeism in terms of *total time lost* (i.e., the number of scheduled days an employee misses). Given that one long illness can drastically affect this absenteeism index, it is clearly not a perfect measure of voluntary absenteeism. In contrast, *absence frequency* (i.e., the total number of distinct absence periods regardless of their duration) is somewhat insensitive to one long illness. Therefore, absence frequency has been used as an indirect estimate of voluntary absenteeism.

This distinction between absence frequency and total time lost should make sense to nurse managers. For example, an employee who missed nine Mondays in a row would have nine absence frequency periods as well as nine total days absent. In contrast, a person who missed nine consecutive days of work would have one absence frequency period but nine total days lost. Intuitively, it seems likely that the first individual was much more prone to being absent voluntarily than the second. In fact, based upon his statistical analysis of absenteeism records, Breaugh (1981) demonstrated that managers' performance appraisal ratings of their employees' attendance were much more closely related to absence frequency periods than to total days lost. Thus, it appears managers really do consider the pattern of the absences more than simply the number of days lost.

Although there are many models of attendance/absenteeism behavior, a revised version of one developed by Rhodes and Steers (1990) is the basis of discussion in this chapter. According to this model (see Figure 17–1), an employee's attendance at work is largely a function of two variables: the individual's ability to attend and motivation to attend.

As can be seen in Figure 17–1, an employee's ability to attend can be affected by such *attendance barriers* as personal illness or injury,

FIGURE 17-1 A DIAGNOSTIC MODEL OF EMPLOYEE ATTENDANCE

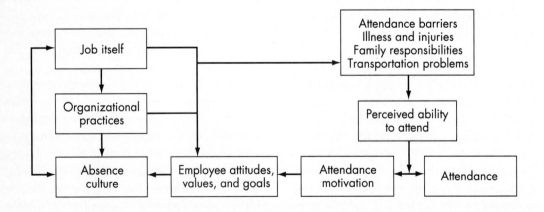

family responsibilities (e.g., a sick child), or transportation problems (e.g., an unreliable automobile). Although it is natural for a manager to view such barriers as resulting in involuntary absenteeism, sometimes this is too simplistic a judgment. For example, an employee who knew she or he had a "sick" car may consciously have not made alternative arrangements to get to work the next day because he or she was *not* motivated to attend. From this example, it should be apparent that some of the distinctions portrayed in Figure 17–1 are not always black and white. It should also be obvious that, in trying to understand employee absenteeism, a manager will have to make assumptions about why the behavior is occurring (i.e., a manager cannot be certain that a person was actually ill).

According to the attendance model, an employee's motivation to attend is affected by four factors: the *job itself, organizational practices,* the *absence culture,* and the *employee's attitudes, values,* and *goals.* In terms of the influence of the job itself (e.g., its duties, challenge, stress, hours) on attendance motivation, obviously, great complexity is involved. However, for our purposes a few summary conclusions taken from Rhodes and Steers (1990) suffice.

In assessing basic job characteristics, it has been argued that employees holding more enriched jobs will be less likely to be absent than those with more mundane jobs. Among the reasons that enriched jobs may increase attendance motivation are because they cause employees to believe that what they are doing is important and because in more enriched jobs other employees are likely to be interdependent on the job holder (i.e., if the job holder doesn't do his or her job, other employees can't do theirs).

The nature of a job not only can influence attendance through its effect on attendance motivation, but also can influence attendance

through its effect on illness and injuries (i.e., attendance barriers). For example, a job that requires heavy lifting (e.g., moving patients from beds to stretchers) may increase the likelihood that a staff nurse will be injured. In a similar vein, a job that exposes a nurse to individuals with highly contagious conditions, such as in an outpatient clinic, may increase the likelihood of illness.

As portrayed in Figure 17–1, organizational practices can also influence attendance motivation. Some health care institutions have absence control policies that influence attendance motivation by rewarding employees for good attendance and/or punishing them for excessive absenteeism. An organization may also be able to increase attendance motivation by carefully recruiting and selecting employees (see Chapter 13 on recruiting and staffing). In addition to affecting attendance motivation, organizational practices may influence an employee's ability to attend. Such organizational activities as offering wellness programs, employee assistance programs, van pools, onsite child care, or coordinating car pools could influence an employee's ability to attend work.

The absence culture of a work unit (or an organization) can also influence employee attendance motivation. Absence culture refers to a "set of shared understandings about absence legitimacy" (Johns & Nicholson, 1982: 136). Some work units have an absence culture that reflects a tolerance for excessive absenteeism. Other units have a culture in which being absent is frowned upon. Although an institution's absence culture can be affected by organizational practices (e.g., the type of people who are hired) and the nature of the jobs involved (e.g., people in higher-level jobs tend to be less accepting of co-workers calling in sick), it is also affected by informal norms that develop among work group members. For example, people in a cohesive work group may develop an understanding that missing work, except for an emergency or a serious illness, is unacceptable. Such an attendance culture is particularly likely to emerge if the employees work in jobs that they see as important (e.g., providing direct patient care) and if an employee being absent causes a hardship for co-workers (e.g., forced overtime, being called in on a day off).

Although features of the job itself, organizational practices, and a work unit's absence culture can all have a direct effect on employee attendance motivation, these factors can also interact with an employee's attitudes (e.g., job satisfaction), values (e.g., personal work ethic), or goals (e.g., desire to get promoted). If a person who seeks variety in a position works in a job that does not provide much variety, the employee may become dissatisfied and thus more likely to abuse sick leave. Employee attitudes, values, and goals can also have a direct effect on attendance motivation. For example, a staff nurse with a high personal work ethic or who has a goal of getting promoted should be more highly motivated to attend work than a nurse who lacks such a work ethic.

Although the model in Figure 17–1 does not single out supervision as a factor influencing attendance motivation, it clearly is an important variable (Rhodes & Steers, 1990). A nurse manager can influence the nature of a staff nurse's job (e.g., the degree of responsibility the person is given), the consistency with which organizational practices are applied (e.g., are sanctions enforced for abuse of sick leave), and a work unit's absence culture (e.g., by stressing the importance of good attendance). Another factor that can influence attendance motivation but that is not singled out in the attendance model is the labor market. To the extent that the job market (e.g., the local employment market for nurses) leads an employee to perceive it would be easy for him or her to find an equivalent job if he or she lost or disliked the current one, one would expect a lower level of attendance motivation than if market conditions were less favorable. This has been happening during the nursing shortage.

Although no feedback arrows are included in the attendance model, clearly the model assumes that an employee's attendance behavior is influenced by his or her past experiences. For example, if an employee's perfect attendance in the previous year was not rewarded, we might expect the employee's attendance motivation to decrease in the coming year. In a similar vein, if a co-worker with an outstanding record received a promotion, one would expect that peers who value a promotion and who witnessed this performance-reward linkage would be more motivated to attend work in the upcoming year.

Four points should be emphasized about the attendance model. First, both ability and motivation to attend must be present for maximum employee attendance. Second, the importance of each element of the attendance model is not the same for each employee. Some staff nurses may desire a position that affords promotion potential, be greatly influenced by their unit's attendance culture, or be bothered by reporting to an authoritarian nurse manager; others may not. Third, although research on employee absenteeism has not been systematically reviewed, considerable research supports the basic elements of the attendance model (see Rhodes & Steers, 1990). Finally, this model should provide a useful framework for nurse managers as they attempt to understand why staff nurses are absent and what might be done about it. In the section that follows, several variables in the attendance model are addressed in more detail.

MANAGING EMPLOYEE ABSENTEEISM

The attendance model in Figure 17–1 is useful not only for understanding why absenteeism occurs but also for developing strategies to control it. Some causes of absenteeism, such as transportation difficulties or child care problems, may be beyond the direct control of nurse managers. The manager, however, should try to do what she or he can, either in interactions with staff nurses or by attempting to get the health care institution to change policies that may be interfering with a nurse's ability or motivation to attend work. On the other hand, a manager must be careful that the steps taken do not go so far as to discourage the legitimate use of sick leave. Clearly, one does not want sick nurses coming to work and exposing patients and co-workers.

Although the attendance model makes it clear that several possible factors can result in absenteeism problems, it is important for nurse managers to systematically diagnose the key factors leading to absenteeism in their units. In doing so, they may need to gather information from several sources, including subordinates, the human resource department, other nurse managers, and higher level supervisors. In investigating absenteeism, studying absence patterns can be particularly informative. Among the questions a study of absenteeism data can answer are: (a) is absenteeism equally distributed across staff nurses, (b) in comparison to other units in your hospital, does your unit have a high absenteeism rate, (c) are most absences short or long in duration, and (d) does the absenteeism have a consistent pattern (e.g., occur predominantly on weekends? shortly before a person quits?)? The usefulness of answering these questions will become clearer as we discuss specific strategies for controlling absenteeism.

After reflecting upon the factors that affect the ability of staff nurses to attend work, many nurse managers conclude there is nothing they can do to influence this key variable. This may be an overly pessimistic reaction. While there may be little that a manager can directly do to affect ability to attend, there may be several actions the organization can take. For example, to lessen child care problems, an institution could set up or sponsor a child care center. Milkovich and Gomez (1976) found that the presence of day care facilities was inversely related to absenteeism. To lessen transportation problems, a health care institution could provide shuttle buses or coordinate car pools. To reduce illness, health fairs, exercise programs, and stress reduction classes could be offered (Latham & Napier, 1984). Given that alcoholism and drug abuse are widely recognized as important causes of absenteeism (Rhodes & Steers, 1990), it may be prudent for an institution to offer access to an employee assistance plan. Nurse managers should attempt to influence their institution to consider offering these types of programs. Such influence attempts are more likely to be successful if a group of nurse managers (or conceivably managers from throughout the institution) coordinate their actions.

In addition to these institutional actions, a nurse manager, through coaching or counseling, may be able to influence a staff nurse's ability to attend. For example, through discussions with a staff nurse, a nurse manager may develop a plan for reducing illness or solving child care problems. The manager's own creativity can expand the list of such actions.

Clearly, the best way for nurse managers to control absenteeism is by affecting their staff's motivation to attend. Based upon the attendance model, nurse managers need to influence characteristics of the nursing job, organizational practices, the absence culture, or the attitudes, values, and goals of their subordinates. Among the absenteeism management strategies that a nurse manager might consider are (a) enriching the staff nurse job by increasing its responsibility, variety, or challenge; (b) reducing job stress (e.g., by providing more timely and more concrete information); (c) creating a norm of excellent attendance (e.g., by emphasizing the negative impact of a nurse not coming to work); (d) enhancing advancement opportunities (e.g., by providing developmental experiences so that the best employees are promotable); (e) improving co-worker relations (e.g., by considering co-worker compatibility when scheduling work and/or creating work teams); (f) trying to select employees who will be satisfied with and committed to their jobs; (g) providing a good role model (i.e., the nurse manager rarely uses sick days); (h) discussing the employee's attendance during the performance appraisal interview; (i) rewarding good attendance with salary increases and other rewards; and (j) enforcing absenteeism control policies (e.g., carrying through on employee discipline when it is merited because of an attendance problem). Given that the aforementioned strategies for influencing attendance motivation have been addressed in detail in other chapters in this book, they are not discussed further in this section.

ABSENTEEISM POLICIES

Although there are exceptions, in most health care institutions employees accrue paid sick days—typically, one sick day for every month employed. Unused sick days accrue across time to some maximum number (e.g., 60 days). Typically, if an employee leaves the hospital with accumulated sick leave or days above the maximum, the person simply loses it. Although such a policy may seem reasonable, it may actually encourage unwanted behavior. For example, once a nurse has reached the maximum limit for accrued sick days, the person may see no reason for not using sick days that would otherwise be lost. Such a policy also encourages absenteeism on the part of employees who know they will be leaving the organization (e.g., those about to retire, change jobs). Knowing they will receive nothing for unused sick leave, exiting employees tend to use up their allotment of paid sick days prior to leaving.

Recently, a few progressive institutions have taken a close look at their absenteeism policies and subsequently have realized they have not been motivating good attendance. In attempting to reward attendance, these organizations have taken a variety of different tacks. For example, some institutions have allowed sick days to accumulate without an upper limit. Then, when an employee leaves the institution, she or he is paid for sick days that have not been used (e.g., one-half day's pay for each unused sick day). Some institutions have allowed retiring employees to add unused sick days to days worked, enabling retirement at an earlier date. Panyan and McGregor (1976) examined the effectiveness of paying (i.e., $10.00) for each unused sick day and found over a 35 percent drop in absenteeism the first year. Over the next three years, absenteeism averaged less than 50 percent of the rate prior to this new policy. In another study, Schlotzhauer and Rosse (1985) examined the effects of allowing hospital employees to convert unused sick leave to either additional vacation days or pay. They report that absenteeism fell 32 percent as a result of this attendance incentive.

As health care institutions have gradually come to realize that employees will use sick days for carrying out personal business, another innovative approach for managing absenteeism, substituting "personal days" for unused sick days, has been tried. The problem that arises with not giving personal days is twofold. Employees are "forced" to lie (i.e., say they are sick when they are not) to carry out what they see as legitimate activities (e.g., attending a conference with their child's teacher). In addition, their manager has no warning and therefore may have difficulty covering for the "sick" employee. By substituting personal days for sick days, the employee no longer has to lie and the nurse manager may have time to plan for a replacement. In moving to a policy that incorporates the use of personal days, an institution typically allocates fewer paid sick days but adds personal days. For example, instead of 12 sick days, an employee may annually receive nine sick days and three personal days. With the availability of personal days, a staff nurse can inform the nurse manager in advance of the need for a personal day off. In many cases, the two of them can arrive at a day off that is optimal for both of them.

Although uncommon, a few organizations have experimented with special financial incentives such as cash bonuses or other prizes as a reward for good attendance. Some institutions have actually established lotteries for rewarding good attendance, where chances of winning the lottery are tied to one's attendance record. For example, Stephens and Burroughs (1978) designed two incentive systems for six nursing units in a hospital. In the first system, individuals were eligible for the lottery ($20 for every 20 employees eligible) if they had no unscheduled absences for a three-week period. In the second system, to be eligible nurses had to be at work on eight randomly chosen, unannounced days over three weeks. Stephens and Burroughs (1978) found both incentive systems to be equally effective, with the incentive being linked to a 40 percent drop in absenteeism.

Obviously, changing an institution's paid sick leave policy is beyond the control of the nurse manager. However, a concerted effort by an organized group of nurse managers can be effective in getting their personnel department to initiate such changes. Simply stated, the innovations that have been discussed reward good attendance. Considering the high costs of absenteeism, these changes can be quite cost effective.

Most health care institutions have formal policies concerning how much absenteeism is allowable. Once this limit is reached, prescribed disciplinary steps are outlined. In disciplining an employee, it is important that the nurse manager follow the discipline policy carefully. The effectiveness of discipline as a strategy for reducing absenteeism is limited. Most discipline policies only take effect after several days have been missed. Not surprisingly, most employees know what this critical number of days is and are careful not to exceed it. In effect, the nurse manager is left with an absenteeism problem but not one that she or he is able to address through the use of discipline.

A SYSTEMS PERSPECTIVE

Although several strategies for improving employee attendance have been discussed, it should be emphasized that there are no panaceas to absenteeism. The nurse manager is cautioned to avoid a "quick fix" approach at all costs. Rather, what is needed is a systems perspective. The nurse manager (and the personnel department) needs to view absenteeism within the context of the whole work environment. One obvious first question is: "Is there an absenteeism problem?" As has already been discussed, one should never have a goal of zero absenteeism. Not only is such a goal unrealistic (the nurse manager will lose credibility), but also it can ultimately lead to sick nurses coming to work. If after comparing the absenteeism in the unit to other relevant comparison data (e.g., rates in other units, other hospitals) a manager perceives an absenteeism problem, then she or he should investigate why the absenteeism is occurring. Such an investigation can involve conversations with others (e.g., higher level supervisors, absence-prone nurses) as well as an examination of absence patterns (e.g., does most absenteeism occur in the month before an employee quits?). Based upon the results of such an investigation, the nurse manager should have a better understanding of how to attempt to manage absenteeism.

As has been noted throughout this chapter, many of the managerial actions addressed in other chapters are relevant to the control of absenteeism. For example, in recruiting employees, the use of a realistic job preview should increase the congruence between job characteristics and employee values and expectations. Similarly, basing merit pay and advancement opportunities on an employee's overall performance appraisal rating (which is partly based on attendance) will motivate better attendance. Also, leadership skills are important in getting the institution to change policy to lessen absenteeism (e.g., providing payment for unused sick days).

It is important to address two specific issues, the use of personal characteristics and past behavior, relevant to employee selection. Although personal characteristics (e.g., marital status, having child care responsibility) have been linked to higher absenteeism rates, for legal reasons, a nurse manager should not base a hiring decision upon such personal characteristics. It is difficult to argue that every person within a category (e.g., married females with children) is likely to be prone to absenteeism. On the other hand, the past behavior of a specific job candidate is potentially valuable information. Several authors (e.g., Breaugh, 1981) have demonstrated that absenteeism tendencies tend to be quite consistent. Although the reasons that some

individuals have a higher level of absenteeism year after year are unclear (e.g., some people may be more susceptible to illness, others may have less of a work ethic), it is acceptable to use a person's past behavior as a predictor of his or her future behavior. Given the consistency of absenteeism behavior, managers should seek prior absenteeism information to aid in making hiring decisions. An applicant's previous absenteeism record may be acquired by written or telephone reference checks.

A multitude of factors affect employee attendance. Some are beyond the control of nurse managers, but others can be directly or indirectly influenced. The nurse manager's goal should be to do what is possible to alleviate this serious employee problem.

◆ TURNOVER

Although turnover rates differ among health care institutions, it is widely accepted that health care and, in particular, nursing, has one of the highest turnover rates in the United States. In the 1980s, the yearly turnover rate in health care institutions averaged between 18 and 25 percent according to the Bureau of National Affairs. In a recent study of four hospitals, Jones (1990) reported an average turnover rate of 27 percent.

As with absenteeism, it is difficult to estimate the actual dollar cost of nursing turnover. However, given the numerous expenses incurred in hiring a new nurse (e.g., recruiting, selection, orientation, on-the-job training) and temporarily replacing a nurse who quits or is fired (e.g., paying other nurses to work overtime or filling the vacancy with a temporary replacement), the costs are certainly sizable. Jones (1990) estimated the cost of a nurse quitting as being $3,000 or more.

Given its pervasiveness and its cost, nursing turnover clearly needs to be better understood and more effectively controlled. To facilitate such understanding and control, it is important that turnover be both clearly defined ("the cessation of membership in an organization by an individual who received monetary compensation from that organization") and differentiated (Mobley, 1982). For too long, turnover has been thought of in simplistic terms and seen as universally "bad." Such a primitive view of turnover is not helpful to managers as they attempt to deal with this costly problem. Rather, varieties of turnover need to be differentiated: Did the employee leave of his or her own accord or was the person asked to leave? Was the departed individual's performance exceptional or mediocre? Will the departed nurse be easy or difficult to replace? Questions such as these have only recently been asked by health care institutions. Yet, until they are answered, it is difficult to establish whether the institution truly has a turnover "problem" and, if so, what can be done about it.

The discussion in this chapter focuses mainly on voluntary turnover. If a health care institution finds a significant amount of involuntary turnover (i.e., employees being terminated), then it needs to carefully examine the way it recruits, selects, trains, and motivates employees. These topics are addressed in detail in other chapters in this book.

MEASUREMENT ISSUES

As with absenteeism, before a supervisor can hope to "manage" turnover, she or he must understand its causes. However, to arrive at such an understanding, the nurse manager must appreciate the complexity of many of the measurement issues involved in studying turnover. One of the first questions that needs to be answered

is: "Was the turnover voluntary or involuntary?" Although this may seem like an easy question to answer (i.e., did the nurse quit?), it often isn't. For example, some employees are given a chance to resign prior to being terminated. Thus, the question becomes: "If a nurse quits prior to being terminated, is this voluntary or involuntary turnover?" To add to the complexity, although a given manager may know that a staff nurse was pressured into quitting, the human resource department may not have this information. Thus, if turnover studies are conducted in the future, the situation described above is likely to be categorized as voluntary turnover. In addition to the complexity of determining if turnover was voluntary or involuntary, two other measurement-related issues (determining the reasons for the turnover and determining whether it was functional) also need to be addressed.

Traditionally, organizations have attempted to determine the reason(s) for voluntary turnover through two sources. Generally, the exiting employee's supervisor is asked why the employee is leaving and an exit interview with the departing employee is conducted by someone in the human resource department. Although such an approach for determining the cause of voluntary turnover is certainly straightforward, its validity has been questioned. Hinrichs (1975) has shown that the reasons given by departing employees in their exit interviews differ greatly from their responses to surveys completed several months after leaving the organization. Hinrichs argues that, because future employers often ask for reference information from prior employers, exiting employees provide "safe" responses (e.g., "a better opportunity came along") during an exit interview. In summarizing his results, Hinrichs found it was rare that departing employees would say anything negative about an organization they were leaving or about their immediate supervisor.

Although this tendency for departing employees to make safe responses is understandable, it makes it difficult to determine why turnover is occurring. To gather more useful information, a health care institution may need to utilize surveys that are sent to former employees several weeks after they have resigned. These former employees will need to be assured that their responses will not influence any future reference information the hospital furnishes on them but rather will only be used to help the institution diagnose why nurses are leaving. Another way to attempt to discover the cause of nurse turnover is through the use of interviews with the former employee's co-workers. Co-workers often know why an employee left.

In evaluating the impact of an employee leaving, it is useful to recognize that turnover is either functional or dysfunctional (Dalton, Krackhardt & Porter, 1981) for the institution. Losing a nurse who is an excellent performer is a greater loss than losing a mediocre performer. Similarly, if a nurse can be easily replaced, the loss to the institution is less than if she or he is hard to replace. Thus, a nurse manager needs to be particularly concerned about turnover when the nurses who are leaving are of high quality and difficult to replace (i.e., dysfunctional turnover). In contrast, if poorly performing nurses who can be easily replaced resign, the institution may actually benefit from the turnover (i.e., functional turnover).

Managers need to disregard the myth that all turnover is bad and replace it with an appreciation of the numerous factors that should be involved in determining whether turnover is a problem meriting attention. In the section that follows, we briefly discuss several factors that should be considered in making such a determination. More detail on turnover measurement issues may be found in Cavanagh (1989) and Parasuraman (1989).

CONSEQUENCES OF TURNOVER

In discussing the consequences of turnover, authors have traditionally focused on the financial costs to the organization (e.g., hiring expenses). Although turnover obviously involves real costs to the organization, this traditional perspective is too narrow; turnover also can have undesirable effects on patients, co-workers, and others. And, as discussed earlier, voluntary turnover is not always undesirable. Anyone with work experience can remember some individual (e.g., a co-worker, a supervisor) whose departure would have significantly improved the organization's functioning. In evaluating the consequences of turnover, a nurse manager (and the institution) must remember that voluntary turnover can have costs and/or benefits. In addition, it should be remembered that what may be seen as a desirable departure by some (e.g., the nurse manager) may be viewed as a loss by others (e.g., a subset of co-workers).

Whether turnover is seen as functional or dysfunctional, there still are costs to the institution in replacing a nurse. For example, there are acquisition costs (e.g., the cost of recruitment and selection), learning costs (e.g., formal instruction, on-the-job instruction), and separation costs (e.g., a loss of efficiency prior to separation, separation pay). For a more detailed presentation of the factors and respective costs involved in employee separation and replacement, refer to Cascio's *Costing Human Resources* (1987).

However, turnover has consequences that go far beyond direct dollar costs. Turnover can have a number of repercussions among other nurses who worked with the departed nurse. Steers and Stone (1982) suggest:

> Turnover can be interpreted by co-workers as a rejection of the job and a recognition that better job opportunities exist elsewhere. For those who remain, ways must be found to reconcile their decision to stay in the light of evidence from others that the job may not be good. As a result, those who remain may re-evaluate their present position in the organization and, as a result, may develop more negative job attitudes (p. 483).

In addition, nurses who remain may have to work longer hours (overtime) or simply work harder to cover for a departed nurse; this can cause both physical and mental strain and may result in additional departures. Thus, one often finds a "turnover spiral" (Staw, 1980). If temporary replacements are used, problems can still result as the workflow of the unit is disturbed and communication patterns within the unit are disrupted. Turnover, and the resultant decreased number of nurses, may also cause the institution to postpone, cancel, or not pursue potentially profitable new ventures. An institution may have to delay opening new clinics or services or, in some cases, may actually have to close existing units.

There are, as suggested earlier, several possible desirable consequences of turnover, especially if the departed nurse was a poor performer. Steers and Stone (1982) state that among these possible desirable outcomes are:

> the possibility of increased performance brought about by recently trained and enthusiastic employees, the possibility that long-running conflicts between people will

be reduced or eliminated through attrition, increased chances for promotion and transfer for those who remain, and the possibility for increased innovation and adaptation brought about by the introduction of fresh ideas (pp. 483–484).

To this list of desirable consequences could be added three additional outcomes: the opportunity for overtime (i.e., some nurses desire voluntary overtime as a way to increase wages), the stimulation of needed policy changes (i.e., as a result of losing a "star performer" an institution may be stimulated to change a problematic policy), and the avoidance of layoffs (i.e., natural attrition may lessen or eliminate the need for forced reduction of staff during times of economic recession).

Although a detailed discussion of the consequences of turnover is beyond the scope of this chapter, the abbreviated discussion provided should make clear the numerous issues that need to be considered in attempting to determine whether a given turnover rate actually is a "turnover problem." If the nurse manager decides that she or he has a turnover problem, then action should be initiated. The turnover model introduced in the next section should be a useful vehicle for helping the manager diagnose the cause of voluntary turnover and subsequently actively manage it (e.g., attempt to reduce the overall turnover rate, influence who is resigning).

A MODEL OF EMPLOYEE TURNOVER

Several models have been developed to explain the turnover process (e.g., Mobley, 1982; Parasuraman, 1989; Price & Mueller, 1981). Each has relative strengths and weaknesses. However, a revised version of a model developed by

March and Simon (1958) is particularly useful for the nurse manager (see Figure 17–2). This model is not unduly complex, yet it portrays the major factors that affect voluntary turnover.

According to the model, voluntary turnover is a direct function of a nurse's perceptions of both the ease and the desirability of leaving the hospital. Perceived ease of movement depends upon the nurse's personal characteristics (e.g., education, area of specialization, age, marital status, having contacts at other hospitals, and ownership of a car) as well as economic conditions (e.g., number of job openings at other hospitals, non–health care institutions hiring nurses for nursing or non-nursing positions).

As with ease of movement, perceptions of the desirability of movement can be affected by sev-

eral factors. Two important ones are the existence of job alternatives within the health care institution and a nurse's attitudes toward his or her job and the organization. To the degree a nurse perceives that other work opportunities (positions) exist within the institution, voluntary turnover should be reduced. That is, a nurse may be able to leave her or his current position by means of a lateral transfer, promotion, or demotion. Thus, if a nurse was having problems with one of his or her co-workers, it may be possible to transfer to a new unit. To some degree, a nurse manager may be able to facilitate alternative job opportunities (e.g., helping a nurse transfer) as a way to reduce voluntary turnover.

Employee attitudes (e.g., job satisfaction, organizational commitment) can also affect per-

FIGURE 17–2 A MODEL OF VOLUNTARY EMPLOYEE TURNOVER

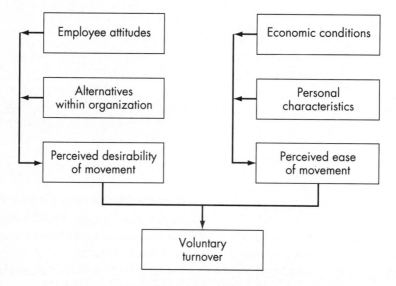

Adapted from J.G. March and H.A. Simon, *Organizations* (New York: John Wiley & Sons, 1958), pp. 90-106. Used by permission.

ceived desirability of movement. A number of studies have shown that the greater an employee's satisfaction level or level of organizational commitment, the lower the probability of the individual quitting. Job satisfaction is affected by various facets of the work environment, including relationships with the nurse manager, other staff nurses, nurse aides, patients, and physicians, as well as the shift worked (e.g., day vs. evening, rotating vs. fixed) and compensation level.

In dealing with turnover, managers need to be aware of three important considerations. First, voluntary turnover can be caused by several factors, only some of which can be influenced by the nurse manager. Second, the manager needs to assess why nurses are leaving; this may be done in cooperation with the human resource department. Figure 17–3 presents a list of several possible causes of turnover. Typically, an institution determines the reasons for turnover by means of exit interviews. However, as noted earlier, the use of "exit questionnaires" (mailed several weeks after a resignation) and interviews with remaining co-workers often provide more accurate data on turnover causes. Finally, the nurse manager must realize that any action taken to reduce voluntary turnover may have other unintended ramifications. The nurse manager should carefully think through a strategy for dealing with turnover prior to implementing it.

STRATEGIES FOR CONTROLLING TURNOVER

The turnover model presented in Figure 17–2 provides a useful organizing framework for deriving strategies to control turnover. The nurse manager's goal should be to do what is within her or his direct and indirect control to reduce dysfunctional voluntary turnover. (As discussed

earlier, a manager may actually welcome functional turnover such as a problem nurse quitting.) Direct measures of control include those in which the nurse manager exerts influence directly, as in interactions with the staff. Indirect turnover control measures include the manager's participation with others (e.g., other nurse managers, other department heads) in changing institutional policies.

From the model depicted in Figure 17–2, it is obvious that if a nurse manager wants to decrease voluntary turnover, she or he can focus upon decreasing staff nurse perceptions of desirability of movement or ease of movement. Each variable is in turn affected by other variables. There is relatively little the nurse manager or the institution can do to influence economic conditions (e.g., whether other institutions are hiring) that affect perceived ease of movement. Therefore, attention should be focused on personal characteristics. For example, a nurse manager, in coordination with the human resource department, may be able to develop a profile of a "long tenure" staff nurse. Although a detailed discussion of how to develop a profile for selecting such long-term nurses is beyond the scope of this chapter (see Chapter 13), a logical predictor would be a nurse's previous turnover record. In fact, it was recently documented that tenure on a previous job was an excellent predictor of how long one stayed in his or her next position (Breaugh & Dossett, 1989).

Although a nurse manager's potential for influencing perceived ease of movement is somewhat limited, the manager can have a substantial impact upon the desirability of movement. For example, she or he can facilitate or hinder movement within the institution. Thus, if a staff nurse is "burned out" from working on an oncology floor, one option is to allow a transfer to another unit. Unfortunately, many nurse managers hinder or even prohibit such a transfer (particularly if the potential transferee is an excellent performer); she or he does not want to lose a good nurse. However, this perspective is shortsighted. If the staff nurse cannot transfer to another unit (intraorganizational mobility), she

---

FIGURE 17–3 CATEGORIES OF REASON FOR TURNOVER

Dissatisfaction

Wages–amount
Wages–equity
Benefits
Hours or shift
Working conditions
Supervision–technical
Supervision–personal
Co-workers
Job security
Job meaningfulness
Use of skills and abilities
Career opportunities
Policies and rules
Other: _____

Alternatives

Returning to school
Military service
Government service
Starting own business
Similar job: same industry
Similar job: other industry
Different job: other industry
Voluntary early retirement
Voluntary transfer to subsidiary
   (loss of seniority)
New position:
   Organization
   Position
   Location
   Earnings

Living conditions

Housing
Transportation
Child care
Health care facilities
Leisure activities
Physical environment
Social environment
Education opportunities
Other: _____

Organization initiated

Resignation in lieu of dismissal
Violation of rules, policy
Unsatisfactory probation period
Attendance
Performance
Layoff
Layoff: downgrade refused
Layoff: transfer refused
End of temporary employment

Personal

Spouse tranferred
To be married
Illness or death in family
Personal illness
Personal injury
Pregnancy

Other

Transfer to: _____
Leave of absence from: _____
On loan to: _____
Retirement
Death

Adapted from W.H. Mobley, *Employee Turnover: Causes, Consequences, and Control* (Reading, MA: Addison-Wesley, 1982), p.38.

or he will often leave the institution entirely (interorganizational mobility). Nurse managers must realize that facilitating transfers within the institution is essential.

Employee attitudes (e.g., job satisfaction, organizational commitment, intrinsic motivation) can be influenced by the nurse manager both directly and indirectly by such actions as providing a realistic job preview (see Chapter 13), enriching or redesigning the staff nurse's job (see Chapter 8), facilitating upward and downward communication (see Chapter 7), linking rewards and performance (Chapter 8), developing work group cohesiveness (see Chapter 5), helping resolve interpersonal conflicts (see Chapter 23), and providing training and educational opportunities (see Chapter 14).

Although the appropriate strategy for addressing nursing turnover will vary depending upon the unique circumstances of the work unit, it is very important that the nurse manager try to do something (be proactive). Landstrom, Biordi, and Gillies (1989) found that 88 percent of the RNs who left their jobs reported that "an appropriate managerial intervention early in their leave-taking decision process would have halted their decision to leave" (p. 23).

A SYSTEMS PERSPECTIVE

Employee absenteeism and turnover have been referred to as withdrawal behaviors because they allow an employee to leave the workplace, one temporarily and one permanently. In many cases, these withdrawal behaviors share a common cause, job dissatisfaction. Given this common cause, it is not surprising that many effective strategies for reducing absenteeism (e.g., providing child care, improving supervisory behavior, coordinating car pools, offering stress management workshops, creating a cohesive work group) also have a positive effect on turn-

over. Therefore, in this section we quickly cover themes that have already been discussed vis-a-vis absenteeism and emphasize issues that are somewhat unique to turnover.

As with absenteeism, the nurse manager must avoid the temptation to look for a quick fix in dealing with turnover. In addition the manager must recognize that what appears to be a simple change (e.g., trying to enrich the job of a high performing nurse) may not be. For example, providing additional duties to enrich a nurse's job may lead to complaints of favoritism from other nurses or the human resource department worrying about assigning duties that are not outlined in the job description. Such potential difficulties should not cause a nurse manager to revert back to status quo behavior. Rather, the manager needs to anticipate such potential problems and deal with them (e.g., be able to justify the differential treatment through the use of performance appraisal data; have the affected nurse agree to the additional duties in writing).

As has already been discussed, the nurse manager wants to create an environment that rewards nurse performance. Obviously, this calls for careful attention being given to the performance appraisal process (e.g., careful documentation) and, when possible, the use of merit pay. However, the nurse manager should go beyond the use of money. The manager wants to do everything in her or his power to reward top-performing nurses for their efforts. Such a performance-oriented climate increases the likelihood of functional turnover (i.e., poorly performing nurses quitting) and decreases the probability of dysfunctional turnover. To be effective, the nurse manager needs to view turnover in terms of what is good for the institution not just for herself or himself. For example, the nurse manager may need to allow a star performer to transfer to another unit rather than risk the loss of this nurse to another health care institution (although many nurse managers do not think of it, if every manager facilitated transfers, each would be as likely to gain a star performer as to lose one).

Work scheduling (i.e., fixed vs. rotating shifts, flexible work hours, job sharing) is a particularly important area not only because of its relationship to voluntary turnover, but also because of its frequent linkage to unionization attempts (it should not be surprising that working conditions that lead to turnover can also motivate interest in unionization). In a *Wall Street Journal* article (February 3, 1987) it was reported that approximately 10 percent of all registered nurses are unionized and that two key causes of this unionization were staff shortages and rotating work schedules. In another *Wall Street Journal* article (January 27, 1987), the use of flexible work schedules and job sharing as ways to recruit and retain nurses at Children's Hospital in Stanford, California, was described. Over 90 percent of the 200 nurses there worked nontraditional schedules. According to the hospital's nursing director, these innovative work schedules have had positive impacts upon both nurse recruitment and retention. Although going to work schedules (i.e., fixed shifts, flexible hours, job sharing) that are seen as more advantageous by staff nurses obviously involves costs (e.g., coordination time, paperwork), such schedules also provide clear benefits. Most nurses prefer fixed shifts. If possible, nurses also prefer flexible hours. And, for many nurses with child care responsibility, job sharing provides a perfect means for remaining in health care and, at the same time, fulfilling parental responsibilities.

Before implementing such innovative work schedules, considerable planning (e.g., cost-benefits analysis) clearly needs to take place. Unfortunately, many health care institutions, even those that are having trouble recruiting and retaining nurses, simply dismiss such schedules out of hand. As with a number of the strategies for reducing turnover and absenteeism discussed in this chapter, a single nurse manager is unlikely to be able to change an institution's policy concerning work schedules. However, if several managers coordinate their efforts, change is more likely to occur. To increase their likelihood of a successful influence attempt, the group of managers may need to build a persuasive case for the program they are suggesting (e.g., document the success of job sharing at other hospitals, cost out the possible financial gain—often part-time nurses are paid at a lower rate and do not receive pension benefits).

Sometimes a nurse manager may simply need to adapt to a high turnover rate. Even if this is the case, the manager may be able to lessen potential problems by doing two things. First, the nurse manager may want to "manage" beliefs about why a nurse left. Sometimes, the reason is unclear and the hospital grapevine will often provide an inaccurate and a less than attractive reason from the institution's perspective (e.g., she left for $1.05 more an hour at a competitor institution). Second, the nurse manager may be able to provide the personnel department with her or his preferred list of replacement workers. One health care organization keeps an up-to-date list of former nurses who will fill in on an occasional basis. Such former employees are more familiar with organizational procedures and thus can handle things more efficiently.

As with absenteeism, a nurse manager wants to do everything she or he can to lessen the problem of turnover. Sometimes this involves coordinating her or his efforts with other managers to change institutional policy. The strategies outlined in this chapter have been shown to be effective in reducing turnover. However, not all are equally applicable to all situations. As a manager, the nurse must be able to analyze situational factors and determine what is appropriate for her or his particular set of circumstances. For example, flexible work hours may be suitable for a clinic but not for an around-the-clock operation. By being creative, nurse managers not only can reduce the overall turnover rate, but they can also have an influence on which nurses leave by providing incentives for the exceptional nurse to stay and by doing less to retain mediocre nurses.

SUMMARY

◆ Historically, health care institutions have had serious problems with excessive employee absenteeism and turnover. Fortunately, there is much the nurse manager can do to actively manage their occurrence.

◆ In this chapter, models describing employee attendance behavior and turnover behavior are presented. These models should help a nurse manager understand why these withdrawal behaviors occur and develop strategies for managing them.

◆ To deal with an absenteeism or a turnover problem, it is important that a nurse manager have a systems perspective, investigate why the withdrawal behavior is occurring, and communicate to staff nurses and the personnel department the problems created by the withdrawal behavior.

◆ In viewing absenteeism and turnover, the nurse manager should not fall into the trap of expecting zero absenteeism or viewing all turnover as dysfunctional.

BIBLIOGRAPHY

Breaugh, J. A. (1981). "Predicting Absenteeism from Prior Absenteeism and Work Attitudes." *Journal of Applied Psychology,* 66: 555–560.

Breaugh, J. A., and Dossett, D. L. (1989). "Rethinking the Use of Personal History Information." *Journal of Business and Psychology,* 3: 371–385.

Bureau of National Affairs. (1988). *Bulletin to Management.* Washington, D.C. Bureau of National Affairs, (March 10).

Cascio, W. (1987). *Costing Human Resources.* Boston: Kent Publishing.

Cavanagh, S. J. (1989). "Nursing Turnover: Literature Review and Methodological Critique." *Journal of Advanced Nursing,* 14: 587–596.

Dalton, D., Krackhardt, D., and Porter, L. (1981). "Functional Turnover." *Journal of Applied Psychology,* 66: 716–721.

Hinrichs, J. (1975). "Measurement of Reasons for Resignation of Professionals: Questionnaire versus Company and Consultant Interviews." *Journal of Applied Psychology,* 60: 530–532.

Johns, G., and Nicholson, N. (1982). "The Meaning of Absence." In: *Research in Organizational Behavior.* Staw, B. M., and Cummings, L. L. (editors). Greenwich, CT: JAI Press.

Jones, C. B. (1990). "Staff Nurse Turnover Costs: Measurements and Results." *Journal of Nursing Administration,* 20: 27–32.

Landstrom, G. L., Biordi, D. L., and Gillies, D. A. (1989). "The Emotional and Behavioral Process of Staff Nurse Turnover." *Journal of Nursing Administration,* 19: 23–28.

Latham, G., and Napier, N. (1984). "Practical Ways to Increase Employee Attendance." In: *Absenteeism.* Goodman, P., Atkin, R., et al. (editors). San Francisco: Jossey-Bass.

March, J., and Simon, H. (1958). *Organizations.* New York: Wiley.

Milkovich, G., and Gomez, L. (1976). "Day Care and Selected Employee Work Behaviors." *Academy of Management Journal,* 19: 111–115.

Mobley, W. (1982). *Employee Turnover: Causes, Consequences, and Control.* Reading, MA: Addison-Wesley.

Panyan, S., and McGregor, M. (1976). "How to Implement a Proactive Incentive Plan: A Field Study." *Personnel Journal,* 55, 460–463.

Parasuraman, S. (1989). "Nursing Turnover: An Integrated Model." *Research in Nursing and Health,* 12: 267–277.

Price, J., and Mueller, C. (1981). "A Causal Model of Turnover for Nurses." *Academy of Management Journal,* 24: 543–565.

Rhodes, S., and Steers, R. (1990). *Managing Employee Absenteeism.* Reading, MA: Addison-Wesley.

Schlotzhauer, D., and Rosse, J. (1985). "A Five-Year Study of a Positive Incentive Absence Control Program." *Personnel Psychology,* 38: 575–585.

Staw, B. M. (1980). "The Consequences of Turnover." *Journal of Occupational Behavior,* 1: 253–273.

Steers, R., and Rhodes, S. (1978). "Major Influences on Employee Attendance: A Process Model." *Journal of Applied Psychology,* 63: 391–407.

Steers, R., and Stone, T. (1982). "Organizational Exit." In: *Personnel Management.* Rowland, K., and Ferris, G. (editors). Boston: Allyn and Bacon.

Stephens, T., and Burroughs, W. (1978). "An Application of Operant Conditioning to Absenteeism in a Hospital Setting." *Journal of Applied Psychology,* 63: 518–521.

Taunton, R. L., Krampitz, S. D., and Woods, C. Q. (1989). "Absenteeism-Retention Links." *Journal of Nursing Administration,* 19: 13–21.

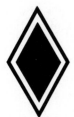

C H A P T E R   18

NURSING ASSOCIATIONS AND COLLECTIVE BARGAINING

National labor law initially excluded most hospital employees. The Wagner Act (298 U.S. 238), passed in 1935, excluded public employees, so all state and local hospitals operated by governmental units were exempt from coverage. The Wagner Act did not specifically exclude private/nonprofit hospitals; in fact, the National Labor Relations Board (NLRB), which is charged with enforcing the Wagner Act, initially claimed jurisdiction over these institutions. In 1947, however, the Taft-Hartley amendment to the Wagner Act did exempt private, nonprofit health care facilities from federal collective bargaining laws (Public Law 101, 80th Congress, June 23, 1947). Furthermore, the NLRB declined to exert jurisdiction over proprietary (privately owned, for profit) hospitals until 1967. But in 1974 the Wagner Act was amended again and the Taft-Hartley exclusion was lifted so that federal labor legislation was extended to private, nonprofit hospitals, nursing homes, health maintenance organizations, health clinics, and other health care institutions in addition to all proprietary health care facilities.

The 1974 health care amendments were not enacted without reason. The health care industry now employs more than five million people. As an economic activity, health care has increased enormously. From 1947 to 1974, hospitals became very complex organizations, and rising expenditures far exceeded inflation in most years. Also, in spite of technological advances, health care has remained very labor-intensive and rapid growth has brought with it a host of employee relations problems.

♦ HEALTH CARE LABOR RELATIONS

Any hospital owned and operated by a nongovernmental agency is now subject to jurisdiction under U.S. labor law. However, a major question remains: "What is a private/nonprofit health care institution?" Frequently, health care institutions are operated by private organizations, but public agencies own the assets. NLRB rulings seem to indicate that the body that employs and directs the management, rather than the owner of the physical assets of the facility, determines whether a health care facility comes under the NLRB's jurisdiction. Consequently, if a private organization is responsible for day-to-day operations, the institution is covered by U.S. labor law.

The Service Employees International Union, the National Union of Hospital and Health Care Employees, and the American Nurses Association and its constituent state nurses' associations are the major organizations recognized as collective bargaining agents. Nurses are also represented by other organizations such as the National Education Association; the American Federation of State, County, and Municipal Employees (AFL-CIO); and the United Food and Commercial Workers International Union (AFL-CIO) (Fossum, 1988). Researchers who have examined union activity in health care institutions predict that unions will continue to grow in representation of employees and that the number of occupational groups represented will also increase (Throckmorton & Kerfoot, 1989). However, unionization overall in America is declining.

The Wagner and Taft-Hartley acts were enacted 11 years apart but are now combined into the Labor Management Relations Act of 1947. The Wagner Act was pro-labor and the Taft-Hartley Act was pro-administration. The Wagner Act, as amended, establishes the National Labor Relations Board, which consists of five members appointed by the president and confirmed by the senate. This board administers all the provisions of the law.

Section 7 is the heart of the original Wagner Act and reads:

> Employees shall have the right to self organization, to form, join, or assist labor organizations, to bargain collectively through representatives of their own choosing, and to engage in other concerted activities for the purpose of collective bargaining or other mutual aid or protection, and shall also have the right to refrain from any or all of such activities except to the extent that such right may be affected by an agreement requiring membership in a labor organization as a condition of employment as authorized in Section 8(a)(3) (Wagner Act, 298 U.S. 238, 1935).

This section indicates that all employees covered by the act shall have the right to decide whether to join a union or not unless they are covered by a closed shop agreement, which requires union membership as a condition of employment, or a union shop agreement, which requires union membership after employment (i.e., 60 days after hire). The former is only found in the construction industry, while the latter is common.

Section 8 of the Wagner Act, as amended, specifies actions of employers and unions that are considered unfair labor practices. For employers these are (a) assisting or dominating any labor organization; (b) discriminating in hiring, assigning, or other terms of employment on the basis of union membership; (c) penalizing or discriminating against an employee for charging an employer with a violation of the act; and (d) refusing to bargain in good faith with the union over issues of wages, hours, and conditions of employment.

The union unfair labor practice provisions are: (a) unions may not coerce employees in the exercise of their Section 7 rights; (b) unions cannot demand or require that an employer violate anything in the act; (c) unions cannot engage in or encourage individuals to strike or to refuse to handle some type of product where the object is to accomplish any of the following: to cease handling nonunion products, force an employer to bargain with an uncertified labor organization, require excessive initiation fees, force an employer to pay for services not rendered, or picket to force recognition; and finally, (d) unions must bargain in good faith with management over wages, hours, and conditions of employment. "Good faith" has a precise definition because of numerous NLRB rulings, but, basically it means that if one party proposes, the other counterproposes. (See Allen and Keavenly [1988: 258–261] for a discussion of good faith bargaining. This is also a good reference for all labor law issues.)

SPECIAL BARGAINING ISSUES FOR HEALTH CARE INSTITUTIONS

The 1974 health care amendments stipulate special procedural regulations for health care in order to minimize the prospect of work interruptions and harm to patients. For example, in most labor situations, it is relatively easy for internal union organizers to have access to employees. In health care institutions, however, this is not the case. In 1976, the NLRB held that a no-solicitation rule prohibiting union organizing activities from any area of the institution where patient contact was possible was overly broad. On appeal, however, the Tenth Circuit Court reversed the NLRB and held that the needs of patients outweigh the organizing rights of employees. So employees or organizers may be banned from organizing in any area to which patients or residents may have access. Passive activities, however, like wearing union membership pins, are approved.

There are also different requirements in negotiations where health care facilities are involved. The party wishing to change the terms of an existing contract is obliged to notify the other party, in writing, within 90 days and not less than 60 days prior to the expiration date of the agreement. Neither party may strike or lock out until this 90-day period has elapsed or the contract has expired, whichever is later. Consequently, there is considerable time for the institution to make alternate arrangements before any strike.

Until 1984, the NLRB held that bargaining units in health care institutions would be structured along occupational lines. Although there had been attempts to place registered nurses in mixed units with other categories of personnel before 1984, the nurses usually ended up in a separate bargaining unit. Technical employees, including licensed practical nurses, X-ray technicians, and laboratory technicians, tended to be grouped into a distinct unit, as did maintenance and service employees, and office and clerical employees. Physicians, when organized, were also in a separate professional unit.

In 1984, the NLRB ruled that maintenance employees at Memphis' St. Francis Hospital could not organize a separate unit. Up to 1984, the NLRB had used a traditional "community of interest" test for determining bargaining units and had allowed up to seven separate units in health care institutions, including one for RNs. The St. Francis case meant that only one or two (professional and nonprofessional) units would be allowed in health care institutions.

In March 1987, however, the U.S. Court of Appeals for the District of Columbia reversed the NLRB's St. Francis decision. This decision returns the process of organizing units in institutions to one similar to that which existed before 1984.

In March 1989, the NLRB announced a rule that allows separate bargaining units for differ-

ent professions in hospitals. This rule was appealed and in April 1991 the Supreme Court affirmed the rule (American Hospital Association v. NLRB, 1991). This decision allows the formation of separate units for RNs.

Unionization seems to be more prevalent in large cities, in larger institutions, in federally controlled institutions, and in institutions located in the Northeast and West. Fewer religious or proprietary institutions are organized. Fewer nurses than other health care employees are unionized.

EFFECT OF UNIONIZATION IN HEALTH CARE

Numerous studies have attempted to measure the effects of health care unionism on wages, employment, and ultimately on costs (Fossum, 1988). One study found that the annual salary of registered nurses is from 4 percent to 7 percent higher for those nurses represented by a bargaining agent; another study showed slightly less than 7 percent (Link & Landon, 1975). However, unionization tends to be geographically specific, and wages in the Northeast and California (where nurses are more heavily unionized) are higher regardless of unionization. In terms of total compensation, aggregating across unionized health care occupations, the union to nonunion differential is about 8 percent.

Given the relative wage gains that seem to be brought about by hospital unionization, the next question is whether there is a relative reduction in the numbers of workers under contract who are employed. There is evidence supporting a reduction, but it is quite modest. Since traditionally it was easy to pass costs on to patients, a significant decrease in employment of the higher cost unionized employees was not evident. Today, with institutions receiving fixed fees (due to DRGs) for services, it is impossible to imagine that they would not meet their costs by reducing staff numbers in response to increased cost per staff member. Also, institutions do substitute among occupational work groups in response to relative wage changes among them. Studies have shown that where LPNs have unionized and their wages have gone up faster than RNs, there tends to be an increase in the proportion of RNs in nursing service (Fossum, 1988).

There are few studies showing the impact of unionization on health care costs. One study has shown that unionization may increase relative average costs per patient day in a short-term general hospital by about 3.8 percent (Miller, Becker & Krinsky, 1979). However, with only a single study, this can only be an estimate. It is highly likely that a certain amount of the cost of unionization is passed on to patients, a certain amount is made up by lesser employment of higher wage employees, and that possibly there is some increase in RN efficiency because of certain work rules demanded in union contracts—for instance, how long breaks last. Consequently, the costs and benefits of collective bargaining probably are almost equal.

◆ WHY INDIVIDUALS JOIN UNIONS

A health care organization is not greatly different from any other industrial organization. It is labor-intensive, and most health care workers work in large, impersonal organizations. This creates a dependency relationship, because the worker must rely on the organization for both a job and a living wage. An authority relationship is created in the workplace, giving the employer control over the workers' job security, tenure, and wages. Organization by the worker therefore presents a credible threat to the employer;

it tends to equalize the economic relationship and rationalize the employment relationship.

In essence, the worker attempts to control the labor market so the organization cannot purchase labor without paying a certain minimum wage, asking the union to supply that labor, or both. The union wants to guarantee job security and income while negotiating rules and procedures against arbitrary employer actions. Collective rather than individual bargaining increases the strength of the individual worker. The essence of unionism in this country is that collective action increases workers' bargaining power. Job security and wages can be negotiated to a much higher level than the free market alone. Without this counterforce against employers, pay would be less for that relative amount of labor.

Professional associations act much like craft unions in that they attempt to control the requirements for entry to—and thus the numbers entering—the profession. State licensing laws and educational requirements for professionals also help control the market.

A union shop clause means that employers may hire whom they please but, within a specified period (usually 30–60 days), the new employee must join the union and maintain his or her membership or face discharge. Most individuals in the United States join unions because of a union shop contract; however, this is not prevalent in health care, where most union membership is voluntary.

◆ NURSES, UNIONS, AND PROFESSIONAL ASSOCIATIONS

Many people believe that collective bargaining is a new movement in nursing, but the fact is that nurses have been concerned with their economic and general welfare for some time. In 1893, nursing leaders established their first organization, the American Society of Superintendents of Training Schools for Nurses, one of whose purposes was a commitment to promote the general welfare of nurses (Miller, 1980). The Nurses' Associated Alumnae of the United States and Canada was formed four years later to provide a national association for all nurses rather than just those interested in education. This association became the American Nurses Association (ANA) in 1911.

In the early 1900s, working conditions and salaries for nurses were extremely poor. The nation was in a general economic depression and the health care system reflected the lack of growth found in other sectors of the economy. Nurses' working conditions were abysmal: long hours, no fringe benefits, and substandard wages. Just prior to the collapse of the economy in 1929, some nurses began to recognize that protest and collective action were necessary if the conditions of the nurse were to improve. In 1928, ANA incorporated into its legislative policy specific references to the general welfare, health, and education of nurses.

In 1945, Shirley Titus, then the executive director of the California Nurses Association, chaired a committee to study the employment conditions of nurses; as a result of the findings of this committee, ANA adopted what was called the Economic Security Program. However, just as this program began to make progress, ANA adopted a no-strike policy in 1950—a policy that was rescinded some years later. At the time, though, this position, along with the passage of the Taft-Hartley Act in 1947, which excluded nonprofit hospitals from any legal obligation to bargain with their employees, left the nurses with virtually no power to bring about change in their working condi-

tions or salaries. The only options available were work stoppages, mass resignations, informational picketing, or individually leaving a work situation. None of these activities, however, was very influential in bettering the situation of the nurse in general.

In 1974, the health care amendments referred to earlier made it possible for nurses to use legal sanctions if necessary to ensure bargaining related to conditions of employment. Since the passage of these amendments, many state nurses associations (SNAs) have qualified as legal bargaining agents for nurses. In addition, ANA changed its structure in 1982 to become a federation of state nurses' associations—a change that has rendered the state associations more direct representation of their member nurses. It remains to be seen how this structured change will affect nurses' collective bargaining activities. Many unions, including the Teamsters, the Meatpackers, and the American Federation of Teachers, are also seeking to organize nurses in the workplace.

Collective bargaining looks increasingly attractive to nurses because of their growing frustration about the inability to practice nursing as they believe it should be practiced, to influence their working conditions, or gain improved personnel policies and benefits. The National Commission on Nursing, after an extensive literature review and public hearings, found that nurses are meeting this frustration in several ways: they leave nursing, they seek another position in the same or different health care agency, they endure their present position, or they seek some form of collective action by joining a union or seeking to have a state nurses association represent them (National Commission on Nursing, 1983). Historically, the use of the SNA as a bargaining agent has been a very divisive issue among nurses within the professional organization and among employing agencies. Some nurses believe that the professional organization should not serve as a labor organization, that this dualism represents a conflict of professional purposes and standards. Others believe that there is no conflict, that the promotion of nurses' economic security and general welfare is a major responsibility of the organization. This continues to be a major issue dividing ANA members.

Another major difficulty in the representation of nurses by SNAs is the conflict regarding membership of supervisory personnel in the association. How can a nurse manager or supervisor who is helping administer a union contract belong to the same organization that serves as bargaining agent for the nurses who are her subordinates? An apparent conflict exists over the nurse manager's divided loyalty. Proponents of SNAs as collective bargaining agents suggest that collective bargaining is only one responsibility of the professional organization and that nurses in administration *can* belong to the same organization. Opponents argue otherwise.

A few SNAs have been charged with violating federal labor laws because association board members have held hospital administrative positions. However, the NLRB has consistently ruled that associations are *not* in violation of labor law when these board members are "insulated" from labor relations activities. When they are not "insulated," and thus control finances of the organization and give local units collective bargaining advice, federal appeals courts have ruled that those associations *are* in violation of federal labor law (Lorenz, 1982). Furthermore, where there is a clear conflict of interest the NLRB has revoked the SNA's certification as sole agent (*NLRB v. North Shore Univ. Hosp.*, 724 F.2nd, 269, 2nd Cir., 1983, 259 NLRB 852). This creates a dilemma for SNAs, which, in following this NLRB ruling, may be in violation of ANA membership rules when they change their bylaws excluding administrators from holding office in the organization. In summary, NLRB and federal appeals decisions have upheld the supervisory nurse's right to belong to the professional association so long as she or he does not participate in the administration of any aspect of the organization that assists collective bargaining activities.

♦ THE NURSE MANAGER'S ROLE

The nurse manager in an institution where the nurses are organized and the parties have negotiated a contract participates in administering the union contract in several ways. The contract will always specify wages, hours, and working conditions; it may specify other items such as union security (e.g., dues deducted from pay checks) and grievance procedures. Most of these items will be handled by the personnel office. The nurse manager, however, actively helps administer the grievance procedures. Besides issues relating to discipline, this entails handling grievances at the first and second steps of the grievance procedure.

Grievances can usually be classified as (a) caused by misunderstanding, (b) caused by intentional contract violations, or (c) caused by symptomatic problems outside the scope of the labor agreement. Grievances caused by a misunderstanding usually stem from circumstances surrounding the grievance, a lack of familiarity with the contract, or an inadequate labor agreement. Self-interest is the usual motivation for using the grievance procedure in an attempt to protect one's perceived, contractual rights. This type of grievance is inevitable even in the most mature, efficient labor/management team. Intentional violation of a contract usually is an effort to capitalize on ambiguous contract language or past practice. Symptomatic grievances are the most difficult to identify and prevent. These grievances are simply a means for the employee to show dissatisfaction or frustration and have three basic causes: (a) personal problems, (b) union politics, and (c) unfavorable contract language. This category describes grievances that stem from the human element in the management/labor relationship.

Any grievance procedure used will be negotiated and clearly described in the labor agreement. Most likely, it will contain a series of progressive steps and time limits for submission/resolution of grievances.

THE GRIEVANCE PROCESS: AN EXAMPLE

The employee talks informally with her or his direct supervisor, usually as soon as possible after the incident has occurred. A representative of the bargaining agent is allowed to be present. The following steps comprise the typical grievance process.

STEP 1. If the grievance is not adjusted in the informal discussion, a written request for the next step is given to the immediate supervisor within 10 workdays. A written response must be received within five workdays. The employee, supervisor, and agent will be present for any discussion.

STEP 2. If the response to Step 1 is not satisfactory, a written appeal may be submitted within 10 workdays to the director of nursing or her or his designee. The employee, agent, grievance chairperson, and the director of nursing or designee can be present for discussion. Again, written response will be provided in five workdays subsequent to these meetings. In most bargaining units the positions of agent and grievance chairpersons are separated. Generally, the grievance chairperson is an officer in the bargaining unit.

STEP 3. The employee, agent, grievance chairperson, director of nursing, and director of personnel meet for discussions. The 10- and five-day time limits for appeal and answer are again observed.

STEP 4. This final step is arbitration, which is invoked when no solution suggested is acceptable. An arbitrator who is a neutral third party is selected and is present at these meetings. The submission of a grievance may be required in 15 days after Step 3 is completed.

Often a statement included in each of the steps states that if the time limits are not observed by one party, the grievance may be considered resolved and further action barred. The contract also usually specifies how an arbitrator is selected.

Beletz offers some suggestions that may be helpful in handling grievances.

1. The objective of the grievance procedure is not to achieve conquest. You do have to work with one another after resolution of the grievance, so treat each other with courtesy and respect.

2. Don't threaten or bluff. On the other hand, this is not an unheard of tactic. Some people use it all the time. If you have investigated properly, you will be able to spot this strategy.

3. Don't withhold facts or information relating to the grievance. This rule is implicit to good faith in bargaining.

4. *Do not,* whatever your position, exhibit internal disagreements or disputes. Both the bargaining unit and the management team must present a solid front when faced with one another.

5. Expediency is a must; delaying tactics serve only to heighten emotions. However, allow time for consideration of all of the facts.

6. Don't blame the other side for taking advantage of your mistakes. Learn from them and don't repeat them the next time.

7. Stay objective. Emotionalism usually leads to further problems.

8. Evaluate and anticipate the other party's position and possible response. The implementation of decisions or the filing of grievances may require planned strategy.

9. Utilize all the resources available. Seek guidance from those higher in administrative positions.

10. Never refuse to meet with the grievant's representatives. The right to representation is one of the advantages of being under the auspices of a collective bargaining unit.

11. The bargaining unit representative, though in a unique position, is not immune from reprimand or discipline. When not involved in bargaining unit activities, the agent is an employee, responsible to the rules and regulations of the institution, and the employer has the right to a full day's work and an acceptable level of performance. However, while handling grievances, the employee/agent is not really considered an employee. She or he is considered the representative and advocate of the employee who filed the grievance.

12. On occasion, discussions in settling grievances become quite heated and emotional. Neither party has to tolerate personal abuse. The meeting should be adjourned and rescheduled at a time when talks can continue on a more objective level.

13. Whether one is a supervisor or an agent, when first contacted regarding a grievance, the grievance may be denied based on the feeling that none of the aforementioned violations have occurred. This does not limit the employee from pursuance of the grievance and seeking redress at the next step in the procedure.

14. Do not submit to emotional appeals as to what is fair. The contract is the sole determinant of what is fair; if necessary, a neutral third party will be utilized to interpret the contract. What one person considers fair may not necessarily be seen in the same light by the other.

15. Be prepared to give or take acceptable compromises and alternative solutions within the framework of the contract, no matter which party suggests them.

16. Know the strengths and weaknesses of the issue for either side.

17. Integral to bargaining are solutions that may also accommodate future changes and needs. Therefore, you must think ahead.

18. Pat formulas do not settle grievances or solve problems. A formula would negate the needed judgment and flexibility that are so necessary to grievance handling.

19. Know where your bottom line is for compromise.

20. Observe the time limits. If you do not, the bargaining unit may lose the right to continue the grievance to the next level or both the bargaining unit and management may lose in an eventual arbitration.

21. It is wise to remember that once a grievance is filed, it may chain-react and almost any imaginable outcome may end up as the solution. However, a carefully written grievance should obviate this possibility.

22. When adjusting a grievance, knowledge is very important. As with any interaction between people, your statement is colored by your temperament and is interpreted by the other party in accordance with his or her own temperament.

23. Gloating over a "win" is human; just remember that you may "lose" the next one; don't become overconfident.

24. One of the most important points in grievance handling is being a good detective. Get all the facts and information, witnesses, and documentation. Find out whether any similar situation ever occurred and what the decision was (Beletz, 1977).

THE GRIEVANCE HEARING.   In actually hearing the grievance in an informal hearing, remember these key behaviors, as set forth by Trotta.

1. Put the grievant at ease. Do not interrupt or disagree with her or him. Let the grievant have her or his say.

2. Listen openly and carefully. Search for what the employee is trying to say. Take notes.

3. Discuss the problem with her or him calmly and with an open mind. Avoid arguments, avoid antagonizing the employee, and avoid the urge to win. Negotiate.

4. Get her or his story straight. Get all the facts. Ask logical questions to clarify doubtful points. Distinguish between fact and opinion.

5. Consider the grievant's viewpoint. Do not assume she or he is automatically wrong.

6. Avoid snap judgment. Do not jump to conclusions. But be willing to admit mistakes.

7. Make an equitable decision, then give it to the grievant promptly. Do not pass the buck (Trotta, 1976).

♦ LABOR RELATIONS IN CANADA

In Canada, collective bargaining rights are extended to all but a very few workers. Although there are differences among provinces, the exceptions generally include certain professionals, employees whose work is of a confidential nature, and employees whose work is defined as managerial. Public sector employees, such as civil servants, teachers, and nurses, were granted most of the same collective bargaining rights, including the right to strike, as private sector employees in the wake of changing public attitudes and enabling legislation in the late 1960s and early 1970s (Muir, 1974). Certain essential service workers such as police officers and firefighters usually are not permitted to strike and are required to settle their disputes by compulsory arbitration. Overall, in Canada the proportion of unionized workers in the workforce is higher than in the United States. Over 35 percent of the workforce (exclusive of agricultural workers) in Canada are members of unions, compared to

less than 20 percent in the United States (Fossum, 1989).

Under the Canadian constitution, the regulation of employer-employee relations falls primarily within provincial jurisdiction. However, federal government employees, territorial workers, and workers in certain industries that cross provincial and national boundaries are entitled to bargain collectively under federal labor laws. Canada consists of 10 provinces and two territories. These are governed by 11 sets of labor laws: one federal and 10 provincial. Despite this diversity, the legislation is relatively similar across Canada, having been modeled originally after labor legislation in the United States as discussed earlier in this chapter.

There are some major differences, however, between the U.S. and Canadian approaches to labor legislation. Carter (1982) has identified four. These are (a) the certification process, (b) strike restrictions, (c) compulsory grievance arbitration, and (d) recognition of the right to union security. Each of these has implications for the first-line nurse manager.

CERTIFICATION

The certification process is a mechanism that gives the union legal status and the rights accorded by labor legislation. Additionally, it ensures that only one union is authorized to represent a certain group of employees. To obtain exclusive bargaining rights for nurses, a trade union must apply to the appropriate labor relations board, providing evidence that it represents the majority of a group of employed nurses. The trade union could be any one of a variety of organizations—for example, a professional nursing association, an exclusive "craft" union for nurses, or an industry-wide employees' union. In the United States, employee vote is used to establish that a trade union is truly authorized by the group of employees it claims to represent. In Canada, such elections are the exception rather than the rule. Moreover, the employer is prohibited from attempting to dissuade employees from joining unions. A union may submit a complaint of unfair labor practice to the labor board should the employer attempt to interfere in the union organization process.

Labor boards are official tribunals specifically established to administer the labor laws. They are empowered to oversee all aspects of labor relations, including approval of applications for certification and assisting parties in the resolution of disputes. The labor boards generally consist of equal numbers of union and management representatives, and government appointees.

A union can also obtain collective bargaining rights by seeking voluntary recognition as a bargaining agent from the employer or employer's association. The rights of nurses to engage in collective bargaining are unrestricted. However, like many of their colleagues in the United States, Canadian nurses have been disinclined to obtain assistance from or to join established trade unions, preferring to work through their professional associations or, more recently, to establish independent unions.

STRIKE RESTRICTIONS

Strikes are generally regarded as the ultimate economic sanction that can be exercised by a union. Although strikes are legally permitted as a means of bringing pressure on an employer to make concessions at the bargaining table, various legal restrictions control the use of the strike weapon in Canada. Strikes are not allowed for the purpose of gaining recognition as a bargaining agent. With the exception of the province of Saskatchewan, strikes are not allowed while a collective agreement is in effect. Strikes may be

used during the process of negotiating a contract, but certain mediation and conciliation procedures must usually be followed first. A strike vote must be taken before a union is entitled to strike, and a formal notice of strike must be given to the employer.

At present, strikes by health care workers are permitted in all provinces except Prince Edward Island, Newfoundland, Ontario, and Alberta. Collective bargaining impasses in these three provinces must ultimately be settled through the process of compulsory arbitration. There have been three province-wide strikes by hospital nurses since 1977 in Alberta. However, in June 1983, the Progressive Conservative government amended the labor laws to prohibit strikes by all hospital workers in the province. In Ontario, strikes by hospital workers have been outlawed since 1965. Public health nurses are entitled to strike, however. On one occasion, public health nurses went on strike to back up their demand for compulsory arbitration for the resolution of interest disputes.

COMPULSORY GRIEVANCE ARBITRATION

Because strikes are illegal if held during the lifetime of a collective agreement (except in Saskatchewan), the parties must make provision for the peaceful resolution of disputes that arise out of the interpretation, administration, or alleged violation of the agreement. The labor statutes usually provide mandatory provision for arbitration should the agreement fail to include such a procedure. If the parties cannot settle a dispute about a grievance, they may jointly appoint a single arbitrator or separately appoint nominees to a tribunal consisting of a union representative, a management representative, and a neutral chairman chosen jointly by the two nominees.

The decision of a majority of the arbitration board is binding.

Appeals may be lodged through the courts by either party when there has been an error at law, when the arbitration board has exceeded its jurisdiction, and in certain other circumstances. The powers of the arbitration board are usually specified in the legislation; in general, an arbitrator may not modify the provision of a collective agreement. He or she may, however, be entitled to reduce the severity of a disciplinary penalty imposed on a grievant.

UNION SECURITY

Unions in Canada are permitted to bargain for their own financial security and, accordingly, nursing unions have negotiated what is known as the Rand Formula into their contracts. This ensures that all nurses who benefit directly from the provisions of the collective agreement must contribute union dues through payroll deduction, irrespective of their involvement in union activities or their willingness to consider themselves union members. The Rand Formula ensures a continuous and predictable income for the union. This feature of labor relations differs significantly from the United States system in which some jurisdictions have introduced right-to-work laws, curtailing the ability of unions to negotiate union security clauses.

◆ HISTORICAL REVIEW OF COLLECTIVE BARGAINING BY CANADIAN NURSES

The Canadian Nurses Association (CNA) accepted the principle of collective bargaining in 1944, the same year in which the Canadian government introduced its influential Wartime Labor Relations Regulations (Carter, 1982). At

that time, the prevailing method for influencing the terms and conditions of employment consisted of the circulation of recommended salaries and personnel policies by provincial nursing associations to their members and to employers. This proved ineffectual because the recommended terms and conditions of employment were not binding on anyone; while other institutional workers resorted to collective bargaining in increasing numbers, the salaries for registered nurses barely kept ahead of salaries for nursing assistants and nursing orderlies. Even so, it was more than 20 years after the CNA took its stand on collective bargaining that the major thrust toward large-scale union organization in nursing occurred.

The first Canadian nursing union seems to have been l'Association des Gardes-Malades Catholiques Licenciées, established in the city of Quebec in 1927, evidently as a result of attempts by the clergy to restrict hospital nursing to Roman Catholic nurses (Michaud, 1980). Nineteen years later (1946), on the other side of the country, the Registered Nurses' Association of British Columbia was granted recognition as a bargaining agent under the provincial Labor Relations Act and began a very active and effective collective bargaining program for its members (Cormick, 1969).

Another nine years elapsed before any further event of much significance took place. Then, in 1965, in the Province of Alberta, the Calgary General Hospital Staff Nurses' Association obtained certification under provincial legislation and signed its first collective agreement with its hospital board. The Alberta Association of Registered Nurses had by this time hired an employment relations officer to assist the membership in forming staff nurse associations in hospitals and health agencies and to provide educational programming in labor relations and collective

bargaining. All other provincial nursing associations soon followed suit, as part of a broader social movement in which employees in the public sector accepted collective bargaining as a respectable method of improving their socioeconomic status.

The diversity of provincial legislation and the reluctance of nurses and their professional associations to obtain certification as trade unions led to the use of a variety of forms of collective bargaining. For instance, several provincial nursing associations entered into procedural agreements with provincial hospital associations, obtaining voluntary recognition as bargaining agents and negotiating terms and conditions of employment on a province-wide basis. The appropriateness of the professional nursing association serving as a bargaining agent, however, was debated from the earliest days of collective bargaining by nurses. Many officers of provincial nursing associations were drawn from the ranks of nursing management and, from the perspective of a labor relations board, both the bargaining unit and the bargaining agent were very probably dominated by the "employer." Paradoxically, in many cases, the nursing leaders were responsible for steering their professional nursing associations toward collective bargaining, even though they themselves were ineligible for membership in the collective bargaining unit according to the law.

RELATIONSHIPS BETWEEN PROFESSIONAL ASSOCIATIONS AND NURSES' UNIONS

A legal challenge to the composition of the professional nursing association as bargaining agent came eventually in the Province of Saskatchewan when another union, the Service Employees International Union, objected to the certification of a local affiliate of the Saskatchewan

Registered Nurses' Association on the grounds that it was "company dominated." The battle was fought all the way to the Supreme Court of Canada, which in 1973 upheld the decision of the Saskatchewan Labor Relations Board to deny certification to the professional association (News, 1973).

Nursing associations in other provinces, assuming that similar legal challenges would be launched, immediately began to modify their constitutions and bylaws to establish semiautonomous collective bargaining subdivisions within their organizational frameworks. The emergence of autonomous socioeconomic subdivisions of the professional nursing associations proved to be an interim phase in the evolution of collective bargaining in the nursing profession in Canada. Gradually, one after another, the staff nurse divisions of the professional associations broke away to become fullfledged nursing unions devoted exclusively to labor relations activities. Members of staff nurse divisions became union members in every sense of the word and were thus obliged to pay union dues as well as professional association fees. (A unique situation now exists in Ontario where the affairs of the nursing profession are distributed among three associations: the Ontario Nurses' Association [the union], the Registered Nurses' Association of Ontario [the professional association], and the Ontario College of Nurses [the registration and disciplinary body].)

The development of independent nursing unions that are unaffiliated with the trade union movement has been a very distinct feature in the Canadian nursing profession, indicating the importance to nurses of remaining in full control of their own socioeconomic affairs. Today each province has both a professional nursing association and a nursing union, with the exception of Prince Edward Island, where the professional

association remains the collective bargaining agent for registered nurses. In the Province of Quebec nurses are represented by a diversity of unions. There are unions composed of French-speaking and bilingual nurses and even an association of middle management nurses who have limited negotiating power. Nurses in Quebec are also represented by other unions having a broad spectrum of health care workers among their members.

SUMMARY

- The 1974 health care amendments to the Wagner Act brought health care employees under U.S. labor law. This also includes public-owned institutions administered by a private firm.

- Several unions and state nursing associations represent nurses.

- The Wagner Act defines the rights of individuals in collective bargaining, outlines union/institution unfair labor practices, establishes the NLRB, and provides for remedies.

- Collective bargaining is different in health care in order to provide protection for patients or residents. Most bargaining units are structured along occupational lines.

- The effects of unionization on health care costs have been negligible. There is little research showing effects on nurses and nursing practice.

- Nursing units often act like craft unions. State associations often represent nurses.

This causes conflict because the association then has contact with labor and administration.

♦ The nurse manager's major responsibility in collective bargaining is to help administer the contract. Hints are provided to help handle grievances.

♦ Labor relations in Canadian nursing differ significantly from relations in the United States, with most nurses belonging to collective bargaining units.

♦ There is a wide variety in union organization, activity, and law in various Canadian provinces.

♦ A union becomes the legal representative of a group of employees in Canada by the process of certification granted by a labor relations board.

♦ Unions that represent nurses in Canada may be the professional association or an independent union organization. Nurses may belong to both organizations.

BIBLIOGRAPHY

Allen, R. E., and Keavenly, T. J. (1988). *Contemporary Labor Relations*. Reading, MA: Addison-Wesley.

American Hospital Association v. NLRB et al. 111 S. Ct. 1539 (1991).

Becker, E. R., Sloan, F. A., and Steinwald, B. (1982). "Union Activity in Hospitals: Past, Present and Future." *Health Care Financing Review*, 3: 4, 11.

Beletz, E. (1977). "Some Pointers for Grievance Handlers." *Supervisory Nurse*, 8(August): 56.

Carter, D. D. (1982). "Collective Bargaining Legislation in Canada." In: *Union-Management Relations in Canada*. Anderson, J., and Gunderson, M. (editors). Don Mills, Ont.: Addison-Wesley.

Cormick, G. W. (1969). "The Collective Bargaining Experience of Canadian Registered Nurses." *Labor Law Journal*, 20(10): 670.

Fossum, J. A. (1988). *Labor Relations*. 2d ed. Dallas, TX: Business Publications.

Henry, K. H. (1984). *The Health Care Supervisor's Legal Guide*. Rockville, MD: Aspen Publications.

Hunt, J. W. (1979). *Employer's Guide to Labor Relations*. Washington, DC: Bureau of National Affairs.

Link, C. R., and Landon, J. H. (1975). "Monopsony and Union Power in the Market for Nurses." *Southern Exon Journal*, 41(4): 644.

Lorenz, F. J. (1982). "Nursing Administration and Undivided Loyalty." *Nursing Administrative Quarterly*, 6(2): 67.

Luttman, P. (1982). "Collective Bargaining and Professionalism: Incompatible Ideologies?" *Nursing Administrative Quarterly*, 6(Winter): 21.

Michaud, A. (1980). "The Evolution of Nurses' Unions vis-a-vis Professional Associations." Unpublished paper presented to the Annual Meeting of the Canadian Nurses' Associations, Vancouver, June 24.

Miller, R. U. (1980). "Collective Bargaining: A Nurse Dilemma." *American Operating Room Nurse Journal*, 31(7): 1195.

Miller, R. U., Becker, B. E., and Krinksy, E. B. (1979). *The Impact of Collective Bargaining on Hospitals*. New York: Praeger.

Muir, J. D. (1974). "Canada's Experience with the Right of Public Employees to Strike." In: *Contemporary Issues in Canadian Personnel Administration*. Jain, H. C. (editor). Scarborough, Ont.: Prentice-Hall of Canada.

National Commission on Nursing (1983). *Summary Report and Recommendations*. Chicago: American Hospital Association, April.

News. (1973). *Canadian Nursing*, 69(8): 9, 12.

NLRB v. North Shore University Hospital; 724 F.2nd, 269; 2nd Cir., 1983, 259 NLRB 852.

Public Law 101, 80th Congress, June 23, 1947.

Sain, T. R. (1984). "Effects of Unionization." *Nursing Management*, 15(1)(January): 43.

Sargis, N. M. (1985). "Collective Bargaining: Serving the Common Good in a Crisis." *Nursing Management*, 16(2): 123–127.

Throckmorton, T., and Kerfoot, K. (1989). "Labor Relations: Theory, Research, and Strategies." In: *Dimensions of Nursing Administration*. Henry, B., et al. (editors). Boston: Blackwell Scientific.

Trotta, M. S. (1976). *Handling Grievance: A Guide for Management and Labor*. Washington, DC: Bureau of National Affairs.

Wagner Act, 298 U.S. 238, 1935.

P A R T 4

BASIC SURVIVAL SKILLS IN NURSING

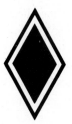

C H A P T E R 19

BUDGETING AND RESOURCE ALLOCATION

The economic climate for the future of health care is uncertain, and with competition for funds increasing, financial resources are becoming scarce. Since the nursing department budget can account for as much as half of an institution's total expenses, there continues to be significant pressure on this department to increase efficiency and effectiveness. For nursing to respond to the pressures and the uncertainty, nurse managers at all levels must become proficient in the budgeting process. Many nurse managers, though already familiar with this process, have not developed the skills necessary to project costs based on current and anticipated needs. The monitoring aspects of budget control are even less understood. Yet, it is the nurse manager on the unit level who is in the best position to predict trends in census and acuity, as well as supply and equipment needs. This chapter presents the conceptual framework of budgeting, to relate the resources necessary to provide patient care to the dollars required to sustain it. Examples are presented to facilitate understanding this relationship.

Budgeting is the process of planning and controlling future operations by comparing actual results with planned expectations. A budget is a detailed plan that communicates these expectations and serves as the basis for comparing them to actual results. As such, it can never be definite or absolute. The budget shows how resources will be acquired and used over some specific time interval; its purpose is to allow management to project activities into the future so that the objectives of the organization are coordinated and met. It also helps to ensure that the resources necessary to achieve these objectives are available at the appropriate time or that operations are carried out within the resources available. Last, a budget helps management control the resources expended.

Budgeting is performed by business, government, and individuals. In fact, nearly everyone budgets, even though he or she may not identify the process as such. A budget may exist only in an individual's mind, but it is nonetheless a budget. Anyone who has planned how to pay a particular bill at some time in the future has a budget. Although it is very simplistic, that plan accomplishes the essential budget functions. One now knows how much of a resource (money) is needed and when (in six months) it is needed. Note that the "when" is just as important as the "how much." The money has to be available at the right time.

◆ PLANNING AND CONTROL

A *budget* helps management plan and control the distribution of resources within the organization. It is a written statement of what resources—money, time, and people—will be needed to provide specific services or products over a specified amount of time.

PLANNING

Planning involves reviewing the established goals and objectives of the nursing unit, the nursing department, and the institution for the next fiscal year. Financial projections are then developed. A budget forces managers to look into the future and may thus help them identify problems and take corrective steps before the problem becomes unmanageable. Planning moves the budget, organizational or individual, from a haphazard reaction method of management to a formal, controlled method. With a budget, the manager spends less time reacting to unanticipated problems and more time on productive endeavors.

As part of the budgeting process, planning

has two additional advantages: improved communication and functional coordination.

COMMUNICATION. Operating budgets are prepared for the entire organization, yielding the master budget, and therefore all levels of management are involved and the organization's goals are communicated to them. The process of compiling, reviewing, and revising data for the budget opens lines of communication between subordinates and superiors and among managers of those departments whose operations are related and interdependent.

COORDINATION. Without a coordinated budget system, each department may operate without regard to what any other department is doing or to the organization's objectives. Obviously, this lack of coordination results in inefficiency and increasing costs. The operating budget becomes the master plan of action for the entire organization, reflecting the coordinated efforts of all levels of management. This helps the organization operate smoothly and efficiently so that particular goals and objectives are met.

CONTROL

Not only is a budget a planning tool to help management establish future objectives and decide how they are to be achieved, it is also a tool to control what is going on. *Control* involves the steps taken by management to ensure that the objectives are met and that all parts of the organization are working in a manner consistent with organizational policies. Controlling is the process of comparing actual results with the results projected in the budget. By measuring the differences between the projected and the actual results, management is better able to make modifications and corrections. Controlling, then, depends on planning. Without a plan, there is no way to compare actual versus planned or anticipated performance. A *profit and loss statement* is a formal document generated by the finance department, showing budgetary expectations, actual results, and the difference (see Figure 19–1). The difference between budget and actual performance is called a *variance*.

It is unlikely that the projected and actual results will be the same. Some variance is to be expected, and management must decide how much variance will occur before an explanation is required. For example, anything under 4 percent, or $500, is acceptable; thus, only variances over that percentage or dollar amount would be examined.

◆ BUDGETARY CONCEPTS AND CONSIDERATIONS

RESPONSIBILITY ACCOUNTING

The basis for budgeting is the concept of *responsibility accounting:* Each manager's performance is judged by how well those items directly under his or her control are managed. To judge a manager's performance in this way, the costs and revenues over which he or she has control must be carefully scrutinized and classified. The effect of responsibility accounting is to personalize the accounting system; this is essential to effective planning and control.

Responsibility accounting is based on three premises: (a) that costs can be organized according to levels of management responsibility; (b) that the costs that are charged to a manager be controllable at that level of management; and (c) that timely budget data can be generated as a basis for evaluating performance.

A formalized system to ensure accountability to budgetary controls is shown in Figure 19–2.

FIGURE 19–1 EXAMPLE OF A FORM IN WHICH MONTHLY EXPENDITURES FOR AN AREA OF RESPONSIBILITY ARE LOGGED AND SENT TO THE NURSE MANAGER FOR REVIEW

Units of Service (patient days)		Current Month Actual	Current Month Budget		YTD Actual	YTD Budget
NAT CLS	**Account description**	**Current month**			**Year-to-date**			**Average unit cost**		
		Ac-tual	Bud-get	Vari-ance	Ac-tual	Bud-get	Vari-ance	Ac-tual	Bud-get	Vari-ance
100	Inpatient revenue									
10	Management									
20	Technician & specialist									
30	Registered nurses									
40	Licensed vocational nurses									
50	Aides & orderlies									
60	Clerical									
90	Other salaries									
100	Paid vacation									
110	Paid holiday									
120	Paid sick leave									
180	FICA tax									
250	Other professional fees									
320	Sutures and surgical needles									
330	Surgical packs									
340	Surgical supplies									
370	IV solutions									
380	Other medical care materials & supplies									
390	Cleaning supplies									
400	Office supplies									
410	Employee wearing apparel									
420	Instrument & minor equipment									
430	Other minor equipment									
440	Laboratory supplies									
450	Repairs & maintenance									
460	Purchased services									
470	Dues and subscriptions									
500	Rentals									
510	Outside education & travel									
520	Other expenses									
	Total direct expenses									

FIGURE 19–2 VARIANCE REPORT

Cost Center _____
Month _____ Year _____

	Current month actual	Current month budget	$ Difference ( )	% Difference ( )
UNITS OF SERVICE				
Revenue (100)				
Expense (Nat. Class)				
Salaries (10,20,30,40, 50,60,90)				
Benefits (100,110,120)				
Other professional Fees (250)				
SUBTOTAL				
Medical supplies (320,330, 340,370,380,440)				
Non-med. supplies (390,400)				
Employee wearing apparel (410)				
Equipment (420,430)				
Repairs & maint. (450)				
Purchased services (460)				
Rentals (500)				
Dues & subscript. (470)				
Outside education & travel (510)				
Other expenses (520)				
TOTAL EXPENSE				

Explanation of all variances in excess of ± 4% & $500.00. Use parentheses ( ) to indicate unfavorable variances. Adapted from Children's Hospital, Los Angeles, Dept. of Nursing.

This form can be completed monthly by nurse managers using information obtained from the profit and loss statement. The key to controlling a variance is timely review and making prompt modifications. Documentation, done on a monthly basis, forms the support for future planning.

MOTIVATIONAL ASPECTS

When used properly, the budget can be an effective way to motivate employees. Thus, the most effective budgets are those employees help to develop; such a process helps ensure that the budgets represent fair standards for evaluating employees' work. Also, job satisfaction can result from achieving the goals and objectives of the organization set forth in the budget. In contrast, an improperly developed or administered budget can cause friction among the employees and management.

For the budgeting process to be a motivational tool, management must recognize that the budget is not perfect; if the actual results do not match the projected ones, this does not necessarily represent poor performance by the employees. Management may have made mistakes in judgment and prediction, and not all circumstances can be foreseen. Therefore, changes and modifications are sometimes necessary. Top management is responsible for communicating the proper attitude toward the budget to lower levels of management. The budget is a tool and, to be effective, it must not be viewed as infallible. The budget should be used as a positive instrument to aid in establishing operating goals, measuring operating results, and isolating areas that need extra attention. Administration of a budget program requires a great deal of insight and sensitivity from management. Lower level managers will not respect the budget if they believe that top management is not committed to

it or is using it to intimidate. The ultimate objective must be to develop an awareness that the budget is designed to be a positive aid in achieving both individual and institutional goals.

BUDGET PERIOD

The planning horizon for budgeting may vary from a year or less to many years, depending on the objectives and the uncertainties involved. Budgets covering the acquisition of land, buildings, and equipment have long-time horizons and may extend 5, 10, or 20 years or more into the future. Obviously, such budgets will not be as detailed as one set up for only a year hence.

Nursing unit budgets are usually developed to cover the one-year period that corresponds to the organization's fiscal year. Most organizations then divide the one-year budget into four quarters and each quarter into the separate three months.

ZERO-BASE BUDGETING

Zero-base budgeting requires managers to start from zero budget levels every year; it has been given a good deal of attention. Managers are required to justify all costs as though they were being initiated for the first time. No cost is viewed as continuing into the future. Traditionally, proposed budgets have been justified on an incremental basis: The manager starts with last year's budget and adds to or subtracts from it according to projected needs, objectives, and the inflation rate or consumer price index.

This latter system can reward a manager for overutilizing dollars since next year's budget is based on last year's figures, allowing adjustments in units of service. It can also penalize prudent managers who do not use all allocated dollars within the months preceding the development of the next fiscal year's budget.

Zero-base budgeting, in contrast, attempts to

get back to such basic questions as why does this activity or department exist and what should be its goals and objectives. It requires that established programs maintain their productivity. Although zero-base budgeting requires much time and is costly, in some situations its use is justified.

FLEXIBLE BUDGETING

Flexible budgets allow management to adapt to changes in activities and unplanned costs once the fiscal year has begun. Patient census, activity mix, and the use of supplies can change suddenly in today's economic environment. Expenses based on a fixed patient census will not reflect actual productivity. A flexible budget takes into account actual costs of personnel and supplies per unit of service and compares that to the actual units of service. Variance results are then compared against a flex standard rather than a budgeted one. Let's look at total supplies used on one nursing unit for one month:

	Supplies		
Actual	Flex Budget	Budget	Variance
$2,500	$2,200	$2,400	<$300>

The above supply budget is based on 600 patient days/month. The anticipated expense would be $2,400. The supply cost per unit of service (per patient day) is $4 ($2,400 ÷ 600). However, during one month, instead of the predicted 600 patient days, 550 patient days occurred. Thus, the expected supply cost (flex budget) would be $2,200 (550 × $4). The actual dollars spent were $2,500. In this example, actual supply costs were $300 over what was expected (flex budget). Flexible budgets, like other budgetary systems, require the manager to investigate negative variances.

THE OPERATING BUDGET

The *operating budget* tells management how much money it will cost to maintain the routine operations of the organization during the fiscal year. Each nursing unit generates an operating budget that combines requirements for personnel, benefits, supplies, and other items necessary to operate the unit, which is defined as a cost center. A *cost center* is the smallest functional unit that generates costs within the organization. Cost centers may be revenue producing, such as laboratory and radiology, or non–revenue producing, such as environmental services and administration. Each nursing unit is usually considered a cost center. In all but a few institutions nursing is not directly reimbursed for its services. Nursing service costs are usually included in the room rate. Formulation of the operating budget should begin several months before the beginning of the next fiscal year to provide sufficient data and time for planning.

UNITS OF SERVICE

Nearly all institutional budgets are derived in some way and to some extent from the forecast of patient occupancy rates, acuity levels, or some other activity standard. A unit of service is the budgetary concept on which expenses are based. Environmental service departments use square footage, the dietary department uses meals served, the emergency room uses patient visits, labor and delivery uses number of deliveries, and nursing care units use patient days. Patient days reflect the number of days that any one patient is in the hospital. Thus, a census of 20 patients per day for 365 days equals 7,300 patient days a year. Other health care settings, such as home health care agencies, use indices appropriate to their services (e.g., number of home visits). Units of service are predicted on past trends and changes in the services provided.

For example, new staff, physicians, additional operating rooms, and inpatient procedures converting to outpatient care are just a few changes that can significantly increase or decrease units of service.

CAPITAL EXPENDITURE BUDGET

The capital expenditure budget is established to fund the purchase of major equipment or architectural renovations. It is a planning process that should occur throughout the fiscal year and culminate at budget preparation time. Each nurse manager should keep a chronological list of all capital items purchased. Reference to the dates of purchase will help in replacement planning, as equipment wears out.

Each institution has its own definition of capital, but there are usually two common criteria: The item must be above a certain cost and have a life expectancy greater than a set time period. For example, a hospital may define capital as any item that costs over $500 or has an expected life of greater than one year. Some institutions also define a capital purchase as two or more items of the same specifications that together exceed a fixed dollar amount. (For example, one bedside chair = $250. The unit will purchase two chairs under the capital budget for a cost of $500.) When considering a capital purchase the nurse managers should consider these questions:

How will it affect volume/workload?

How will it affect patient days/revenue?

Is the supply budget impacted?

Will additional space be needed?

Are other departments affected?

Capital items are usually requested on forms designed for that purpose (see Figure 19–3). Included in the capital request are cost estimates

of installation, delivery charges, and service contracts. The justification for each item should be well documented. The purchasing and accounting departments can help the nurse manager obtain information about depreciation time span, salvage value, age of equipment, and the like. These data, coupled with clinical information, aid in the preparation of the request. Since institutions usually set aside a fixed amount for total capital purchases, a well-documented request helps the decision maker determine need.

Other aspects of the operation such as personnel or supply budgets must be considered. For example, if monitoring equipment is being requested, the cost of EKG paper and electrodes should be determined, documented, and included in the supply budget. Likewise, the need for additional nursing and non-nursing personnel to operate the new equipment, training of personnel already on hand, or possibly the need for additional nursing hours per patient day should be quantified, documented, and included.

Capital expenditure budgets can be difficult to develop due to rapid changes in technology; however, by working closely with the medical staff and nursing staff and keeping current with internal changes and external trends, nurse managers can be effective in anticipating capital needs.

◆ SUPPLY AND EXPENSE BUDGET

The supply and expense budget funds the non-capital equipment and supplies needed to operate a nursing unit. It includes such items as medical-surgical supplies, pharmacy items, and paper and office supplies, in addition to other

FIGURE 19-3 CAPITAL ITEM REQUEST FORM

Priority Listing #

1. Department _____ Nursing _____

   Location _____

2. Cost Center Title _____

3. Cost Center Number _____ 6062 _____

4. 5 Physiologic Monitor (ECG & Respiratory)
   Request Title and Quantity

5. 78833B
   Model No., Type, Catalog No., Size, etc.

6. Hewlett-Packard
   Potential Vendor, Tel. No. or Vendor Location
   (Alternate Vendor, if Available)

JUSTIFICATION:

Current monitors are constantly down for repair. This
model is outdated and has been phased out. With the
type of patients that are admitted to this unit, we need
a more sophisticated and reliable system to monitor
continuously the cardiac and respiratory status of sick
infants. This is phase II of the planning for replacement in a systematic approach. We have 12 more
monitors to be replaced over the next 3 years.

If more space is needed, please turn over.

PURCHASING'S COMMENT	ELECTRONIC/ENG'S COMMENT

BUDGET USE ONLY
Budget Request # _____
Equipment Cost $ _____
R & C Cost $ _____
Total Cost $ _____

Estimated:

7. Equipment Cost $5,705.70 ea x 5 = $28,000

8. R & C Cost _____

9. Tax _____ $1,854.35 _____

10. Freight _____

11. UL Approval _____

12. Other _____

13. Total Costs _____ $30,682.35 + freight _____

14. Related New Operating Costs:

    a. Salaries (No. of FTE) _____
    b. Non-Wage
       Supplies _____
       Repair & Maint. _____

15. Reason for Request:

    [X] Patient Care

    [ ] Non-Patient

    [X] Replacement of Equipment Specify ID
    # F-13-576, F13-577, F13-575,
    F13-584, F13-580

    [ ] Enhancement of Existing Equip.

    [ ] Comply with Statutory Mandate

    [ ] Expanding or New Program

    [ ] Will Increase Revenue or Cut Expenses

    [ ] Other

16. Funding source, if any, other than hospital
    funds:

    1. Grant/Account # _____
    2. Contract/Account # _____
    3. Special Fund # _____
    4. Other/Account # _____

17. Projected Month of Purchase _____
18. Person to Contact _____
    (please print)

Date	Exten.	Division Head
Date	Exten.	Department Head

operating expenses such as rentals, maintenance costs, and service contracts.

An essential tool used in developing this budget is a report or statement of expenses. Such a statement, if prepared at the end of each accounting period (usually a month), should include the amount budgeted, the amount actually spent, and a year-to-date total. This information should be available for each expense category, such as medical-surgical supplies or pharmacy, and for the unit total, as shown previously in Figure 19–2.

The first step in developing the supply budget is to analyze the previous expense statements to determine any trends that could be significant in forecasting for the coming year. Changes in supply requirements or utilization can result from volume changes, a change in patient mix, a change in the type of patients, a new piece of equipment, or change in procedure. Of course, such changes can occur for numerous other reasons as well; these need to be considered on a unit-by-unit basis and quantified as accurately as possible.

Supply budgets also need to be adjusted for inflationary impact, and adjustment guidelines are usually provided by the purchasing department. For instance, the purchasing department may predict a 5 percent increase in all pharmacy costs and a 4 percent increase in all other categories.

To budget for the next year, assuming no major changes (e.g., in census, acuity, or new services), would require only an adjustment for inflation. Using medical supplies as an example, the amount to be budgeted is calculated using the cost-per-patient-day figures. However, now it is anticipated that due to the purchase of new equipment, additional EKG paper and electrodes will be required. The cost of paper and electrodes is estimated to be an additional $180

per month in the medical-surgical supply expense account, and the inflationary impact is expected to be 4 percent. For the first six months of this year, the expenses for medical-surgical supplies were $17,982, or $2,997 per month. To plan for additional supplies, we should budget the previous $2,997 per month plus $180 plus 4 percent, which would yield $3,117 per month.

Nurse managers must be familiar with expense account categories and the items in each one so current expenses can be properly analyzed and the impact of future changes can be accurately predicted.

MONITORING THE SUPPLY AND EXPENSE BUDGET

The supply and expense budget is monitored in much the same way as the personnel budget, using monthly expense statements as the tool. Again, the first step is to determine whether there are significant variances and, if so, to determine the cause so that corrective action can be taken.

In determining causes for variations, the activity level of the unit should be examined for any relationship to the variance. If a variance in supply costs is due to increased use of an item because of an unanticipated increase in census, there is a legitimate reason for the variance and corrective action may not be indicated. However, if the variance is due to improper utilization of supplies, then a plan to correct the situation should be developed. From time to time the nurse manager may find it necessary to make staff aware of budget overruns and ask for their assistance in conserving supplies and equipment. The important thing is to evaluate the situation carefully so appropriate steps, if indicated, may be taken.

Reports received from the accounting department should include information about all supplies received from the inhouse ordering systems and those received from out-of-hospital purchases. Supply costs should be shown and the nurse manager can then determine if appropriate charges to the unit's cost center were made. The nurse manager must have a clear understanding of those charges that are patient charge items and those that are unit charges. Some institutions charge the nursing unit for patient charge items that are used by the unit but accidentally not charged to the patient. The nurse manager must then develop a mechanism for tracking "lost charges" and a plan to improve revenue capture. Some managers find that by placing a patient charge card in the patient's room as well as in the supply area, nurses are more likely to put patient charge stickers on the cards.

♦ PERSONNEL BUDGET

The personnel budget (also referred to as the salary or manpower budget) is an especially important part of the budgeting process. It can account for as much as 90 percent of the total nursing service budget. It includes the salaries of all nursing staff, as well as compensation for such things as vacation time, sick leave, holidays, overtime, differentials, merit increases, and orientation and education time. Nurse managers at the unit level are the best sources for determining staffing requirements. Staffing requests should be developed with as much objective information as is available.

RELEVANT COMPONENTS
When computing the personnel budget, you must take into consideration the following significant factors:

1. Units of service

2. Mix in patient acuity

3. Required hours of nursing care

4. Fixed and variable staffing

5. Technological changes

6. Changes in medical practice

7. Regulatory requirements

8. Support services

9. Plans for the next year

UNITS OF SERVICE. Personnel budget needs are based initially on the projected units of service. This projection is usually made by the institution's financial department in collaboration with the department of nursing. The bed capacity of a nursing unit as well as the actual rate of occupancy should be considered. These data should be analyzed for any identifiable trends or patterns. As a general rule, if the occupancy rate is 90 percent or greater, the census can probably be considered fairly stable, with relatively little variation from day to day. However, the lower the occupancy rate, the greater the possibility for daily variation, which then creates the need to look more closely for patterns or trends.

Consider a 30-bed nursing unit with a 65 percent occupancy rate. In this case, it would be important to know if the census is evenly distributed over the time period or if there are discernible patterns or fluctuations. The distribution can be fairly equal, with a census of 19–20 patients per day, or there could be a very high census on weekdays with a very low census on weekends. Such a distribution of patient population will significantly affect the staffing patterns and the personnel budget.

MIX IN PATIENT ACUITY. The acuity levels of the various patients on the unit at any given time must also be considered. A patient classification system is a valuable tool in measuring the complexity of care needed by patients and in categorizing patients according to the level of care required over a specified period of time. Such systems can be beneficial in objectively defining staffing needs and supporting staffing requests. While a nurse manager can probably predict staffing needs fairly accurately with subjective data, it is difficult to support staffing and budgetary needs without objective evidence. Thus, it becomes important to base future personnel requirements on the amount of nursing care that patients actually need, rather than the amount of care actually provided. In situations of understaffing, patients do not receive the required hours of nursing care. Unless data reflect the hours indicated as well as the actual hours provided, labor projections will be false.

Classification systems vary for different nursing areas. Numerous patient classification systems are available today, ranging from the simplest to very comprehensive management information systems. All of these, however, should enable classification of patients according to the level of nursing care required, not on time actually spent delivering the care. Tools must minimize subjectivity and demonstrate validity and reliability if they are to accurately predict nursing work load.

REQUIRED HOURS OF NURSING CARE.

The first step in calculating staffing need for a given unit is to predict patient days by level of acuity. This information can be obtained from the census information and patient classification data. Assume, for instance, a 30-bed medical-surgical unit with an average census of 26 patients per day per month. On the basis of trend analysis, the average daily patient distribution is budgeted from historical data and may be displayed in this manner.

Level of care (from lowest acuity [I] to highest [IV])	Number of patients per day
I	5
II	17
III	3
IV	1
	26

The next step is to determine the hours of nursing care required for this particular mix of patients on the basis of an (assumed) patient classification system that utilizes the following standard hours of care needed by each patient for each acuity level:

Level	Hours per patient day
I	5.0
II	6.0
III	8.0
IV	12.0

To determine the daily hours of nursing care required, multiply the number of patients of each type by the standard hours of care required.

Total hours of care required in a 24-hour period is divided by the average daily census
$(163 \div 26 = 6.269)$

Thus, given a stable patient census and mix, the direct hours of nursing care per patient day would be 6.30 (see Table 19.1).

FIXED AND VARIABLE STAFFING.

Fixed staffing does not change as volume changes. The nurse manager, clinical nurse specialist, nurse educator, unit secretaries, monitor technicians, and a charge nurse on each shift are examples of individuals that may be needed regardless of the patient census and/or acuity. The inclusion of one or more of these individuals in the nursing hours per patient day (NHPPD) varies by institution.

Direct caregivers, who include registered nurses, licensed vocational nurses, and nurses aides, are examples of individuals whose numbers will vary depending on the census.

TECHNOLOGICAL CHANGES. Changes in technology that could affect the number or type of personnel required should be considered. For example, an intensive care unit that is about to purchase more sophisticated monitoring equipment may need additional staff due to the increased complexity of care, or, if the unit does not have enough registered nurses to manage the new equipment, an increase in their numbers should be considered when the staffing pattern and resulting budget are developed.

CHANGES IN MEDICAL PRACTICE. Changes in medical practice may create needs for different types of personnel, additional personnel, or a change in personnel mix. A signifi-

cant increase in the use of hyperalimentation, for example, might increase the nursing care and staff requirements significantly. Also important is whether the ratio of RNs to support personnel is appropriate to provide the type of care required with hyperalimentation. The development of a home hyperalimentation program would require increased patient care hours and may necessitate hiring a clinical nurse specialist as program coordinator.

REGULATORY REQUIREMENTS. The complexity of health care services provided to patients, the increasing acuity of hospitalized patients, and the growing recognition that quality of care affects outcomes has resulted in increasing attention to nursing requirement regulations for health care institutions. The Joint Commission on Accreditation for Healthcare Organizations (JCAHO) and various state

TABLE 19-1 STANDARD LABOR HOURS BUDGET
(for the period January 1 through December 31)

Classification	Patients per day	Hours per patient day	Hours of care per 24 hours
Level I	5	5.0	25
Level II	17	6.0	102
Level III	3	8.0	24
Level IV	1	12.0	12
Total	26		163

guidelines often require the number and/or level of nursing personnel required on specific units.

SUPPORT SERVICES. Support services such as environmental services, dietary services, radiology, and the laboratory should be considered with regard to the level of support they are now providing, how that support affects staffing levels, and whether any changes in these services are anticipated.

PLANS FOR THE NEXT YEAR. To accurately predict staffing requirements, institutional, nursing division, and nursing department goals for the coming year should be set first. These should include, at least, projections of activity level and any new programs or services.

Careful evaluation of these factors is the key to realistic planning. Such evaluation enables an accurate forecast to be made for the coming year, and this, in turn, is essential in developing staffing and budgetary requirements. The nursing executive is an essential resource at institution budget sessions; she or he can identify the impact of these areas on nursing's overall budgetary needs for patient care.

STAFFING PATTERNS

Using the recommended hours of care as a guideline, nurse managers can distribute those hours over all shifts by developing a staffing pattern. In addition to the previously mentioned relevant components of a personnel budget, other factors should be considered such as personnel mix, hours of work, distribution of workload, and delivery system.

PERSONNEL MIX. Personnel mix includes the number of personnel currently available at each skill level (RN, LVN, or aide), as well as the skill level recommended due to patient acuity.

HOURS OF WORK. Whether 8-hour, 10-hour, 12-hour, or other flexible scheduling is used, work shifts affect the staffing pattern, as well as the number of personnel needed.

DISTRIBUTION OF WORKLOAD. The nurse manager must analyze the workload distribution over the shifts and determine how the staffing should be distributed. This decision-making process needs to be individualized to particular patient requirements. Two possible alternatives are: (a) 35 percent of the staff allocated to all three shifts or (b) 45 percent on days, 30 percent on evenings, and 25 percent on nights. A 12-hour staffing pattern might allocate 60 percent of the staff on days and 40 percent on nights. The key is flexibility. Things can change from month to month or shift to shift. Initial projections merely serve as a guide.

DELIVERY SYSTEM. The method of delivering care (primary, team, differentiated practice, or functional nursing) also affects the staffing patterns.

POSITION CONTROL

The position control is the list of approved labor positions for the department. The positions are displayed by category of personnel (e.g., nurse manager, RN, LVN) as well as the number of full-time equivalents (FTEs). An FTE is a full-time position that can be equated to 40 hours of work per week or 80 hours per pay period. In institutions where nurses work 12-hour shifts, 72 hours per pay period may constitute one FTE.

An FTE is the equivalent of 2,080 paid hours per year (40 hours per week × 52 weeks per year = 2,080 hours). For a 36-hour workweek, one FTE = 1,872 hours (36 × 52 = 1,872). Paid hours include productive time (hours actually worked) plus nonproductive time (vacation, holiday, sick). The amount of nonproductive time actually built into each FTE varies with each organization. For purposes of budgeting, the nonproductive time is an expense that must be covered by additional paid productive hours.

THE FTE BUDGET. Using a hypothetical 26-bed unit where all staff work 8-hour shifts, the number of variable nursing staff needed on duty for 24 hours can be determined in the following manner.

The required nursing hours were determined to be 163 hours per 24 hours. The budgeted hours per patient day 6.369 (NHPPD) $\times$ 26 patients is 163.

Thus, 163 $\div$ 8-hour shifts = 20.3, the variable FTEs required per day. Since each nurse works eight hours a day, five days per week, additional FTEs (over 20.3) will be required to cover days off:

163 $\times$ 365 (days per year) = 59,495 (paid hours required in 1 year)

59,495 $\div$ 2,080 = 28.6 FTEs (required for the personnel budget)

For a nursing unit staffed totally by nurses who work 72 hours per pay period on 12-hour shifts, the FTEs required would be higher:

59,495 (total required hours) $\div$ 1,872 (paid hours) = 31.78 FTEs

One FTE can be filled by one person or any combination of personnel. For example, one nurse may work 24 hours per week and two other nurses each may work 8 hours per week (24 + 8 + 8 = 40).

The fixed positions required for the nursing unit are added into the overall position control. Since fixed positions are not usually replaced when off, each position is simply budgeted as 1.0 FTE. An exception may occur with unit secretaries. On some nursing units they are counted

as variable labor and their FTE comes out of the NHPPD. In other nursing units, unit secretaries may be needed seven days a week and yet they are excluded from the NHPPD count. Their FTE complement is considered separately.

Once unit staffing requirements have been determined, the required FTEs need to be compared to the available resources. When FTEs needed do not match the position control either by available numbers or necessary mix, the nurse manager considers budget requests for new positions or a change in mix.

DIFFERENTIALS AND OVERTIME

The budget for differentials for evenings and nights is calculated by multiplying the hours by the differential rate. For example, based on an average daily census of 26, a manager of a nursing unit that needs four RNs each on evenings and nights would multiply the differential rate on each shift by 8 and then multiply that number by 4:

Evening differential = $1 per hour
$1 per hour $\times$ 8 hours per shift = $8 per shift per nurse
$8 $\times$ 4 nurses = $32 per day additional needed budget dollars
$32 $\times$ 365 days a year = $11,680 a year

Night differential = $2 per hour
$2 $\times$ 8 hours = $16 per shift per nurse
$16 $\times$ 4 nurses = $64 per day additional needed budget dollars
$64 $\times$ 365 days = $23,360

Total additional budget dollars for differential = $35,040

An overtime budget is established to cover situations that cannot be anticipated, such as fluctuations in workload or temporary shortages of staff due to illness or other reasons. Overtime is calculated by determining the historical average number of hours of overtime worked and multiplying by 1.5 times the hourly rate. Thus, if the average number of overtime hours is expected to be 8 hours per week, the overtime rate is $18, or $12 × 1.5. The weekly overtime costs are then $144, and the annual cost is $7,488.

When trends are used to predict overtime, nurse managers should consider whether the amount of overtime used in the past was really justified and whether the level predicted is really appropriate. It may be possible to reduce overtime by adjusting the staffing schedule. Overtime dollars may be able to be decreased due to filled positions.

Nurse managers must calculate the number of per diem staff and registry staff used by calculating the hours and figuring the FTE complement.

4,160 per diem hours, 4160 ÷ 2080 = 2 FTEs

3,000 registry hours, 3000 ÷ 2080 = 1.44 FTEs

These FTEs need to be budgeted at their prevailing rates unless census predictions are less than the past year and/or vacant positions are filled.

Nursing units on 12-hour shifts need to account for the last four hours of each shift as overtime dollars. Whether this figure is accounted for within the overtime dollar figures, as well as within the overall salary projections, depends on the institution.

BENEFITS

To complete the personnel budget, benefits are figured as a percentage of the average yearly salary. In most institutions, vacation pay, holiday pay, sick leave, insurance premiums, workman's compensation, and any other benefits, such as life insurance or child care, usually average around 17 percent to 27 percent.

At this point, accumulation of data for the personnel budget should be complete. In summary, the first step is to project the activity for the coming year in terms of patient days and acuity of illness. The daily hours of care required for the projected mix of patients are then calculated using the hours of care. A staffing pattern is then developed, and the required variable and fixed FTEs are determined. The final steps include calculating differentials, overtime, and indirect labor costs.

MONITORING THE PERSONNEL BUDGET

Constant monitoring is necessary to ensure that expenses remain within the projected budgetary limits. This calls for the use of monthly expense statements, which include the amount budgeted for the month, the amount actually spent, and year-to-date information. Figure 19–4 illustrates such a statement.

The monthly report should be analyzed for significant variances. The causes for variances should then be determined and corrective action should be taken where indicated. In most cases, it is acceptable to be underbudget unless the dollar amount is significant—this might indicate improper planning.

The areas of variance that require most effort in problem identification are those that are overbudget where the variance is significant. To be significant means to be over some percentage set by management, such as 5 percent. In Figure 19–4, for instance, the RN salaries are significantly overbudget, and the reason for the variance should be explored carefully. Some questions to ask are: Was the patient activity during the period at the expected level or greater? Were the hours actually worked the number planned? Were the salaries as anticipated? Did the vacancies increase and were positions filled by a higher hourly wage? Were unworked hours, vacation, sick time, holiday pay, and so on as expected? The important point to determine is whether the variations were due to inappropriate planning or to unanticipated activity or expense that was beyond control.

As stated earlier, personnel costs represent the major portion of the total nursing service budget, and this requires that significant attention be paid to managing human resources. Lack of attention to this fact can affect the personnel budget indirectly or directly: indirectly through such factors as high turnover rates or high sick-leave time; directly by poor scheduling techniques or improper monitoring and use of overtime.

SUMMARY

♦ Budgeting is the process of planning future operations and controlling operations by comparing actual results with planned expectations.

♦ A budget is a detailed plan used to communicate these expectations and serve as the basis for comparing them to actual results.

♦ The organizational budget represents a series of interrelated budgets for all activities of the organization.

♦ Planning and control are two separate functions of the budget.

♦ Planning involves establishing future goals and objectives and the steps necessary to achieve those goals.

♦ Controlling is the process of comparing actual results with planned or budgeted results. By measuring these differences, management is better able to make modifications and corrections.

♦ A total unit budget includes a personnel budget, a supply and expense budget, and a capital expenditure budget.

FIGURE 19–4 MONTHLY PERSONNEL EXPENSE STATEMENT

Expense	Current Month–June			Year-to-Date (6 Months)		
	Actual	Budget	Variance	Actual	Budget	Variance
Management	3,200	4,000	800	22,200	24,000	1,800
Technician & specialist	2,855	2,855	0	15,421	17,130	1,709
Registered nurses	57,911	53,974	(3937)	179,479	181,929	2,450
Licensed vocational nurses	4,321	7,058	2,737	17,166	26,559	9,393
Aides & orderlies	0.00	0.00		0.00	0.00	
Clerical	3,813	3,650	(163)	22,420	21,900	(520)
Total	72,100	71,537	(563)	256,686	271,518	14,832

◆ The personnel budget is influenced by patient census, activity levels, technological changes, and changes in medical practice and clinical services.

◆ A unit personnel budget can be developed by (a) predicting patient days, (b) determining hours of nursing care required for this patient mix, (c) distributing hours required over all shifts, (d) developing a staffing pattern considering available personnel mix, and (e) converting patient care hours needed to budgeted costs.

BIBLIOGRAPHY

Arndt, C., and Huckabay, L. M. D. (1975). *Nursing Administration: Theory for Practice with a Systems Approach*. St. Louis, MO: C. V. Mosby.

Cleland, V. (1982). "Relating Nursing Staff Quality to Patient Needs." *Journal of Nursing Administration,* 12: 32.

Dale, R., and Mable, R. J. (1983). "Nursing Classification System: Foundation for Personnel Planning and Control." *Journal of Nursing Administration,* 13: 10.

Donovan, H. M. (1975). *Nursing Service Administration: Managing the Enterprise*. St. Louis, MO: C. V. Mosby.

Finkler, S. A. (1984). *Budgeting Concepts for Nurse Managers*. Orlando, FL: Grune and Stratton.

Hillestad, E. A. (1983). "Budgeting: Functional or Dysfunctional?" *Nursing Economics,* 1(3)(November/December): 199.

Huttmann, B. (1984). "Selling Your Budget." *RN,* 47: 25.

Kirby, K. K., and Wiczai, L. J. (1985). "Implementing and Monitoring Variable Staffing." *Nursing Economics,* 3(4)(July/August): 216–222.

Knight-Sheen, J. P. (1983). *The Medrec Calculator: A New Way to Plan for Nurse Staffing*. San Antonio, TX: Medrec.

McLane, A. M. (1987). "Classification of Nursing Diagnosis." In: *Proceedings of the Seventh Conference*. St. Louis, MO: C. V. Mosby.

Rotkovitch, R. (1981). "The Nursing Director's Role in Money Management." *Journal of Nursing Administration,* 11(11, 12): 13.

Stevens, B. J. (1980). *The Nurse as Executive*. 2d ed. Wakefield, MA: Contemporary Publications.

Stevens, B. J. (1981). "What Is the Executive's Role in Budgeting for Her Department?" *Journal of Nursing Administration,* 11: 22.

Strasen, L. (1987). *Key Business Skills for Nurse Managers*. Philadelphia: J. B. Lippincott.

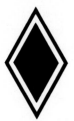

MANAGING AND INITIATING CHANGE

Change is inevitable, if not always welcome. Change is necessary for growth, although it often produces anxiety and fear. Even when planned, it can be threatening because change is the process of making something different from what it was. There is a sense of loss of the familiar, the status quo. This is particularly true when change is unplanned or beyond human control. And even when the change is expected and valued, a grief reaction still may occur. Those who manage and initiate change often encounter resistance from those experiencing unease and, possibly, symptoms of anxiety and grief.

Although nurse managers should understand and anticipate these reactions to change, they need to develop and exude a different approach, a positive aura for change. They can view change as a challenge and encourage their colleagues to participate. They can become uncomfortable with the status quo and find comfort in taking risks. The health care system is changing, with or without nurses' contributions. Leaders initiate change; followers survive it. Nurse managers must become skilled in implementing change introduced by administration. But they should work to get nurses into administration, not just nursing administration, and on the board—nurses who are as comfortable in the boardroom as they are at the bedside. Nurse leaders must initiate the changes they believe are necessary to strengthen nursing practice, provide quality care, and create a better system.

◆ CLIMATE FOR CHANGE

The health care system is in the midst of unprecedented change in a climate of uncertainty. Much of this change is economically driven. The government, insurance companies, employers, labor unions, and the public are exerting external pressure to control spending and redirect health care from expensive inpatient to more cost-effective outpatient care. The major payers of health care agree that more attention must be given to prevention and self-care. They are pressuring for disease-prevention programs and better management of resource consumption.

Health care organizations must change internally if they are to weather these pressures. To survive they must be focused yet flexible (Kanter, 1989). Restructuring is an ongoing activity. Health care institutions are expanding their outpatient services and adding new programs for health promotion. They are developing new patient care delivery systems to maximize efficiency and quality, while controlling the patient's length of stay. These changes require modifications in technology, personnel, and structure. In today's economic environment, organizational change is essential for adaptation; creative change is mandatory for growth.

This climate for change produces new opportunities for nurses. The demand for nurses has become insatiable. Increasingly, institutions are investing resources to retain nurses and improve the work environment. Nursing's long-standing call for greater autonomy in the workplace is receiving serious attention. Those working in hospitals find top-level management is listening to suggestions for environmental change that will increase nurse satisfaction. Innovation is "in." The participatory approach is popular because status quo management will not work when a whole system is in transition. Transitional times demand new ways of thinking, creative strategies, and fresh options.

Nurses outside health care institutions are forging new roles. Many are accepting case management roles to help employers discourage excessive resource consumption. Some are opening their own businesses in home health care and preventive health programs. As third-party payers of health care push for options to expensive disease-oriented institutional care, opportunities arise for innovative nurses. Whether they practice independently, work in bureaucracies, or form their own organizations, today's nurses need to understand, manage, and produce change.

◆ NURSE AS CHANGE AGENT

The notion of the "nurse as change agent" is not new. A change agent is one who works to bring about a change. The nurse often acts as an "insider," a change agent who is part of the system being altered (usually the unit she or he manages). But nurses can also be "outsiders," or consultants for change in other systems. Nurses have been prepared for the former more than the latter. In either case, though, there has never been a better time for the nursing profession to take the initiative. As the largest health profession, nurses make the health care system run. They have concrete ideas about how to make it run better.

Although many patients are admitted to institutions for technological intervention, they remain for 24-hour nursing care. To a large extent, nurses control length of stay. Their expertise and organization can determine the cost and quality of care an institution offers. On the one hand, nursing represents the biggest slice of the institutional budget. On the other hand, the quality of nursing care is a "differential advantage" for the organization. An institution known for its excellent nursing care has a competitive edge. Nurses who can suggest changes to control costs, improve quality, or offer new services will be change agents in great demand in institutions.

Outside institutions, nurse change agents can move the health care system from a medical to a nursing model. Fueled by businesses' interest in holding down the cost of illness care by encouraging employees to promote healthy living, nurses can create new niches in the business world. They can develop and manage prevention programs. They can case manage employees' health problems by linking them to existing services. They can create the gap-filling services consumers will require as they are left to care for themselves, outside institutions. In addition, nurses are the most logical problem solvers for creating cost-effective ways to care for the elderly.

Changes will continue at a rapid pace with or without nursing's expert guidance. However, nurses, like organizations, cannot afford to merely "survive" changes. If they are to exist as a distinct profession that has expertise in solving "human responses to actual or potential health problems" (ANA, 1980: 3), they must be proactive in shaping the future. The opportunities exist now for nurses, especially those in management positions, to change the system about which they so often complain.

◆ CHANGE WITHIN A SYSTEMS FRAMEWORK

Most nurses work in organizations. As described in Chapter 2 modern organizational theory conceptualizes the organization as a complex social system within the suprasystem of society (Kast & Rosenzweig, 1970). It is an integrated whole of mutually dependent parts that exchange information and energy through semipermeable boundaries (Chinn, 1969). There is also constant interaction with the environment. Because this dynamic interaction change is inevitable, a change in one part of the system produces change throughout the system. Although change is considered necessary for growth, integrative processes are required to achieve system viability and goal achievement.

A successful organization achieves organization equilibrium, or a balance among the forces operating on it and within it. Dynamic equilibrium occurs when an organization responds to change by shifting to a new balance or by modifying its goals (Chinn, 1969). Every system experiences stresses, strains, and conflicts, produced in part by the opposing forces of the system's maintenance and adaptive mechanisms. Maintenance mechanisms prevent change from occurring too rapidly while adaptive mechanisms work to keep the system changing over time. The significance of these forces cannot be overemphasized, for the scope and pace of organizational change depend on how they are managed. While managers work to reduce tension, relieve stress (see Chapter 10), and resolve conflict (see Chapter 22), they must do so cautiously or pay "the price of overlooking the possibility of increasing tensions and conflict to facilitate creativity, innovation and social change" (Chinn, 1969: 301).

There are several advantages in using the systems frame of reference to understand and manage change. First, it mandates integrative thinking. The change agent must analyze the system and system-environment boundaries, mechanisms, and flow of information and energy. At the same time, the change agent must always recognize that the whole is greater than the sum of its parts. This complex and comprehensive approach precludes the search for simple causal relationships. Instead, the manager searches for the multiple, interacting variables that facilitate and restrict system changes. The importance of external (environmental) variables is examined in relation to internal variables.

The systems framework also directs attention to the hierarchical arrangement of the system's subsystems. Understanding this hierarchy facilitates coordination of communication and activities (see Chapter 7), and thus the change agent can assess the transactions taking place at all levels of the system. This assessment begins with the suprasystem: Management of change begins with those who have an overall view, because effective managers know external forces have a pervasive effect on the whole system. They know the search for organizational problems and solutions does not begin and end on the unit, in the department, or even within the organization itself. Often, change outside the system holds the greatest promise, if not the greatest challenge. For example, nurse staffing and recruitment problems include such suprasystem variables as state regulatory ceilings on hospital expense budgets, which restrain substantive professional nurse salary increases; reductions in federal financial support for professional nurse education; and Medicare's hospital payment scheme, based on medical diagnostic categories that do not factor in the intensity of nursing care required. These variables are only a few of the environmental factors influencing the education and recruitment of nurses whose job is to give intensive care to large caseloads of "general medical patients" in institutions. They point out the need to make change in the suprasystem known as the health care delivery system.

These issues are serious and demand attention from nurse managers who have a macro-perspective and change agent skills. Reshaping the health care delivery system necessitates political action. Governmental policies influence the financing, structure, content, and process of delivering health care. Nurses must become comfortable with and sophisticated in formulating policy beyond their unit or institution. What nurses can legally do, what care third-party payers will reimburse, and even how nurses dispose of syringes are policy issues decided in the political arena. Though nuances vary according to the political body (e.g., legislature, regulatory boards, departments), the political process is the change process.

At the organizational, departmental, and unit levels, creative change also begins with this macro-perspective. Nurse change agents start by thinking broadly. Looking at the sociopolitical and economic picture, they check the pulse of the external environment, competing organizations, the board of directors, and the professions. What is the climate? What are the trends? What does the consumer want and need? What does the nursing profession propose? Combining ideas from unconnected sources (Kanter, 1983) causes innovative thinking to "percolate." The more "fluid" the vertical and horizontal organizational boundaries, the better communication is from top-down, bottom-up, and lateral directions. Creative ideas flow best from managers who think big, brainstorm ideas, and stimulate "grassroots" staff talents.

◆ THE PROCESS OF CHANGE

Whether it is environmental, systemwide, or unit-based, the change process involves strategies. This process can and should be learned by all nurses, especially managers. The nurse manager needs to develop a system of integrative thinking that demands that problems be looked at as a whole. Skill in applying change theory is a valuable management tool inside or outside the institutional setting. The change process based on this theory is a problem-solving process, much like the nursing process. Different experts identify different numbers of steps or stages in the change process. The number of steps is unimportant. What is important is un-

derstanding what the change agent needs to do and why. The process is dynamic and fluid. As you become experienced with change, the sense of that "flow" becomes incorporated into your repertoire of nursing skills. Those who can master the nuances of communication skills can become "change masters" (Kanter, 1983).

The problem-solving change process described in this chapter synthesizes classical change theory and current nursing, sociological, psychological, and organizational thought. However, the nurse educated to manage and initiate change should know the theoretical foundation for the change process she or he implements. Therefore, key aspects of selected change theories are summarized in the following section; then a seven-step process is delineated with examples. Readers are encouraged to consult primary references for a fuller understanding of each. These theoretical views have many similarities, but the unique insights of each are also rich sources of current approaches to change.

◆ CHANGE THEORIES

LEWIN'S FORCE-FIELD MODEL

Lewin (1951) provides a social-psychological view of the change process. He sees behavior as a dynamic balance of forces working in opposite directions within a field (such as an organization). *Driving forces* facilitate change because they are pushing participants in the desired direction. *Restraining forces* impede change because they are leading participants in the other direction. To plan change, one must analyze these forces and shift the balance in the direction of change through a three-step process: *unfreezing, moving,* and *refreezing.* Change occurs by adding a new force, changing the direction of a force, or changing the magnitude of any one force. Basically, strategies for change are aimed at increasing driving forces, decreasing restraining forces, or both.

Lewin's force-field model and an example are diagrammed in Figure 20–1. This scheme shows a system's opposing driving and restraining forces of change. These forces, part of the system's maintenance and adaptive mechanisms, are balanced at the present, or status quo, level. To achieve change, first an imbalance must occur between these driving and restraining forces (as in the example). This imbalance unfreezes the present patterned behavior. Behavior moves to a new level, at which the opposing forces are brought into a new state of equilibrium. Once participants integrate the new patterns of behavior into their personalities and relationships with others, a refreezing takes place. The new level becomes institutionalized into

FIGURE 20–1 LEWIN'S FORCE-FIELD MODEL OF CHANGE

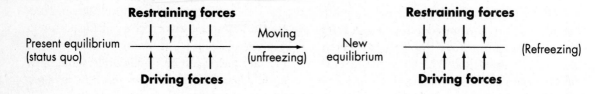

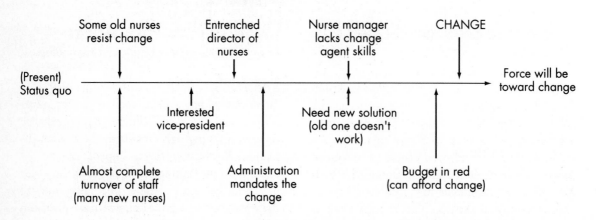

K. Lewin, *Field Theory in Social Science* (New York: Harper & Row, 1951, p. 158).

formal and informal behavioral patterns.

Lewin's change strategies fall within his three-step process. They are:

1. Unfreeze the existing equilibrium. Motivate participants by getting them ready for change. Build trust and recognition for the need to change. Actively participating in problem identification and generating alternate solutions helps to thaw attitudes.

2. Move the target system to a new level of equilibrium. Get participants to agree that the status quo is not beneficial to them. Encourage "cognitive redefinition" by helping them view the problem from a new perspective. Stimulate identification by linking their views to those of a respected or powerful leader who supports the change. Help them scan the environment to search for relevant information.

3. Refreeze the system at the new level of equilibrium. Reinforce the new patterns of behavior. Institutionalize them through formal and informal mechanisms (policies, communications channels, etc.).

Lewinian thinking is fundamental to the views of later theorists. Clearly, it is a behavioral approach that nurses find consistent with their theoretical understanding of humans. The image of people's attitudes thawing, becoming more fluid, shifting to a desired state, and then refreezing is conceptually useful. This symbolism helps to keep theory and reality in mind simultaneously.

LIPPITT'S PHASES OF CHANGE

Lippitt et al. (1958) extend Lewin's theory to a seven-step process and focus more on what the change agent must do than on the evolution of change itself. They emphasize participation of key members of the target system throughout the change process, particularly in the planning stages. Communication skills, rapport building, and problem-solving strategies underlie their phases.

1. Diagnose the problem. Involve key people in data collection and problem solving.

2. Assess the motivation and capacity for change. Assess financial and human resources and constraints. Analyze the structure and function of the organization. Identify and prioritize possible solutions.

3. Assess the change agent's motivation and resources. Identifying this self-assessment phase is an important contribution. One's own commitment to change, energy level, future ambitions, and power bases must be considered. Starting a change and dropping it midstream can waste valuable personal energy and undermine the confidence of colleagues and subordinates.

4. Select progressive change objects. Develop the action plan, evaluation criteria, and specific strategies.

5. Choose a change agent role. The change agent can act as cheerleader, expert, consultant, or group facilitator. Whichever role is selected, all participants should identify it so that expectations are clear.

6. Maintain the change. Communication, feedback, revision making, and coordination are essential components of this phase.

7. Terminate the helping relationship. The change agent withdraws from the selected role gradually as the change becomes institutionalized.

Those who must continually implement in-

novation need to have the authority and accountability to do so.

HAVELOCK'S MODEL

Havelock (1973) describes a six-step process,
also a modification of Lewin's model. It is included here only briefly. Havelock emphasizes
the unfreezing or planning stage, which he defines as (a) building a relationship, (b) diagnosing the problem, and (c) acquiring resources.
This stage is followed by the moving stage: (d)
choosing the solution and (e) gaining acceptance. Refreezing is referred to as (f) stabilization and self-renewal. Havelock describes an
active change agent as one who uses a participative approach.

ROGERS'S DIFFUSION OF INNOVATIONS

Rogers (1983) takes a broader approach than
Lewin, Lippitt, or Havelock. His five-step
innovation-decision process details how an individual or "decision-making unit" passes from
"first knowledge of an innovation" to confirmation of the decision to adopt or reject a new
idea (1983: 20). His framework emphasizes the
reversible nature of change because participants
may initially adopt a proposal but later discontinue it, or the reverse—they may initially reject
it but adopt it at a later time. This is a useful
distinction. If the change agent is unsuccessful in
achieving full implementation of a proposal, she
or he should not assume the issue is dead. It can
be resurrected, perhaps in an altered form or at
a more opportune time. However, if it is accepted, one also cannot assume permanence.

Rogers's five steps to the diffusion of innovation are:

1. Knowledge. The decision-making unit is
   introduced to the innovation and begins to
   understand it.

2. Persuasion. A favorable (or unfavorable) attitude toward the innovation forms.

3. Decision. Activities lead to a decision to
   adopt or reject the innovation.

4. Implementation. The innovation is put to
   use and reinvention or alterations may
   occur.

5. Confirmation. The individual or decision-
   making unit seeks reinforcement that the decision was correct. If there are conflicting
   messages or experiences, the original decision may be reversed.

Finally, Rogers stresses two important aspects of successful planned change: Key people
and policy makers must be interested in the innovation and committed to making it happen.

SUMMARY OF THEORETICAL PERSPECTIVES

These models of change are not the only ones
that exist. They are classic formulations that
overlap despite differences in perspective (see
Figure 20–2). A seven-step eclectic approach
based on the nursing process abstracts the common points and identifies those significant for
the nurse change agent. Insights from current
experts of innovation are integrated into this
model.

◆ THE SEVEN STEPS TO PLANNED CHANGE: AN ECLECTIC APPROACH

The nursing process arose in the 1950s when
nurses sought a framework for problem solving
patient care. The process of assessment, planning, implementation, and evaluation now
structures nurses' thinking and care delivery; it

is second nature to the professional nurse. Essentially, managing change follows the same path as the nursing process: assessment, planning, implementation, and evaluation (see Figure 20–3). However, since many nurses are less comfortable with change than with patient care, these steps are subdivided and extended into seven steps. Much emphasis is placed on the assessment phase of change for two reasons. First, without thorough data collection and analysis, planned change will not proceed past the "wouldn't it be a good idea if we . . ." stage. Second, nurses often are not familiar with the kind of data they need to collect or with the method by which to analyze those data to manage and initiate change.

A situation is presented to illustrate the steps in the change process. It involves staff nurse participation in institutional discharge planning. Readers are also encouraged to identify a situation relevant to their own practice or management role. For example, nurses in private practice might consider how to obtain hospital admitting privileges. Nurse managers could substitute the initiation of an improved patient classification system (see Chapter 19) to link patient acuity levels to staffing patterns.

ASSESSMENT

1. IDENTIFY THE PROBLEM OR THE OPPORTUNITY. Opportunities demand change as much as (or more than) problems do. They are often overlooked by managers who manage but do not lead: Change is often planned to close a *performance gap*, a discrepancy between the desired and actual state of affairs. Performance gaps may arise because of problems in reaching performance goals or because new goals have been created. Be it a problem or an opportunity, it must be identified clearly. If the issue is perceived differently by key persons, the search for

FIGURE 20–2 COMPARISON OF CHANGE MODELS

Lewin	Lippitt	Havelock	Rogers
1. Unfreezing	1. Diagnose problem 2. Assess motivation 3. Assess change agent's motivations and resources	1. Building a relationship 2. Diagnosing the problem 3. Acquiring resources	1. Knowledge 2. Persuasion 3. Decision
2. Moving	4. Select progressive change objects 5. Choose change agent role	4. Choosing the solution 5. Gaining acceptance	4. Implementation
3. Refreezing	6. Maintain change 7. Terminate helping relationship	6. Stabilization	5. Confirmation

solutions becomes confused. Start by asking the right questions, such as:

a. Where are we now? What is unique about us? What should our business be?

b. What can we do that is different from and better than what our competitors do?

c. What is the driving stimulus in our organization? What determines how we make our final decisions?

d. What prevents us from moving in the direction we wish to go?

e. What kind of change is required?

This last question generates integrative thinking on the potential effect of change on the system. Organizational change involves modifications in the system's interacting components: technology, structure, and people. The introduction of new technology may necessitate changes in the structure of the organization. The physical plant will be altered if new services (e.g., open-heart surgery) are added. Relationships among the people who work in the system change when the structure is changed. New units are opened; others close. New rules and regulations, new authority structures, and new budgeting methods are structural changes. They, in turn, change staff needs, requiring people with different skills, knowledge bases, attitudes, and motivations. No matter what the opportunity or problem, behavioral change—or "people change"—is the most challenging.

Given the transitional state of the health care system, nurse managers need to develop creative insights to address problems, discover opportunities, and avoid status quo management. Creative insight involves looking at old problems in a fresh way from many different perspectives. Past history is not used as a guide for solutions. The manager concentrates on moving beyond the habitual, comfortable ways of experiencing a phenomenon to arrive at new insights and new

FIGURE 20–3 SEVEN STEPS OF PLANNED CHANGE: AN EXTENSION OF THE NURSING PROCESS

Nursing Process	Change Process
Assessment	1. Identify the problem or opportunity 2. Collect data 3. Analyze data
Planning	4. Plan the change strategies
Implementation	5. Implement the change
Evaluation	6. Evaluate effectiveness 7. Stablize the change

possibilities (Hickman & Silva, 1984). Problems can become opportunities for change that not only will solve the immediate problem but also can help reshape and stimulate the system.

Situation: Discharge Planning. An example of creative insight in defining a problem occurred in a medium-size medical center. Upper management had identified a staffing problem that they solved by using temporary agency nurses, pulling staff from one floor to float to another, and requesting nurses to remain on duty for an additional eight hours (for overtime pay). However, the pediatric unit supervisor saw the problem differently. After conferencing with her staff, she perceived that the staffing levels indicated upper management's unwillingness to give the staff control, accountability, and respect. The problem, in her view, was inadequate staffing due to mismanagement of human resources. Nurses who are experts in the care of children resent being pulled to a unit that does not require this expertise or to a unit that requires an expertise the child care specialist does not have. During periods of frequent pulling, these nurses were more likely to call in sick.

With this problem in focus, ideas were generated. The problem was refashioned into an opportunity to create a "children's center," a decentralized unit encompassing pediatric and pediatric intensive care services. The proposal was to staff and manage this unit autonomously with collaboration between the unit supervisor and the pediatric nurses under her jurisdiction. No nurses would float in or out of this unit. Rather, a contingency schedule was developed to provide staff coverage for sick calls from within. Such a schedule provided a stable plan for adequate human resources to maintain optimal client care and, at the same time, promote collegial relationships and accountability. It also lowered overtime costs. Nurses were less likely

to call in sick needlessly when they knew their colleagues would be required to cover for them. The depersonalization of coverage is eliminated.

2. COLLECT DATA. Once the problem or opportunity has been clearly defined, the change agent collects data external and internal to the system. This step is crucial to the eventual success of the planned change. All driving and restraining forces are identified so the driving forces can be emphasized and the restraining forces reduced. It is imperative to assess the political pulse. Who will gain from this change? Who will lose? Who has more power and why? Can those power bases be altered? How?

The nurse manager can best assess the political climate by examining the reasons for the present situation. Who is in control that may be benefitting now? The ego involvement, commitment of the involved people, and personality likes and dislikes are as important to assess as the formal organizational structures and processes. The innovator has to gauge the potential resistance.

The costs and benefits of the proposed change are obvious focal points. The nurse manager also needs to assess resources—especially those the manager can control. A manager who has the respect and support of an excellent nursing staff has access to a powerful resource in today's climate. Current research findings are also helpful data in the change process.

Situation. To introduce her proposal for a decentralized unit with autonomous staffing prerogatives, the pediatric unit supervisor had to collect data to support her arguments. Examples of external data included state, regional, and local supply and demand statistics for general and pediatric nurses; consumer demand for expert pediatric nursing services; staffing policies from competing institutions; and research data regarding motivation of professional employees.

Internal data were derived from different system levels (organizational, group, and personal). At the organizational level, the supervisor examined the hospital's philosophy, goals, and marketing plans. She sought evidence that the hospital would benefit from marketing a Children's Center with a stable staff of specialist nurses. There was no competing focus, which would have been the case if administration had long-range plans to market a different unit. At the group and personal levels, the supervisor consulted her own staff and discussed the ideas with nurses from other specialized units. If the staff had been organized in a bargaining unit, she would have had to investigate the bargaining unit's negotiated staffing policies and potential support for the idea. The goal was to collect data to support the idea that this change matched the goals, norms, and values of the organization and its members. As a nurse leader, this supervisor was also interested in demonstrating how this idea reflected the goals and values of the nursing department and the profession.

Quantitative data help document needed change. Historical staffing and turnover data for this unit were compiled. Records were kept demonstrating higher absenteeism during periods of frequent pulling. Incident reports of unit and non-unit members documented the higher quality of care provided by seasoned specialists as opposed to temporary nurses. Finally, she estimated the cost savings expected from not hiring temporary nurses.

3. ANALYZE DATA. The kinds, amounts, and sources of data collected are important, but they are useless unless they are analyzed. The change agent should focus more energy on analyzing and summarizing the data than on running around collecting it. The point is to flush out resistance, identify potential solutions and strategies, begin to identify areas of consensus, and build a case for whichever option is selected. When possible, a statistical analysis should be made; it is worth the effort, especially when the change agent will need to persuade persons in power who are comfortable with financial analyses, statistics, and probabilities. Themes from the data can be pulled out and threaded together to make a cogent case. These should be presented succinctly using bar graphs and charts.

PLANNING

4. PLAN THE CHANGE STRATEGY. Planning the who, how, and when of the change is a key step. What will be the target system for the change? Members from this system should be active participants in the planning stage. The more involved they are at this point, the less resistance there will be later. Lewin's unfreezing imagery is relevant here. Present attitudes, habits, and ways of thinking have to soften so members of the target system will be ready for new ways of thinking and behaving. Boundaries must melt before the system can shift and restructure.

This is the time to "rock the boat" by making people uncomfortable with the status quo. The seeds of discontent are planted by introducing information that may make people feel dissatisfied with the present and interested in something new. This information comes from the data collected (e.g., research findings, quantitative data, and surveys of clients or staff). The proposed change should be couched in comfortable terms as far as possible. Anxiety about the new change should be minimized.

Managers need to plan the resources required to make the change and establish feedback mechanisms to evaluate its progress and success. Establish control points with people who will provide the feedback. Work with these people to set specific goals with time frames. Develop operational indicators that signal success or failure in terms of performance and satisfaction.

Situation. Potential control points and indicators for the Children Center's proposal might be stated as:

a. Within six months, the nurse manager will develop a contingency schedule in collaboration with staff nurses, on a monthly basis.

b. Within eight months, there will be a 20 percent decline in sick-outs.

c. Within 10 months, the staff will meet with upper management to report the effect of the new staffing policy on their professional identity and sense of control.

d. Within 12 months, the unit supervisor will submit a recommendation to continue or discontinue the staffing policy based on such evidence as staff turnover, sick-outs, and use of agency personnel.

IMPLEMENTATION

5. IMPLEMENT THE CHANGE. The plans are put into motion (Lewin's moving stage). Interventions are designed to gain the necessary compliance. The change agent creates a supportive climate, acts as energizer, obtains and provides feedback, and overcomes resistance. Managers are the key change process actors. They use implementation tactics "to install planned changes, whether they be novel or routine" (Nutt, 1986: 233). The specific activities undertaken to induce organizational change constitute the method of change (Katz & Kahn, 1978). Depending on the change strategy se-

lected (see the next section), the method might include giving a lecture or forming task forces. Some methods are directed toward changing individuals in an organization while others are directed toward changing the group.

Methods to change individuals. The most common method used to change individuals' perceptions, attitudes, and values is information giving (Katz & Kahn, 1978; Nutt, 1986). External expert consultants or internal organization staff persons prepare and disseminate the information, usually in a top-down communication flow. Providing information is prerequisite to change implementation, but it is inadequate alone unless the lack of information is the only obstacle to effecting change. Information provision does not address the motivation to change.

Training combines information giving with practice in skills. As a socialization strategy, it is more of a system maintenance mechanism than an adaptation mechanism. Training typically shows people how they are to perform in a system, not how to change it. Counseling or psychotherapy is most effective for the troubled organization member or the person who holds a powerful organization position. Selection, placement, or termination of key people may be useful tactics for altering the forces for or against change.

Methods to change groups. Some implementation tactics use groups rather than individuals to attain compliance to change. The power of an organizational group to influence its members depends on its authority to act on an issue and the significance of the issue itself. The greatest influence is achieved when group members discuss issues that are perceived important and make relevant, binding decisions based on those discussions. Research on the use of sensitivity groups has not demonstrated effectiveness in implementing organizational change, most likely because these groups are not necessarily composed of members who occupy closely related positions in the organization. A more successful strategy has been the use of survey feedback, in which organizational groups who do share closely related positions discuss issues as an "organizational family."

Individual and group implementation tactics can be combined. Whatever methods are used, participants should feel their input is valued. They should be rewarded for their efforts. Some people are not always persuaded a change is beneficial before it is implemented. Some undergo "cognitive dissonance," which means behavior changes first and attitudes are modified later to fit the behavior. In this case, the change agent should be aware of participants' conflict and reward the desired behaviors. It may take some time for attitudes to catch up.

Situation. The pediatric supervisor recognized that she was initiating a unit-level change that would have systemwide implications. Both individual and group methods of change were needed. Providing "fact sheets" to her own unit members heightened their interest and offered a common ground for later discussion. To reduce resistance from other supervisors, she met informally with them one by one. Her tactic was to change attitudes by appealing to their professional values. Group meetings followed in which she suggested a trial program and requested participation in developing guidelines for contingency scheduling. She began to screen staff nurse applicants as to their desire for autonomy. Additionally, she persuaded the director of nurses and the nurse recruiter to visit another institution that had already instituted a similar policy in its critical care unit.

EVALUATION

6. EVALUATE EFFECTIVENESS. At each control point, the established operational indicators (step 4) are monitored as planned. The change agent determines if presumed benefits were achieved from a financial as well as a qualitative perspective. The extent of success or failure is determined and explained. Unintended consequences and undesirable outcomes may have occurred.

For example, the unit manager in the case study might obtain evidence that the new Children's Center attracts clients and retains expert staff. She would also need to measure staff satisfaction. It is possible the staff resent covering for one another and that conflict is brewing.

7. STABILIZE THE CHANGE. The change is extended past the pilot stage and the target system is refrozen. The change agent terminates the helping relationship by delegating responsibilities to target system members. The "energizer role" is still needed to reinforce the new behaviors through positive feedback. A degree of permanency is cultivated by writing formal policies and making sure staff repeat the new behavior frequently.

♦ CHANGE AGENT STRATEGIES

Regardless of the setting or proposed change, the seven-step change process should be followed. However, specific strategies can be used, depending on the amount of resistance anticipated and the degree of power the change agent possesses. The three classic models of strategies were first described by Bennis, Benne, and Chinn (1969). They remain useful categories to consider in deciding which strategies the change agent should select under the circumstances.

POWER-COERCIVE

Power-coercive strategies are based on the application of power by legitimate authority, economic sanctions, or political clout. For example, changes are made through law, policy, or financial appropriations. Those in control enforce changes by restricting budgets or creating policies. Those who are not in power may not even be aware of what is happening. Even if they are aware, they have little power to stop it. The change process continues through the seven steps just detailed, but there is little, if any, participation of the target system members. Resistance is handled by authority measures: Accept it or leave.

The federal government's enactment of the prospective payment system for Medicare clients' hospitalizations was a power-coercive strategy for changing the economic incentives. The institution is not paid for a client's care based on the number of days hospitalized. Rather, the institution receives a predetermined fee based on the client's DRG (diagnosis-related group) regardless of the length of stay.

Power-coercive strategies are useful when a consensus is unlikely despite efforts to stimulate participation throughout the change process. When much resistance is anticipated, time is short, and the change is critical for organizational survival, this group of strategies may be necessary. A vice-president of nursing, for example, might have to exert legitimate authority to appoint a specific person to be a unit supervisor because the unit is leaderless during a critical time (a local epidemic of measles). Although the professional autonomy of the unit's members would be better served if they were given the opportunity to interview and evaluate a candidate, organizational and unit survival needs might supersede this goal for the short run.

Of course, the potential negative consequences of this unilateral approach cannot be ignored. If the unit members have been practicing in a decentralized framework and value the accustomed autonomy, they are not likely to react positively. Resistance to the appointed leader and decreased morale can be expected. These strategies should not be used lightly or often if the nurse manager wishes to foster a climate of openness to change.

EMPIRICAL-RATIONAL

In the *empirical-rational model* of change strategies, the power ingredient is knowledge. The assumption is that people are rational and will follow their rational self-interest if that self-interest is made clear to them. It is also assumed that the change agent who has knowledge has expert power to persuade people to accept a rationally justified change that will benefit them. The flow of influence moves from those who know to those who do not know. New ideas are invented and communicated or diffused to all participants (like Rogers's "diffusion of innovation"). It is a matter of educating and disseminating information. Once enlightened, rational people will either accept or reject the idea based on its merits and consequences.

Because people do not always respond rationally, this strategy should not be used alone (Haffer, 1986). However, empirical-rational strategies are often effective when little resistance exists to the proposed change and it is perceived as reasonable. Introduction of new technology that is easy to use, cuts nursing time, and improves quality of care would be accepted readily after inservice education and perhaps a trial use. The change agent can direct the change. There is little need for staff participation in the early steps of the change process although input is useful for the evaluation and stabilization stages. The benefits of change for the staff and perhaps research findings regarding client outcomes are the major driving forces. Well-researched, cost-effective technology can be implemented through this group of strategies.

NORMATIVE-REEDUCATIVE

In contrast to the rational-empirical model, *normative-reeducative strategies* of change rest on the assumption that people act in accordance with social norms and values. Information and rational arguments are insufficient strategies to change people's patterns of actions; the change agent must focus on non-cognitive determinants of behavior as well. People's roles and relationships, perceptual orientations, attitudes, and feelings will influence their acceptance of change.

In this mode, the power ingredient is not authority or knowledge, but skill in interpersonal relationships. The change agent does not use coercion or nonreciprocal influence, but collaboration. Members of the target system are involved throughout the change process: People must participate in their own reeducation if they are to be reeducated at all. Change, or reeducation, is a normative change as well as cognitive and perceptual change, and participation in groups is an essential change strategy (Bennis, Benne & Chinn, 1969).

Normative-reeducative strategies are well suited to the creative problem solving needed in nursing and health care today. The change agent consciously uses the change process based on theories of change that emphasize a human relations approach. Members of the target system are involved throughout the change process.

Value conflicts from all parts of the system are brought into the open and "worked through" so change can progress.

With their firm grasp of the behavioral sciences and communication skills, nurses are comfortable with this model. In most cases, the normative-reeducative approach to change will be effective in reducing resistance and stimulating personal and organizational creativity. The obvious drawback is the time required for group participation and conflict resolution throughout the change process. When there is adequate time or when group consensus is fundamental to successful adoption of the change, the manager is well advised to adopt this framework. Examples include changing from a team to a primary nursing system (or the reverse) or initiating a new service.

◆ CHANGE AGENT SKILLS

Making changes is not easy, but it is a mandatory skill for managers. Successful change agents demonstrate certain characteristics that can be cultivated and mastered with practice. Among these are:

1. The ability to combine ideas from unconnected sources

2. The ability to energize others by keeping the interest level up and demonstrating a high personal energy level

3. Skill in human relations; well-developed interpersonal communication, group management, and problem-solving skills

4. Integrative thinking; the ability to retain a "big picture" focus while dealing with each part of the system

5. Sufficient flexibility to modify ideas when modifications will improve the change, but persistent enough to resist nonproductive tampering with the planned change

6. Confidence and the tendency not to be easily discouraged

7. Realistic thinking

8. Trustworthiness; a track record of integrity and success with other changes

9. Ability to articulate a "vision" through insights and versatile thinking

10. Ability to handle resistance

◆ HANDLING RESISTANCE

Why do people resist change? A generalized resistance stems from fear of losing the comfort of the familiar, no matter how inadequate it is. There is comfort in clinging to the present and uncertainty about the consequences of change. Change can threaten those with vested interest in the status quo. People view new ideas with selected perceptions: "How will this change affect me?"

For example, the change may represent a social loss when the organization is restructured and social relationships altered. Decentralization may abolish positions and decrease promotion opportunities, an actual or potential economic loss to some people. A union may resist change that threatens job security for some of its members, even if other members or the organization as a whole will benefit. Even the inconvenience of learning new behaviors can be at the root of resistance.

The change agent should anticipate, ameliorate, and use resistance to change. Look for resistance. It will be lurking somewhere, perhaps where least expected. It can be recognized in such statements as:

1. "We tried that before."

2. "It won't work."

3. "No one else does it like that."

4. "We've always done it this way."

5. "We can't afford it."

6. "We don't have the time."

7. "It will cause too much commotion."

8. "You'll never get it past the board."

9. "Let's wait awhile."

10. "Every new boss wants something new to do."

11. "Let's start a task force to look at it . . . put it on the agenda."

Expect resistance and listen carefully to who says what, when, and in what circumstances. Verbal resisters are easier to deal with than "closet" resisters. Look for nonverbal signs of resistance such as poor work habits and lack of interest in the change.

Resistance has positive and negative aspects. On the one hand, resistance forces the change agent to be clear about why the change is needed. The agent must know the change inside and out because she or he must defend it against challengers. The positive part of resistance is the sharper focus and problem solving it encourages. It prevents the unexpected. It forces the change agent to clarify information, keep the interest level high, and answer the question, "Why is this change necessary?" Resistance is a stimulant as much as it is a force to be overcome. It may motivate the target system to do better

BOX 20-1

Hickman and Silva (1984) offer exercises for removing blinders to insight.

1. Write down one new idea a day for a month. It can pertain to work, research, professional activities, family, or leisure, but it must be new. Consider some action on each idea (discuss it with colleagues, experiment with it), or implement it.
2. Break out of the mold. Do something unexpected, even "against the rules." Learn to tolerate ambiguity.
3. Routinely look at things differently. Read a book on creativity or attend a creativity seminar. See Steele and Maraviglia, *Creativity in Nursing* (1981), for example, and many others. Do not stick to nursing references. Try *A Whack on the Side of the Head,* by Roger von Oech (1983).

4. Engage in wild thinking. Build in time for "unfettered thinking" in your meetings (supervisors' meetings, for example)—at least one hour several times a month.
5. Make things complex and ambiguous. Every day for an month, choose one problem or situation and look for multiple meanings, rich possibilities. Break it apart and put it back together in a different way. Check out all the angles.

The practice of divergent thinking prepares you to use the process almost automatically in day-to-day situations, such as in solving a difficult problem. Refer to Chapter 11 for a more detailed discussion of creativity in decision making.

---

what it is doing presently, so it does not have to change. In this case, resistance can produce a change in behavior.

On the other hand, resistance is not always beneficial, especially if it persists beyond the planning stage and well into the implementation phase. It can "wear down" supporters and redirect system energy from implementation of the change to dealing with resisters. Morale can suffer.

When handling resistance, the change agent must first be sure that she or he wants to reduce it. Resistance can be used to sharpen decisions, for example, and eventually gain consensus. If it is necessary to minimize it, do not personalize the resistance. Remain rational, stick to the problem-solving change process, and proceed with the following guidelines.

1. Communicate with those who oppose the change. Get to the root of their reasons for opposition.

2. Clarify information and provide accurate feedback.

3. Be open to revisions but clear about what must remain.

4. Present the negative consequences of resistance (threats to organizational survival, compromised client care, etc.).

5. Emphasize the positive consequences of the change and how the individual or group will benefit. However, do not spend too much energy on rational analysis of why the change is good and why the arguments against it do not hold up. People's resistance

frequently flows from feelings that are not rational.

6. Keep resisters involved in face-to-face contact with supporters. Encourage proponents to empathize with opponents, recognize valid objections, and relieve unnecessary fears.

7. Maintain a climate of trust, support, and confidence.

8. Divert attention by creating a different "disturbance." Energy can shift to a "more important" problem inside the system, thereby redirecting resistance. Alternatively, attention can be brought to an external threat to create a "bully phenomenon." When members perceive a greater environmental threat (such as competition or restrictive governmental policies), they tend to unify internally.

9. Follow the "politics of change."

♦ POLITICS OF CHANGE

Energy is needed to change a system. Power is the main source of that energy. Although few nurses use coercive power sources, they do rely on information, expertise, and possibly positional power to persuade others. They should be "politically astute" by using these classic "political" strategies.

1. Analyze the organizational chart. Know the formal lines of authority. Identify informal lines as well (see Chapter 7 on communication).

2. Identify the key persons who will be affected by the change. Pay attention to those immediately above and below the point of change.

3. Find out as much as possible about these key people. What are their "tickle points"? What interests them, gets them excited, turns them off? What is on their personal and organizational agendas? Who typically aligns with whom on important decisions?

4. Begin to build a coalition of support before you start the change process. Identify those key people who will most likely support your idea and those who are most likely to be persuaded easily. Talk informally with them to "flush out" possible objections to your idea and potential opponents. What will the costs and benefits be to them—especially in political terms? Can your idea be modified in ways that retain your objectives but appeal to more key people?

This information helps the change agent develop the most "sellable" idea or at least pinpoint probable resistance. It is a broad beginning to the data collection step of the change process and has to be fine-tuned once the idea is better defined.

The politics of change continue through all the steps of the change process. The astute change agent keeps one ear to the ground at all times to monitor power struggles. All change agents must follow the cardinal rule: Don't try to change too much too fast. But the savvy change agent develops a sense of "exquisite timing" by pacing the change process according to the political pulse. For example, the change agent unfreezes the system during a period of coalition building and high interest, while resistance is low or at least unorganized. The change agent may stall moving the project beyond a pilot stage if resistance solidifies or gains a powerful ally. In this case, the change agent exercises mechanisms to reduce resistance. If resistance continues, she or he may consider two options:

(a) the change is not workable and should be modified to meet the strongest objections (compromise) or (b) the change is fine-tuned sufficiently but change must proceed now and resistance must be overcome. If the last option is selected, energy is focused on overcoming resistance. Supporters are mobilized, and constant, consistent pressure is exerted to move ahead.

How the change agent uses the politics of change depends on whether she or he is an "insider" or "outsider." Someone who is part of the system being changed knows that system, has a stake in the outcome, and is familiar with the people, language, and politics. However, being an insider can restrict one's ability to move freely throughout the system. The agent may be "locked" into certain roles, authority structures, and expectations. Perspective may be limited. An outsider offers a fresh perspective and is independent of internal policies but is unfamiliar with the system, people's values, and personal agendas. Either agent can accomplish change, but she or he must assess and use the politics of change differently.

EXERCISE TO STIMULATE CREATIVE THINKING

Having "vision" is not mysterious. It is hard work. The "discipline of innovation" (Drucker, 1985) involves a deliberate, conscious search for innovative opportunities. Nurses can become innovators. To do so, they cannot cling to the status quo but must nurture the risk takers in their midst. This is not the time to rely solely on logic and pragmatic, careful, small steps toward solutions to the complex problems we face. Nurses cannot continue to do more with less and do it well. They have to do it differently.

SUMMARY

♦ Whether managing in a hospital, health maintenance organization, industry, or community health setting, the nurse manager links together subsystems of an organization to meet organizational objectives. In this role, the nurse must deal with change because it is inherent in an open system.

♦ Inevitable conflicts and stresses occur as the organization strives to adapt and grow in a changing environment.

♦ Whether the nurse manager is managing or initiating change, she or he must have knowledge and skill in the change process within a systems framework. The manager has to analyze the many interrelating factors that influence the system's response to change. If she or he is to "manage" change conceived by top management, the nurse manager may not become involved until the late planning and implementation stages. Nonetheless, the change agent has to understand how to "move" a change plan, how to use and reduce resistance, and how to evaluate outcomes before "stabilizing" the change.

♦ A seven-step process for implementing change includes identification, data collection and analysis, strategy planning, implementation, evaluation, and stabilization.

♦ Nurses will continue to implement change. They can choose to survive it or manage it. The challenge is to expand their influence by initiating change at all levels of the health care system.

◆ Nurses must think creatively and act accordingly. They need to be connected with their colleagues.

◆ The professional association is a forum for the exchange of new ideas and experiences in change. Ideas from disconnected sources can combine, percolate, and produce innovation.

◆ There are many strategies for effectively implementing change.

BIBLIOGRAPHY

American Nurses Association (ANA). (1980). *Nursing: A Social Policy Statement*. Kansas City, MO: ANA.

Bennis, W., Benne, K., and Chinn, R. (editors). (1969). *The Planning of Change*. 2d ed. New York: Holt, Rinehart & Winston.

Chinn, R. (1969). "The Utility of Systems Models and Developmental Models for Practitioners." In: *The Planning of Change*. 2d ed. Bennis, W., Benne, K., and Chinn, R. (editors). New York: Holt, Rinehart & Winston. Pp. 297–312.

Drucker, P. (1974). *Management: Tasks, Responsibilities, Practice*. New York: Harper & Row.

Drucker, P. (1985). "The Discipline of Innovation." *Harvard Business Review*, 63(3)(May–June): 67–72.

Drucker, P. (1985). *Innovations and Entrepreneurship*. New York: Harper & Row.

Haffer, A. (1986). "Facilitating Change: Choosing the Appropriate Strategy." *Journal of Nursing Administration*, 16(4) (April): 18–22.

Havelock, R. (1973). *The Change Agent's Guide to Innovation in Education*. New Jersey: Educational Technology Publications.

Hickman, C., and Silva, M. (1984). *Creating Excellence: Managing Corporate Culture, Strategy and Change in the New Age*. New York: New American Library.

Kanter, R. M. (1983). *The Change Masters: Innovation for Productivity in the American Corporation*. New York: Simon and Schuster.

Kanter, R. M. (1989). *When Giants Learn to Dance*. New York: Simon and Schuster.

Kast, F. E., and Rosenzweig, J. E. (1970). *Organization and Management: A Systems Approach*. New York: McGraw-Hill.

Katz, D., and Kahn, R. (1978). *The Social Psychology of Organizations*. 2d ed. New York: Wiley. Chap. 19.

Lancaster, J., and Lancaster, W. (1982). *The Nurse as Change Agent*. St. Louis, MO: C. V. Mosby.

Lewin, K. (1951). *Field Theory in Social Science*. New York: Harper & Row.

Lippitt, R., Watson, J., and Westley, B. (1958). *The Dynamics of Planned Change*. New York: Harcourt, Brace.

Nutt, P. (1986). "Tactics of Implementation." *Academy of Management Journal*, 29(2): 230–261.

Rogers, E. (1983). *Diffusion of Innovations*. 3d ed. New York: Free Press.

Schermerhorn, J. R., Jr. (1984). *Management for Productivity*. New York: Wiley.

Steele, S., and Maraviglia, F. (1981). *Creativity in Nursing*. Thorofare, NJ: Charles B. Slack.

von Oech, R. (1983). *A Whack on the Side of the Head*. New York: Warner Brothers.

C H A P T E R 21

QUALITY ASSURANCE AND RISK MANAGEMENT

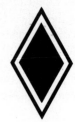

In today's highly competitive health care environment, health care institutions, administrators, physicians, and nurses are accountable for the quality, marketability, and cost of health care. Limited resources of both manpower and dollars make the role of the nurse manager an incredible challenge. Nurse managers' understanding of the concepts of quality assurance will enhance their role in implementing and evaluating standards of care; nurse managers implementing this as part of their role will assist the institution to be marketable as well as competitive.

Nurse managers actively participate in risk management programs. An active role in risk management contributes to the institution by identifying and decreasing potential liability that in effect will ultimately maintain or decrease the cost of health care. A manager active in quality assurance as well as risk management assumes responsibility for the quality of nursing practice, containing costs, and attracting patients to the institution.

The accountability of health care institutions, physicians, and nurses has changed drastically in the past decade. This is due largely to the increased number of successfully litigated claims and the increased dollar amounts awarded in the settlements and to the legislative and judicial decisions that have put responsibility for patient safety on health care providers, both individuals and institutions.

◆ HISTORY OF QUALITY ASSURANCE

The process of systematic evaluation of health care is not new; quality assurance activities date back to Florence Nightingale. She urged that all nursing care being rendered be evaluated. During the Crimean War, Nightingale reported statistics on the mortality of British soldiers in comparison to civilians before and after some of her innovative nursing practices. She reported that the patient outcome mortality rate decreased by 2 percent in a six-month period at one military hospital (Nutting and Dock, 1907). She communicated her findings and received public support. The government interest in health care accountability resulted in the regular evaluation of hospital care; these efforts eventually contributed to similar health care being delivered to soldiers and civilians.

Patient outcomes were also evaluated by the medical profession. Through the studies of Doctor Armory Grove in the early twentieth century, support for a classification system for different diseases was developed along with standards as to when to medically revisit and assess individuals who fell under specific classifications (Bull, 1985).

In the late 1940s and early 1950s, the general public became more aware of organizing, planning, and evaluating methods of health care services. In 1952, the Joint Commission on Accreditation of Hospitals (now the Joint Commission on Accreditation of Healthcare Organizations, or JCAHO) was founded; it provides standards for accreditation. The American Nurses Association (ANA) in 1959 published its *Functions, Standards and Qualifications for Practice,* and the National League for Nursing published *What People Can Expect of a Modern Nursing Service.* All of these efforts helped form professional and public expectations about adequate care.

In the 1960s, the general public was concerned about consumer protection, human rights, and the right to health care. It was then that the federal government started financing health care through the enactment of Medicare and Medicaid. The ANA created a division of nursing practice, which was charged with the responsibility to develop standards for practice. These standards were then to be utilized to develop a quality assurance program. The ANA also developed a schematic model for the quality assurance process. The nursing profession, on its own initiative, assumed that its responsibility was to be accountable to patients for providing, evaluating, and improving patient care, through the utilization of the ANA standards and model.

Several landmark decisions have had their impact on accountability. In a 1965 case, *Darling v. Charleston Community Memorial Hospital,* the Illinois Supreme Court found the hospital liable for the care of a young athlete whose leg was amputated following complications from a fracture.* The court found the hospital negligent in two areas: (a) by the nurses' failure to inform the physician or hospital regarding the onset of complications and (b) by not protecting the patient from incompetence of the physician. Decisions in similar cases have been based on this precedent of corporate responsibility for providing a system to monitor patient care and to correct deficiencies in quality. In addition, hospitals and other not for profit institutions (including schools and churches) lost their charitable immunity through a Supreme Court decision in 1969. Since that time, hospitals have experienced a steady increase in litigation, insurance premiums, and dollar settlements.

Negligence, known as an "unintentional tort" in civil law, is the largest area of malpractice litigation. Health care institutions sustain liability in two categories of negligence: custodial (environmental) and professional (Lanham &

Orlikoff, 1981). *Custodial* negligence refers to environmental conditions that result in falls or other such injuries. Financial loss from custodial negligence is generally low, although the number of claims is high. *Professional* negligence refers to patient injury due to the quality of care given or the absence of care when it was indicated. Both types of negligence are preventable (Dixon et al., 1980).

As a consequence of increasing litigation, malpractice insurance premiums have skyrocketed, pushing institutional costs even higher. Some insurance carriers now require institutions to develop risk management programs as a condition for coverage.

The federal government amended the Social Security Act in 1972 to mandate professional review of health care delivery through the Professional Standards Review Organization (PSRO) which evaluated the quality of existing health care and determined whether the health care offered met professional standards and whether it was provided in an appropriate health care setting. JCAHO, in its initial quality assurance standards, required audits of care delivered.

In 1975, JCAHO increased the number of multidisciplinary audits required and nursing became a major contributor in the evaluation of charts. Currently, JCAHO requires the nursing department to examine a nursing care problem quarterly, document its assessment of the problem, develop and implement a plan for correction, and evaluate the effectiveness of the action taken. Thus, JCAHO requirements acknowledge the nursing profession's earlier efforts for organized quality assurance.

Early in the 1970s, Norma Lang developed the model currently utilized for quality assurance. Instruments for measuring nursing care were developed, but limited data generated from quality assurance studies were published. The

---

*211 N. E. 2d 53, 33 Ill. 2d, 326 (1965), cert. denied 383 U.S. 946, 16 L. Ed. 2d 209, 86 S. Ct. 1204 (1966).

process and outcomes instruments developed included Slater's Rating Scale of Nursing Competence, which measures the competence of the nurses; the Quality Patient Care Scale (Qual-Pacs), which measures the quality of nursing care concurrently; and the Medicus tool, which evaluates structure, process, and outcome components of nursing care, with the emphasis being on process. On January 1, 1977, Florida became the first state with a law requiring hospitals, regardless of size or type, to have a program designed to reduce risks, including an incident review committee (Federation of American Hospitals manual, 1977). Then, on January 1, 1980, the Joint Commission on Accreditation of Healthcare Organizations' requirements for risk management and quality assurance went into effect.

During the early 1980s, JCAHO revised their standard for evaluating nursing care by stating that care needed to be evaluated objectively against pre-established standards and criteria. They further stated that results needed to be analyzed to determine the problem areas in nursing practice and a plan had to be developed to correct practice deficiencies. A method to reevaluate the effectiveness of the corrective action was also necessary. Again, in 1990, JCAHO revisited the nursing standards and reconfirmed the idea that nursing develop and evaluate standards of nursing practice.

A risk-free health care setting is impossible. Systematic action to reduce risks, however, is not only possible but essential. A risk management program must be established because the disturbing trends that have given rise to the hospital liability problem will persist and probably worsen. Rising insurance premiums, record settlements, rising patient expectations, less reluctance on the part of patients and their families to sue faceless institutions and rarely seen specialists, and more pressure for quality assurance are forces that are not going to go away.

As the cost of health care has escalated and as the federal government has become increasingly involved in paying for health care, there is increased pressure to ensure that services rendered are necessary and that services provided meet nationally recognized standards of care. Further, both the federal government and other third-party payers (insurance carriers) are insisting that services be provided at the lowest possible cost. This is a change from prior times when any services needed were provided without much concern about the cost—the government or insurance company would pay after the cost had been incurred. Today, the prospective payment system demands that costs be contained within the DRG allotment and thus, quality, cost-effective care becomes essential.

Controlling costs is discussed in Chapter 5 on productivity and in Chapter 19 on budgeting and resource allocation. This chapter focuses on assuring quality and managing risk.

◆ QUALITY ASSURANCE

Accountability is operationalized by what is known in health care as quality assurance. *Quality assurance* describes all activities related to establishing, maintaining, and assuring high-quality care for patients. It includes assessment of patient care and correction of problems identified.

Quality assurance can be voluntary or mandatory. Nursing practice that conforms to the ANA *Standards of Nursing Practice* is a voluntary form of quality assurance. When the institution meets the state board of health requirements, quality assurance is mandatory. (Theoretically, it is voluntary for institutions to meet the JCAHO standards for accreditation, but without accreditation they will not be reimbursed by third-party payers [Medicare, insurance carriers].)

Quality assurance is the method by which performance of care is evaluated for effectiveness. Standards for appropriate care are established and provide the basis upon which potential risk can be assessed. Then, measures taken to reduce that risk are begun. Quality assurance is the foundation of any risk management program.

QUALITY ASSURANCE PROCESS

Quality assurance is the systematic process of evaluating the quality of care given in a particular unit or institution. It involves setting standards, determining criteria to meet those standards, data collection, evaluating how well the criteria have been met, making plans for change based on the evaluation, and following up on implementation for change.

SETTING STANDARDS. The nursing profession itself has designated generic standards of nursing practice (the American Nurses Association *Standards of Nursing Practice*). In addition to these general standards, each institution and each patient care unit must designate standards that are specific to the patient population served. These standards are the foundation upon which all other measures of quality assurance are based. An example of a standard is: Every patient will have a written care plan.

DETERMINING CRITERIA. After standards of performance are established, criteria must be determined that will indicate if the standards are being met and to what degree they are met. Just as with standards of care, criteria must be general as well as specific to the individual unit. One criterion to demonstrate that the standards regarding care plans for every patient are being met would be: A nursing care plan is developed and written by a registered nurse within 12 hours of admission. This criterion, then, provides a *measurable* indicator to evaluate performance.

DATA COLLECTION. The actual collection of data is the third step in quality assurance. Sufficient observations and random samples are necessary for producing reliable and valid information. A useful rule is that 10 percent of the institutional patient population per month should be sampled. The devised tool to collect data should leave as little room for interpretation by the data collector as possible. Data collectors need to be taught the purpose of quality assurance along with the principles of data collection. Furthermore, research shows that consistent performance in collecting data over an extended period is difficult, so all collectors' data should be compared regularly to determine continuing reliability.

Data collection methods include patient observations and interviews, nurse observations and interviews, and review of charts. Flow sheets and kardexes are also resources from which to assemble information about past and present conditions.

A policy should outline guidelines of the reporting of quality assurance data so it is clear who in the organization needs to receive quality assurance information. The policy also should state at what level in the organization the analysis of the different criteria is to take place, to whom these analyses and recommendations are to be reported, who is responsible for implementing the recommendations, and who is responsible for follow-up. Unless definite policies are established, the system may fail and changes in nursing practice are not likely to occur.

EVALUATING PERFORMANCE. Several methods can be used to evaluate performance. These include reviewing documented records, observing activities as they take place, examining patients, and interviewing patients, families, and staff. Records are the most commonly used source for evaluation because of the relative ease of their use, but they are not as reliable as direct observations. It is quite possible to write in the patient's chart activities that were not done or to not record those things that were done. Further, the chart only indicates that care was provided; it does not demonstrate the quality of that care. In the previous example, records would be examined to determine if care plans were written on each patient within 12 hours of admission and, if so, that standards had been met. Other criteria would be used to measure the quality of the care plan, such as, "Every care plan will include patient education appropriate to the patient's medical diagnosis, nursing diagnosis, interventions planned, and discharge planning." Then, the care plan would be checked to see if it contained these components.

MAKING PLANS FOR CHANGE. Since no performance standards can be met perfectly at all times, quality assurance planning must include methods for correcting deficits. First, the unit and/or institution must determine how much deviation from the standard is acceptable before changes are made. If 45 out of 50 patients admitted have a care plan recorded within 12 hours of admission and the other 5 have recorded care plans within the next 6 hours, is this deviation acceptable? If not, then how should this be corrected? Is the unit short-staffed? Have there been an unusually large number of admis-

sions recently? Are a number of new graduates being oriented on the unit? Plans for correcting deficiencies in performance are the responsibility of the nurse manager and, after collecting all pertinent information about possible causes, the nurse manager should consult with staff and/or the supervisor and make plans for correcting the performance deficit.

FOLLOW-UP. Following up on how effective changes have been in improving performance is the final, but very necessary, step in the quality assurance process. Many times, quality assurance programs fall short of doing what it is they are designed to do—assure quality of care—because they only record performance and plan to improve it. If, in the example described, the nurse manager found that the next 50 patients had care plans recorded within 12 hours, then the performance had improved relative to that standard. If it had not improved, then another approach would need to be taken or, possibly, the criterion should be evaluated for appropriateness for that unit.

MONITORING NURSING CARE

In addition to the individual patient care activities described, another component of quality assurance is the ongoing monitoring of nursing care. Several methods are used to monitor nursing care. These include the nursing audit, peer review, utilization review, and patient satisfaction.

NURSING AUDIT. A nursing audit can be retrospective or concurrent. A *retrospective* audit is conducted after a patient's discharge and involves examining records of a large number of cases. The patient's entire course of care is evaluated and comparisons made across cases. Recommendations for change can be made from the perspective of many patients with similar care problems and with the spectrum of care considered.

A *concurrent* audit is conducted during the patient's course of care; it examines the care being given to achieve a desirable outcome in the patient's health and evaluates the nursing care activities being provided. Changes can be made if they are indicated by patient outcomes.

PEER REVIEW. Peer review occurs when practicing nurses determine the standards and criteria that indicate quality care and then assess performance against these. In this case, nurses are the "experts" at knowing what the indicators of quality care are and when such care has been provided. Their expertise is especially useful in complicated cases; sometimes more than one expert's opinion is used for comparisons.

UTILIZATION REVIEW. Utilization reviews are based on the appropriate allocation of resources and are mandated by the JCAHO. Such a review is not specifically directed toward nursing care, but it may provide information on nursing practices that will require further investigation.

PATIENT SATISFACTION. Most institutions have a method to determine patients' satisfaction with their care. The usual method is a questionnaire the patient is asked to fill out either before leaving the institution or after returning home. Although patient satisfaction is very important, standards of professional care are often not indicated due to the fact that the consumer's knowledge of expert care is limited. However, the patient is quite aware of receiving care in a timely fashion and of the many variables in the environment that contribute to recovery. Patient satisfaction should be used as one of several indicators of quality.

Once standards have been set, criteria established, and methods for evaluating adherence to the standards determined, the institution is prepared to examine its risk in relation to its accountability. Risk management programs in health care institutions involve two important areas: patient and/or family incident review, and employee and visitor safety. Since nursing is involved most with patient care, this chapter emphasizes a risk management incident program for patients, their families, or both.

◆ A RISK MANAGEMENT PROGRAM

Risk management follows the current trend of adapting business strategies to institution management; it is the institutional parallel to product liability prevention in industry. Risk management is a planned program of loss prevention and liability control. Its purpose is to identify, analyze, and evaluate risks, followed by a plan for reducing the frequency and severity of accidents and injuries. Risk management is a continuous daily program of detection, education, and intervention.

Risk management calls for a team approach involving all departments of the institution. It must be an institution-wide program with board of directors' approval and input from medicine, nursing, and other professional departments. Input from medicine and nursing is received through several mechanisms: annually, through review by the medical quality assurance committee or the policy procedure committee, and through the review by the medical and nursing administrative staff. The program must have high-level commitment, including that of the chief executive officer and the director of nursing service.

A risk management program includes the following activities.

1. *Identifying* potential risks for accident, injury, or financial loss. Formal and informal communication with all institutional departments and inspection of facilities are essential to identifying problem areas.

2. *Reviewing* present institution-wide monitoring systems (incident reports, audits, committee minutes, oral complaints, patient questionnaires), evaluating completeness, and determining additional systems needed to provide the factual data essential for risk management control.

3. *Analyzing* the frequency, severity, and causes of general categories and specific types of incidents causing injury or adverse outcomes to patients. To plan risk intervention strategies, estimating the possible loss associated with the various types of incidents is needed.

4. *Reviewing and appraising* safety and risk aspects of patient care procedures and new programs.

5. *Monitoring* laws and codes related to patient safety, consent, and care.

6. *Eliminating or reducing* risks as much as possible.

7. *Reviewing* the work of other committees to determine potential liability and recommend prevention or corrective action. Examples of such committees are infection, medical audit, safety/security, pharmacy, nursing audit, and productivity. In many institutions the quality assurance and risk management committees and programs have been combined.

8. *Identifying* needs for patient, family, and personnel education suggested by all of the foregoing and implementing the appropriate educational program.

9. *Evaluating* the results of a risk management program.

10. *Providing* periodic reports to administration, medical staff, and the board of directors.

The establishment of a risk management program starts at the top. The institution's board of directors directs the administrator to establish the program and commits the necessary resources. The administrator then appoints a risk management committee, whose members are responsible for the overall planning and decision making that are involved in risk management. However, for effective implementation, a risk manager should be appointed to manage the day-to-day operation of the program.

Membership on the risk management committee should be interdisciplinary, with representatives from medicine, nursing, medical records, legal counsel, education, and insurance claims. Typical members of a risk management committee would be:

1. A risk manager

2. Nursing representatives
   Nursing service administrator
   Nurse manager representative
   Staff nurse representative

3. Medical staff representatives

4. Related committee chairs
   Quality assurance
   Utilization review
   Infection control
   Pharmacy and therapeutics
   Operating room

5. Patient accounts representative

6. Legal counsel (ex-officio)

7. Others by invitation
   Education and training coordinator
   Insurance claims representative

The chair can be any member of the committee. Typically, the chair is a member of administration or the risk manager. The committee's purpose is to develop and promote appropriate measures to minimize risk to patients and institutional personnel and to carry out the risk management activities listed above. The committee develops risk management policies and guidelines for handling critical incidents. It establishes programs for increasing staff awareness, detection, education, and proper reporting of risk potential and incidents.

THE RISK MANAGER

The risk manager administers the program and serves as the liaison between administration, the risk management committee, and other related committees and departments. This person usually also serves as the liaison between insurance company representatives, institution attorneys, and others. The risk manager should report to the chief administrator and should have a clearly defined role in the organizational structure of the institution.

There is no typical profile for risk managers. They come from a variety of backgrounds, including administration, law, nursing, former quality assurance coordinators, and former claims representatives from insurance companies. They need effective communicative skills, evaluative skills (such as those learned in research methodology), should be able to develop positive interpersonal relationships, and must exhibit leadership and team-building skills.

The responsibilities of the risk manager include, but are not limited to, the following.

1. Schedules meetings and prepares agenda for risk management committee (if risk manager is the chair; if not, helps with agenda).

2. Reviews incident reports daily; investigates as needed; takes action or refers to appropriate physician, nurse manager, or committee; follows up with patient and family as appropriate.

3. Monitors data collection mechanisms such as incident report summaries.

4. Visits periodically the patients and their families who are at high risk, since individual concern for patients is the single most effective way to reduce litigiousness. High risk patients include those on long-term care or ones with repeated admissions, transfers from intensive care to general units and vice versa, night emergency room admissions, and postoperative patients.

5. Summarizes litigation on a periodic basis, including dollar outcome.

6. Prepares monthly incident report summary.

7. Develops, with help of risk management committee members, staff education programs.

The risk management organizational model shown in Figure 21–1 illustrates the relationship among units in a risk management program.

◆ NURSING'S ROLE IN RISK MANAGEMENT

In the institutional setting, nursing is the one department involved in patient care 24 hours a day; nursing personnel are critical to the success of a risk management program. The chief nursing administrator must be committed to the program. His or her attitude will influence the staff and their participation. After all, it is the staff, with their daily patient contact, who actually implement a risk management program.

High risk areas in hospitals fall into five general categories: (a) medication errors, (b) complications from diagnostic or treatment procedures, (c) falls, (d) patient or family dissatisfaction with care, and (e) refusal of treatment or to sign consent for treatment. Nursing is involved in all areas, but the medical staff may be primarily responsible in cases involving refusal of treatment or of consent to treatment.

Medical records and incident reports serve to document institutional, nurse, and physician accountability. However, it has been estimated that for every reported incident, 35 are unreported. If records are faulty, inadequate, or omitted, the institution is more likely to be sued and more likely to lose (Dixon et al., 1980). Incident reports are used to analyze the severity, frequency, and causes of incidents within the five risk categories. Such analysis serves as a basis for intervention.

INCIDENT REPORTS

Accurate and comprehensive reporting on both the patient's chart and in the incident report is essential to protect the institution and the care givers from litigation. Incident reporting is most often the nurse's responsibility. Reluctance to

FIGURE 21-1 RISK MANAGEMENT ORGANIZATIONAL MODEL

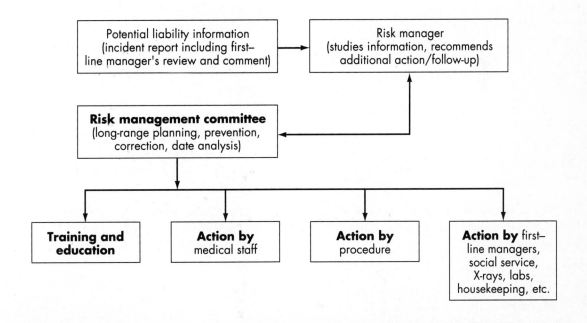

report incidents is usually due to fear of the consequences. This can be alleviated by two techniques: (a) staff education programs that emphasize objective reporting, omitting inflammatory words and judgmental statements; and (b) a clear understanding that the purpose of the incident reporting process is for documentation and follow-up and that the report will not be used, under any circumstances, for disciplinary action.

A reportable incident should include any unexpected or unplanned occurrence that affects or could potentially affect a patient or family member. The report is only as effective as the form on which it is reported, so attention should be paid to the adequacy of the form as well as to the data it calls for (Duran, 1980). Figure 21–2 is a sample incident report form.

The suggested process of reporting incidents involves the following steps.

1. *Discovery.* Physicians, nurses, patients, families, or any institutional employee or volunteer may report actual or potential risk.

2. *Notification.* The risk manager receives the completed incident form within *24 hours* after the incident. A telephone call may be made earlier, to hasten follow-up in the event of a major incident.

3. *Investigation.* The risk manager or representative investigates the incident immediately.

4. *Consultation.* The manager consults with physician, risk management committee member, or both.

5. *Action.* The manager should clarify any misinformation to the patient or family, explaining exactly what happened. The patient should be referred to the appropriate source

for help and for compensation for any needed service; the latter should be offered, if indicated.

6. *Record.* The manager should be sure that all records, including incident reports, follow-up, and action taken, if any, are filed in a central depository.

SOME EXAMPLES

The following are some examples of actual events in the various risk categories.

Medication errors, including administration of intravenous fluids. It is a reportable incident when a medication or fluid is omitted, given to the wrong patient, given at the wrong time or in the wrong dosage, or given by the wrong route. Administration of the wrong medication or fluid is also reportable.

Patient A. Weight was transcribed wrong from emergency room sheet. Medication dose was calculated on incorrect weight; therefore, patient was given double the dose required. Error discovered after first dose and corrected. Second dose omitted.

Patient B. Tegretol dosage written in Medex as "Tegretol 100 mg chewable tab— 50 mg p.o. B.I.D." Tegretol 100 mg given p.o. at 1400. Meds checked at 1430 and error noted. 50 mg Tegretol should have been given. Doctor notified. Second dose held.

Patient C. During rounds at 3:30 P.M. found D/5/ISO/M hanging. Order was D/5W. Fluids last checked at 2:00 P.M. Changed to correct fluid. Doctor notified.

Diagnostic procedure. Any incident occurring before, during, or after such procedures as blood sample stick, biopsy, X-ray, lumbar punc-

FIGURE 21-2 INCIDENT REPORT FORM

PATIENT INCIDENT REPORT

NUMBER **00520**

PATIENT

PATIENT NAME					
ADDRESS					
HOSPITAL NO.	ROOM NO.	HOME PHONE NO.	AGE	SEX ☐M ☐F	DATE ADMITTED

REASON FOR HOSPITALIZATION ▶

ATTENDING PHYSICIAN   CHARGE/ PRIMARY NURSE ▶

LIST MEDICATIONS WITHIN LAST 6 HOURS, IF PERTINENT: ▶

INCIDENT FACTS

ACTIVITY ORDERS	ADJUSTABLE BED HEIGHT	BEDRAILS	TYPE OF INCIDENT	
☐ RESTRAINTS	☐YES ☐ NO	☐ UP	☐ MEDICATION	☐ PATIENT MOVEMENT
☐ BEDREST	POSITION	☐ DOWN	☐ DIAGNOSTIC PROCEDURE	☐ PATIENT/PARENT ATTITUDE
☐ UP c̄ ASSISTANCE	☐HIGH ☐ LOW	☐ NONE	☐ PATIENT TREATMENT	☐ MEDICO-LEGAL
☐ UP s̄ ASSISTANCE				

EXACT LOCATION OF INCIDENT: ▶

	DATE	TIME	SHIFT	☐ DAY ☐ EVE ☐NIGHT

DESCRIPTION BY PERSON PREPARING REPORT ▶
(use separate sheet if necessary)

NAME OF PERSONS PRESENT AT TIME OF INCIDENT (include employees)   ADDRESS   PHONE

MEDICAL

WAS PERSON INVOLVED EXAMINED BY A PHYSICIAN IN HOSPITAL?	☐ YES ☐ NO	DATE	TIME	WHERE

EXAMINING PHYSICIAN'S NAME ▶   ANY APPARENT INJURY ☐ YES ☐ NO   X-RAY ORDERED ☐ YES ☐NO

SIGNATURE OF PERSON PREPARING REPORT **X**   TITLE   DATE

IMMEDIATE FOLLOW-UP ▶

FOLLOW-UP AT DISCHARGE ▶
(if pertinent)

X

(Signature)   PATIENT CARE MANAGER

Form No. 1036 Rev. 2/80

A form used by St. Louis Children's Hospital, Missouri. Used by permission.

ture, or other invasive procedure is categorized as a diagnostic procedure incident.

Patient A. When I checked the IV site, I saw that it was red and swollen. For this reason, I discontinued the IV. When removing the tape, a small area of skin breakdown was noted where tape had been. There was also a small knot on the medial aspect of the left antecubital above the IV insertion site. Doctor notified. Wound dressed.

Patient B. When I was turning Mrs. Jones, she complained of a burning sensation. A rash was noted over both buttocks. Pad under patient heavily saturated. Changed bed linen and powder applied to patient's buttocks.

Medical-legal incident. If a patient or family refuses treatment as ordered and prescribed or refuses to sign consents, the situation is categorized as a medical-legal incident.

Patient A. After a visit from a member of the clergy, patient indicated he was no longer in need of medical attention and asked to be discharged. Physician called. Doctor explained potential side effects if treatment were discontinued. Patient continued to ask for discharge. Doctor explained "against medical advice" (A.M.A.) form. Patient signed A.M.A. form and left at 1300 without medications.

Patient B. Patient refused to sign consent for bone marrow. States side effects not understood. Doctor reviewed reasons for test and side effects three different times. Doctor informed the patient that without consent he could not perform the test. Offered to call in another physician for second opinion. Patient agreed. After doctor left, patient signed

consent, still indicating lack of understanding of the side effects.

Patient or family attitude toward care. When a patient or family indicate general dissatisfaction with care and the situation cannot be or has not been resolved, then an incident report is filed.

Patient A. Mother complained that she had found child saturated with urine every morning she arrived (around 0800). Explained to mother that diapers and linen are changed at 0600 when 0600 feedings and meds are given. Patient's back, buttocks, and perineal areas are free of skin breakdown. Parents continue to be distressed. Discussed with primary nurse.

Patient B. Mr. Smith obviously very angry. Greeted me at the door complaining that his wife had not been treated properly in our emergency room the night before. Waited to speak to someone from administration. Was unable to reach the administrator on call. Suggested Mr. Smith call administrator in the morning. Mr. Smith thanked me for my time and assured me that he would call the administrator the next day.

◆ ROLE OF THE NURSE MANAGER

A risk management system allows the institution to act on the root causes of liability claims. It identifies individuals, areas, and procedures that are deficient. It spots communication failures immediately and allows the institution to remedy a breakdown before an angry patient or family files a claim. The nurse manager plays the key role in the success of any risk management program.

A patient incident or a patient's or family's expression of dissatisfaction regarding care not only indicates some slippage in quality of care, it also indicates potential liability. A distraught, dissatisfied, complaining patient is a high risk; a satisfied patient or family is a low risk. A risk management or liability control program should therefore emphasize a personal approach. Many claims are filed because of a breakdown in communication between the health care provider and the patient. In many instances, after an incident or bad outcome, a quick, simple visit or call from an institution representative to the patient or family can soothe tempers and clarify misinformation.

For instance, Stephanie's parents wrote a letter indicating that they discovered a needle sticking out of their child's foot about four days after discharge. The nurse manager called the mother to discuss Stephanie's present condition and follow-up. The mother informed her that Stephanie was fine and expressed pleasant surprise about the follow-up call. Although the nurse manager asked the mother to send her the piece of needle and (after consultation with administration) offered to make an appointment for Stephanie to be seen at no charge, she never heard from the mother again. A subsequent letter from the mother thanked the nurse manager for "caring."

David received an overdose of preoperative medication. The child suffered some ill effects and his surgery was cancelled and rescheduled for a later date. The nurse manager discussed with the parents what had happened and committed a staff member to observe the child closely until there was absolutely no possibility of his being in any danger. Several weeks later

the family wrote a letter thanking the nursing staff for the care and special attention.

In both situations, prompt attention and care by the head nurse protected the patients involved and may have averted a potential liability claim. The important factors in these successful endings are obvious: recognition of the incident, quick follow-up and action, personal contact, and immediate restitution (where appropriate). It is estimated that 90 percent of patients' concerns can and should be handled at the unit level. When that first line of communication breaks down, however, the first-line manager needs a resource—usually the risk manager or nursing service administrator.

KEY BEHAVIORS

Handling a patient's or family member's complaints stemming from an incident can be very difficult. These confrontations are often highly emotional, and the patient or family member must be calmed down, yet satisfied. Sometimes just an opportunity to release the anger or emotion is all that is needed. Figure 21–3 shows a set of key behaviors that may be used to defuse a complaint from a patient or family member.

The first three key behaviors have to do with *listening* to the person to defuse the situation. Arguing or interrupting only increases the person's anger or emotion. After the patient or family member has had his or her say, then an attempt can be made to solve the problem by asking what is expected in the form of a solution. The nurse manager or other institution representative should then explain what can and cannot be done and try to negotiate with the injured party an agreement on a solution. It is important to be specific. Vague resolutions of problems may only lead to more problems later on if expectations for solution and time-table differ.

The nurse manager must also be sure that all incidents are properly documented. The documentation on the incident form should be detailed, including all the factors relating to the incident as demonstrated in the previous examples. The documentation in the chart, however, should be only a statement of the *facts* and of the patient's physical response; no reference to the incident report or words like *error* or *inappropriate* should be used. When a patient receives 100 mg of Demerol instead of 50 mg as ordered, the proper documentation in the chart is, "100 mg of Demerol administered. Physician notified." The remainder of the documentation should include any reaction of the patient to the dosage such as "Patient's vital signs unchanged." If there is an untoward reaction, a

---

FIGURE 21-3 KEY BEHAVIORS FOR HANDLING COMPLAINTS

♦ Listen openly.

♦ Do not speak until the person has had his or her say.

♦ Avoid reacting emotionally (don't get defensive).

♦ Ask for his or her expectations about a solution to the problem.

♦ Explain what you can and cannot do to solve the problem (if appropriate).

♦ Agree on specific steps to be taken and specific deadlines.

Adapted from P.J. Decker, *Health Care Management Microtraining* (St. Louis, MO: Decker & Associates, 1982). Used by permission.

---

follow-up note should be written in the chart, giving an update of the patient's status. A note related to the patient's reaction should be written as frequently as the status changes and should continue until the patient returns to his or her previous status.

DOCUMENTATION

Documentation in the incident report form, however, should indicate all factors related to the incident. There are sections in Figure 21–2, for instance, asking for "immediate follow-up" and "follow-up at discharge." These sections are ordinarily completed by the nurse manager. Thus, in the case of the patient with tissue change around the IV site, the nurse manager's immediate follow-up included notifying the physician and caring for the skin around the IV. At the time of the patient's discharge, the entry in the "follow-up at discharge" space read as follows: "The space around the IV site is healing well. Mother given appointment to follow-up clinic in seven days to check site and healing process. Will report status at that time and continue follow-up as needed."

The chart must never be used as a tool for disciplinary comments or action or expressions of anger. Notes such as, "Incident would never have occurred if Doctor X had written the correct order in the first place," or, "This carelessness is inexcusable," are totally inappropriate and serve no meaningful purpose. Carelessness and incorrect orders do indeed cause errors and incidents, but the place to address and resolve these issues is in the risk management committee or in the nurse manager's office, not the patient chart.

A CARING ATTITUDE

It is also the nurse manager who sets the tone on the unit that contributes to a safe and low risk environment. Situations that contribute to patient incidents and eventually legal problems are mistrust, misinformation, guilt (and thus the need to blame others), confusion, conflicting stories, and, ultimately, gross negligence. Except for gross negligence, the most common cause for legal action is an unfriendly, uncaring attitude on the part of institution staff.

Compare the very different outcomes for two similar, actual incidents. The report on *Patient A* read: "Upon the patient's return from X-ray, it was noted that the skin around the IV site was very puffy from obvious leaking of dye into the tissue. After three days the skin sloughed." A note by the physician in the chart at discharge indicated that the patient would require plastic surgery in the future. No incident report was filed, however, nor was there any indication of any discussion with the patient. Six weeks after the patient's discharge the hospital received a letter from an attorney, indicating that an intent to sue had been initiated by the patient.

The report on *Patient B* was similar, to begin with: "IV infiltration in X-ray." In this case, however, an incident report was filed as soon as the patient returned from X-ray and it was noted that the dye had infused into the tissue. The nurse manager requested on the incident report that it be returned to her for follow-up. The risk manager was notified and returned the incident report to the nurse manager. The two of them then discussed going to the patient, along with the physician, to discuss the possibility of a slough and, if indicated, to provide the patient with appropriate referral and treatment. The nurse manager, the risk manager, and the physician did discuss the situation with the patient. Three days after the infusion, there was an indication of skin sloughing and the physician determined that plastic surgery might be required in the future. Arrangements for future treatment

were made with the patient. The family took no legal action.

Analysis of these two incidents strongly suggests that it was the nurse manager's quick and appropriate action in the second case that made the difference in outcome. If an unfriendly, uncaring attitude is the cause of most legal suits, what are the implications for the nurse manager? Take the example of the mother who was distressed about her baby's condition each morning she arrived. If no personal response or follow-up had been made and the patient's treatment had not met the mother's expectations, her first reaction might have been, "This is another example of careless, sloppy care." But, when the situation is handled with personal follow-up, an opposite reaction can be expected. When the mother complained about the child's care, the staff nurse and the nurse manager, rather than being defensive, discussed the complaint and established a plan of action, including explanation of the nurse's routine, checking the baby immediately, and correcting the situation. Most important, the nurse changed the routine to accommodate the mother's concern.

When the man complained to the nurse manager that he did not think his wife had received appropriate care during the night, the nurse manager might very well have said, "That's not my problem. I didn't work last night." Instead, the manager indicated with whom he should discuss his problem and gave him that person's phone number. If the nurse had simply disclaimed responsibility, it would have added fuel to the man's anger, but, when his concerns were listened to and he was given an appropriate referral, his anger was dissipated.

The nurse manager might also be involved in other activities of the risk management program, such as determining staff educational needs and participating in programs designed to meet those needs, or in establishing protocols for classifying patients at risk—for example, for falls. Whatever activity is pursued in a risk management program, the nurse manager's participation is critical to its success.

◆ EVALUATION OF RISK MANAGEMENT

Identifying and reducing risks involves close monitoring and analysis of incident reports. Incident reports that include statements of blame should be discussed. A risk management program needs support and participation from all staff. To elicit their commitment, the use of incident reports must be limited to risk reduction only. This policy must be emphasized and practiced.

A risk management program requires resources and, in times of budget reductions, it may be one of the first to be cut. However, risk management is directed toward reducing losses; it is a case of spending money to save it. Return on the investment takes time, however, and it is difficult to estimate what might have been lost. Comparison with past data is of course one way, but that is based on the premise that future loss can be assumed from past loss figures. Over time, a risk management program can be cost-effective as well as provide a safer environment for patients.

An additional benefit of a risk management program may be an increase in positive attitudes toward the institution on the part of both employees and the community. When implemented in a spirit of concern and responsibility, a risk management program can be a visible means of responding to patient needs. Institutions, physicians, and nurses have had their share of negative press in the past—sometimes with good reason. The courts, insurance carriers, and legislative action have mandated that institutions respond to patient demands. Risk management meets this obligation.

Risk management makes sense. It improves the quality of patient care and reduces liability claims. It represents the outstanding characteristic of health care professionals: care and concern for people. It provides the best care possible at the most reasonable cost.

SUMMARY

◆ Accountability in health care institutions has prompted the recent development of quality assurance and risk management programs.

◆ Quality assurance is the method by which performance of care is evaluated for effectiveness.

◆ A quality assurance program is the basis for managing risk.

◆ The key ingredients in a successful patient risk management program are an organized program of incident reporting; review and follow-up; a risk management program, including a risk manager and committee with well-defined objectives; nurse managers who support the risk management program; and, most important, a friendly, caring environment as perceived by the patient and his or her family.

◆ Steps in reporting incidents have been described, as well as suggested behaviors in handling a dissatisfied or angry patient and family. Differences between documenting on the incident form and the patient's chart were discussed.

♦ Risk management is a recent development and the literature is just beginning to be available. Suggested reading in this area appears in the bibliography.

BIBLIOGRAPHY

American Nurses' Association. (1973). *Standards of Nursing Practice.* Kansas City, MO: American Nurses' Association.

Brooten, D. A., Hayman, L., and Naylors, M. D. (1978). *Leadership for Change: A Guide for the Frustrated Nurse.* Philadelphia: J. B. Lippincott.

Brown, B. L., Jr. (1979). *Risk Management for Hospitals: A Practical Approach.* Gaithersburg, MD: Aspen Publishing.

Bull, M. (1985). "Quality Assurance: Its Origins, Transformation and Prospects." In: *Quality Assurance.* Meisenheimer, C. G. (editor). Rockville, MD: Aspen Publishing. P. 3.

Decker, C. M. (1985). "Quality Assurance: Accent on Monitoring." *Nursing Management,* 16(11): 20–24.

Dixon, N. E., et al. (1980). *Quality, Trending and Management for the 80's: A Hospital-Wide Quality Assurance Program.* Chicago: American Hospital Association.

Duran, G. S. (1980). "On the Scene: Risk Management in Health Care." *Nursing Administration Quarterly,* 5: 19.

Federation of American Hospitals. (1977). "FAH Manual Outlines Control Programs on Risk Management for Hospital Use." *Review,* 10: 17.

Kraus, G. P. (1986). *Health Care Risk Management: Organization and Claims Administration.* Owings Mills, MD: National Health Publications.

Lanham, G. B., and Orlikoff, J. E. (1981). "Full Coverage of Issues Reflects Importance of Risk Management." *Hospitals,* 55: 165.

Monahan, M. L. (1987). "Quality Assurance and Nursing." In: *Medical Surgical Nursing: Concepts and Clinical Practice.* Phipps, W., Long, B., and Woods, N. (editors). St. Louis, MO: C. V. Mosby. Pp. 113–123.

Nutting, M. A., and Dock, L. L. (1907). *A History of Nursing.* New York: Putnam. P. 142.

Poteet, G. W. (1983). "Risk Management and Nursing." *Nursing Clinics of North America,* 18(3): 457–465.

Ulrich, B., Fredin, N., and Cavouras, C. A. (1986). "Assuring Quality through a Professional Practice Approach." *Nursing Economics,* 4(6): 277–287.

C H A P T E R   22

DEALING WITH CONFLICT

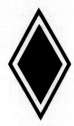

Conflict is present in all aspects of life and in all organizations due to the complexity of organizational relationships, the interactions among the members of the organization, and their dependence on one another. The presence of conflict does not necessarily mean a negative process is occurring. Conflict is neutral, but the results of conflict can be constructive or destructive. Poorly managed conflict can create distance and distrust among employees in an organization and lead to lowered productivity. Well-managed conflict can stimulate competition, identify legitimate differences within organizations, and serve as a powerful motivator.

This chapter discusses the phenomenon known as conflict and presents a model of conflict and various conflict resolution techniques that are applicable to nursing. It is important for nurse managers to understand this process, the conditions that lead to conflict, and the means to resolve conflict for their units to perform effectively.

♦ IMPORTANCE OF CONFLICT

Dealing with conflict has become increasingly important to administrators in health care institutions. This is in part due to the increasing complexity of delivering health care, the rising expectations of those delivering and receiving health care, the changing role of nurses, increased competition among health care institutions, pressure from Medicare, increased government regulations, and the threats posed by legal action.

Conflict is viewed as not only inevitable but as a natural condition and necessary if people and organizations are to change. Conflict is both functional and dysfunctional to individuals and organizations. Some of the positive and negative aspects of conflict are noted below.

POSITIVE ASPECTS OF CONFLICT

Even though conflict is inevitable in organizations, it does not have to be destructive. There can be many positive consequences of conflict. For one, it provides heightened sensitivity to problems. Conflict can serve as a stimulus in developing new facts or solutions; when there is disagreement about the choice of a solution to a problem, a novel solution is often discovered. Some conflict in organizations can be useful in that it can help deal with the cost versus benefit issue facing every organization. For example, disagreements over patient care can cause the parties in conflict to become more aware of the tradeoffs, especially costs versus benefits, of a particular service or technique. Conflict helps people recognize legitimate differences within an organization or profession and serves as a powerful motivator. In fact, conflict over the past 25 years has led to a number of positive changes both for nursing and the status of women (Brooten, Hayman & Naylors, 1978: 18).

NEGATIVE ASPECTS OF CONFLICT

Conflict can result in the conflict's being suppressed, which does not resolve the conflict and may cause severe consequences in the future. Conflict often leads to aggressive behavior on the part of those individuals or groups in conflict. Groups placed in "win-lose" competition have the tendency to increase the in-group/out-group bias between them (Sherif & Sherif, 1961) and to increase the evaluation of their own group while decreasing their evaluation of the other group. The groups become more cohesive and task oriented while in conflict. Communication between the groups decreases and each group views the other as an enemy, therefore making it very difficult for the groups to work together in the future.

♦ WHAT IS CONFLICT?

Conflict can be viewed from both a behavioral and a process standpoint. From a *behavioral standpoint* conflict is defined as "a perceived condition that exists between parties (e.g., individuals, groups, departments) in which one or more of the parties perceive (a) goal incompatibility and (b) some opportunity for interfering with the goal accomplishment of others" (Albanese, 1981: 458). From a *process standpoint* conflict can be defined as what occurs when real or perceived differences exist in the goals, values, ideas, attitudes, beliefs, feelings, or actions of two or more parties (individuals or groups). Conflict exists when two or more mutually exclusive goals, values, ideas, attitudes, beliefs, feelings or actions occur:

1. Within one individual (intrapersonal)

2. Between two or more individuals (interpersonal)

3. Within one group (intragroup)

4. Between two or more groups (intergroup)

♦ COMPETITION VS. CONFLICT

Conflict is not the same as competition. Competition has some of the elements of conflict in that goal attainment by one unit prevents the other unit from achieving its goals, but competition follows basic rules and is not typically associated with anger and hostility. Filley (1975: 2) defines *competitive conflict* as a victory for one side at a loss for the other side. The process by which the conflict is resolved is determined by a set of rules. The goals of each side are mutually incompatible, but the emphasis is on winning, not the defeat or reduction of the oppo-

nent. When one side has clearly "won," the competition is terminated.

Disruptive conflict, on the other hand, does not follow any mutually acceptable set of rules and does not emphasize winning. The parties involved are engaged in activity to reduce, defeat, or eliminate the opponent. This type of conflict takes place in an environment charged with fear, anger, and stress. For example, an intern on night call may demonstrate disruptive conflict by refusing to answer pages, turning off the beeper, or by belittling nurses for calling with "minor" problems. Nurses react to this type of behavior with their own disruptive behavior: frequent, "by the book," middle-of-the-night phone calls to get back at the offending intern. A more subtle example of disruptive behavior would be a failure to extend minor work-saving courtesies to an unpopular intern. Disruptive conflict can, in unusual circumstances, result in irrational, disruptive, or violent behavior.

♦ THE CONFLICT PROCESS MODEL

Filley's model of conflict resolution provides a generalized format for examining conflict behavior in relation to the nurse manager's job. This model provides a framework that helps explain how and why conflict occurs and, ultimately, how one can minimize conflict or resolve it with the least amount of negative aftermath.

Filley suggests that conflict and its resolution develop according to a specific process. This process begins with certain preexisting conditions (antecedent conditions). The parties are influenced by their feelings or perceptions about the situation (perceived or felt conflict), which initiates behavior (manifest behavior). The conflict is either resolved or suppressed (conflict resolution or suppression), and in the aftermath new attitudes and feelings between the parties evolve (see Figure 22–1).

Antecedent conditions are conditions that have been shown to exist in a conflict situation. These conditions are not necessarily the cause of conflict but have been associated with increased rates of conflict and may propel a situation toward conflict. For the nurse manager these include incompatible goals, differences in values and beliefs, task interdependencies (especially asymmetric dependencies where one department is dependent on the other but not vice versa), unclear/ambiguous roles, competition for scarce resources, differentiation or distancing mechanisms, proximity, and unifying mechanisms.

NATURE OF GOALS AND THEIR IMPORTANCE TO CONFLICT

The most important antecedent condition to conflict is *incompatible goals*. As discussed in Chapter 3 goals are desired results toward

FIGURE 22–1 CONFLICT PROCESS

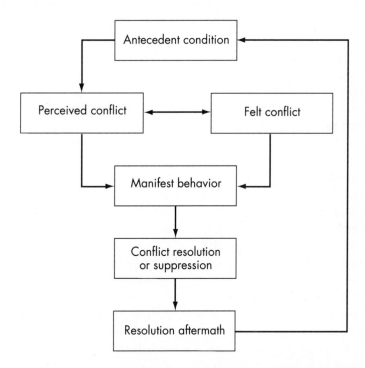

Adapted from A.C. Filley, R.J. House and S. Kerr: *Managerial Process and Organizational Behavior*, (A.C. Filley, University of Wisconsin, Madison, Wisconsin, 1976, p. 72). Used by permission.

which behavior is directed. Even though in health care institutions the common goal is achieving the highest quality patient care given the resources, conflict in goals is inevitable as individuals often view this from different perspectives. In addition, individuals and organizations have multiple goals that change over time. A health care organization may have specific goals to achieve the best possible care for the patient and control costs to stay within budget, while at the same time provide intrinsically satisfying jobs for its employees. These multiple goals will frequently conflict with each other, creating a situation in which decisions have to be made regarding the relative priorities of these conflicting goals. This issue of priority setting can be one of the most difficult but at the same time important activities a health care administrator must face. Goals are also important because they become the basis for allocating resources in organizations and, therefore, are an important source (antecedent) of conflict in the organization.

Similarly, individuals experience goal conflicts due to multiple goals and the inability to achieve each goal. Individuals allocate scarce resources such as their time on the basis of the goal priority and, therefore, might achieve one goal at the expense of achieving others. Interference with goal attainment is the source of conflict, whether it is because of multiple (and mutually incompatible) personal or departmental goals.

An example of goal conflict in nursing is the dichotomy between nursing education and nursing service. This issue can best be described as a conflict between groups with differing goals. Nursing education teaches the practice of nursing based on a conceptual foundation. Nurse managers who employ new graduates have criticized the lack of clinical experience in the educational program (Brooten, Hayman & Naylors, 1978: 60). They want to hire nurses who will need a minimum of orientation and be able to function independently as quickly as possible.

OTHER ANTECEDENT CONDITIONS

Roles are defined as the expectations of each regarding one's own and others' behavior. *Unclear roles* occur when one or more parties have related responsibilities that are ambiguous or overlapping. The nurse manager might experience conflict in her responsibility as administrator versus her role as staff member. Similar to this are unclear or overlapping job descriptions or assignments. For example, there could be conflict over such mundane issues as the responsibility of the nurse versus transporters in sending a patient to another department or moving a patient from bed to chair.

Competition for scarce resources could be internal (among different units in the institution) or external (among different institutions). Internally, competition for resources could involve the assigning of staff from one unit to another or the stockpiling of supplies, such as linen or wheelchairs, by one unit. Externally, institutions may compete for patients due to reduced occupancy rates. Recently, competition for resources has become a conflictive factor between nurses and physicians. Physicians have challenged the role of nurse practitioners, charging them with practicing medicine without a license, on the basis of legal interpretations of medical and nursing practice acts.* While these charges are publicly touted to promote patient care, many of the involved parties believe they really stem from economic concerns and are intended to reduce competition for health care services.

Differences in values and beliefs is a frequent contributor to conflict in health care institu-

---

Sermchief v. Gonzales, 660 S. W. 2d 683 (Mo. banc 1983), pp. 683–690.

tions. Values and beliefs result from the socialization processes that individuals experience. Conflicts between physicians and nurses, or between nurses and administrators, or even among nurses with associate degrees versus diplomas versus baccalaureate degrees often come from differences in values and beliefs. The last division raises conflict over which education is the best preparation for practice.

Task interdependency is a potential source of conflict in health care institutions. The three levels of functional interdependence are pooled interdependence, sequential interdependence, and reciprocal interdependence (Thompson, 1967). *Pooled interdependence* exists when units are relatively independent of each other—they are members of the same organization and draw their budgets and other resources from a common pool. An example in a health care unit might be the interaction between the finance department and the nursing department. Direct interaction seldom occurs, and managing the relationship between these units is not difficult. *Sequential interdependence* is where the output of one unit is the input of another unit, where the tasks of the first unit need to be performed before the second unit can perform its task. This is similar to the relationship between support groups such as admissions, discharge, and nursing. Functional nursing involves sequential interdependence. Sequential interdependence can become a particularly difficult situation when the dependent unit is of higher status—for example, when a nurse has to wait for housekeeping services. *Reciprocal interdependence* is where the output from each unit becomes the input of the other unit and vice versa. The relationship between the nurse and the physician is typically reciprocal in nature, as are the relationships among shifts; among the LPN, NA, and the RN; and between units such as radiology and the medical-surgical unit. Team nursing, primary nursing, and differential practice are also examples of reciprocal interdependencies.

Distancing mechanisms or *differentiation* serve to divide a group's members into small distinct groups, thus increasing the chance for conflict. This tends to lead to a "we-they" distinction. Examples might be opposition between intensive care nurses and floor nurses, night versus day shifts, and nursing aides versus registered nurses. One of the more frequently seen examples is distancing between physicians and nurses. Differentiation among subunits is also due to differences in structure. Many administrative units are very bureaucratic in nature, nursing units are structured on a more professional basis, while the staff physicians have even a different structure, and the nonstaff physicians, who are entrepreneurs, are relatively independent from the health care unit.

Unifying mechanisms occur when a greater intimacy develops or when unity is sought. All nurse managers might be expected to reach consensus over an issue but experience internal conflict as they find themselves forced to accept a position as a group, while individually they may not be wholly committed to the group's position. The most classic example of a unifying mechanism is the relationship between husband and wife. As intimacy increases, issues arise that would not normally cause conflict in a casual relationship but do affect these closer relationships. A nurse manager's friendship with a staff member may lead to this type of conflict.

Conflict commonly seen in the health care environment is *structural* conflict. This conflict evolves from the relationship between members of organizations. These relationships (superior to subordinate, peer to peer) provoke conflict due to inadequate communication, competition for resources, opposing interests, or a lack of shared perceptions or attitudes. A nurse manager (superior) stimulates conflict between herself or himself and a staff member (subordinate) in reprimanding the staff member for some inappropriate act. If the nurse manager is unable to communicate to the staff member why the act was unacceptable, opposing interests develop and the conflict is sustained. In this situation, positional power is often imposed. Positional power refers to the authority inherent in a certain position—for example, the director of nursing service has greater positional power than a nurse manager.

OTHER ASPECTS OF THE CONFLICT PROCESS

Perceived and felt conflict are parts of the conflict process that explain how conflict may occur when the parties involved view the situations or issues from differing perspectives or misunderstand each other's position, or when positions are based on limited knowledge. Perceived conflict refers to each party's perception of the other's position. It is a logical and impersonal set of conflicting conditions present between two or more parties. Felt conflict refers to the feelings of opposition within the relationship of two or more parties. It is characterized by mistrust, hostility, and fear.

To demonstrate how this process may work, consider this situation. Nurse manager Jones and surgeon Smith have worked together for years. They have mutual respect for each other's ability and skills and communicate frequently. When their subordinates clash, they are left with conflicting accounts of a situation where the only agreed-upon fact is that a patient received less than appropriate care. Now consider the same scenario if the nurse and doctor have never dealt with each other or if one feels that the other will not approach the problem construc-

tively. In these situations, the attitudes and feelings of the nurse and physician are critical.

In the first situation, because of their positive regard for each other's abilities, nurse and physician believe they can constructively solve the conflict. The nurse does not feel the physician will try to dominate, while the physician respects the nurse manager's managerial ability. With these preexisting attitudes, the physician and nurse can remain neutral while assisting their subordinates to solve the conflict. In the second situation, the nurse and physician may approach the situation differently. If each assumes the other will defend her or his subordinates at all costs, communication will be inhibited. The conflict is resolved by domination of the stronger person, either in personality or position. One wins; the other loses.

Manifest behavior is the action that results or what happens. Overt action may take the form of aggression, competition, debate, or problem solving. Covert action may be expressed by a variety of indirect tactics such as scapegoating, avoidance, or apathy.

The final stages of the conflict process are suppression or resolution and the resulting aftermath. *Suppression* occurs when one person or group defeats the other. Only the dominant side is committed to the agreement and the loser may or may not carry out the agreement. *Resolution* occurs when a mutually agreed-upon solution is arrived at and both parties commit themselves to carry out the agreement. The optimal solution to conflictive situations is to manage the issues in a way that will lead to a solution wherein both parties see themselves as winners and the problem is solved. This leaves an aftermath that will affect future relations and can influence feelings and attitudes. In the example of conflict between the nurse manager and the physician, consider the difference in the aftermath and how future issues would be approached if both parties felt positive about the outcome, as compared to future interactions if one or both parties felt they had lost.

♦ GROUP PROCESSES

Groups are often a source of conflict in organizations. Understanding why groups form and how they influence behavior in organizations is important for a nurse manager and is discussed in Chapter 12. Nursing groups are often highly cohesive with powerful norms as to how group members should behave. These norms are often a source of either intragroup or intergroup conflict.

INTRAGROUP CONFLICT

Intragroup conflict can occur when group norms or standards are violated or changed. For example, in an organization undergoing decentralization, nurse managers might be expected to change in various ways, such as pursuing graduate education or wearing street clothes and a lab coat instead of a conventional uniform. This change might conflict with group norms and could stimulate internal conflict for nurse managers who have perceived themselves differently. Groups often develop norms relative to how hard a person is expected to work, making it more difficult for the nurse manager to influence productivity. Another potential intragroup conflict problem that a nurse manager must deal with would be the introduction of new members into a cohesive group. The nurse manager must make sure the new members are accepted and made part of the group.

INTERGROUP CONFLICT

Intergroup conflict arises between groups with differing goals, the achievement of which by one group can occur only at the expense of the other.

These types of conflicts can range from small day-to-day problems to broader issues. For example, administration's goal is to control salary expenses, while nursing's goal is to upgrade staffing with a resultant increase in salary costs. A smaller day-to-day issue might be when the radiology department wants patients sent to X-ray in gowns without metal snaps on the sleeve because the snaps show on the film. Nursing staff prefer these snaps because they make it easier to change gowns on patients receiving intravenous fluids. Neither side wants the bother of changing gowns prior to X-rays and believes the other should do this task.

INTRAORGANIZATIONAL CONFLICT

Conflict between groups, departments, or divisions of an organization is often a consequence of the degree to which these units are differentiated from one another. According to Lawrence and Lorsch (1967), differentiation between units may be due to differences in *structure, time orientation, interpersonal orientation,* or *subenvironment orientation.* For example, some units in hospitals such as food service and housekeeping tend to have more mechanistic structures, while financial services and accounting might have a bureaucratic structure, and units such as nursing are structured on a more professional basis. In terms of time orientation, research units might have long-time orientations while the emergency room would be an example of a unit with a short-time orientation. Some units in a hospital such as personnel or public relations might have strong interpersonal orientations, while laboratories might have strong task orientations. The final dimension of differentiation is subenvironment orientation. Administrative units such as finance would have an orientation toward the economic environment, while units such as radiology would have a more technical or scientific subenvironmental orientation.

The more differentiated units are the greater the potential for conflict, especially if these units must work together to perform their tasks or one unit is highly dependent on the other unit. Similarly, conflicts may occur between staff units—those units providing support services—and line units—those units providing specific care and services to patients. The manner in which a health care institution is departmentalized or how units are physically located can be sources of conflict. As noted before, resource allocations and different goals may also be sources of intraorganizational conflict.

♦ COMMUNICATION PROBLEMS

Marriner (1979) identifies conflicts originating from senders (those initiating the communication—see Chapter 8), groups, and individuals. Sender conflict can be either intra- or intersender. Intrasender conflict occurs when one sender gives conflicting instructions to another—the director of nursing, for instance, demands that the floor be adequately staffed but forbids the use of paid overtime. Intersender conflict occurs when two conflicting messages are received from differing sources. This might occur when staff is encouraged by the risk manager to report medication errors, while the nurse manager follows up with discipline over the error. The nurse is caught between conflicting messages from two sources. The nurse is encouraged to "tell all" to help the institution protect itself, but by doing so may be subjected to disciplinary action. In the case of a "not so serious error," the nurse may rationalize that the error did not cause any

harm, so why subject herself or himself to potential discipline just to report the error.

♦ CONFLICT MANAGEMENT

The management of conflict is an important part of the nurse manager's job. A number of techniques can be used to manage conflict; some are more effective than others. One method of conflict management is *suppression*. This could even include the elimination of one of the parties in the conflict through transfer or termination. The opposite of suppression is a form of conflict resolution that stresses harmony or a "don't rock the boat" attitude. One party is dominated by the other without resistance. In the past, nurses have been subordinate to physicians and were taught to follow physicians' orders without question.

Some of the other, less effective techniques for managing conflict include withdrawing, smoothing, avoiding, forcing, and competing, though each mode of response is useful in given situations. *Withdrawal* from the conflict simply removes at least one party, thereby making it impossible to resolve the situation. The issues remain unsolved and feelings about the issue may resurface inappropriately.

Smoothing is accomplished by complimenting one's opponent, downplaying differences, and focusing on minor areas of agreement, as if little disagreement exists. Smoothing may be appropriate in dealing with minor problems but, in response to major problems, it produces the same results as withdrawing.

Avoiding is similar to withdrawal, except the participants never acknowledge that a conflict exists. Avoidance is the conflict resolution technique often used in highly cohesive groups that are engaged in "groupthink." The group avoids disagreement because they do not want to do anything that may interfere with the good feelings they have for each other (Janis, 1972).

Forcing is a method that yields an immediate end to the conflict but leaves the cause of the conflict unresolved. A superior can resort to issuing orders, but the subordinate will lack commitment to the demanded action. Forcing may be appropriate in life or death situations but is otherwise inappropriate.

Competing is an all-out effort to win, regardless of the cost. Competing, like forcing, may be needed to prevail in situations involving unpopular or critical decisions.

Negotiation, collaboration, compromise, and confrontation are generally more effective modes of responding to conflict. *Negotiation* involves a give-and-take on various issues among the parties. It is used in situations in which consensus will never be reached. Therefore, the best solution is not often achieved. Negotiation often becomes a structured, formal procedure, as in collective bargaining.

Collaboration implies mutual attention to the problem that utilizes the talents of all parties. In collaboration, the focus is on solving the problem, not defeating the opponent; the goal is to satisfy both parties' concerns. Collaboration is useful in situations where the goals of both parties are too important to be compromised.

Compromise is used to divide the rewards between both parties. Neither gets what he or she wants. Compromise can serve as a backup to resolve conflict when collaboration is ineffective. It is sometimes the only choice when opponents of equal power are in conflict over two or more mutually exclusive goals. Compromising is also expedient when a solution is needed rapidly.

The *confrontation* technique is similar to the collaboration technique and is considered the most effective means for resolving conflicts.

This is a very problem-oriented technique, where the conflict is brought out into the open and attempts are made to resolve it through knowledge and reason. Lawrence and Lorsch (1967) refer to this mode using aphorisms such as "by digging and digging the truth is discovered" and "seek 'til you find and you'll not lose your labor." The goal of this conflict resolution technique is to achieve win-win solutions.

GROUP CONFLICT RESOLUTION

Filley (1975) identifies three basic strategies for dealing with conflict according to the outcome: win-lose, lose-lose, and win-win. In the *win-lose* outcome, one party exerts dominance, usually by power of authority, and the other party submits and loses. Forcing, competing, and negotiation are techniques that are likely to lead to win-lose competition. Majority rule is another example of the win-lose outcome, especially within groups. It may be a satisfactory method of resolving conflict, however, if various factions vote differently on different issues and the group functions over time so that members win some and lose some. Win-lose outcomes often occur between groups. A potential negative consequence of this is that frequent losing can lead to the loss of cohesiveness within groups and diminish the authority of the group leader.

In the *lose-lose* method, neither side wins. The settlement reached is unsatisfactory to both sides. Often, avoiding, withdrawing, smoothing, and compromising lead to lose-lose outcomes. One compromising strategy involves using bribes to influence another's cooperation in doing something he or she dislikes. For example, the nurse manager may promise a future raise in an attempt to coerce a staff member to work an extra weekend. Using a third party as arbitrator can lead to a lose-lose outcome. Since an outsider may want to give something to each side, neither gets what is desired. Often either a win-lose or a lose-lose outcome occurs. This is common in arbitration of labor-management disputes. Another strategy that may help a lose-lose or win-lose outcome is resorting to rules. The outcome is left to chance (whatever the rules say), and confrontation is avoided.

The win-lose and lose-lose methods share some common characteristics.

1. The conflict is a personal "we-they" conflict rather than a problem-centered focus. This is very likely to occur when two cohesive groups that do not share common values or goals are in conflict.

2. Parties direct their energy toward total victory for themselves and total defeat for the other. This can cause long-term problems for the organization.

3. Each sees the issue from her or his own point of view rather than as a problem in need of a solution.

4. The emphasis is on outcomes rather than definition of goals, values, or objectives.

5. Conflicts are personalized.

6. Conflict-resolving activities are not differentiated from other group processes.

7. There is a short-run view of the conflict, with settlement of the immediate problem as the goal rather than resolution of differences (Filley, 1975: 25).

Win-win methods focus on goals and attempt to meet the needs of both parties. The common techniques of conflict resolution that lead to win-win outcomes are collaboration and confrontation. Two specific win-win strategies are consensus and integrative decision making. Consensus involves attention to the facts and to the position of the other parties and avoidance

of trading, voting, or averaging, where everyone loses something. The consensus decision is often superior to even the best individual one. This technique is most useful in a group setting.

Integrative decision-making methods focus on the means of problem solution rather than the ends and are most useful when the needs of the parties are polarized. Using integrative decision-making methods, the parties jointly identify the value needs of each, conduct an exhaustive search for alternatives that could meet these needs of each, and then select the best alternative. Like the consensus methods, integrative decision making focuses on defeating the problem, not each other.

The group consensus technique is sensitive to the seven characteristics of the win-lose and lose-lose outcomes listed above. If these factors are present as the parties attempt to resolve the issues, all of the involved parties will not be committed to the solution. In this situation, a win-win outcome is unlikely. True consensus occurs when the problem is fully explored, the needs and goals of the involved parties are understood, and a solution that meets these needs is agreed upon.

Integrative problem solving is a constructive process that emphasizes that the parties jointly identify the problem and their needs. They explore a number of alternative solutions and come to consensus on a solution. The focus of this group activity is to solve the problem and not to force, dominate, suppress, or compromise. The group works toward a common goal in an atmosphere that encourages the free exchange of ideas and feelings.

PERSONAL CONFLICT RESOLUTION STYLES

Individuals have particular styles for resolving conflicts. Even though these might not be used in every situation, there are tendencies to behave in these ways. You can assess your own response to conflict by ranking the following questions. Place a 5 beside the sentence you think is most like yourself (your real you), a 4 beside the next, then 3, 2, and 1, respectively.

Conflict Questionnaire

___ A. When conflict arises, I try to remain neutral.

___ B. I try to avoid generating conflict, but when it does appear, I try to soothe feelings to keep people together.

___ C. When conflict arises, I try to find fair solutions that accommodate others.

___ D. When conflict arises, I try to cut it off or to win my position.

___ E. When conflict arises, I try to identify reasons for it and seek to resolve underlying causes. (Blake, Mouton & Tapper, 1981: 9)

These common styles of conflict resolution are shown in Figure 22–2, the nurse administrator grid. The five styles of conflict resolution used by nurse managers and the corresponding letter from the exercise above are avoider (A), friendly helper (B), compromiser (C), tough battler (D), and problem solver (E).

According to Blake, Mouton, and Tapper (1981: 56) the nurse manager who uses the "avoider" style (1,1) in conflict situations tends to remain neutral, withdraws from the situation, delays responding to the conflict situation, or may even given the appearance of being busy to keep others from bringing her or him into the conflict. Unfortunately, the issue doesn't go away and remains unresolved, and feelings about the issue may resurface inappropriately. Often this style leads to the conflict being taken to someone higher up.

The "friendly helper" nurse manager (1,9) dreads conflict because it threatens warmth and approval (Blake, Mouton & Tapper, 1981: 39). Therefore, conflicts are smoothed over so that the nurse manager can get back into a closer supportive relationship with others.

Avoiding, withdrawing, and smoothing have been followed in the nursing profession, with its heritage of an emphasis on obedience and submissiveness. These strategies may still be useful techniques, such as when other issues are more important, and the current issue is trivial by comparison; the potential for disruption is greater than the benefits of resolution; or time is needed for emotions to stabilize and a perspective to be regained, but generally these techniques are not as useful as the techniques listed below.

The "tough battler" nurse manager (9,1) feels that she is losing control when conflict occurs and tends to respond with anger and attempts to use power to win any conflicts (Blake, Mouton & Tapper, 1981: 20). This frequently causes suppression of the conflict, because others are denied any chance to react and wish to avoid the wrath of the nurse manager. There is some evidence to indicate that the tough battler tends to win frequently in conflicts with friendly helpers who want to smooth over the conflict quickly (see Figure 22–3).

The "compromiser" nurse manager (5,5) starts with the assumptions that no person or department ever has its exclusive way, extreme positions promote conflict and should therefore be avoided, and steady progress comes from compromising (Blake, Mouton & Tapper, 1981: 72–74). This nurse manager uses tact and diplomacy and seldom tries to confront conflict because that could cause someone to win and someone to lose. This technique involves a give-and-take on various issues among the parties. Often the solution selected is the one that is politically safe, salable, or workable.

The "problem solver" nurse manager (9,9)

recognizes that conflict may delay or prevent the achievement of organizational and personal goals, but she or he also recognizes that conflict can frequently lead to innovation, creativity, and the development of new ideas (Blake, Mouton & Tapper, 1981: 93). The nurse manager recognizes that though conflict may be inevitable, it might also be resolvable. Therefore, she

FIGURE 22–2 THE NURSE ADMINISTRATOR CONFLICT GRID®

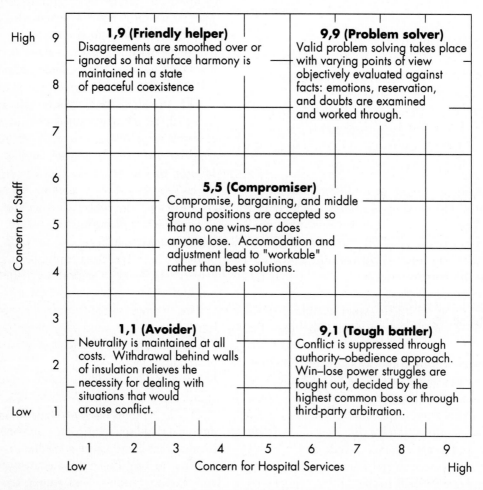

1,9 (Friendly helper)
Disagreements are smoothed over or ignored so that surface harmony is maintained in a state of peaceful coexistence

9,9 (Problem solver)
Valid problem solving takes place with varying points of view objectively evaluated against facts: emotions, reservation, and doubts are examined and worked through.

5,5 (Compromiser)
Compromise, bargaining, and middle ground positions are accepted so that no one wins—nor does anyone lose. Accomodation and adjustment lead to "workable" rather than best solutions.

1,1 (Avoider)
Neutrality is maintained at all costs. Withdrawal behind walls of insulation relieves the necessity for dealing with situations that would arouse conflict.

9,1 (Tough battler)
Conflict is suppressed through authority–obedience approach. Win–lose power struggles are fought out, decided by the highest common boss or through third-party arbitration.

Concern for Staff (High 9, 8, 7, 6, 5, 4, 3, 2, Low 1)

Concern for Hospital Services (1 Low, 2, 3, 4, 5, 6, 7, 8, 9 High)

Adapted from R. Blake, and J. Mouton, "The Fifth Achievement," *Journal of Applied Behavioral Management,* 6, (1970): 413-426. Used by permission.

tries to anticipate conflict, and when it does occur she confronts the conflict and tries to find out its causes and the optimal way to deal with it. Collaboration is often a technique used by the problem-solving nurse manager. Collaboration implies a mutual attention to the problem that utilizes the talents of all parties. In collaboration, the focus is on solving the problem, not defeating the opponent; the goal is to satisfy both parties' concerns. Collaboration is useful in situations where the goals of both parties are too important to be compromised.

Though problem solving is the preferred means by which nurse managers should deal with conflict, Figure 22–3 shows that the problem solver loses about 50 percent of the conflicts with the tough battler (Cummings, Harnett & Stevens, 1971). It is important for the organization to reward the problem-solving style of conflict resolution, train individuals in how to use this style, and discourage the tough battler style. As noted before, however, this technique is difficult to use by nurse managers because confrontation has been discouraged for women, and even more so for nurses, by society's traditional mores.

CONFLICT INTERVENTION

Nurse managers may be involved in resolving conflict on several different levels. They may be participants in the conflict either as individuals, as supervisors, or as representatives of a unit. In fact, they must often initiate conflict by confronting staff, individually or collectively, when a problem develops. They may also serve as mediators or judges to conflicting parties. There could be a conflict within the unit, between parties from different units, or between internal and external parties (e.g., a nursing instructor from an outside school has a conflict with staff on a particular unit). Whatever the nurse manager's position in the conflict situation, the process needed to resolve conflict is essentially the same and is consistent with the problem-solving technique discussed before.

FIGURE 22–3 ESTIMATED OUTCOMES OF THE COMBINATIONS OF CONFLICT STYLE IN BARGAINING

	Tough battler	Friendly helper	Problem solver
Tough battler	Stalemate 80%	Battler wins 90%	Battler wins over 50%
Friendly helper	X	Stalemate 80%	Problem solver wins
Problem solver	X	X	Quick agreement

Adapted from A.C. Filey, R.J. House, and S. Kerr, Managerial Process and Organizational Behavior. Used by permission.

It is important for the nurse manager and other participants in conflict resolution to be realistic regarding the outcome. Often those inexperienced in conflict negotiation expect unrealistic outcomes. When two or more parties hold mutually exclusive ideas, attitudes, feelings, or goals, it is extremely difficult, without the commitment and willingness of all concerned, to arrive at an agreeable solution that meets the needs of both.

Conflict resolution begins with a decision regarding if and when to intervene. The nurse manager should make sure the parties know when she or he is likely to intervene. Failure to intervene can allow the conflict to get out of hand, while early intervention may be demotivating to the parties, causing them to lose confidence in themselves and reduce risk-taking behavior in the future. Some conflicts are so minor, particularly if they are between only two people, that intervention is not necessary and the situation may be better handled by the two people. This might provide a developmental experience and improve their abilities to resolve conflict in the future. On the other hand, where there is potential for considerable harm to result from the conflict, the nurse manager must intervene.

Sometimes the nurse manager may postpone intervention purposely, to allow the conflict to escalate, since increased intensity can stimulate the participants to seek resolution. The manager can escalate the conflict even further by exposing the participants to each other more frequently without the presence of others and without an easy means of escape. Participants are then forced to face the conflict between them. Giving the participants a shared task or shared goals not directly related to the conflict may help them understand each other better and increase their chances to resolve their conflicts by themselves. Using a method such as this one is useful only if the conflict is not of high intensity, if the participants are not highly anxious about it, and if the manager believes that the conflict will not decrease efficiency of the department in the meantime.

If a nurse manager decides to intervene in a conflict between two or more parties, mediation techniques are very applicable. She or he must make decisions as to when, where, and how the intervention should take place. Routine problems can be handled in either the superior's or subordinate's office, but serious conflicts should take place in a neutral location unless the parties involved in the conflict are of unequal power. In this case, the setting should favor the disadvantaged participant, thereby equalizing their power.

The time and place should be one where distractions will not interfere and adequate time is available. Since conflict resolution takes time, the manager must be prepared to allow sufficient time for all parties to explain their points of view and arrive at a mutually agreeable solution. A quick solution often resorted to by inexperienced managers is to impose positional power. This could result in a win-lose outcome, leading to feelings of elation and eventual complacency on the part of the winners and loss of morale on the part of the losers.

The following are some of the basic rules on how to mediate a conflict between two or more parties.

1. Protect each party's self-respect. Deal with a conflict of issues, not personalities.

2. Do not put blame or responsibility for the problem on the participants. The participants are responsible for developing a solution to the problem.

3. Allow open and complete discussion of the problem from each participant.

4. Maintain equity in the frequency and duration of each party's presentation. A higher status person tends to speak more frequently and longer than a lower status person. If this occurs, the mediator should intervene and ask the lower status person for response and opinion.

5. Encourage full expression of positive and negative feelings within an accepting atmosphere. The novice mediator tends to discourage expressions of disagreement.

6. Make sure both parties listen actively to each other's words. One way to do this is to establish the ground rule that requires each person to summarize the comments of the other prior to stating her or his own position.

7. Identify key themes in the discussion and restate these at frequent intervals.

8. Encourage the parties to provide frequent feedback to each other's comments. Each must truly understand the other's position.

9. Assist the participants in developing alternative solutions, selecting a mutually agreeable one, and developing a plan to carry it out. All parties must be agreeable to the solution for successful resolution to occur.

10. At an agreed-upon interval, follow up on the progress of the plan.

11. Give positive feedback to participants regarding their cooperation in solving the conflict.

Conflict resolution is a difficult process, consuming both time and energy. Management and staff must be concerned and committed to resolving conflict by being willing to listen to others' positions and to finding agreeable solutions.

OTHER CONFLICT MANAGEMENT TECHNIQUES

Many other techniques besides personal intervention can be used to resolve conflict and are consistent with the problem-solving approach. Some of these include changing or clarifying goals, developing superordinate goals, and holding confrontation meetings. Other techniques that also may be effective include appeals to the hierarchy, negotiating and providing cooling off periods, establishing liaison persons, restructuring by buffering and decoupling, and dividing the resources so each party can partially achieve their goals (Hunger, 1976). In addition, groups can be rewarded for contributions to the organization and for cooperating with other groups. Rotation among groups and sharing resources also can be useful. These techniques are particularly useful in dealing with intergroup or intraorganizational conflict. Although the nurse manager frequently does not have direct responsibility for resolving these types of conflicts, it is important that she or he understand the nature of these conflicts and some of the techniques that can be used to resolve them.

SUMMARY

♦ The nurse manager must recognize that conflict is inevitable in productive organizations.

♦ Conflict in health care organizations frequently results from different goals, different values and beliefs, competition for scarce resources, task interdependencies, and/or group processes.

♦ Conflict can be disruptive or can be used constructively to promote change.

♦ The nurse manager should ask whether the conflict is disruptive and, therefore, is keeping the conflicting parties from accomplishing organizational and/or personal goals.

♦ If the conflict is disruptive, then the nurse manager should ask what methods might be used to deal with the conflict.

♦ Should the nurse manager intervene in the conflict personally or should the nurse manager involve other parties, including her or his supervisor?

♦ The five styles of conflict resolution used by nurse managers to intervene in conflicts include the avoider, the friendly helper, the compromiser, the tough battler, and the problem solver. Though there are situations where each of these styles can be effective, the most effective style of conflict resolution is the problem-solver style.

♦ Consistent with the problem-solving approach is the technique of mediation.

♦ Other means that can be used to resolve conflicts include superordinate goals, confrontation meetings, structural changes, negotiation and compromise, and buffering devices or dividing resources so each party can partially achieve its goals.

BIBLIOGRAPHY

Albanese, R. (1981). *Managing: Toward Accountability for Performance.* Homewood, IL: Irwin.

Beckhard, R. (1967). "The Confrontation Meeting." *Harvard Business Review,* 45(March–April): 149–155.

Blake, R. R., Mouton, J. S., and Tapper, M. (1981). *Grid Approaches for Managerial Leadership in Nursing.* St. Louis, MO: C. V. Mosby.

Brooten, D. A., Hayman, L., and Naylors, M. D. (1978). *Leadership for Change: A Guide for the Frustrated Nurse.* Philadelphia: J. B. Lippincott.

Cummings, L. L., Harnett, D. L., and Stevens, O. J. (1971). "Risk, Fate, Conciliation and Trust: An International Study of Attitudinal Differences among Executives." *Academy of Management Journal,* 14: 285.

Douglass, L. (1983). *The Effective Nurse: Leader and Manager.* 2nd ed. St. Louis, MO: C. V. Mosby.

Feldman, D. C. (1984). "The Development and Enforcement of Group Norms." *Academy of Management Review,* 9: 47–53.

Filley, A. C. (1975). *Interpersonal Conflict Resolution.* Glenview, IL: Scott, Foresman.

Filley, A. C., House, R. J., and Kerr, S. (1976). *Managerial Process and Organizational Behavior.* Glenview, IL: Scott, Foresman.

Hunger, J. D. (1979). "An Analysis of Intergroup Conflict and Conflict Management." In: *Management Pragmatics.* Webber, R. A. (editor). Homewood, IL: Irwin. Pp. 353–358.

Hunger, J. D., and Stern, L. W. (1976). "An Assessment of the Functionality of the Superordinate Goal in Reducing Conflict." *Academy of Management Journal,* 19(4) (December): 591–605.

Janis, I. L. (1972). *Victims of Group-Think: A Psychological Study of Foreign Policy Decisions and Fiascos.* Boston: Houghton Mifflin.

Klein, S. M., and Ritti, R. R. (1984). *Understanding Organizational Behavior.* 2nd ed. Boston: Kent.

Lawrence, P. R., and Lorsch, J. W. (1967). "Differentiation and Integration in Complex Organizations." *Administrative Science Quarterly,* 12(1)(June): 1–47.

Marriner, A. (1979). "Conflict Theory." *Supervisor Nurse,* 10(April): 12.

Sherif, M., Harvey, O. J., White, B. J., Hood, W., and Sherif, C. W. (1961). *Intergroup Conflict and Cooperation: The Robbers' Cave Experiment.* Norman, OK: University Book Exchange.

Sherif, M., and Sherif, C. W. (1969). *Social Psychology.* New York: Harper & Row.

Silber, M. B. (1984). "Managing Confrontations: Once More into the Breach." *Nursing Management,* 15(4)(April): 54.

Thomas, K. W. (1976). "Conflict and Conflict Management." In: *Handbook of Industrial and Organizational Psychology.* Dunnette, M. D. (editor). Chicago: Rand McNally. Pp. 889–935.

Thompson, J. D. (1967). *Organizations in Action.* New York: McGraw-Hill.

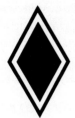

POWER
AND
POLITICS

As a nurse, do you want power? Do you need power? Do you have power? Are you politically savvy? Should you be more involved in the politics of nursing and health care? These are essential questions for nurses to consider. While many nurses may believe their work should be apolitical, failure to recognize the politics of patient care and nursing management can result in poor quality of care for the patient and frustration for the nurse (Mason, 1985).

As the United States attempts to address a critical shortage of nurses, it has become apparent that the retention and effective utilization of nurses depends on their inclusion and active participation in groups that are responsible for developing institutional and health policy (Secretary's Commission on Nursing, 1988). It is also incumbent upon nurses to take leadership roles in transforming the health care system to ensure access to quality health care. This can only be done if nurses develop their power base and political skills.

This chapter presents a framework for political action, identifies sources and uses of power, discusses strategies for effective political action, discusses the role of marketing in developing power and politics, and applies the principles of power and politics to the practice of the staff nurse, the role of the nurse manager, and the role of nurse leaders in the community.

♦ A FRAMEWORK FOR POLITICAL ACTION

Although most people associate the word "politics" with government, it pertains to every aspect of life that involves some competition for the allocation of scarce resources or influencing of decision making. As such, it is relevant to what nurses do in their daily practice, whether as a staff nurse, clinical nurse specialist, or nurse manager. And what nurses do in their everyday practice is influenced by, and in turn influences, what governments do, what professional organizations do, and what communities do. Although the spheres are discussed separately here, it is important to recognize that what one does or does not do in one sphere can have an effect on the other spheres and the nurse's overall political power.

POLITICS IN THE WORKPLACE

Politics in the workplace is often regarded with disdain, as reflected in the remark, "She plays politics." This is often used to imply that the individual got what he or she wanted because of personal connections, rather than on merit. And yet, would that same person want a chief nurse administrator who did not understand or use politics in her or his role as an advocate for nursing within the institution? Ehrat (1983) pointed out that politics is inherent in health care delivery because health care involves multiple special interest groups all competing for their piece of a limited pool of resources. A group's failure to recognize this fact ensures that the group's ability to influence decision making within the institution will be limited.

POLITICS IN GOVERNMENT

Politics, in the sphere of government, influences who gets what kind of health care, where, and why. Although nursing has traditionally embraced the concept of equality in relation to who gets health care, at least 37 million Americans are uninsured and may be denied access to health and nursing care—at least certain kinds of care. In 1990, the United States was still not guaranteeing the approximately $1,500 per mother for "high touch, low-tech" prenatal care, but was ensuring that very low birth weight infants born to mothers who did not get prenatal care would receive extensive high-tech care in neonatal intensive care units at an average of $167,000 per infant (Institute of Medicine, 1988).

POLITICS IN FINANCING

Which individuals qualify to be patients cared for by a nurse in an institution is to a certain extent determined by the politics of health care financing in this country. Financing also influences where patients receive their care. In metropolitan regions of the country, one can find at least two tiers of health care—one for the poor (the public hospital, the well child clinic) and one for the middle and upper classes (the private institution and private physician). While public health care institutions and agencies can often provide excellent care, they frequently are underfinanced and have limited resources (staff, equipment, medications, etc.) for providing care.

POLITICS IN THE ORGANIZATION

Once a patient gets into the hospital bed, the kind and quality of nursing care he or she receives can also be influenced by politics. For example, the nurse may not find the time to sit with the elderly patient who needs to be fed but will unquestioningly take the time to give the tube feeding that the physician has now ordered (and which will be reimbursed) for a patient who is not eating. The politics of this situation involve what values and policies the institution and third party payers have embraced: In this case, nursing care requiring a physician's order—and particularly care that involves a technical procedure—is valued, expected, and reimbursed before humanistic, low-tech, personal care. Are nurses involved in defining the mission and philosophy of the institution or

third party payers? They should be. Are nurses participating as equals in committees that set institutional policy? They should be. This is political action.

Something as mundane as which health care providers have reserved parking spaces, a reserved dining room, or the largest offices (or any office!) becomes an important symbol of the power and influence of particular groups. The resources available for nurses to provide safe, effective patient care also reflect the power of nursing within the institution. For example, staff nurses on a general medical-surgical floor may waste precious time trying to locate one of the unit's two electronic thermometers that are available for taking temperatures. Why does the floor have only two electronic thermometers? Most institutions do not purchase the thermometers—the manufacturers often give them to the institution for free because the company makes its profit from the thermometer sheaths that must be replaced with each use and are made specifically for the company's thermometer. Why will the institution spend money on expensive diagnostic equipment (such as a nuclear magnetic imager) but not on relatively inexpensive equipment that would facilitate cost-effective utilization of the nurses' time? In institutions where nurses have a high degree of power and influence, the nurse manager controls the unit's budget and is able to negotiate for necessary time-saving equipment.

Policy can be defined as: "the principles that govern action directed towards given ends. The concept denotes action about means as well as ends and it, therefore, implies change: changing situations, systems, practices, behavior" (Titmus, 1974: 23). Whether in government or the workplace, nurses need to bring their valuable expertise and perspectives to the places where policies are made. While individual nurses can and should participate in developing institutional and health care policy, professional nursing organizations provide a mechanism for nurses to collectively influence policy. Most nursing organizations, such as the American Nurses Association, its constituent state nurses associations, the National League for Nursing, and the specialty nursing organizations, monitor and influence governmental legislation and regulations.

The primary focus for many of these organizations is furthering nurses' practice in a variety of ways. For example, nursing organizations on local, state, and national levels collaborated to prevent the implementation of the American Medical Association's proposal for a Registered Care Technician (RCT) in the late 1980s. The AMA proposed that an RCT could provide bedside patient care that the nursing organizations believed required the preparation and skill of a registered nurse. Organized nursing's successful effort to protect its practice and ensure quality of care delivered to the public was preceded by years of work by state nurses associations to update state laws that defined the scope of nursing practice, i.e., nurse practice acts. Nursing organizations also monitor governmental regulations and patterns of institutional policies that can jeopardize nursing practice and have worked to secure adequate reimbursement of nursing services.

Increasingly, these associations are also playing a major role in developing and influencing broader health and social policies that influence the quality of health care and the health of communities. The American Nurses Association participates in a variety of coalitions for developing a national policy on long-term care, securing the rights of employees to take an unpaid leave of absence from work to care for a sick family member or new child, and framing a na-

tional health care plan to ensure access to cost-effective health care services.

For many of these nursing organizations, the increasing attention that they are giving to broader health care issues came about as a result of the political action of many of their members who believed that nurses' voices should be heard on these larger issues. These nurse members developed resolutions that addressed these issues and lobbied for their passage at the business meetings of their organizations. Just as politics determines the officers, rules, and policies of government, it also determines the shape and focus of nursing organizations. These organizations are an important forum for nurses to learn, develop, and apply their political skills.

POLITICS IN THE COMMUNITY

The workplace, governments, and organizations all interact with the community, whether local, regional, national, or international. One nurse found that her leadership in a community effort to eliminate improper garbage dumping in her town enabled her to develop important connections to government officials on both the local and state levels. It also brought her to the attention of her hospital administrator in a positive and powerful way. The administrator knew that she had done excellent work with the issue and had developed both a fine reputation in the community and significant connections to other persons of influence. For many nurses who have children, an important forum for developing their political skills and power is the school's PTA or school board. Her or his identity as a nurse in these groups can and should be made known. The connections developed here can be used to further other purposes in other spheres in the future.

This framework suggests that nurses need to understand the connections between what they do in their everyday work and what takes place in the rest of the community, nation, and world. Such a macroscopic view is particularly needed for the nurse manager. While the nurse manager is rightfully concerned about how the unit is functioning, he or she must recognize that it does not function in a vacuum. Understanding and considering the broader context in which the unit is functioning makes the difference in whether the nurse manager is seen as visionary, whether the unit is on the cutting edge of nursing practice, and whether the unit sets the standard for excellence in the institution.

◆ POLITICS: THE ART OF INFLUENCING

Politics is influencing, especially the allocation of scarce resources (Mason & Talbott, 1985). These resources include money, time, personnel, or materials. Politics is a means to an end, a means for influencing events and the decisions of others (Stevens, 1980). Nurses who renounce politics are essentially saying they do not want to influence the events in their everyday work.

Politics is an interpersonal endeavor. It involves skills of communication and persuasion. Nurses' skills in communication make them particularly effective in political activities. Nurses understand the importance of rapport and how to create meaningful connections with people. They understand the importance of time in developing these connections. They also understand the need to appeal to the other person's needs and interests if the goal is going to be reached. At a "Nurses Night" telephone bank to solicit support for a congressional candidate, the candidate's manager told the nurse organizer of the event, "You nurses are wonderful at this! I was listening to one nurse talking on the phone

with a man who I thought must be her uncle or someone she knew well—it was a stranger, but they were talking like they were old friends!"

Politics is a collective endeavor. It often requires the support and action of many to bring effective politics to bear on a situation or issue. Furthermore, working with others for political action can be invigorating, more creative, and simply more effective since there are more people to do the work and provide the emotional support that may be needed to sustain long-term political action. And it is also more fun to celebrate victories with a group! The politically astute nurse develops and carefully uses a support base that crosses the hierarchical lines of each sphere. In the workplace, this means developing connections to other nurses, the maintenance people, top administrators, the social work department, physicians, and other workers at all levels of the organization. Certainly, this takes time, but it can and should be a part of the nurse's everyday work. For example, greet and speak to the person who is cleaning the floor every morning, sit with different people at lunch, and invite the new director of medicine for a cup of coffee. It involves going to professional nursing meetings and sharing your business card with those whom you meet. It involves providing support for others' agendas, knowing that they may be able to support you on an issue in the future. And it involves being able to organize and mobilize groups of nurses and coalitions of diverse groups. It is helpful to have a target list of people with whom you would like to connect to build your support base, remembering that the secretary to the chief officer in the organization may be one of the most powerful persons in the organization by virtue of his or her ability to control access to the chief officer.

Politics is also about analysis and planning.

Just as the nursing process requires a thorough assessment, good politics arises from a careful and insightful political analysis of the situation, issue, or problem. A political analysis includes assessing the structure and functioning of the sphere in which you are operating. What is the organizational structure? What are the formal and informal lines of communication? Who holds the legitimate power? Who holds the informal power? What are the stated and unstated missions and agendas of the organization? What individuals are involved in the issue or situation (remembering that from a systems perspective, one change in the system can have far-reaching effects in the rest of the system)? What are the values, interests, beliefs, priorities, and agendas of these players? What connections and power bases do they have? What is the current context of the situation or issue? What is the climate for change? What outside forces might be influencing the situation or potential solutions or changes? What recent events might influence how others view the situation and their openness for change?

A good political analysis also includes a thorough assessment of the issue or problem itself. Why does the issue exist? What are the contributing factors? Who is affected by the issue? Do efforts need to be devoted to creating an audience who are interested in the issue? What beliefs and feelings do people hold about the issue? Are more data needed about the issue?

Effective political action usually involves good planning. Based on the analysis just outlined, a group that was trying to influence an issue or situation would brainstorm about alternative solutions and evaluate their risks and benefits. But it would also develop a plan for introducing its alternative and persuading others to support its position. Political analysis provides information about who can be counted on

to play what role in this process. For example, who should introduce the alternative to the person with the formal authority to make the decision about whether to adopt it or not? Sometimes, the most politically astute approach is not to have the originator of the alternative introduce it, but rather the individual who is most likely to be accepted by the decision maker(s). Is collective action needed? What coalitions need to be formed? The political analysis also will suggest strategies related to timing. Should the alternative be proposed now or in two months? Should it be proposed as a pilot project or demonstration project? Should it be gradually phased in or implemented fully at one time? Should group pressure be brought to bear now or later? Timing is often crucial to the effectiveness of the political action. People usually are more willing to accept something as a trial or test. Pilot projects also enable those affected to adjust to the change.

Politics is also about images. Do people think you can make the change? Do people think the change will be harmful to them? Do people trust you? Do people identify positively with the coalition involved? Your future ability to be politically effective may hinge on the image that others have of you or of the issue. For example, it is well known that when a workers' contract is settled in a collective bargaining dispute, both the union and management sides try to come out of the negotiations with the appearance of having won the most. Even losses can be seen as victories, particularly if the effort resulted in the mobilization and empowerment of nurses so that the whole group's power and likelihood of future success are enhanced. Defining the message you want others to receive and effectively marketing that message can create the image that is needed to further your political agenda.

Some of these guidelines for effective political

action stem from long-standing political tenets that are very often based upon how men have operated in politics. Machiavelli's *The Prince* is the classic example of cutthroat strategies for getting what one wants. The nursing literature has given attention to learning how to "swim with the sharks," and certainly, nurses need to be aware of how the game of politics is traditionally played. However, work by feminist scholars is suggesting that many women may be uncomfortable with cutthroat, Machiavellian politics. It is important for nurses to think about the ethics of their politics and whether they can bring a new ethic to bear in the nursing sphere of influence. This is particularly relevant to understanding what power is, how to get it, and how it can be used and abused.

♦ USING POWER TO INCREASE YOUR PROFESSIONAL INFLUENCE

To manage patient care successfully and to be more effective, nurses must understand the concept and importance of power. Then, they must be willing to acquire power. By developing a power base, one has the potential for maximum influence. The willingness to use power increases a nurse's ability to acquire the resources needed to improve patient care (Carter, 1988).

Regardless of when, why, and where care takes place, power centers around an individual's ability to influence others or the behavior of others. Power also is defined as the potential to achieve goals. Bennis and Nannus (1985) suggest that power is the basic energy needed to initiate and sustain action translating intention into reality. To acquire power, maintain it effectively, and use it skillfully, nurses must be aware

of the sources and types of power that they will use to influence and transform patient care.

Power can be acquired through a variety of sources (Benner, 1984; Ferguson, 1985; French & Raven, 1960; Stevens, 1983). Reward, coercive, referent, legitimate, charismatic, and expert power are defined and discussed in Chapter 9. In addition, there are two other bases of power:

Connection or network power is developed through relationships with other people. Both the quantity and the quality of these relationships can determine how much power is derived from this source. Ferguson (1985) suggests that nursing as a profession has a right to and need for collective or collaborative power. Developing connections and networks can further this collective power.

Informational power is the possession and judicious sharing of valued information that another individual desires. Informational power is related to connection power since what information one has may depend on one's networks and access to information. One's reputation as a reliable confidant can influence access to valued information. On the other hand, someone who is known to be a gossip will be given only the information that others want made public.

Despite an increase in pride and self-esteem that comes with using power and influence, some nurses still consider power unattractive. The image of power associated with aggression and coercion remains ever popular. In a profession that prides itself on care and compassion, power is viewed as alien. How then is the disparity between power as good versus power as bad resolved?

Several authors have noted that women and

nurses are not as comfortable with power-grab-bing, which has been the traditionally accepted means of relating to power for one's own self-interests and use (Mason et al., 1991; Miller, 1976; Wheeler & Chinn, 1989). Rather, women and nurses tend to be more comfortable with power-sharing and empowerment: power "with" rather than power "over" others. While nurses need power to ensure that patients have access to cost-effective quality nursing care, nurses can transform health care organizations by bringing a vision of power acquisition and usage that embraces equality and caring.

In a health care environment driven by com-petition and cost, nurses offer the necessary knowledge and expertise to influence health care reform and reimbursement. To transform the notion that power is good and can be used to gain, maintain, and expand resources, nurses need to combine the various sources of power presented in Chapter 19 and here and apply them to the advancement of excellence in nurs-ing practice. Promoting the positive effects of power can sustain nursing's power base in the health care arena and foster quality patient care. To use power to change and improve patient care is to recognize that power is natural and desirable.

Nursing must perceive power for what it re-ally is—the ability to mobilize and focus energy and resources. What better position can nurses be in but to assume power and influence to face new problems and responsibilities in reshaping nursing practice to adapt to environmental changes? Power is the means, not the end, to seek new ways of doing things in this uncertain and unsettling time of health care delivery. Sur-vival in this turbulent health care environment calls for nursing's knowledge and expertise to initiate and sustain influence at all levels of care: the workplace, government, financing, organi-zations, and community.

♦ MARKETING: IMAGE AS POWER

A major source of power for individual nurses and for the profession is possessing an image of power. Even if one does not have actual power from other sources, the perception by others that one is powerful bestows a degree of power. The same is true for the profession as a whole. If the public or legislators see the profession of nursing as powerful, the profession's ability to achieve its goals and agendas is enhanced.

Kotler (1984) states that "an image is the sum of beliefs, ideas, and impressions that a person has of an object" (p. 57). Images emerge from interactions and communications with others. If nurses present themselves as caring and compas-sionate experts in health care through their in-teractions and communications with the public, then a strong, favorable image develops for both the individual nurse and the profession. Nurses, as the ambassadors of care, must understand the importance and benefit of positive therapeutic communications and image. Developing a posi-tive image of power is important for both the individual and the profession.

Individual nurses can promote an image of power by a variety of means.

1. Appropriate introduction of self through name selection, eye contact, and handshak-ing can immediately establish you as a pow-erful person. If nurses introduce themselves by first name to Dr. Smith, the physician, the

nurses have immediately set forth an unequal power relationship unless the physician uses his or her first name. While women are not socialized to initiate handshakes, it is a power strategy that is routine in male-dominated circles, including health care organizations. In Western cultures, eye contact conveys a sense of confidence and connection to the individual to whom one is speaking. These seemingly minor behaviors can have a major impact on whether the nurse is perceived as competent and powerful.

2. Appropriate attire can symbolize power and success. While nurses may believe that they are limited in choice of attire by uniform codes set by institutions, it is in fact the presentation of the uniform that can hold the key to power. For example, a nurse manager needs a powerful image both with unit staff and with administrators and other professionals who are setting institutional policy. An astute nurse manager might wear a suit to work on the day of a high-level interdisciplinary committee meeting, rather than a uniform. Certainly attention to details of grooming and uniform selection can enhance the power of the staff nurse as well.

3. Conveying a positive and energetic attitude can send the message that you are a "doer" and someone to be sought out for involvement in important issues. Chronic complaining conveys a sense of powerlessness, whereas, the problem solver and optimist promotes a "can-do" attitude that suggests power and instills confidence in others.

The concern with images of power has extended to the profession as a whole. A recent survey demonstrated that the American public has more confidence, trust, and favorable regard for nurses than for physicians and institution administrators (Mason et al., 1991). The national nursing organizations plan to capitalize on this finding by using it to lobby for increasing the public's access to nursing care.

As the health care provider closest to the client, nurses best understand clients' needs and wants. Nursing is present upon the first client contact and thereafter for 24 hours per day, seven days a week, to assess and monitor care. By capitalizing on the special relationship that nurses have with clients, nurses can use the principles of marketing to enhance their position and image as professional care givers.

Kotler and Clarke (1987) describe marketing as "the analysis, planning, implementation, and control of carefully formulated programs designed to bring about voluntary exchanges of values with target markets for the purpose of achieving organizational objectives" (p. 5). Nursing must market its professional expertise and ability to achieve the objectives of health care organizations. From a marketing perspective, nursing's goal is to ensure that identified markets (e.g., clients, physicians, other health professionals, community members) have a clear understanding of what nursing is, what nursing does, and what it is going to do. In doing so, nursing is seen as a profession that gives expert care with a scientific knowledge base. Nursing care is often seen as an earmark or indicator of an organization's overall quality. Regardless of the setting, quality nursing care is something that is desired and valued. Through understanding clients' needs and preferences for programs that promote wellness and maintain and restore health, nurses become the organization's competitive edge to enhancing revenues. Marketing an image of expertise linked with quality and cost will position nursing powerfully and competitively in the health care marketplace.

♦ APPLICATION OF POWER, POLITICS, AND MARKETING TO MANAGING NURSING CARE

The delivery of nursing services occurs at many levels in health care organizations. The effectiveness of that care delivery is linked to the application of power, politics, and marketing. For the staff nurse, the politics of bedside care involves the art of influencing the allocation of scarce resources, be it equipment, supplies, time, or personnel, for the delivery of nursing care. To maintain access to the resources needed for patient care, nurses must connect to the whole organization and beyond, not just their own nursing unit. Staff nurses need to understand that they belong to a complex organization that is continually confronted with limited resources and is in competition for those resources. With this understanding in mind, staff nurses can use their power when the limitations interfere with and place restrictions on patient care. Whether the restrictions come in the form of limited supplies, money, or time, nurses can use their power and the political skills of artful negotiation, collaboration, and networking to obtain the necessary resources to provide care. Speaking on behalf of patient care, access, and quality is what drives the politics of nursing care.

What happens in the workplace both depends upon and influences what is happening in the larger community, professional organizations, and government. The effective nurse manager understands the connections among these spheres and uses them to the advantage of nursing, patients, and the health care organization. Developing influence in each of these three spheres takes time and an overall plan of action. It is suggested that the nurse develop a longrange plan for doing so. While the nurse's first priority should be to establish influence in the workplace, she or he can gradually increase connections and influence in the other spheres and, later on, even make these other spheres a priority for further development.

The professional organization provides an opportunity for developing political skills that can be used both in the association and in the other spheres. Obviously, the first step is to join a local and state nurses' association and/or a specialty organization. Attending meetings provides an opportunity to network with other influential nurses and to become known within the organization. Professional organizations depend upon volunteer effort to accomplish their mission. Volunteering for one of the many committees that these organizations usually have gives the nurse the opportunity to learn more about how the organization operates and to influence its actions and decisions. Seeking a leadership position with the committee provides additional influence and visibility. Such visibility is often needed if you are interested in serving on the major policy making body of the organization, the board of directors.

Serving in these various capacities provides the nurse with the opportunity to develop some political skills, influence, and connections. However, most organizations also provide opportunities for the general membership to influence the organization's direction and decisions. This is usually done through making and passing motions at a regular meeting and/or through resolutions brought forth for action at the annual business meeting (often held in conjunction with the annual convention of the association).

Whether in committee, at a board meeting, or at a membership meeting, securing passage of motions and resolutions requires an understanding of formal and informal political processes. Support must be garnered for the motion or resolution. Just getting the item on the agenda may require a formal motion or some behind-the-scenes pressure on the individual who controls the agenda. Once an item is on the agenda, it is important to make sure people are prepared to speak in favor of the motion or resolution (or in opposition, if that is preferred). Since the image of power can be as important as actual power, some people will not bring a motion or resolution forward unless there is a certainty of passage. This may mean contacting people before the meeting and garnering their support for the motion. On the other hand, raising the issue may be an important first step in a long-range plan to secure support. It is not uncommon for someone to "float" an issue or motion at one meeting to get a sense of the nature and strength of opposing arguments so preparations can be made to reduce the opposition in the future. Additionally, the issue may be so important to some individuals that their convictions dictate that concerns about power images be put aside. Regardless, the politically astute nurse will reflect on these options.

The government provides the most widely accepted arena for political participation. This participation can be grouped into two categories: (a) lobbying and (b) electioneering. However, these categories are interrelated, particularly in terms of developing connections and relationships with policy makers in the executive and legislative branches of government.

It is important to recognize which level of government has the power to decide which is-sues. For example, defense of the nation is the responsibility of the federal government, but licensure and regulation of professions is the purview of the states. Demarcations of responsibility are not always clear and may overlap, as occurs with administration of the Medicaid program, which is jointly determined by the federal and state governments.

Getting on the agenda of policy makers in government often requires both that the issue be within their purview and that the issue be of concern to the public or important to the welfare of the state, town, or nation. Just as one must market an issue in the workplace, getting on the agenda of governmental policy makers may require marketing skills that include effective use of the media. The importance of media contacts throughout the policy process in government should not be underestimated. Creating such connections can come from personal or social contacts, writing letters (particularly complimentary ones!) to journalists and reporters in response to their work on a topic, and providing reporters with ideas, leads, or information about a good story. Professional organizations and health care agencies/institutions often have public relations staff who can help shape a story for the media or develop a marketing strategy for getting on the agenda or selling the issue to the public or policy makers.

Being able to influence governmental policies is facilitated by having connections with the policy makers. The first step is finding out who these people are. The local board of elections or League of Women Voters usually provide this information by telephone. The second step is to begin to establish relationships with these elected officials. This is done by writing letters to them, visiting them, attending functions that they sponsor, attending their fundraisers, and working in their elections. In all of these activities, it is important to identify oneself as a nurse and by name repeatedly. Most state nurses associations and Leagues of Women Voters provide concrete information about letter writing and grassroots lobbying. It is most important to have frequent contact that can strengthen the connection. One New York public official frequently tells people to keep a stack of postcards handy and drop one in the mail to the public official with your thoughts on current issues they may be addressing or ought to address.

It is also important for nurses to recognize the power of their expertise in the sphere of government. Legislators, in particular, are usually not experts on health care and nursing. Nurses are. Nurses can offer to advise their legislators on nursing and health care matters. If the legislator does not have a health policy advisory committee, the nurse can offer to initiate one. Additionally, nurses can and must share their everyday work experiences with policy makers, who need to hear about the patient who was kept in the hospital, at the expense of the state, because there were no nursing home beds available or no housing available. They need to hear about the staffing shortages, the effects of excessive paperwork required by the state on the amount of time nurses can spend at the bedside, and the condition of crack-addicted newborns. They also need to hear about ideas for solving these problems, such as the effect of bedside computers on the amount and quality of time the nurse spends with the patient, or the impact of the prenatal care program where nurses successfully provide outreach and services to high risk pregnant women.

The nurse's expertise needs to be shared with the legislator's staff, who may be the key people deciding which position the legislator should take on an issue. And it should be shared with members of the executive branch of govern-

ment. This branch includes elected officials, such as a mayor, governor, or treasurer. It also includes appointed officials and staff, such as the commissioner of health or the director of the state board for nursing and the staff in their departments.

The more outside support you have for an issue, the better. This requires building coalitions with the public and interdisciplinary groups. Organizations such as the National Organization for Women and the Gray Panthers provide potential alliances for nursing and health care issues. Certainly, you must be able to organize and mobilize the nursing community around the issue. That means being able to mobilize the nursing staff on your unit or in your agency or being able to call on professional nursing organizations to provide support.

The electoral process provides an opportunity for nurses to promote candidates for public offices who are supportive of nursing and quality health care. It also enables the nurse to develop relationships with elected officials that provide important access to policy makers. Although incumbents currently have the advantage in most races, it is important for nurses to put their efforts behind candidates whose positions support quality health care and nursing. Weighing a candidate's positions on these and other issues is the first step in the selection process. On the federal and state levels, political action committees (PACs) of nursing organizations make collective decisions about candidates to endorse and to support financially and in other ways. The ANA-PAC does this for the American Nurses Association, and most state nurses associations have PACs for state races. Financial and volunteer support for candidates endorsed by these groups provide opportunities for nursing's collective voice to be recognized and heard. PAC endorsement does not guarantee that the legislator will vote as nurses want once elected, but it does enable access to the legislator.

Once the nurse selects the best candidate to support, the next step is to participate in the campaign. This participation may range from telling a friend about the candidate to attending a fundraiser or organizing a "Nurses Night" at campaign headquarters. Getting other nurses to donate a couple of hours each to the campaign can be a valuable contribution. Campaigns are costly and require enormous volunteer effort. The kinds of efforts needed are varied. Some require the interpersonal skills that nurses have developed from their work. Others require patience, such as stuffing envelopes. Mobilizing many nurses to make small contributions to the campaign has made the difference in some candidates getting elected (Ford-Roegner, 1985).

Increasingly, nurses are recognizing that the best way to influence health policy is to become a policy maker. This may mean running for political office (perhaps beginning with the local school board or town council) or getting appointed to a task force or commission that is developing policy. For example, the mayor may form a commission to develop a policy for the city on a local response to the AIDS crisis. Appointment of one or more nurses to this commission may depend on whether nurses participated in the mayor's campaign, the power of the local nurses association, the power image of nurses in the community, the understanding of the mayor's appointments staffer, a nurse on the mayor's staff who can lobby for such an appointment, or a personal connection to the mayor. Whatever the means, nurses can and must monitor such appointments and ensure that qualified nurses receive them.

Community support for quality nursing and health care comes in many forms that can in-

clude legislation, financial support, volunteer effort, and mobilization of public opinion. Government officials are often key players in the community as a whole. The area's representative to the U.S. Congress can influence local matters as well as national ones. Similarly, the chief operating officers of health care organizations are often recognized as leaders in the community. Power in the community as a whole also may lie in the hands of the mother who became concerned about the garbage dump next to the school and was able to organize and mobilize the community to take action. Mothers Against Drunk Driving (MADD) is an example of local, grassroots activity that now has become a national organization with considerable political influence.

Effective politics in the community, as in the workplace and government, requires an analysis of the informal power structures and processes. Who are the key players? Who can mobilize large segments of the community as needed? What are the values and beliefs of the community? Where are the places of action in the community? Is the community organized? The president of the local merchants' association may be able to mobilize members of that association to call for more community-based drug programs or to provide financial support for the pediatric nursing unit's project to initiate an educational and support group for families of chronically ill children. The PTA may be a power voice on educational and child health policies. The local Rotary Club or churches may be important sources of community support and action.

Efforts may be needed to get the community organized. Community organizers know that this is best done through an issue that is very important to the everyday lives and well-being of community members. Quality of life issues might include whether the neighborhood clinic is open in the evening, whether immediate and long-term supports are available to victims of rape, whether meals-on-wheels programs are available for the homebound elderly, and whether drug treatment programs are available in the community. Organizing and mobilizing community support requires being visible in the community and being recognized as someone who is concerned about the welfare of the community itself. This can most easily be done by getting involved in a community group or with a community issue that is of personal or professional importance. Nurses who are also parents may find that participating in the PTA or day care advisory committee is an important place for their involvement. The maternal-child nurse may prefer participating in the health committee of the community planning board that is working on developing a plan for a shelter of homeless families. Or the nurse may attend a community meeting that is addressing the opening of a group home for the mentally retarded and actively share both her or his expertise as a nurse and her or his opinion as a community member. The opportunities for involvement are endless. They enable nurses to develop political skills and connections, participate in community decisions, and contribute to the quality of their own lives and the lives of neighbors.

SUMMARY

♦ To use power and politics to change and improve patient care benefits the achievement of nursing's goals of autonomy, economic independence, and professional status.

♦ Nursing must perceive power for what it really is—the ability to mobilize and focus

energy and resources. What better position can nurses be in but to assume responsibilities for reshaping nursing practice to adapt to environmental changes?

♦ Power is the means, not the end, to seek new ways of doing things in this uncertain and unsettling time of health care.

♦ Survival in this turbulent health care environment calls for nursing's knowledge and expertise to initiate and sustain influence at all levels of care: the workplace, government, financing, organization, and community.

BIBLIOGRAPHY

Benner, P. (1984). *From Novice to Expert: Excellence and Power in Clinical Nursing Practice.* Menlo Park, CA: Addison-Wesley.

Bennis, W., and Nannus, B. (1985). *Leaders.* New York: Harper & Row.

Ehrat, K. S. (1983). "A Model for Politically Astute Planning and Decision Making." *Journal of Nursing Administration,* 13: 29–35.

Ferguson, V. D. (1985). "Two Perspectives on Power." In: *Political Action Handbook for Nurses: Changing the Workplace, Government, Organization and Community.* Mason, D., and Talbott, S. (editors). Menlo Park, CA: Addison-Wesley. Pp. 88–93.

Ford-Roegner, P. (1985). "Voter Participation and Campaigning." In: *Political Action Handbook for Nurses: Changing the Workplace, Government, Organization and Community.* Mason, D., and Talbott, S. (editors). Menlo Park, CA: Addison-Wesley. Pp. 398–410.

French, J., and Raven, B. (1960). "The Bases of Social Power." In: *Studies in Social Power.* Cartwright, D. (editor). Ann Arbor, Research Center for Group Dynamics, Institute for Social Research, University of Michigan.

Institute of Medicine. (1988). *Prenatal Care: Reaching Mothers, Reaching Infants.* Washington, DC: National Academy Press.

Kanter, R. B. (1989). *When Giants Learn to Dance.* New York: Simon and Schuster.

Kotler, P. (1984). *Marketing Management: Analysis, Planning, and Control.* 5th ed. Englewood Cliffs, NJ: Prentice-Hall.

Kotler, P., and Clarke, R. N. (1987). *Marketing for Health Care Organizations.* Englewood Cliffs, NJ: Prentice-Hall.

Maraldo, P. (1985). "Politics Is People." In: *Political Action Handbook for Nurses: Changing the Workplace, Government, Organization and Community.* Mason, D., and Talbott, S. (editors). Menlo Park, CA: Addison-Wesley. Pp. 81–87.

Mason, D. (1985). "The Politics of Patient Care." In: *Political Action Handbook for Nurses: Changing the Workplace, Government, Organization and Community.* Mason, D., and Talbott, S. (editors). Menlo Park, CA: Addison-Wesley. Pp. 38–52.

Mason, D., Costello-Nickitas, D., Scanlan, J., and Magnuson, B. (1991). "Empowering Nurses for Politically Astute Change in the Workplace." *Journal of Continuing Education in Nursing,* 1(22): 5–10.

Mason, D., and Talbott, S. (editors). (1985). *Political Action Handbook for Nurses: Changing the Workplace, Government, Organization and Community.* Menlo Park, CA: Addison-Wesley.

Miller, J. B. (1976). *Toward a New Psychology of Women.* Boston: Beacon Press.

Secretary's Commission on Nursing. (1988). *Commission on Nursing: Final Report.* Washington, DC: U.S. Department of Health and Human Services.

Stevens, B. J. (1980). "Power and Politics for the Nurse Executive." *Nursing and Health Care,* 1(4): 208–210.

Titmus, R. M. (1974). *Social Policy.* New York: Pantheon Books.

Wheeler, C. E., and Chinn, P. L. (1989). *Peace and Power: A Handbook for Feminist Process.* 2nd ed. New York: National League for Nursing.

A PRAGMATIC VIEW OF NURSING MANAGEMENT

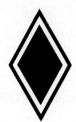

Throughout this book we have presented the most current knowledge available in nursing management. Now, however, we offer some practical advice—the kind of "hands-on" advice seldom found in a textbook but that is the knowledge passed on by an experienced manager to a novice. We think you will find it useful and a fitting conclusion to the book.

◆ TRANSITION

Transition from a clinical nursing role to that of nurse manager calls for learning and practicing an entirely new set of skills. Imagine this: Your interview for nurse manager was a week ago and today is your first day on the job. You drive to work down a country road, through a little town, onto a major highway, and into the city. You park in a maze of other cars and arrive at your worksite. When you walk into the nursing administrator's office, she points out the window at an 18-wheel truck and says, "Drive it. Your trip will be 2,000 miles. It's a challenge. You'll feel achievement every day. You will have a seasoned driver to ride with you, but you must do the driving. Good luck."

Driving that truck and making a transition to a management position have much in common. You know the basic road rules, how a truck runs, and how to read a road map and you have a sense of the right direction. However, learning new skills, new knowledge, and new driving techniques is something else.

So it is with nursing management. You know the basic concepts, you know how the organization runs, and you know how to give good nursing care. However, the skills of management are different.

◆ SOCIALIZATION FOR THE NURSE MANAGER ROLE

Position is a collectively recognized category of persons for whom there are common attributes, common behaviors, or common reactions of others toward them; *role* is the set of prescriptions defining what the behaviors of position members should be. Whoever fills a position is expected to perform the role in essentially the same way as any other person. This constancy allows organizations to remain stable over time.

In real organizational life, however, each person's performance is unique. Learning to express uniqueness appropriately within the confines of organizational bureaucracy is one of the greatest challenges for position holders (nurse managers, in this case). One aspect of uniqueness is how nurse managers respond to others' messages about how they should perform. These messages often are conflicting. For example, what the director expects, what the staff expects, what the nurse executive expects, and what a family expects all may be different. Resolving these conflicting messages in a mutually agreeable manner is essential to surviving in the position.

Clinical nursing is the main focus of nursing education and management courses offered in baccalaureate nursing programs usually do not have the needed depth to prepare someone for the nurse manager role adequately. At the associate degree level, even less management content is included. Yet students graduate and within several weeks are managing groups of people. In a few years or so, many have joined the management team.

Today, the tendency is still to promote nurses with good clinical skills into management positions on the assumption that they also will have good management skills. These nurses are committed to the organization and know the system well, but are unskilled in management theory, research, and strategies. The same may be true of their assistant directors of nursing, and so on. Also, many institutions do not provide a structured and comprehensive orientation to the new role. Nurse managers generally "go to bat" with institution administrators who have extensive management preparation like other chief executive officers in business or industry. Therefore, socialization for nurse managers too often occurs on a day-to-day, trial-and-error basis. Consequently, health care, at its most critical point, frequently must depend on those least prepared to manage it.

Fortunately, today's masters programs in nursing administration are producing better prepared managers. Careful selection of a program is essential because some do not teach all management principles sufficiently. Also, selection of a work institution that provides a comprehensive nurse manager orientation such as that described by Werkheiser et al. (1990a, 1990b) may improve your socialization into the nurse manager role.

It is not uncommon for new nurse managers with baccalaureate and even masters degrees, but little management experience, to find themselves in a position of managing, or working for, other nurses without comparable academic credentials but with years of experience. This can create problems for both parties and new nurse managers must be sensitive to the possibly troublesome implications of the situation. It is similar to what is called the "boot ensign" relationship in the military, where persons who have just completed officer's training and have little practical experience find themselves working with highly seasoned and experienced enlisted persons.

Problems arise when new nurse managers start making changes and exercising authority without drawing on the background and experiences of their staff and their boss. Both are going to resent newcomers who make such statements as, "I frankly don't see how you functioned before I got here." If you find yourself in the "boot ensign" position, try not to come on too strong with your boss, peers, or staff. Even if you see situations in dire need of changing, wait until you've gained the staff's confidence before making drastic changes. Don't criticize or disparage anything the prior nurse manager did. Instead, present yourself as wanting to build on the previous manager's contributions. You need your staff's and boss's respect and support to make improvements.

None of this is meant to imply that advanced nursing or management education is not valued. Quite the contrary: You must acquire new knowledge continuously just to survive and be effective in the complex and demanding field of health care. If you are fortunate enough to have advanced formal education or unique past experiences, treasure them. The trick is to use your knowledge in a way that does not offend or belittle others.

◆ IDENTIFICATION WITH MANAGEMENT

What happens when a nurse becomes a manager for the first time? Consider the following example. Nurses on Ms. Robbins's unit say that when Ms. Robbins became nurse manager, she "changed"; Ms. Robbins thinks *they* changed.

They are both right—the relationship between them changed. No longer is Ms. Robbins responsible only for individual patient care, she now is responsible for the operation of the entire unit. She must see that patients on her unit receive the best care her staff can provide; that all staff are working to the best of their ability; and that adequate resources, such as equipment and supplies, are available. Furthermore, she must identify with management so that she can carry out organizational goals on her unit as if they were her own. Her responsibility has shifted to the organization as a whole. This shift to a wider view can be perceived by the staff as an abandonment of staff values. Ms. Robbins can minimize this perception by keeping her staff informed and by involving them in formulation and implementation of unit goals that dovetail with organizational goals.

It is not uncommon to hear a new nurse manager say, "*They* want us to do . . ." or "*They* have interpreted the policy to mean . . . ." The emphasis is on the pronoun "they" as opposed to "we." If Ms. Robbins identifies with management, she sees her responsibilities as intertwined with those of her boss and other managers in the nursing department. When her boss makes a decision, Ms. Robbins shares in the decision. This does not mean she rubberstamps all of her boss's decisions. She may be very concerned about possible negative implications and is responsible for bringing these concerns to her boss. If, after concerns are discussed, the decision stands, it becomes a joint commitment. Ms. Robbins's follow-through and communication to those she manages will be based on a posture that says, "*We* want this," not, "*They* want this." This cohesive communication conveys clear expectations and is one foundation for good nursing management.

♦ CAREER OR JOB?

Nurses who decide to be managers must reflect on the fact that while they have taken on a career that is defined clearly in a business sense, they also must retain their professional nursing values. A career may be defined as any lifelong work characterized by commitment, personal growth, and increasing levels of responsibility. Careers are very different from jobs. One difference lies in the way one is paid. A job pays for hours worked, whereas in a career one is paid for what one has accomplished, regardless of hours worked.

Managers must internalize and value this career concept for both personal effectiveness and work satisfaction. Generally, nurses do not enter management with a well-defined sense of what is being asked of them or what this means in terms of a career. Career effectiveness emerges after one begins to think this way, but nurse managers also must have ambition, political savvy, and management skills. None of these qualities should be considered "bad" or morally reprehensible. Nurses must have *ambition* to be powerful. They must be *astute politically* to be effective managers, and they must be *proficient managerially* to deal with corporate issues, people, and money. A career orientation to nursing management may well be the highest priority for nursing in the decades ahead. It certainly will be a high priority for institution administrators, boards, and consumers.

Astute institution administrators and governing boards are beginning to realize that nurses are among the most significant controllers of cost. They also realize that effective nurse managers can make clear to staff the need for cost containment and enlist staff support in achieving this goal. Failure to inform staff and elicit their cooperation will result in organizational failure.

♦ POLITICS

Politics—which is *not* a dirty word—refers to an inclusive complex of relationships within an organization, including the latter's norms, values, culture, the way things are done, and what is and is not acceptable. Politics can be seen, then, as using situations, people, and resources in an astute but honest and ethical manner. As a nursing manager on the way up the ladder, you must decide if you *want* to play. The process is the same as joining a professional organization, social group, or tennis club. There are ways to act and not to act within any given group. If you play, you're in; if not, you're out. You never will fit perfectly into any organization, but the closer the better.

Nurse managers who advance rapidly in their careers usually have discovered where the opportunities are. They know what the real power positions are and what is needed to take advantage of opportunities. They're aware, too, of what education is needed, what support groups are effective, and what image is acceptable. That's the political side. It goes without saying, however, that they also need to be committed nurses and effective, efficient managers.

In a study comparing nursing administrators and first-level nurse managers, Heineken (1985) found that administrators believed more than did first-level nurse managers that (a) power is equated with political skill and (b) control over others is necessary to acquire and retain power and autonomy. If upper level administrators and first-level managers differ in their perceptions of both the importance of politics and values about power, the difference undoubtedly will be re-

flected in distorted communication, conflict, and lack of unity. Such differences must be addressed if nursing personnel are to work together. From a practical standpoint, successful nurse managers have learned that politics are played every day in every situation, especially at work; they are willing to participate in the game. See Chapter 23 for more on power and politics.

To know the system within which work is done may at first elude new managers, then puzzle, and, with effort and tutoring, become a revelation. Complex organizational relationships, both formal and informal, bombard new managers with deadly force. Traditional nursing and patient care values may conflict with new information, and frequently the neophyte is ill-prepared to cope with the results.

Having a sense of flow of information, approvals, and actions within a given health care organization takes energy and time. Nurses must know the pieces of the organization and how they fit together, yet each organization is different, so this cannot be learned from a book. Success in plotting a course depends on reconnaissance. Managers must be excellent in environmental reconnaissance both within the institution and outside it. Rarely do new nurse managers enter jobs having studied organizational dynamics in depth, desirable though it may be.

Nurse managers must set out to learn all they can of management theory and then recognize that one theory cannot explain every situation. Managers must be eclectic, selecting the concepts that, when put into action in a particular situation, will yield the best results. Managers should seek out anything in psychology, business, accounting, anthropology, and so on that will help them explain the situation and identify an appropriate direction. The effective manager is flexible!

♦ KEEPING UP WITH TRENDS

For nurse managers, understanding trends and keeping track of them are essential skills. They need to develop a strong sense of where they are and where the world may be taking them. Trends in three general areas—societal, health care, and nursing—should be watched carefully, as they will generate a frame of reference for plotting a course. In *Megatrends*, Naisbitt (1982) examines social changes and suggests that several states seem to be bellwethers, or leaders, in societal change. California, Washington, Colorado, Connecticut, and Florida fall into this group, closely followed by Minnesota and North Carolina. Keep an eye on what nurses in these states are doing in relation to the following societal trends or shifts in direction: movement from an industrial society to an information society, from emphasis on sickness to prevention and wellness, and from small nuclear families to greater numbers of single-parent families and dual-career families; movement to a more casual social style, to more women working, to more career options for women, to new definitions of roles for both women and men, and to faster communication; movement from mainstream economy to alternatives; movement to superorganizational structures and to limited career mobility in organizations (people will keep the jobs they now have); and movement from hierarchy to networking.

These societal trends will affect changes in health care profoundly. Nurse managers must regard the understanding and tracking of health care trends as a priority. Figures 24–1 and 24–2 show some health care and nursing trends to watch.

As a nursing manager you will be called upon by colleagues and others to translate these trends into action on a day-to-day basis. Careful and consistent reading in publications such as *Nursing Economics, Nursing Outlook, Wall Street Journal, Harvard Business Review, Inc.,* and *Fortune* will put you in a position to affect

---

FIGURE 24–1 CURRENT HEALTH CARE TRENDS

♦ Domination of health care industry by cost-conscious business people.

♦ Multihospital systems, to include international corporations.

♦ Complex legal and collaborative arrangements.

♦ Rationing of health care as a result of reimbursement and legislative issues.

♦ Shift from centralization to decentralization.

♦ Explosion in use of different technologies, such as barcodes, fax machines, and robotics.

♦ Extension of health care services originating in the organizational (health care institution) system.

♦ Services once provided in institutions now being "bled out" to others.

♦ An increasingly older population needing health care, with concomitant increase in length of stay.

♦ More attention to complex ethical issues such as "pulling the plug" or extension of life.

♦ Patient teaching as a major product line for hospitals.

♦ Majority of physicians will be employed by chains or in group practices associated with chains.

♦ Rapid growth of managed care systems.

♦ Increasing concern about access to care.

high-quality patient care by communicating needs efficiently in a futuristic perspective. Finally, to be on top of current trends, there are three more imperatives.

1. *You must know computers.* Managers cannot work without information.

2. *You must be business-oriented.* Health care is big business.

3. *You must think in long-range terms.* Before today is over, your world will have changed.

FIGURE 24–2 CURRENT NURSING TRENDS

♦ Increasing corporate-mindedness of nurses.

♦ Recognition that nursing is a major revenue producer in the institution.

♦ Third-party reimbursement for nurses and nursing services.

♦ Growth in fees-for-service at both group and individual levels.

♦ Major manpower distribution problems and patterns.

♦ Joint practice issues between physicians and nurses.

♦ Increasing demands for and on nursing managers.

♦ Fewer caregivers in proportion to the population.

♦ Goal of all-RN staffing abandoned with an accompanying increase in the use of LPNs.

♦ Increasing emphasis on high-quality basic and continuing education for professional nurses.

♦ Increasing entrepreneurship of nurses.

♦ COLLEAGUES, MENTORS, AND SPONSORS

As nurse managers assess their effectiveness, promotion potential, and security, one very crucial issue must be evaluated: What types of colleagueship, mentorship, and sponsorship are occurring? (They're not the same thing.) Colleagues, mentors, and sponsors are those very important persons who provide support, advice, and depth to us in our career development. They provide an informal system that works like this: Whenever you need advice or help, someone you know or have known over time assists you in reaching an objective or decision. The relationship generally is based on respect and trust between individuals. Your need is another person's opportunity to return a favor. The informal system rests frequently on personal long-standing relationships and unspoken obligations. Informal systems rarely are discussed openly.

COLLEAGUES

The three major players in an informal system are colleagues, mentors, and sponsors. *Colleagues* are professional peers who share values, purpose and position and present reality; they give support in the worst and best of times. You can develop a sense of colleagueship with other nurse managers by supporting each other in decisions or issues, especially when confronted by others. Identify areas of agreement and disagreement among your group of nurse managers. Use the areas of agreement to present a united front. Use the awareness of areas of disagreement to prevent the group from being divided and conquered. Set up support groups and decision-making plans among yourselves.

MENTORS

A *mentor* is a wiser and more experienced person who guides, supports, and nurtures a less experienced person. Shapiro, Haseltine, and Rowe (1978) assert that women who want to get ahead in a profession need more than a role model; they need a system of mentors and sponsors. The mentor relationship is characterized by a present orientation: It is for today and what must be done now. A mentor teaches the manager how to do a job. A mentor need not be a supervisor or one titled in the organization. Mentors tell you what you need to know and show you how to do it. They trust you with a job by giving assignments that are important, test limits, and provide learning. Mentors help by talking to you. They introduce you to people with whom you will move. Having a mentor instills greater personal satisfaction, increased self-confidence, and enhanced self-esteem. The relationship usually is intensely personal and rarely is hidden.

Mentors are usually the same sex as the protégé, eight to 15 years older, highly placed in the organization, powerful, and with a need for power. They are knowledgeable individuals who are willing to share their experiences and are not threatened by the protégé's potential for equaling or exceeding them (Hunts & Michael, 1983). Protégés are selected by mentors for several reasons: good performance, loyalty to people and the organization, the "right" social background or a social acquaintance with each other, appropriate appearance, social similarity, opportunity to demonstrate the extraordinary, and high visibility.

Mentor/protégé relationships seem to advance through several stages. The *initiation* stage usually lasts six months to a year, during which the relationship gets started. The *protégé* stage is that in which the protégé's work is not yet recognized for its own merit, but rather as a byproduct of the mentor's instruction, support, and encouragement. The mentor thus buffers the protégé from criticism. (A *breakup* stage may occur from six months to two years after a significant change in the relationship, usually resulting from the protégé's taking a job in another department or institution so that there is a physical separation of the two individuals. It also can occur if the mentor refuses to accept the protégé as a peer or when the relationship becomes dysfunctional for some reason.) The *lasting friendship* stage is the final phase and will occur if the mentor accepts the protégé as peer or if the relationship is reestablished after a significant separation. The complete mentor process usually includes the last stage.

Nurse managers also need to remember that they may become mentors for junior colleagues and staff. Select one or two promising neophytes or junior nurses and share your knowledge of the system, give assignments that are important, and promote learning. This relationship provides growth not only for the protégé, but also for you.

Be aware that a mentoring relationship can have its hazards (Darling, 1985b; George & Kummerow, 1981). Having a mentor can be perceived as favoritism and can cause jealousy and resentment in those who have no mentor. Also, mentoring between opposite sexes can create tension with spouses. Occasionally negative mentoring or "toxic" mentoring can occur. For example, the toxic mentor may be one who is hypercritical or leaves the protégé to flounder in a new situation. In examining the toxic relationship, Darling (1985a: 44) suggests the following:

1. Be sure you look for any potentially destructive patterns you may have carried over au-

tomatically from childhood. Identify the kinds of behaviors that are truly healthy for you and from which you may grow.

2. Identify the stage of your own growth. What now is becoming toxic may have been just what you needed a short time ago. Getting out is a possibility.

3. Try to understand the needs of the other person. Is the mentor responding to overload?

4. If you must ally yourself with a toxic mentor for some valid reasons, (a) build a support network of others and (b) draw on your own internal mentoring resources.

SELF-MENTORING

Several self-mentoring strategies can be used in providing your own guidance and direction in your career. Darling (1985a) offers five activities for self-mentoring.

1. Interact with people. Ask questions, listen, and clarify your understanding.

2. Find and use references. Read books and articles.

3. Observe people who are knowledgeable and have insight.

4. Enroll in educational programs, especially ones that include skill practices.

5. Figure things out for yourself; reflect; work things through.

SPONSORS

The relationship with a sponsor is quite different. It is future-oriented rather than present-oriented. This is a relationship that opens closed doors. A sponsor may be at any high-level position, formal or informal, in the organization or in the community that affects the organization. A sponsor tells you what you need to do to prepare for a leadership role and for career advancement and success. Sponsors trust your ability and they trust you with inside information. They take you along to appropriate places, meetings, or gatherings. At first they may just silently make sure you are there. They help you by talking about you, especially to those who control your career moves. Sponsors make sure you know people who have influence. This relationship may be unidentifiable in that the sponsor chooses to remain silent and unknown. If open, it is a collegial relationship.

HOW TO DEVELOP THE MENTOR OR SPONSOR RELATIONSHIP

1. Don't sit back and wait. Scout around senior management and search out potential relationships. Ask for advice.

2. Look for someone who already has been a mentor or sponsor.

3. Don't choose, or be chosen, by only one mentor or sponsor. Loss of power by that one individual can then mean loss of power for you.

4. Don't expect the relationship to give you all you need to do your job. Be realistic.

5. Keep foremost in your mind the importance of delivering your end of the commitment.

Both mentor and sponsor relationships are fragile and are based upon mutual trust. Nursing managers, recognizing these relationships by identifiable points, can maximize their depth and effectiveness.

◆ GROUPS

People and group performance are critical issues in a nurse management position. The new nurse manager often does not have in-depth information about them. Yet, the organization's expectation is a unit staff that works together for maximum results. There is more about groups in Chapter 5, but here are some hints to keep in mind when leading group discussions:

Set a warm, accepting, and nonthreatening tone.

Foster cooperation in the group.

Establish the purpose and importance of the meeting immediately.

Establish goals and identify major objectives.

Define all terms and concepts.

Allocate time for all decision-making steps.

Lead/discuss so that all members have an opportunity to contribute.

Help integrate the materials and ideas that have been generated.

Have the group generate ideas for solving problems.

Help group members identify the implications of the ideas.

Help the group evaluate the quality of the discussion.

◆ BASIC SURVIVAL SKILLS

Necessary for survival in the world of nursing management are characteristics and a style similar to those of business leaders. Successful nurse managers need to have:

1. A well-developed sense of self-awareness. Each nursing unit reflects characteristics of its leader. Evaluation of your own idiosyncrasies, styles, and motivations will provide some insight into the climate of your unit. Nurse managers live in a world of false cues. Staff will be "dishonest" in an effort to please and to manipulate the climate. The manager frequently is told what she or he is perceived to want to know. The challenge is to make feedback, positive or negative, okay.

2. The ability to manage work, personal, and family life. The higher you go in management and administration, the more involved you become. Feeling as though you are juggling 25 pingpong balls at once will wear you down. Decide which ones to drop. Set your priorities to accomplish what you do best—your professional work. Hire someone else to do the housework or yardwork. Give yourself time to engage in activities that add to a sound, well-rounded life (and reduce the stress that accompanies management.) A well-rounded life makes you more valuable.

3. Multiple interests and well-rounded experiences. Plan for a variety of educational, personal, and cultural experiences. Make opportunities for your staff to see units in

other institutions and other units in your own organization.

4. Interpersonal sensitivity. Listen to verbal and nonverbal cues from your staff. Chances are you are expert at listening to patients; do it with staff, also. Sense "vibes." Focus carefully on the total person who is communicating.

5. The ability to enhance the self-esteem of others. Make sure to praise staff frequently in a sincere manner for their accomplishments. This praise will be especially effective if it is specific and the only focus of the conversation you have with the staff member. Don't tack negative comments onto the end of praise.

6. The courage to take risks. Don't worry about your job! Once managers become too cautious to take risks, their effectiveness is diminished greatly, thereby actually lessening job security. Begin early to network and, if possible, have a potential job offer in your pocket.

7. A competent assistant. Don't give up vacations or other opportunities to revitalize yourself. Mentor and develop staff who can run the show while you are away. One who is "indispensable" cannot be promoted, so always train your replacement.

8. A method for self-criticism and self-discipline. Nurse managers should design a method to move away from the "yearly" evaluation and create methods within the system that will provide accurate peer, medical staff, and consumer feedback as often as possible.

9. A great curiosity. Generally, in health care, we are governed by professional socializa-

tion to think in the scientific mode. Creative thinking thereby is lessened greatly. Learn the joy of a lively mind and play (creativity and play are the same) in your setting.

10. An experiential attitude. Be optimistic. "Let's try" and "let's learn" should be heard often on your unit.

11. An ability to get staff involved in solving problems. Ask staff for ideas in solving problems and don't discount any solution proposed. Try to select one of their solutions; staff will have more investment in adhering to a solution if it is theirs.

12. The tolerance for sustained work. Nursing is seldom if ever an eight-hour day. If that is your expectation or value, remove yourself from the position.

13. A sense of calling or mission. This may sound trite, but successful people have it. Others do not. There is a meaning to work that is a personal commitment.

◆ THE FIRST WEEKS AS A MANAGER

Here are some guidelines for your first weeks on the job, taken from Thompson and Wood's *Management Strategies for Women* (1980).

FIRST DAY ON THE JOB

Do a quick review of the budget. Collect any existing organizational planning documents.

Meet the staff.

Get your office set up for work. Decorate after hours.

Start listing the things you want to accomplish for the organization.

Mark all meetings or deadlines on your calendar.

You're the boss. Get started.

MEETING AND DEALING WITH STAFF

Learn names. Memorize them before you go "on tour."

Meet as many people as possible on a one-to-one basis, starting with key people.

Invite people to your office so they can learn more about you. Include potential antagonists to establish turf.

When establishing relationships, it is 51 percent up to you and 49 percent up to your staff.

Until you know how staff members operate, ask why they made the decisions they did.

Ask for specific help and support. If it is not forthcoming and if your request is reasonable, conduct a performance discussion. Be firm, calm, and clear.

Take corrective action if your staff starts going over your head.

Get involved in hiring key staff members.

Immediately get on top of important issues. Establish a method for keeping track of them.

Begin establishing informal grapevines. The sooner they're working, the better.

INITIAL STAFF MEETINGS

Don't meet in large groups until you're ready. However, don't delay too long.

Do not put substantive or complex issues/ problems on the first agenda if you are not ready to deal with them or cannot orchestrate some solutions. Set the agenda so that you stay in control.

Be as certain as possible that you can deliver on any commitments you may make during the meeting.

Postpone (tactfully) those issues raised by others that you are not prepared to manage. Set a definite time to deal with each, though.

If possible, announce a major decision you've made or an important new policy or procedure.

Don't be overly sentimental in your first remarks to the full group. Be pleasant, firm, and businesslike. At the same time, a little warmth will ease tension.

STRENGTHENING YOUR POSITION IN THE EARLY WEEKS

Relax. You're going to mess up somewhere. Just keep the mistakes small.

If operational plans exist for your area of responsibility, become knowledgeable about them, pick up the reins, and move ahead. If they do not exist, begin planning activities so that you know where you are headed, why, and at what cost.

Get your performance planning and appraisal processes underway as soon as possible. Help your staff to understand where they are headed, why, and at what cost.

Don't be above asking for advice when you need it.

Establish directions and priorities yourself and do the initial detailed work yourself. You can't turn the ship around with someone else doing the steering.

Make a list of people you'll need to know outside the organization. Find ways to get to know them.

If you delegate responsibility on an interim basis, delegate authority on the same basis.

Analyze immediately why something failed.

Study other people who you think are successful. Spend time with them. Talk with them. Borrow their good ideas. Try to figure out why they are successful in the eyes of others.

If you hear about someone who has done something well, find out how he or she made it happen.

DEALING WITH INSECURITIES

Don't jump headlong into tough situations without proper briefing and background. In the early weeks, move cautiously and carefully. It will build confidence for later on.

If some individual really makes you feel insecure or anxious, get to know that person better.

Don't spill your insecurities to everyone. Let them think you have it all together.

Remember that people have greater respect for managers who make mistakes with some degree of decisiveness than managers who never make mistakes because they never lead.

◆ STRATEGIES FOR WORKING WITH YOUR BOSS

Most management concepts related to dealing with staff can be applied to relationships with your boss. Working effectively with your boss is important because your boss directly influences your career and success within the organization. Managing your boss or managing upward, therefore, is a crucial skill for successful nurse managers. To manage upward you must remember that the relationship requires participation by both you and your boss. You will know when you are managing upward successfully because power and influence will be moving in both directions.

One aspect of managing upward is to understand your boss's position from his or her frame of reference. This will make it easier to propose solutions and ideas that the boss will accept. Understand that your boss is a *person* with even more responsibility and pressure than you have. Learn about your boss from a personal perspective: What pressures does she or he face both personally and professionally? How does she or he react to stress? What is her or his background? Where did she or he go to school? This assessment of your boss will allow you to identify ways to reduce her or his stress and avoid "punching the wrong buttons."

Other strategies for managing your boss are:

Give immediate positive feedback for good things that she or he does. Positive feedback is a welcome change.

Never let your boss get a surprise; keep him or her informed.

Always tell the truth.

Find ways to compensate for weaknesses of your boss. Fill in weak areas tactfully. Volunteer to do something the boss dislikes doing.

Be your own publicist. Don't brag, but keep your boss informed of what you achieve.

Keep aware of your boss's achievements.

If your boss asks you to do something, do it well and ahead of deadline if possible. If appropriate add some of your own suggestions.

Establish a positive relationship with the boss's secretary.

INFLUENCING YOUR BOSS

Nurse managers need to approach their boss to influence her or him about all sorts of things. You, for instance, may need your boss's support for purchasing capital equipment, for changes in staffing, or for a new policy or procedure. Timing, rationale, possible objections, and choice of form or format all are important when preparing to make such a request. Timing is critical. Choose an opportunity when your boss has time and appears receptive. Also, consider the impact of your ideas on other events occurring at that time. Figure 24–3 gives guidelines that may help you achieve success in influencing your boss.

Should you present your ideas in spoken or written form? Usually some combination is used. Even if you have a brief meeting and a relatively small request, it is a good idea to follow up with a memorandum detailing your ideas and the plans to which you both agreed. Sometimes the procedure works in reverse. If a written proposal is read by the supervisor prior to a meeting, both of you are familiar with the idea at the start. In the latter case, careful preparation of the written material is essential to sell your ideas. For how to prepare a written proposal, see Chapter 7.

What can you do if, in spite of your careful preparation, your boss says no? First, think through your boss's reasoning and evaluate it. Ask yourself: "What new information did I get from the boss?" "What are ways I can renegotiate?" "What do I need to know or do to overcome objections?" Once these are answered, approach your boss again with the new material. This says that the proposal is a high priority with you and possibly new information may stimulate him or her to reevaluate. If it is important enough, you may want to take it higher. If so, tell your boss whom you would like to hear the proposal. Keep an open mind, listen, and try to meet objections with suggestions of how to solve problems. Be prepared for another no or the possibility of compromise, which is better than no movement at all.

TAKING A PROBLEM TO YOUR BOSS

Certain steps or key behaviors are involved in taking a problem to your boss. You can use these behaviors in taking a problem to your boss as well as when staff come to you with problems. The behaviors are designed to facilitate problem-solving processes. By solving the problem together and, if necessary, by both taking active steps, your and your boss's acceptance of and commitment to the solution is facilitated. Setting a specific follow-up date is important, because it prevents a solution from being delayed or forgotten. Figure 24–4 presents the steps in discussing a work-related problem with your boss.

By utilizing these steps, you ensure that the problem is addressed at a time when both you and your boss are able to devote attention to it. This should maximize the exchange of relevant information, understanding, and ideas.

FIGURE 24–3 GUIDELINES FOR INFLUENCING YOUR BOSS

Capitalize on your boss's strengths.
♦ What strengths and limitations does he or she have?
♦ What information do you have that he or she needs?
♦ What help can the boss provide personally and organizationally?

Be prepared.
♦ Do you know your boss's overall professional priorities or goals?
♦ What concerns or difficulties may he or she be facing?
♦ What excites your boss? What turns him or her off?

Cite benefits.
♦ What's in it for the boss if he or she supports your idea, proposal, or plan?
♦ How will the organization benefit?
♦ What are the short-term and long-term advantages?

Build a strong case.
♦ What policies, precedents, or procedures support what you want to do?
♦ Which of your supporters are valued by your boss for their opinions?
♦ How can you trade on your own expertise or credibility?
♦ What will the consequences be if the proposed idea is not accepted?
♦ What will have to be done later as a result?

Avoid surprises.
♦ Do you need to lay some groundwork with a brief memo or phone call explaining the purpose
  and importance of the meeting?
♦ What are the risks or advantages of hitting the boss cold with your idea, proposal, or plan?

Anticipate resistance.
♦ What aspects of your plan are likely to prompt resistance, such as "costs too much,"
  "takes too long," or "too risky"?
♦ How can you minimize or eliminate potential resistance by the way you manage the meeting?
♦ What data do you need to help overcome resistance?
♦ How will your idea affect morale, turnover, absenteeism? These cost money.

Separate need from "nice to have."
♦ What tradeoffs or compromises are you prepared to make?
♦ What part of your proposal is essential, what part merely desirable?
♦ "Half a loaf is better than none"; which half do you want?

Persist.
♦ How far and how hard are you willing to push to get your idea accepted?
♦ What does past experience tell you about the best timing or sequence for your attempts to influence
  your boss?
♦ Remember: The best ideas or changes seldom are accepted the first time they are proposed.
  If you learn from previously unsuccessful efforts and try again, you improve your
  chances of acceptance.

Adapted from Development Dimensions International, *Leadership and Influence, Part 3* (Pittsburgh, PA: Development Dimensions International, 1986).

◆ WORKING WITH PHYSICIANS

Today's nurse managers are role models and leaders for establishing nurse-physician relationships on their units. Researchers are beginning to document the relationship of nurse-physician communication to patient outcomes. Knaus et al. (1986) found that lower than expected death rates in intensive care units were related to excellent coordination and communi-

cation among the nurse-physician staff. Likewise, Gavett et al. (1985) reported that lack of communication and coordination among health care providers was related to unnecessarily high-cost stays for patients. Nurse managers have critical reasons, then, for setting a positive tone that fosters mutual respect among nurses and physicians on their units.

In today's competitive health care marketplace it also is necessary to view the physician as a nursing service customer. Institutions are competing for patients and physicians are the primary source of patients. The product of nursing service is patient care. Nurse managers who ignore physicians as customers of nursing service may find decreasing occupancy rates (Luciano & Darling, 1985).

What do physicians want? Physicians first want quality staff—nurses, health care workers, and other physicians ("What do . . . ," 1987). Then they want up-to-date facilities and equipment, quality care measurement, and training for nursing personnel. Physicians also want respect and regard patient care as their primary concern (Spitzer, 1988). These are many of the same "things" that nurses want in a work environment.

To support greater collaboration between nurses and physicians and to improve the product of nursing service—patient care—the following strategies are offered.

Establish a collaborative practice committee on your unit composed of equal membership of nurses and physicians. In the meetings, identify problems, develop mutually satisfactory solutions, and learn more about each other. Emphasize similarities and quality care. Start with positive physicians who will support the committee and successful outcomes.

Actively listen and respond to physician

FIGURE 24–4 KEY BEHAVIORS FOR TAKING A PROBLEM TO YOUR BOSS

◆ State your desire to talk about a work-related problem and, if necessary, make an appointment to meet, identifying approximate amount of time needed.

◆ If the suggested time is not convenient, ask when and where would be convenient.

◆ State the problem and explain its effect on work activities.

◆ Listen for restatement of problem or for indication that problem has been understood.

◆ State your willingness to cooperate in any solution to the problem and listen openly to boss's comment.

If necessary, continue:

◆ State alternative or your preferred solution.

◆ Agree on steps each of you will take to solve the problem.

◆ Ask if there is a need to follow up the problem. If so, plan and record a specific follow-up date.

P.J. Decker, *Health Care Management Microtraining* (St. Louis, Mo: Decker and Associates, 1983). Used by permission.

complaints as customer complaints. Create a problem-solving structure. Stop blaming physicians exclusively for communication problems.

Build your staff's clinical competence and credibility. Ensure that your staff has the clinical preparation necessary to meet the unit's standards of care.

Consider yourself and your staff equal partners with physicians in health care.

Respect the physicians as persons and expect that they respect you.

Use every opportunity to increase your staff's contact with physicians and to include your staff in meetings that include physicians. Remember that limited interactions contribute to poor communication.

Serve as a role model to your staff in nurse-physician communication.

Support your staff in participating in collaborative efforts, by words and by actions.

SUMMARY

♦ Transition from a clinical role to nurse manager calls for learning and practicing a new set of skills. Nurses generally are not educated for or socialized to management so they must learn these skills.

♦ Nurse managers must identify with administration so they can carry out organizational goals on their units as if they were their own.

♦ Management is a career that takes ambition, political savvy, and management skills. It also takes keeping up with societal, business,

and legal trends because these trends affect health care.

♦ Nurse managers must understand and be willing to practice organizational politics and must know the route to success in their particular institution.

♦ Nurse managers must know the system in which they work: their institution. What are its goals, values, and priorities? Understanding organizational and management theories is the key to understanding an institution.

♦ Successful nurse managers network, find mentors, increase communication skills, and are visible to administration.

♦ Understanding group dynamics is important. Nurses work in groups and group climate determines productivity.

♦ Successful nurse managers need to have several skills: a sense of self-awareness, ability to manage work and personal/family life, multiple interests, interpersonal sensitivity, ability to enhance self-esteem of others, the courage to take risks, competent assistants, methods for self-criticism and self-discipline, great curiosity, an experiential attitude, ability to involve staff in solving problems, tolerance for sustained work, and a sense of calling.

♦ The first day on the job is critical. Meeting staff and initial staff meetings are important. Learning to deal with insecurities and discovering strategies to deal with your boss are critical.

♦ Nurse managers are critical in setting a positive tone that fosters mutual respect among nurses and physicians on their units.

♦ Being a successful manager means knowing

who you are, what your capabilities are, and working from there. It means growing and gaining strength where you are weak.

♦ Being a successful nurse manager means looking, acting, and thinking as a professional.

BIBLIOGRAPHY

Aydelotte, M. K. (1987). "Nursing's Preferred Future." *Nursing Outlook,* 35: 114–120.

Bajnok, I., and Gitterman, G. (1988). "Nurses as Colleagues and Mentors." *Canadian Nurse,* 84(2): 16–17.

Bartkowski, J. J., and Swandby, J. M. (1985). "Charting Nursing's Course through *Megatrends.*" *Nursing and Health Care,* 6: 375–377.

Berkley, G. (1985). *How to Manage Your Boss.* Englewood Cliffs, NJ: Prentice-Hall.

Bowman, G. W., Warety, N. B., and Greepet, S. A. (1965). "Are Women Executive People?" *Harvard Business Review,* 43: 14.

Cavanaugh, D. E. (1985). "Gamesmanship: The Art of Strategizing." *Journal of Nursing Administration,* 15(4): 38–41.

Chenevert, M. (1985). *Pro-Nurse Handbook.* St. Louis, MO: C. V. Mosby.

Darling, J., and Taylor, R. (1986). "Upward Management: Getting in Step with the Boss." *Business,* 36: 3–8.

Darling, L. A. W. (1985a). "Self-Mentoring Strategies." *Journal of Nursing Administration,* 15(4): 42–43.

Darling, L. A. W. (1985b). "What to Do about Toxic Mentors." *Journal of Nursing Administration,* 15(5): 43–44.

Darling, L. A. W., and McGrath, L. (1983). "Minimizing Promotion Trauma." *Journal of Nursing Administration,* 13(9): 14.

Decker, P. J. (1982). *Health Care Management Microtraining.* St. Louis, MO: Decker and Associates.

Development Dimensions International. (1986). *Leadership and Influence, Part 3.* Pittsburgh, PA: Development Dimensions International.

Gabarro, J., and Kotter, J. (1980). "Managing Your Boss." *Harvard Business Review,* 58: 92–100.

Gambacorta, S. (1983). "Head Nurses Face Reality Shock, Too!" *Nursing Management,* 14(7): 46–48.

Gavett, J. W., Drucker, W. R., McCrum, M. S., and Dickenson, J. C. (1985). *A Study of High Cost Inpatients in Strong Memorial Hospital.* Rochester, NY: Rochester Area Hospital Corporation and University of Rochester.

George, P., and Kummerow, J. (1981). "Mentoring for Career Women." *Training,* (February): vol. 18.

Gleeson, S., Nestor, O. W., and Riddell, A. J. (1983). "Helping Nurses through the Management Threshold." *Nursing Administration Quarterly,* 7(2): 11.

Hegarty, C. (1980). *How to Manage Your Boss.* Mill Valley, CA: Whatever Publishing.

Heineken, J. (1985). "Power: Conflicting Views." *Journal of Nursing Administration,* 15(11): 36–39.

Hunts, D. M., and Michael, C. (1983). "Mentorship: A Career Training and Development Tool." *Academy of Management Review,* 8: 475.

Johnston, P. F. (1983). "Improving the Nurse-Physician Relationship." *Journal of Nursing Administration,* 13(3): 19–20.

Kanter, R. M. (1977). *Men and Women of the Corporation.* New York: Basic Books.

Kerfoot, K. (1989). "Nurse/Physician Collaboration: A Cost/Quality Issue for the Nurse Manager." *Nursing Economics,* 7: 335–336, 338.

Kinsey, D. C. (1990). "Mentorship and Influence in Nursing." *Nursing Management,* 21(5): 45–46.

Knaus, W. A., Draper, E. A., Wagner, D. P., and Zimmerman, J. E. (1986). "An Evaluation of Outcome from Intensive Care in Major Medical Centers." *Annals of Internal Medicine,* 104: 410–418.

Levenstein, A. (1985). "Caught in the Middle." *Nursing Management,* 16(2): 55–56.

Luciano, K., and Darling, L. A. W. (1985). "The Physician as a Nursing Service Customer." *Journal of Nursing Administration,* 15(6): 17–20.

Naisbitt, J. (1982). *Megatrends: Ten New Directions Transforming Our Lives.* New York: Warner Books.

Nornhold, P. (1990). "90 Predictions for the '90s." *Nursing,* 20(1): 34–41.

Notkin, M. S. (1983). "Collaboration and Communication." *Nursing Administration Quarterly,* 8(1): 1–7.

Persons, C. B., and Wieck, L. (1985). "Networking: A Power Strategy." *Nursing Economics,* 3(1): 53–57.

Shapiro, E. C., Haseltine, F. P., and Rowe, M. (1978). "Moving Up: Role Models, Mentors, and the Patron System." *Sloan Management Review,* 19(Spring): 51–58.

Spitzer, R. B. (1988). "Meeting Consumer Expectations." *Nursing Administration Quarterly,* 12(3): 31–39.

Strasen, L. (1987). *Key Business Skills for Nurse Managers.* Philadelphia: J. B. Lippincott.

Stuart, G. W. (1986). "An Organizational Strategy for Empowering Nursing." *Nursing Economics,* 4: 69–73.

Thompson, A. M., and Wood, M. D. (1980). *Management Strategies for Women.* New York: Simon and Schuster.

Toffler, A. (1981). *The Third Wave.* New York: Bantam Books.

Vance, C. N. (1982). "The Mentor Connection." *Journal of Nursing Administration,* 12(4): 7–13.

Veninga, R. L. (1987). "When Bad Things Happen to Good Nursing Departments: How to Stay Hopeful in Tough Times." *Journal of Nursing Administration,* 17(2): 35–40.

Vestal, K. W. (1987). "Managing Upward." *Journal of Pediatric Nursing,* 2(1): 55–57.

Werkheiser, L. K., Negro, P. A., Vann, B. J., Holstad, J. M., Byrd, J. C., and Von Talge, J. (1990a). "New Nurse Managers: Part I—Orientation for the 1990s." *Nursing Management,* 21(11): 56–63.

Werkheiser, L. K., Negro, P. A., Vann, B. J., Holstad, J. M., Byrd, J. C., and Von Talge, J. (1990b). "The New Nurse Manager Resource Peer: Part II." *Nursing Management,* 21(12): 30–33.

"What Do Physicians Really Want from Hospitals?" (1987). *Hospitals,* 61(June 5): 46.